AI-Assisted Computational Approaches for Immunological Disorders

Jen-Tsung Chen
National University of Kaohsiung, Taiwan

IGI Global
Scientific Publishing
Publishing Tomorrow's Research Today

Vice President of Editorial	Melissa Wagner
Director of Acquisitions	Mikaela Felty
Director of Book Development	Jocelynn Hessler
Production Manager	Mike Brehm
Cover Design	Phillip Shickler

Published in the United States of America by
IGI Global Scientific Publishing
701 East Chocolate Avenue
Hershey, PA, 17033, USA
Tel: 717-533-8845
Fax: 717-533-7115
Website: https://www.igi-global.com E-mail: cust@igi-global.com

Library of Congress Cataloging-in-Publication Data

Names: Chen, Jen-Tsung editor
Title: AI-assisted computational approaches for immunological disorders / edited by Jen-Tsung Chen.
Description: Hershey, PA : IGI Global Scientific Publishing, [2025] | Includes bibliographical references and index. | Summary: "This book attempts to propose strategies that hold promise for developing precision medicine and personalized healthcare in major immunological disorders, such as immunodeficiency, autoimmune diseases, allergies, asthma, cancers, and neurological diseases. Additionally, this book proposes ways of AI-assisted diagnosis, disease susceptibility and outcomes, drug and vaccine development, immunotherapy, cell therapy, gene therapy, CRISPR/Cas9, and nanotechnology, in managing diverse immunological disorders"-- Provided by publisher.
Identifiers: LCCN 2025004065 (print) | LCCN 2025004066 (ebook) | ISBN 9798369397251 hardcover | ISBN 9798369397268 paperback | ISBN 9798369397275 ebook
Subjects: LCSH: Immunoinformatics | Artificial intelligence--Medical applications | Immunology--Data processing | Immunologic diseases--Treatment--Data processing | Immunologic diseases--Diagnosis--Data processing
Classification: LCC QR182.2.I46 A437 2025 (print) | LCC QR182.2.I46 (ebook) | DDC 616.07/90285--dc23/eng/20250611
LC record available at https://lccn.loc.gov/2025004065
LC ebook record available at https://lccn.loc.gov/2025004066

British Cataloguing in Publication Data
A Cataloguing in Publication record for this book is available from the British Library.

Table of Contents

Detailed Table of Contents

The integration of artificial intelligence (AI) into healthcare is vital for sustainability. This overview highlights how AI enhances sustainable practices and improves patient care amid rising costs and resource scarcity. Technologies like machine learning (ML), natural language processing (NLP), and predictive analytics streamline operations, boost diagnostic accuracy, and personalize treatment plans. AI's ability to analyze large datasets helps providers make data-driven decisions, improving care quality. It plays a key role in medical imaging, supply chain management, and patient engagement, though challenges like data privacy and algorithmic bias remain. Effective integration requires investments and training. AI optimizes resource allocation and preventive care, especially in telemedicine during the COVID-19 pandemic. Future sustainable healthcare will rely on AI advancements and collaboration among stakeholders.

The goals of this chapter are to review artificial intelligence and big data techniques in precision medicine and corroborate applications of artificial intelligence techniques to solve challenges in immunological disorders. The integration of artificial intelligence in precision medicine has strengthened immunology in biomedical sciences. Precision medicine detects the health outcomes of specific patients. Biomedical studies have shown that clinical research defining the integration of artificial intelligence and precision medicine will present solutions for the challenging issues in precision medicine. This chapter covers various features of artificial intelligence in precision medicine that may nourish biomedical science research. We discuss how artificial intelligence solidifies the technical environment of precision medicine and the application of artificial intelligence methods to analyze biomedical big data of immunological disorders.

The integration of Artificial Intelligence (AI) in immunological disorder diagnosis is transforming medical diagnostics by enabling rapid and accurate decision-making. This chapter explores AI-enhanced

provide a comprehensive overview of the transformative potential of AI in cell therapy while emphasizing the importance of a multidisciplinary approach to overcome existing hurdles and realize its full potential in healthcare.

A groundbreaking advancement in healthcare is the application of AI algorithms to track patients' chronic diseases and vital signs, delivering real-time feedback to medical professionals. Monitoring and treating the symptoms of Oral Lichen Planus (OLP), a chronic inflammatory disorder affecting the mouth's mucous membranes, can be particularly challenging. The purpose of this systematic review is to disclose the most valid and reliable scoring systems suitable for clinical monitoring of disease progression and predicting response to therapy in Oral lichen planus patients.

The tumor immune microenvironment (TIME) plays a crucial role in immunotherapy by shifting the immune response from pro-tumor to anti-tumor, ultimately improving treatment outcomes. In precision medicine, high-throughput molecular profiling, including genomics, transcriptomics, proteomics, and informatics, provides critical insights into tumor biology and immune interactions. These advanced techniques help identify key biomarkers influencing therapy response. TIME comprises tumor-specific antigens, viruses, germline antibodies, and neoantigens, which serve as primary targets for cancer vaccines and immune checkpoint inhibitors (ICBs). Understanding their interactions with the immune system is essential for optimizing treatment strategies. This chapter explores the role of machine learning (ML) in predicting immunotherapy responses by analyzing large datasets to uncover patterns that influence treatment efficacy. By leveraging computational power, ML enhances the precision of immunotherapy, advancing personalized cancer care and improving patient outcomes.

Integrating artificial intelligence (AI) with nanotechnology has revolutionized immunological research by enabling the precise design, optimization, and functionalization of nanoparticles. AI-generated nanoparticles (AIGNPs) exhibit enhanced capabilities in vaccine development, cancer immunotherapy, and autoimmune disease treatment through improved antigen delivery, targeted drug release, and immune modulation. AI-powered models help researchers quickly analyze how nanoparticles behave, interact with immune cells, and determine their compatibility with the body. This speeds up the development of new treatments. But there are still a lot of obstacles. Obstacles still include strict legal requirements, moral dilemmas, and the requirement for extensive experimental support. AI-generated nanoparticles have infinite therapeutic potential once these obstacles are removed. Resolving these issues could result in more precise and personalized cancer immunotherapy, which would revolutionize patient care.

Recent advances in cancer research have revolutionized our understanding of cancer as not merely a disease of uncontrolled cell growth but fundamentally as an immunological disorder where malignant cells evade and suppress immune surveillance. This chapter presents a novel framework for conceptualizing and treating cancer through an integrative approach that combines immunological insights with personalized nutrition and artificial intelligence-driven interventions. The chapter synthesizes current evidence on immunonutrition in oncology, examining specific nutrients and bioactive compounds that enhance anti-tumor immunity. Furthermore, we discuss how artificial intelligence algorithms can be leveraged to develop personalized nutritional protocols based on individual patient parameters, including genetic profiles and immune biomarkers.

Preface

INTRODUCTION

The rapid convergence of artificial intelligence (AI) and biomedical science has opened unprecedented avenues for understanding, diagnosing, and treating immunological disorders. The immune system, inherently complex and deeply individualized, poses substantial challenges in clinical management and research innovation. Yet AI's capacity to manage massive, multi-dimensional datasets with speed and precision has introduced new frameworks for interpreting immunological data, forecasting disease trajectories, and tailoring treatment to individual patients. This edited volume, *AI-Assisted Computational Approaches for Immunological Disorders*, brings together a diverse collection of perspectives, methodologies, and case studies to showcase AI's transformative role in this vital field.

As editor, I have had the privilege of working with leading researchers from across the globe—scientists, clinicians, and technologists whose contributions represent the cutting edge of interdisciplinary collaboration. Across fourteen chapters, this volume explores the integration of machine learning, natural language processing, and big data analytics in topics ranging from sustainable healthcare and personalized medicine to vaccine design, cell therapy, and nanoparticle applications. The volume also addresses ethical and regulatory challenges, reminding us that technological advancement must be coupled with careful consideration of societal impacts. These chapters reflect not only the current state of research but also a forward-looking vision of how AI can elevate immunological science and patient care.

This book is intended for a broad readership: researchers in bioinformatics and immunology, AI developers and data scientists, healthcare professionals, policy-makers, and postgraduate students. The goal is to provide both foundational insights and practical applications, while also encouraging further inquiry into this rapidly evolving domain. By bringing together diverse voices and perspectives, I hope this volume catalyzes continued innovation and cross-disciplinary partnerships that bridge computation and clinical need.

CHAPTER OVERVIEW

Chapter 1: AI Algorithms in Sustainable Healthcare

This chapter explores the transformative role of artificial intelligence (AI) in promoting sustainable healthcare systems. By leveraging machine learning, natural language processing, and predictive analytics, AI enhances diagnostic accuracy, streamlines operations, and supports personalized treatments. The authors discuss how AI contributes to resource optimization, especially in telemedicine, while addressing challenges such as algorithmic bias and data privacy. The chapter underscores the importance of training, investment, and cross-sector collaboration for sustainable, AI-driven healthcare advancements.

Chapter 2: AI Tools and Applications in Managing Immunological Disorders

Focusing on the intersection of AI and precision medicine, this chapter examines how AI techniques address challenges in diagnosing and treating immunological disorders. The authors highlight how AI strengthens biomedical research by enabling the analysis of big data, supporting individualized health outcomes, and reinforcing the infrastructure of precision medicine. This chapter sets the foundation for understanding AI's role in transforming immunology and personalizing patient care.

Chapter 3: AI-Enhanced Diagnosis for Immunological Disorders

This chapter presents AI as a powerful tool in diagnosing immunological disorders through methods such as deep learning, machine learning, and natural language processing. It details the application of convolutional neural networks, support vector machines, and genomic analysis in identifying biomarkers and predicting disease trajectories. The authors also explore the use of big data and federated learning in improving diagnostic precision while addressing the limitations of bias, data heterogeneity, and regulatory issues.

Chapter 4: AI Technologies for Predicting Susceptibility and Outcomes of Immunological Disorders

This chapter discusses how AI technologies analyze clinical, genomic, and environmental data to predict immunological disease susceptibility and outcomes. Techniques like support vector machines, random forests, and clustering models support disease tracking and personalized diagnosis. The authors also address limitations in data quality, interpretability, and clinician trust, emphasizing the need for collaboration and explainable AI to enhance clinical relevance and transparency.

Chapter 5: AI-Driven Drug Discovery, Design and Development in Immunological Disorders

Highlighting the shift from traditional to AI-enhanced drug discovery, this chapter focuses on how AI accelerates the development of therapies for immunological disorders. Through the integration of omics data and patient profiles, AI enables the modeling of complex diseases and the in silico creation of drug candidates. The authors detail the application of AI in autoimmune disease research, efficacy prediction, and patient stratification, offering new avenues for tailored therapeutic development.

Chapter 6: AI-Assisted Vaccine Design and Development in Immunological Disorders

This chapter examines AI's role in revolutionizing vaccine design through immunogen identification, epitope prediction, and multi-omics integration. AI algorithms enable the creation of precise, condition-specific vaccines by analyzing genomic, transcriptomic, and proteomic data. The authors demonstrate how AI supports personalized immunization strategies for complex immunological disorders, addressing challenges in immune profiling and antigen prioritization.

Chapter 7: AI-Driven Precision Medicine and Personalized Healthcare for Immunological Disorders

Emphasizing the heterogeneity of immunological disorders, this chapter explores how AI technologies enable precision medicine and personalized healthcare. The authors explain how AI facilitates individualized treatment by analyzing unique patient characteristics and pathogenetic pathways. The integration of AI with personalized medicine offers targeted therapies and more effective disease management strategies tailored to each patient's immune profile.

Chapter 8: AI-Assisted Cell Therapy: Opportunities and Challenges

This chapter delves into the integration of AI in regenerative medicine, particularly in enhancing the precision of cell therapies. The authors discuss how AI aids in optimizing cell selection, engineering, and treatment customization. They also explore key challenges, such as data validation, privacy, and ethics, advocating for a multidisciplinary approach to realize the full potential of AI-assisted cellular therapies.

Chapter 9: AI Technologies in Autoimmune Diseases: Advances, Limitations and Prospects

Focusing on autoimmune conditions such as Oral Lichen Planus, this chapter reviews the use of AI in disease monitoring and therapeutic prediction. The authors provide a systematic assessment of scoring systems for clinical evaluation and explore how real-time feedback and chronic disease tracking are enhanced by AI. The chapter also addresses ongoing challenges in data reliability and clinical application.

Chapter 10: AI-Assisted Immunology for Precision Cancer Medicine

This chapter explores the application of AI in understanding the tumor immune microenvironment and optimizing immunotherapy in cancer treatment. AI-driven analyses of genomics, proteomics, and immune interactions reveal patterns that influence therapy responses. The authors present how machine learning supports the development of personalized immunotherapies, improving outcomes in precision cancer medicine.

Chapter 11: AI-Generated Nanoparticles in Immunological Research: Opportunities and Challenges

This chapter highlights the role of AI in designing and optimizing nanoparticles for targeted drug delivery and immune modulation. AI-generated nanoparticles offer advancements in vaccine development and cancer therapy by enhancing compatibility and efficacy. The authors address barriers such as regulatory challenges, ethical concerns, and the need for experimental validation, pointing to the transformative potential of AI-nanotechnology integration.

Chapter 12: Reframing Cancer as an Immunological Disorder through Personalized Nutrition and AI Integration

Proposing a novel perspective, this chapter reconceptualizes cancer as an immunological disorder and explores the integration of AI and personalized nutrition in its treatment. The authors discuss how bioactive compounds can enhance immune responses and how AI algorithms develop tailored nutrition plans based on immune biomarkers and genetic data. The approach aims to complement conventional therapies and improve cancer management.

Chapter 13: AI-Driven Decision Support Systems for Immunological Disorders: Bridging Big Data, Omics, and Precision Medicine

This chapter outlines how AI-powered decision support systems harness big data and omics to personalize treatment in immunology. The authors detail the use of AI in identifying biomarkers, guiding therapies, and integrating real-time analytics. Challenges like data quality, algorithmic fairness, and ethical concerns are critically assessed, while the potential of AI to strengthen healthcare resilience and improve immune-related outcomes is emphasized.

Chapter 14: Challenges, Limitations, and Ethical Considerations of AI in Immunology and Healthcare

Concluding the volume, this chapter critically examines the ethical, practical, and scientific hurdles in deploying AI in immunological research and healthcare. Topics include variability in patient responses, algorithmic bias, data governance, and accessibility in low-resource settings. The authors propose adaptive strategies and equitable collaboration frameworks to ensure that AI fulfills its promise of advancing global health equity and immunological innovation.

CONCLUSION

In curating this volume, I have drawn inspiration from the spirit of scientific curiosity and global collaboration that defines this field. The contributors represent a mosaic of expertise and geographic diversity, and their collective work points to a future where AI not only enhances but fundamentally redefines our understanding of immunological health. I am grateful for their insights, diligence, and commitment to advancing science for the greater good. Their efforts are a testament to what is possible when technology and medicine converge in the service of humanity.

Looking ahead, I believe the integration of AI into immunology will continue to expand, shaped by both technological advancements and evolving societal needs. As we face ongoing public health challenges, the need for scalable, intelligent, and personalized healthcare solutions becomes more urgent. AI offers powerful tools, but it is the collaboration among researchers, clinicians, ethicists, and technologists that will ultimately determine its success. This volume is offered as both a record of current achievements and a roadmap for future exploration.

I hope this book stimulates new ideas, partnerships, and research directions. Whether you are a seasoned expert or an emerging scholar, I invite you to engage with the material, question assumptions, and contribute to the evolving dialogue at the intersection of artificial intelligence and immunological science. It is my sincere hope that the insights shared here will inspire continued progress toward a more precise, equitable, and intelligent future in healthcare.

Chapter 1
AI Algorithms in Sustainable Healthcare

Anita Ioana Visan
https://orcid.org/0000-0003-0539-4160
National Institute for Lasers, Plasma, and Radiation Physics, Romania

Irina Gabriela Negut
https://orcid.org/0000-0003-4038-7548
National Institute for Lasers, Plasma, and Radiation Physics, Romania

ABSTRACT

The integration of artificial intelligence (AI) into healthcare is vital for sustainability. This overview highlights how AI enhances sustainable practices and improves patient care amid rising costs and resource scarcity. Technologies like machine learning (ML), natural language processing (NLP), and predictive analytics streamline operations, boost diagnostic accuracy, and personalize treatment plans. AI's ability to analyze large datasets helps providers make data-driven decisions, improving care quality. It plays a key role in medical imaging, supply chain management, and patient engagement, though challenges like data privacy and algorithmic bias remain. Effective integration requires investments and training. AI optimizes resource allocation and preventive care, especially in telemedicine during the COVID-19 pandemic. Future sustainable healthcare will rely on AI advancements and collaboration among stakeholders.

1. INTRODUCTION: UNDERSTANDING AI IN HEALTHCARE

Integrating artificial intelligence (AI) into healthcare systems is increasingly recognized as a pivotal element in the pursuit of sustainability within the sector. As healthcare faces escalating challenges, including rising costs, resource scarcity, and environmental impacts, AI algorithms emerge as a promising avenue for fostering sustainable practices while simultaneously enhancing patient care.

The AI's potential to transform healthcare is underscored by its ability to streamline operations, improve diagnostic accuracy, and personalize treatment plans, thereby addressing the multifaceted challenges that the sector faces today (Secinaro et al., 2021; Al Kuwaiti et al., 2023; Rathore & Rathore, 2023; Ismail et al., 2022).Understanding AI in healthcare requires a comprehensive grasp of its various technologies,

DOI: 10.4018/979-8-3693-9725-1.ch001

which include machine learning, natural language processing, and predictive analytics. These technologies are designed to replicate human cognitive functions, enabling the processing of extensive datasets to identify patterns and generate predictions that inform clinical decision-making (Al Kuwaiti et al., 2023; Rathore & Rathore, 2023). For instance, AI applications can analyze electronic health records (EHRs) to identify trends in patient health, allowing healthcare providers to make data-driven decisions that enhance care quality and operational efficiency. The AI ability to sift through vast amounts of data and extract meaningful insights is particularly crucial in a healthcare landscape that is increasingly data-rich yet resource-constrained (Al Kuwaiti et al., 2023; Rathore & Rathore, 2023; Ismail et al., 2022). The applications of AI in healthcare are diverse and span numerous domains, influencing diagnostics, treatment planning, patient management, and operational efficiencies (Secinaro et al., 2021; Al Kuwaiti et al., 2023; Rathore & Rathore, 2023). For example, AI-driven tools are being utilized in medical imaging to enhance disease detection and predict the progression of conditions through advanced image recognition techniques, particularly in radiology (Al Kuwaiti et al., 2023; Rathore & Rathore, 2023; Ismail et al., 2022). Furthermore, AI's role in operational efficiency is exemplified by its application in supply chain management within healthcare systems, where intelligent algorithms can optimize resource allocation and reduce waste. This multifaceted application of AI improves patient outcomes and contributes to the sustainability of healthcare systems by minimizing unnecessary expenditures and resource use.

The majority of AI medical applications are founded on three primary types of algorithms: natural language processing (NLP), image processing, and reinforcement learning (RL) (Figure 1).

Figure 1. Applications of AI and ML in medical infrastructure

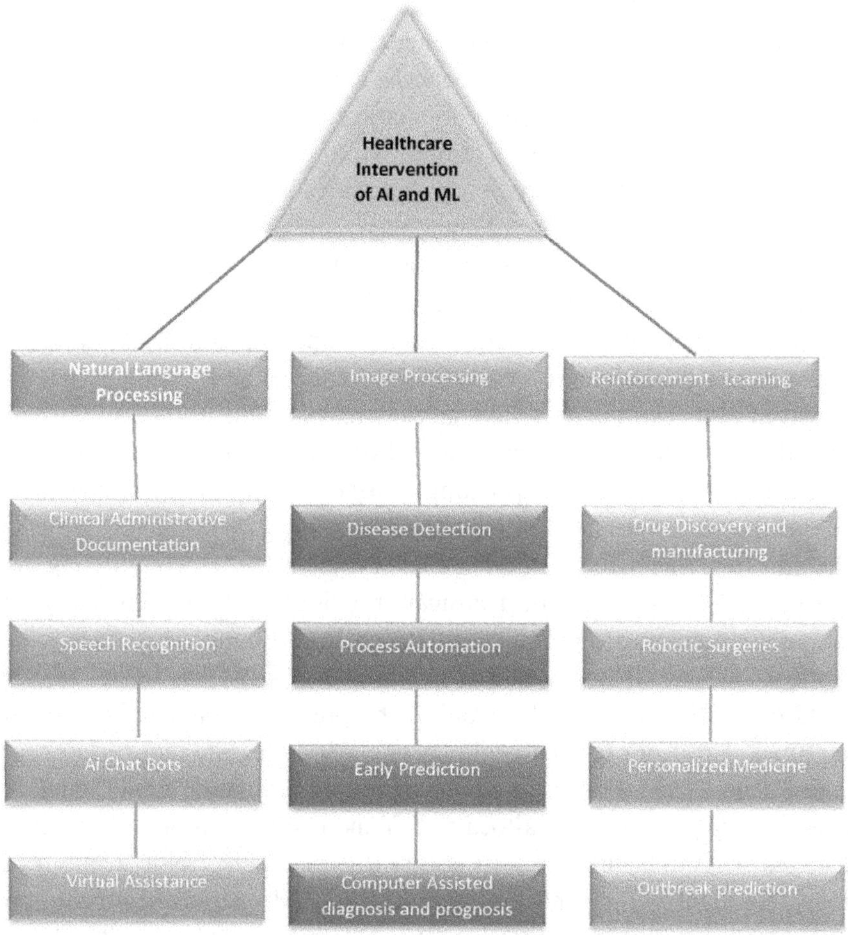

(Kumar et al., 2023)

Machine Learning (ML), a type of AI, uses algorithms that learn from data to get better at tasks over time. In healthcare, ML can analyze large amounts of medical data, like imaging studies and genetic information, to find disease patterns and predict how patients will do. For example, ML techniques can improve how accurately we diagnose illnesses and create more personalized treatment plans (Secinaro et al., 2021); Poalelungi et al., 2023; Aquino et al., 2023). Because ML can process and analyze large datasets, healthcare providers can make better-informed decisions, which can lead to improved patient outcomes (Secinaro et al., 2021; Hoseini, 2023).

NLP technologies are increasingly utilized in healthcare for various applications, including the analysis of clinical notes, patient interactions, and the extraction of meaningful insights from unstructured data. This capability is crucial for improving communication between healthcare providers and patients, as well as for enhancing the efficiency of administrative processes (Secinaro et al., 2021; Hoseini, 2023). NLP can also facilitate the development of virtual health assistants, which can provide patients with timely information and support (Poalelungi et al., 2023; Lee & Yoon, 2021). NLP applications include chatbots and virtual assistants that interpret EHRs and assist in patient interactions, thereby improving communication and operational efficiency. Predictive analytics is another critical component of AI in healthcare, employing statistical algorithms and machine learning techniques to identify the likelihood of future outcomes based on historical data. In healthcare, predictive analytics can help anticipate patient admissions, readmissions, and potential complications, enabling proactive care management (Batra & Reche, 2023), For instance, predictive models can analyze patient demographics, medical history, and treatment responses to forecast which patients are at risk of developing certain conditions, thereby allowing healthcare providers to implement preventive measures (Nor et al., 2020). By identifying patterns that may be indicative of diseases, AI can enhance diagnostic accuracy and speed (Ding et al., 2023). For example, AI systems have been developed to detect early signs of diabetic retinopathy, significantly improving screening processes (Huang et al., 2022). AI can aid clinicians in developing personalized treatment plans based on a patient's unique attributes, including genetics, lifestyle, and health history. This tailored approach can lead to more effective interventions and improved patient outcomes (Yu et al., 2024). AI-driven tools can analyze vast datasets to recommend the most suitable therapies for individual patients, thereby enhancing the precision of treatment (Singi et al., 2022). AI-powered tools can streamline patient management by automating routine tasks, monitoring patient compliance, and providing reminders for medications and follow-up appointments. This enhances patient engagement and supports better healthcare adherence (Williamson & Prybutok, 2024). By utilizing AI to track patient progress and adherence to treatment plans, healthcare providers can intervene early when issues arise, improving overall health outcomes (Pereira et al., 2021). By utilizing AI to track patient progress and adherence to treatment plans, healthcare providers can intervene early when issues arise, improving overall health outcomes.AI can optimize hospital operations by predicting patient flow, managing resources, and reducing wait times. This leads to improved patient experiences and more effective use of healthcare resources (Batra & Reche, 2023). For instance, AI algorithms can analyze historical admission data to forecast peak times, allowing hospitals to allocate staff and resources more effectively. One of the most significant advantages of AI in healthcare is its ability to process electronic health records (EHRs) and other large datasets. By identifying trends in patient health, AI enables healthcare providers to make data-driven decisions that enhance care quality and efficiency (Nor et al., 2020). For example, AI can flag potential health risks in populations, allowing for early interventions and preventive measures that can save lives and reduce healthcare costs. The integration of AI into clinical workflows not only improves patient outcomes but also contributes to the sustainability of healthcare systems by optimizing resource utilization and reducing waste.

Image processing tools, particularly those utilizing convolutional neural networks (CNNs), are pivotal in disease detection, enabling healthcare professionals to diagnose conditions with greater accuracy and speed. CNNs, a class of deep learning algorithms, have transformed the landscape of medical imaging by automating the analysis of complex image data, which traditionally required extensive human expertise. The ability of CNNs to learn hierarchical features from images allows for the effective classification and segmentation of medical images, significantly enhancing diagnostic capabilities in various medical fields (Ergün et al., 2024; Hosny et al., 2018). One of the primary advantages of employing CNNs in medical imaging is their capacity to analyze vast datasets, such as X-rays, MRIs, and CT scans, with remarkable precision. Studies have demonstrated that CNNs can outperform traditional image analysis methods, leading to improved diagnostic accuracy and reduced time for image interpretation (Ergün et al., 2024; Al-Karawi et al., 2024). For instance, a study on the use of deep learning for COVID-19 detection from X-ray images highlighted the effectiveness of CNNs in identifying the disease with high sensitivity and specificity, showcasing their potential in urgent clinical scenarios (Alasasfeh et al., 2021). Furthermore, the integration of CNNs into clinical workflows can alleviate the workload of radiologists, allowing them to focus on more complex cases while relying on AI for routine image assessments (Ergün et al., 2024). The application of CNNs extends beyond mere classification; they are also instrumental in the segmentation of medical images, which is crucial for precise localization of tumors or other anomalies. For example, CNN-based methods have been successfully employed in brain tumor segmentation, where they provide detailed delineation of tumor boundaries, thus aiding in treatment planning and monitoring (Hosny et al., 2018). Additionally, CNNs can be trained to recognize various pathologies, enabling rapid triage of cases based on urgency and severity (Botwe et al., 2021). Moreover, the continuous improvement of CNN architectures and training methodologies has further enhanced their performance in medical imaging tasks. Techniques such as data augmentation, transfer learning, and the use of large annotated datasets have contributed to the robustness and generalizability of CNN models across different imaging modalities (Shorten & Khoshgoftaar, 2019). As a result, healthcare professionals can leverage these advanced tools to make more informed decisions, ultimately leading to better patient outcomes. However, the deployment of CNNs in clinical settings is not without challenges. Issues related to data privacy, the need for high-quality annotated datasets, and the interpretability of AI decisions remain significant hurdles that must be addressed to ensure the safe and effective use of these technologies in healthcare (Neto & Endo, 2023). Additionally, while CNNs can enhance diagnostic capabilities, the importance of human oversight cannot be overstated; expert interpretation remains essential to validate AI-generated results and ensure patient safety (Botwe et al., 2021; Temsah et al., 2024). In conclusion, CNNs represent a transformative advancement in medical image processing, offering significant improvements in disease detection and diagnosis. Their ability to analyze complex image data with high accuracy and speed positions them as invaluable tools in modern healthcare, facilitating timely and effective patient care. As the technology continues to evolve, ongoing research and collaboration between AI developers and healthcare professionals will be crucial to maximize the benefits of CNNs while addressing the associated challenges.

Reinforcement learning applications encompass a wide range of uses, including surgical robotics, drug discovery, and personalized medicine, where RL-driven algorithms can formulate optimal treatment plans based on individual patient data (Rathore & Rathore, 2023; Temsah et al., 2024).

In the realm of surgical robotics, reinforcement learning has been instrumental in developing systems that can adapt and improve their performance over time. RL algorithms enable robotic systems to learn from their interactions with the surgical environment, optimizing their movements and decision-making processes. For instance, RL can be used to train robotic arms to perform intricate surgical tasks with precision, learning from previous surgeries to minimize errors and improve patient safety (Rahmani et al., 2021). The ability of these systems to analyze feedback from their actions allows them to refine their techniques, ultimately leading to better surgical outcomes and reduced recovery times for patients (Shameer et al., 2018).

Reinforcement learning also plays a significant role in drug discovery, where it can streamline the process of identifying potential therapeutic compounds. Traditional drug discovery methods are often time-consuming and costly, but RL can accelerate this process by predicting the efficacy of various compounds based on historical data. By modeling the interactions between drugs and biological systems, RL algorithms can suggest optimal combinations and dosages, thereby enhancing the efficiency of clinical trials (Iovino et al., 2020). This approach not only reduces the time required to bring new drugs to market but also increases the likelihood of successful outcomes in clinical settings (Iovino et al., 2020).

In personalized medicine, reinforcement learning algorithms are particularly valuable for tailoring treatment plans to individual patients. By analyzing a patient's unique genetic makeup, medical history, and response to previous treatments, RL can help clinicians devise personalized therapeutic strategies that maximize efficacy while minimizing side effects (Oh et al., 2022). For example, RL has been utilized to develop dynamic treatment regimes that adapt to a patient's changing condition over time, ensuring that the treatment remains optimal throughout the course of care (Wang et al., 2018). This adaptability is crucial in managing chronic diseases, where patient responses can vary significantly and require ongoing adjustments to treatment plans (Barriga Rodriguez et al., 2020). Moreover, the integration of reinforcement learning with other advanced technologies, such as deep learning and radiomics, further enhances its potential in personalized medicine. By combining these approaches, healthcare providers can gain deeper insights into disease mechanisms and patient responses, leading to more informed and effective treatment decisions (Parekh & Jacobs, 2019). The ability of RL to process large datasets and learn from complex interactions makes it an invaluable tool in the ongoing pursuit of personalized healthcare solutions.

The challenges accompanying the AI implementation in healthcare are significant and multifaceted. These include concerns regarding data privacy, algorithmic bias, and the need for regulatory frameworks that can keep pace with technological advancements (Tsiakas et al., 2018). Moreover, integrating AI into existing healthcare workflows necessitates substantial changes in organizational culture and staff training to ensure that healthcare professionals can effectively leverage these technologies. Addressing these challenges is crucial for realizing the full potential of AI in enhancing patient care and achieving sustainability in healthcare systems (Hassanien & Mononteliza, 2020).

2. CONTRIBUTIONS TO SUSTAINABLE PRACTICES

2.1. Optimizing Resource Allocation

One of the most significant contributions of AI to sustainable healthcare is its ability to optimize resource allocation. By utilizing predictive analytics, AI can forecast patient admission rates, streamline staff scheduling, and manage inventory effectively. This optimization reduces waste and ensures that resources are directed where they are most needed, leading to lower operational costs and a diminished environmental footprint (Abou Ghayda et al., 2024). For example, AI-driven models have been shown to decrease hospital readmissions by tailoring treatment plans to individual patient needs, thereby improving outcomes and reducing healthcare expenses (Movahed & Bilderback, 2024).

The integration of Artificial Intelligence into healthcare systems has emerged as a transformative force, particularly in optimizing resource allocation. The application of AI technologies in healthcare is not merely a trend but a necessity driven by the increasing demand for efficient healthcare delivery amidst limited resources. AI can significantly enhance the efficiency of healthcare operations by analyzing vast amounts of data, predicting patient needs, and optimizing the distribution of medical resources. This subsection will explore the various dimensions of optimizing resource allocation through AI, including its impact on healthcare efficiency, ethical considerations, and the challenges that accompany its implementation. AI's ability to process and analyze large datasets allows healthcare providers to make informed decisions regarding resource allocation. For instance, predictive analytics can identify patient populations at risk, enabling healthcare systems to allocate resources more effectively to those in need. As noted by Yin et al., AI applications in clinical practice have demonstrated the potential to improve decision-making processes, thereby enhancing the overall efficiency of healthcare delivery systems (Yin et al., 2021). Moreover, AI-driven algorithms can streamline operations by predicting patient inflow, optimizing staff schedules, and managing inventory levels, which ultimately leads to reduced operational costs and improved patient outcomes (Guerra, 2024). This is particularly crucial in emergency departments where resource allocation must be dynamic and responsive to real-time demands. The ethical implications of AI in resource allocation cannot be overlooked. As AI systems increasingly influence decisions regarding the distribution of healthcare resources, concerns about fairness, transparency, and accountability arise. Claudy and Graso emphasize that the transition to AI-led decision-making necessitates a thorough examination of algorithmic fairness and the potential biases embedded within these systems (Claudy et al., 2022). Ensuring that AI algorithms are designed to promote equitable access to healthcare resources is paramount, especially in diverse populations where disparities in health outcomes are prevalent. Therefore, it is essential to incorporate ethical frameworks into the development and deployment of AI technologies in healthcare to mitigate risks associated with biased decision-making. Furthermore, the implementation of AI in optimizing resource allocation presents several challenges that must be addressed. As highlighted by Alnasser, uncertainties regarding the effectiveness and value of AI in practice persist, underscoring the need for comprehensive health technology assessments (Alnasser, 2023). Stakeholders must evaluate the economic implications of AI applications and develop implementation guidelines that ensure the responsible use of these technologies. Additionally, the integration of AI systems into existing healthcare infrastructures requires significant investment in technology and training, which can be a barrier for many healthcare organizations, particularly in low-resource settings (Babarinde et al., 2023). The role of AI in enhancing risk management practices within healthcare settings is another critical aspect of optimizing resource allocation. AI-driven predictive analytics can identify potential risks and prioritize interventions, allowing healthcare providers to allocate resources more effectively (Guerra, 2024). For example, machine learning algorithms can analyze historical patient data to predict future healthcare needs, enabling hospitals to prepare and allocate resources accordingly. This proactive approach not only improves patient outcomes but also enhances the overall efficiency of healthcare systems by reducing unnecessary expenditures and resource wastage. Moreover, the application of AI in optimizing resource allocation extends beyond clinical settings to include administrative and operational aspects of healthcare delivery. Secinaro et al. propose a data-driven optimization methodology that determines the optimal number of healthcare staff required to maximize patient productivity (Secinaro et al., 2021). By leveraging AI technologies, healthcare organizations can ensure that they are not overstaffed or understaffed, which can lead to inefficiencies and compromised patient care. This optimization of human resources is crucial in maintaining a balance between cost-effectiveness and quality of care. AI's potential to facilitate better communication and coordination among healthcare providers is also significant in the context of resource allocation. By utilizing AI algorithms to analyze patient data and predict disease outbreaks, healthcare systems can improve the distribution of medical resources, ensuring that they are allocated where they are most needed (Victor, 2023). This capability is particularly relevant in managing public health crises, such as pandemics, where timely and efficient resource allocation can save lives and reduce the burden on healthcare systems. Despite the promising benefits of AI in optimizing resource allocation, there are inherent challenges that must be navigated. The reliance on data-driven decision-making raises concerns about data privacy and security, as sensitive patient information is often involved in AI analyses. As Eshwar points out, regulatory compliance and ethical considerations are paramount in ensuring that AI technologies are used responsibly within healthcare settings (Eshwar, 2023). Furthermore, the need for continuous monitoring and evaluation of AI systems is essential to ensure that they remain effective and equitable over time. In conclusion, the optimization of resource allocation through AI in healthcare presents a multifaceted opportunity to enhance efficiency, improve patient outcomes, and address the challenges of limited resources. While the potential benefits are substantial, it is crucial to approach the implementation of AI with a focus on ethical considerations, economic implications, and the need for robust regulatory frameworks. As healthcare continues to evolve, the integration of AI technologies will play a pivotal role in shaping the future of resource allocation, ultimately leading to a more sustainable and effective healthcare system.

2.2. Enhancing Preventive Care

AI's predictive capabilities extend to preventive care, where it can identify at-risk populations by analyzing data from EHRs, wearables, and social determinants of health (Okolo et al., 2024). By facilitating early interventions, healthcare systems can enhance patient outcomes and minimize the necessity for more intensive, resource-heavy treatments later on. This proactive approach not only improves individual health but also contributes to the sustainability of healthcare systems by reducing the overall demand for resources (Okolo et al., 2024).

AI is greatly improving preventive care in healthcare, leading to better health and smarter use of resources. AI technologies help with early disease detection, personalized health plans, and efficient use of healthcare resources. This section will explain how AI improves preventive care through predictive analytics, patient profiling, and tailored health interventions.

AI improves preventive care mainly through predictive analytics, which helps healthcare providers find at-risk populations before diseases start. By analyzing large datasets, AI algorithms can spot patterns and risk factors for different health conditions. For example, Jansson et al. point out that AI-enhanced scheduling systems can sort patients into high- and low-risk groups, allowing healthcare providers to take preventive actions early (Jansson et al., 2022). This is very important for managing long-term diseases, where early action can change the course of the disease and improve patient outcomes. Moreover, AI's ability to personalize health interventions is pivotal in enhancing preventive care. Chew and Achananuparp emphasize the importance of integrating AI-generated reports with individual demographic and clinical profiles to facilitate self-management among patients (Chew & Achananuparp, 2022). This personalized approach not only empowers patients to take charge of their health but also ensures that healthcare resources are allocated efficiently. For example, AI can recommend specific lifestyle changes or screenings based on an individual's unique risk factors, thereby optimizing the use of healthcare services and reducing unnecessary expenditures. The role of AI in preventive care is further exemplified in elderly care, where early diagnosis and intervention are critical. Yousefi discusses how AI technologies, such as care robots and diagnostic tools, can assist in the early detection of conditions like stroke, thereby enhancing the quality of life and promoting independence among elderly individuals (Yousefi et al., 2023). By providing timely interventions, AI not only improves health outcomes but also reduces the burden on healthcare systems by preventing complications that require more intensive treatment. In addition to individual patient care, AI can enhance preventive care at the population level by identifying trends and outbreaks in real-time. For instance, AI systems can analyze data from various sources, including social media and electronic health records, to predict disease outbreaks and inform public health responses. This capability is essential for managing infectious diseases and ensuring that preventive measures, such as vaccinations and health education campaigns, are implemented effectively. Furthermore, the acceptability of AI technologies among patients is crucial for their successful integration into preventive care strategies. Research by Young et al. indicates that while patients generally accept the use of AI in their care, they desire transparency regarding the effectiveness and application of these technologies (Young et al., 2021). This underscores the need for healthcare providers to communicate the benefits and limitations of AI tools to foster trust and encourage patient engagement in preventive care initiatives. Despite the promising advancements, challenges remain in the widespread adoption of AI in preventive care. Issues related to data quality, algorithmic bias, and the need for robust regulatory frameworks must be addressed to ensure that AI technologies are effective and equitable. As highlighted by Nadarzynski et al., understanding patient hesitancy towards AI applications is essential for developing strategies that enhance acceptance and utilization of these technologies in healthcare (Nadarzynski et al., 2019). In conclusion, AI is poised to revolutionize preventive care by enabling early detection, personalized interventions, and efficient resource allocation. The successful integration of AI into preventive care strategies requires a multifaceted approach that addresses ethical considerations, patient engagement, and the need for continuous evaluation of AI systems. As healthcare systems strive for sustainability and improved health outcomes, leveraging AI technologies will be essential in enhancing preventive care practices.

2.3. Telemedicine and Remote Monitoring

The COVID-19 pandemic has accelerated the adoption of telemedicine, with AI playing a crucial role in this transformation. AI algorithms assist in triaging patients remotely, conducting virtual health assessments, and monitoring chronic conditions through wearable devices (Kale, 2019). This shift not only enhances access to care but also mitigates the carbon footprint associated with patient travel, aligning with sustainability goals (El Morr & Ali-Hassan, 2019). Moreover, remote monitoring facilitated by AI allows for proactive healthcare interventions, tracking vital signs and identifying potential health issues in real-time (Kale, 2019).

The rapid advancements in digital technology, AI, and 5G wireless systems have enabled the introduction of telemedicine in various medical specialties, including ophthalmology (Li et al., 2022). The COVID-19 pandemic has further accelerated the development and adoption of these technologies (Li et al., 2022). Telemedicine offers several benefits, such as improving access to medical services, providing previously unavailable care options, and reducing medical costs (Hwang et al., 2019). In the field of ophthalmology, real-time video consultations between hospital-based ophthalmologists and emergency physicians or other specialists can help emergency patients receive timely evaluations and referrals, improving diagnostic accuracy (Li et al., 2022). Furthermore, the integration of telemedicine with AI-based automated algorithms can provide instant diagnosis of conditions like diabetic retinopathy and reduce the burden on healthcare systems (Rajalakshmi et al., 2021). Telemedicine-based screening with AI grading has been shown to be cost-effective compared to traditional fundus photography-based screening, particularly in urban and rural areas of China (Li et al., 2023). While telemedicine and remote monitoring offer substantial benefits, they also introduce complex ethical dilemmas that need careful consideration. One prominent concern is data sovereignty, especially in cross-border care scenarios. When patients receive care from providers in different countries, it is crucial to address questions about which jurisdiction's data privacy laws apply and how patient data is protected across borders. AI algorithms that process and transmit sensitive patient information must comply with diverse regulatory frameworks to ensure patient rights are upheld. Another ethical challenge arises around equitable access to telemedicine technologies. While telemedicine can improve access for some populations, it may exacerbate disparities for others who lack digital literacy or access to technology. It is important to consider how AI solutions can be designed and implemented to promote inclusivity and avoid unintended discrimination. Finally, the use of AI in remote patient monitoring raises questions about the potential for over-reliance on technology and the impact on the patient-provider relationship. Striking a balance between leveraging AI for efficient monitoring and maintaining the human connection and trust between patients and healthcare professionals is essential (Li et al., 2023). The use of digital fundus cameras and remote interpretation has facilitated larger population coverage of diabetic retinopathy screening and timely referral of those with sight-threatening conditions to ophthalmologists (Rajalakshmi et al., 2021). The benefits of telemedicine and remote monitoring extend beyond ophthalmology. In the context of heart failure, a feasibility study found that providing patients with a digital solution, including lifestyle-change and disease self-care support, a remote symptom monitoring system, and a secure messaging platform between healthcare providers and patients, was well-accepted by patients and showed promising trends in clinical outcomes (Arnar et al., 2022). However, the successful implementation of telemedicine and digital health solutions requires rigorous usability testing, both pre- and post-deployment, to understand the healthcare user journey and ensure that the solutions are tailored to the specific needs and workflows of healthcare professionals and patients (Chokshi & Mann, 2018). Additionally, a supportive organizational and contextual environment is vital for the scalability and sustainability of these digital innovations (Cripps & Scarbrough, 2022). The integration of telemedicine and remote monitoring with AI and other digital technologies has the potential to improve access to healthcare, enhance patient outcomes, and contribute to the sustainability of healthcare systems. However, careful consideration of user needs, organizational support, and the broader contextual factors is essential for the successful and sustainable implementation of these technologies (Mather & Almond, 2022).

2.4. Drug Discovery and Development

The pharmaceutical industry is notoriously resource-intensive, and AI algorithms can significantly streamline drug discovery processes. By predicting molecular interactions and optimizing clinical trial designs, AI reduces the time and resources required for bringing new therapies to market (Udegbe et al., 2024). This acceleration not only shortens the timeline for new treatments but also lessens the environmental impact associated with traditional drug development methods, contributing to a more sustainable healthcare landscape (Kale, 2019).

The use of AI and machine learning (ML) in drug discovery and development is changing pharmaceutical sciences, with the potential to make the creation of new treatments more efficient and sustainable. Traditional drug discovery takes a long time and costs a lot, often more than a billion dollars and up to 15 years to bring a new drug to market (Vella & Ebejer, 2022). AI technologies are becoming powerful tools to speed up different parts of this process, from finding drug targets to conducting clinical trials, which contributes to more sustainable healthcare.

Machine learning algorithms are being used a lot to predict how drugs and targets will interact, improve potential drug compounds, and evaluate the safety and effectiveness of new drugs. For example, a large study comparing different ML methods for predicting drug targets showed that deep learning methods were more accurate than older methods like support vector machines and random forests (Mayr et al., 2018). This ability to accurately predict interactions speeds up the process of finding good drug candidates and also reduces the amount of lab testing needed, saving resources and reducing waste. Moreover, AI's ability to analyze vast datasets from electronic health records and real-world evidence has been instrumental in improving clinical trial designs and eligibility assessments (Vamathevan et al., 2019). By leveraging historical data, AI can identify patient populations that are more likely to respond to specific treatments, thereby enhancing the efficiency of clinical trials and reducing the time and costs associated with drug (Vatansever et al., 2021). This targeted approach not only improves the likelihood of trial success but also aligns with sustainable practices by optimizing resource allocation. In addition to improving the efficiency of drug discovery, AI technologies also facilitate the exploration of previously neglected areas of research. For example, machine learning has been applied to discover antiviral compounds against diseases like yellow fever, which have historically received less attention compared to more prevalent infections such as dengue and Zika (Gawriljuk et al., 2021). This capability to uncover new therapeutic avenues is crucial for addressing global health challenges and ensuring that drug development is responsive to emerging infectious diseases. The application of AI in drug discovery is not limited to predictive modeling; it also encompasses active learning strategies that adaptively refine models based on ongoing experimental results. This iterative process allows researchers to focus on the most promising candidates, thereby minimizing the time and resources spent on less viable option (Reker, 2019). Such active learning frameworks are particularly beneficial in high-throughput screening environments, where the rapid evaluation of numerous compounds is essential. Furthermore, the convergence of AI with other technological advancements, such as robotics and automation, is set to revolutionize the drug discovery landscape. Automated systems can perform repetitive tasks with high precision, while AI algorithms can analyze the resulting data to identify patterns and make predictions (Brown et al., 2020). This synergy not only accelerates the discovery process but also reduces human error, contributing to more reliable outcomes. The challenges associated with drug discovery, including the high attrition rates of candidates during clinical trials, underscore the need for innovative solutions. AI has the potential to address these challenges by enhancing the predictive power of models used to assess drug-like properties, such as absorption, distribution, metabolism, excretion, and toxicity (ADME/T) (Cai et al., 2020). By improving the accuracy of these predictions, AI can help ensure that only the most promising candidates advance through the development pipeline, thereby reducing waste and improving sustainability. Moreover, the application of AI in drug discovery extends to the realm of personalized medicine, where machine learning algorithms can analyze genetic and phenotypic data to tailor treatments to individual patients (Vamathevan et al., 2019). This personalized approach not only enhances therapeutic efficacy but also minimizes adverse effects, contributing to more sustainable healthcare practices by ensuring that treatments are both effective and safe. Despite the promising advancements, the integration of AI into drug discovery is not without challenges. Issues related to data quality, algorithm interpretability, and the need for interdisciplinary collaboration must be addressed to fully realize the potential of AI in this field (Dara et al., 2022; Udegbe et al., 2024). Ensuring that AI models are transparent and interpretable is crucial for gaining the trust of stakeholders, including regulatory bodies, healthcare providers, and patients. In conclusion, the incorporation of AI and machine learning into drug discovery and development processes represents a significant advancement towards more sustainable healthcare practices. By enhancing efficiency, reducing costs, and enabling the exploration of new therapeutic avenues, AI technologies are poised to transform the pharmaceutical landscape. However, ongoing efforts to address the challenges associated with data quality, model interpretability, and interdisciplinary collaboration will be essential to fully harness the potential of AI in drug discovery.

2.5. Personalized Medicine

AI's ability to analyze genetic, lifestyle, and environmental data enables the development of personalized medicine approaches. By tailoring treatments to individual patients, AI can lead to more effective therapies with fewer side effects, ultimately reducing the burden on healthcare systems and minimizing the use of unnecessary treatments (Okolo et al., 2024). This precision in treatment not only enhances patient outcomes but also aligns with the principles of sustainability by ensuring that healthcare resources are utilized efficiently (Udegbe et al., 2024).

The advent of AI has significantly transformed the landscape of personalized medicine, enabling healthcare providers to tailor treatments to individual patients based on their unique genetic, environmental, and lifestyle factors. This shift towards personalized medicine is not merely a trend but a fundamental change in how healthcare is delivered, promising to enhance patient outcomes and optimize resource utilization in a sustainable manner. AI algorithms facilitate the integration of vast amounts of data, including genomic information, clinical histories, and real-time health metrics, to inform more precise and effective treatment strategies (Ahmed & Adil, 2023). One of the most compelling applications of AI in personalized medicine is its ability to analyze data from wearable sensors and other health monitoring devices. For instance, AI-driven tools can process data from electrocardiograms (ECGs) to detect cardiac events, such as acute ST-elevation myocardial infarction (STEMI), with remarkable accuracy (Huang et al., 2022). The development of specialized AI architectures, such as deep Bidirectional Long Short-Term Memory (BiLSTM) models, has demonstrated superior performance in diagnosing cardiovascular conditions compared to traditional methods, thereby enhancing the precision of patient care (Huang et al., 2022). This capability not only improves diagnostic accuracy but also allows for timely interventions, which are crucial in critical care settings. Moreover, AI's role in personalized medicine extends to optimizing treatment plans based on individual patient profiles. By leveraging machine learning algorithms, healthcare providers can predict how patients will respond to specific therapies, thereby minimizing adverse reactions and improving treatment efficacy (Ahmed & Adil, 2023). For example, AI can analyze genomic data to identify patients who are likely to benefit from targeted therapies, such as those used in oncology, where treatments can be tailored to the genetic makeup of tumors (Ahmed & Adil, 2023). This approach not only enhances patient outcomes but also contributes to the sustainability of healthcare systems by reducing the trial-and-error nature of traditional treatment methods. The integration of AI in personalized medicine also addresses the growing complexity of healthcare data. As patient populations become more diverse and the volume of health-related data increases, AI algorithms can help synthesize this information to identify patterns and correlations that may not be immediately apparent to healthcare professionals. This data-driven approach enables clinicians to make informed decisions that are tailored to the specific needs of their patients, thereby enhancing the overall quality of care (Yelne et al., 2023; Gou et al., 2024). However, the successful implementation of AI in personalized medicine is not without challenges. Issues related to data quality, interoperability, and patient privacy must be addressed to fully realize the potential of AI technologies in this field (Hoseini, 2023; Laï et al., 2020). Furthermore, the acceptance of AI-driven solutions by both healthcare providers and patients is crucial for their widespread adoption. Studies have shown that while there is a general enthusiasm for AI in healthcare, there is also a significant level of skepticism regarding its reliability and ethical implications (Stewart et al., 2023). Therefore, fostering trust and ensuring transparency in AI applications are essential for overcoming these barriers. In addition to enhancing individual patient care, AI's role in personalized medicine has broader implications for public health. By enabling more effective disease prevention strategies and early interventions, AI can help reduce the overall burden on healthcare systems. For instance, predictive analytics can identify at-risk populations and facilitate targeted health initiatives, thereby promoting healthier communities and reducing healthcare costs (Ahmed & Adil, 2023). This proactive approach aligns with sustainable healthcare practices by focusing on prevention rather than reactive treatment. Furthermore, the convergence of AI with other technological advancements, such as telemedicine and big data analytics, is set to revolutionize personalized medicine. The ability to deliver personalized care remotely through telehealth platforms, combined with AI's analytical capabilities, allows for continuous monitoring and adjustment of treatment plans based on real-time data (Secara & Hordiiuk, 2024). This integration not only enhances patient engagement but also ensures that care is both accessible and tailored to individual needs, thereby promoting health equity. As the field of personalized medicine continues to evolve, ongoing research and collaboration among stakeholders will be essential to harness the full potential of AI technologies. Interdisciplinary approaches that combine insights from genomics, data science, and clinical practice will be crucial for developing innovative solutions that address the complexities of patient care (Chew & Achananuparp, 2022; Issa et al., 2024). Moreover, educational initiatives aimed at equipping healthcare professionals with the necessary skills to utilize AI tools effectively will play a vital role in the successful integration of these technologies into clinical practice (Issa et al., 2024; Alowais et al., 2023). In conclusion, AI is poised to play a transformative role in personalized medicine, offering the potential for more precise, effective, and sustainable healthcare interventions. By leveraging advanced data analytics and machine learning algorithms, healthcare providers can tailor treatments to individual patients, ultimately improving outcomes and reducing costs. However, addressing the challenges associated with data quality, ethical considerations, and stakeholder acceptance will be critical for realizing the full benefits of AI in this domain.

3. CHALLENGES AND CONSIDERATIONS

Despite the immense potential of AI in promoting sustainable healthcare, several challenges must be addressed. Issues such as data privacy, algorithmic bias, and the need for robust regulatory frameworks are critical to ensuring that AI implementations are ethical, equitable, and effective. The integration of AI into existing healthcare infrastructures necessitates significant investments in technology and training for healthcare professionals, which can be a barrier to widespread adoption. Moreover, the ethical implications of AI in healthcare cannot be overlooked. Patients often express concerns regarding the use of AI technologies, particularly regarding the need for physician oversight and the potential for harm if these systems are not adequately regulated. Engaging the public in discussions about the benefits and risks of AI applications is essential to fostering trust and acceptance among patients and healthcare providers.

The integration of Artificial Intelligence into healthcare systems presents numerous challenges and considerations that must be addressed to ensure successful implementation and sustainability. These challenges can be categorized into several key areas, including ethical concerns, data quality, workforce implications, and technological integration (Table 1).

Table 1. AI challenges in healthcare.

Challenge/Considerations	Description	References
Ethical Considerations	The deployment of AI in healthcare raises significant ethical dilemmas, including issues of bias, accountability, and patient privacy. Ethical frameworks are necessary to guide the responsible use of AI technologies	(Familoni, 2024)
	Ethical frameworks are essential to ensure equitable healthcare outcomes and to mitigate biases in AI algorithms Moreover, the need for transparency in AI decision-making processes is critical to maintain trust among healthcare professionals and patients	(Muley et al., 2023)
Data Quality and Management	High-quality data is crucial for the effective functioning of AI algorithms. Challenges include data privacy concerns, standardization, and interoperability across various healthcare systems	(Hoseini, 2023)
	The quality of data directly affects the performance of AI applications, and inadequate data management can lead to suboptimal outcomes . Furthermore, the integration of diverse data sources is essential to enhance AI's predictive capabilities	(Gama et al., 2022)
Workforce Implications	The introduction of AI technologies can lead to apprehensions among healthcare professionals regarding job displacement and the need for new skill sets	(Mikava & Mamulaidze, 2023)
	There is a prevalent fear of job loss among healthcare workers, which can hinder the acceptance of AI technologies Training and education in AI fundamentals and data analytics are vital for healthcare professionals to adapt to these changes	(Steerling et al., 2023)
Technological Integration	Integrating AI into existing healthcare workflows poses significant challenges, including resistance to change and the complexity of embedding AI tools into clinical practice	(Movahed & Bilderback, 2024)
	Successful implementation requires addressing the technological gaps and ensuring that AI tools complement existing workflows rather than disrupt them . Additionally, fostering collaboration among stakeholders is essential for overcoming integration hurdles	(Movahed & Bilderback, 2024; 84]
Sustainability and Scalability	For AI solutions to contribute to sustainable healthcare, they must be scalable and adaptable to various healthcare settings, including those in low-resource environments. This requires a strategic approach to implementation that considers the diverse needs of different populations and healthcare systems	(Vishwakarma et al., 2023)
Trust and Transparency	Building trust in AI systems is critical for their acceptance by both healthcare providers and patients. This involves ensuring that AI algorithms are transparent, understandable, and aligned with the values and expectations of users. Lack of trust can lead to reluctance in adopting AI technologies	(Chomutare et al., 2022)

The integration of AI in healthcare, while promising significant advancements in efficiency and patient care, also presents a myriad of challenges and considerations that must be addressed to ensure its successful implementation and sustainability. These challenges encompass ethical, technical, and operational dimensions, each of which plays a crucial role in shaping the future of AI in healthcare. One of the foremost challenges is the ethical implications of AI technologies. As AI systems are increasingly utilized for clinical decision-making, concerns regarding bias, accountability, and transparency have come to the forefront. For instance, AI algorithms trained on biased datasets can perpetuate existing disparities in healthcare, leading to unequal treatment outcomes among different demographic groups (Katirai, 2023; Anyanwu et al., 2024). This raises critical questions about the fairness and justice of AI applications in healthcare, necessitating the development of robust frameworks to mitigate bias and ensure equitable access to AI-driven solutions (Coeckelbergh, 2021). Furthermore, the ethical principle of beneficence must be upheld, ensuring that AI technologies enhance patient welfare rather than compromise it (Olorunsogo et al., 2024). In addition to ethical concerns, the technical challenges associated with AI implementation are significant. The complexity of healthcare data, which is often heterogeneous and unstructured, poses a barrier to the effective training and validation of AI algorithms (Yelne et al., 2023). Ensuring data quality and interoperability among various healthcare systems is essential for the successful deployment of AI technologies. Moreover, the rapid pace of AI advancements often outstrips existing regulatory frameworks, creating uncertainty regarding compliance and governance (Lee & Yoon, 2021). This regulatory lag can hinder the adoption of AI solutions, as healthcare providers may be reluctant to implement technologies that lack clear guidelines and oversight. Trust in AI systems is another critical consideration that affects their acceptance among healthcare professionals and patients alike. Research indicates that healthcare workers may exhibit skepticism towards AI technologies, particularly when it comes to accountability and liability in clinical decision-making (Petersson et al., 2022). This lack of trust can impede the integration of AI into clinical workflows, as healthcare professionals may be hesitant to rely on algorithms for critical decisions. Building trust requires transparency in AI operations, including clear explanations of how algorithms arrive at their conclusions and the ability to audit AI systems for accuracy and fairness (Petersson et al., 2022). Moreover, the implementation of AI in healthcare necessitates a cultural shift within healthcare organizations. Healthcare professionals must be equipped with the knowledge and skills to effectively utilize AI tools, which may require significant investment in training and education • (Alowais et al., 2023)

Resistance to change can also pose a barrier, as some healthcare providers may be reluctant to adopt new technologies that disrupt established practices. Fostering a culture of innovation and continuous learning is essential for overcoming these challenges and ensuring that AI technologies are embraced as valuable tools for enhancing patient care (Yelne et al., 2023). Data privacy and security are paramount concerns in the context of AI in healthcare. The use of sensitive patient data to train AI algorithms raises questions about data protection and patient consent (Ogaga & Zhao, 2023). Ensuring compliance with regulations such as the Health Insurance Portability and Accountability Act (HIPAA) in the United States and the General Data Protection Regulation (GDPR) in Europe is critical for safeguarding patient information. Healthcare organizations must implement robust data governance policies to protect against breaches and unauthorized access, thereby maintaining patient trust and confidence in AI applications (Lee & Yoon, 2021). The sustainability of AI technologies in healthcare is also contingent upon their economic viability. While AI has the potential to reduce costs and improve efficiency, the initial investment required for AI infrastructure and training can be substantial (Movahed & Bilderback, 2024). Healthcare organizations must carefully evaluate the return on investment (ROI) associated with AI implementation, considering both short-term costs and long-term benefits. Additionally, the economic impact of AI on the workforce must be considered, as automation may lead to job displacement in certain areas of healthcare (Yelne et al., 2023). Finally, the broader societal implications of AI in healthcare must be acknowledged. As AI technologies become more prevalent, there is a risk of exacerbating existing inequalities in healthcare access and outcomes. Policymakers and healthcare leaders must work collaboratively to ensure that AI solutions are developed and deployed in ways that promote health equity and address the needs of underserved populations (Lee & Yoon, 2021). This requires a commitment to inclusive practices in AI development, ensuring that diverse voices are represented in the design and implementation of AI technologies. In conclusion, while AI holds immense potential to revolutionize healthcare, its successful integration is fraught with challenges that must be carefully navigated. Addressing ethical considerations, technical barriers, trust issues, data privacy, economic viability, and societal implications is essential for realizing the full benefits of AI in sustainable healthcare.

The integration of AI into healthcare demands a multifaceted approach that extends beyond technological innovation. Interdisciplinary perspectives, such as ethical frameworks and policy analyses, are crucial for contextualizing AI within broader societal and environmental sustainability goals. Ethical frameworks, such as the one proposed by Jobin et al., provide guidelines for addressing concerns related to bias, accountability, and transparency in AI decision-making. Policy analyses offer insights into regulatory and governance structures necessary to ensure equitable access to AI-driven healthcare solutions. By incorporating these interdisciplinary perspectives, we can foster the responsible development and deployment of AI technologies, aligning them with the principles of sustainability and societal well-being (Familoni, 2024).

Addressing the regulatory challenges and ethical considerations surrounding AI in healthcare is paramount. Issues of AI accountability and transparency are particularly salient. It is essential to establish clear frameworks that define liability when AI systems make errors and to ensure that the decision-making processes of AI algorithms are transparent and understandable to healthcare providers and patients. This will foster trust and facilitate the responsible adoption of AI technologies in clinical settings (Muley et al., 2023).

By proactively engaging with these challenges, stakeholders can foster an environment where AI technologies enhance patient care while promoting equity and sustainability in healthcare systems.

4. FUTURE DIRECTIONS AND INNOVATIONS IN AI FOR SUSTAINABLE HEALTHCARE

The future of sustainable healthcare is intricately linked to advancements in artificial intelligence (AI) technologies, which are poised to revolutionize the healthcare landscape. Emerging trends and innovative applications of AI, such as machine learning, natural language processing, and computer vision, are rapidly evolving and hold significant promise for enhancing healthcare sustainability. For instance, deep learning techniques have shown proficiency in interpreting complex medical images, leading to faster and more accurate diagnoses while optimizing resource utilization within healthcare systems by minimizing the need for repeat imaging and invasive procedures (Lee & Yoon, 2021; Choudhury & Asan, 2020). This optimization is crucial as it correlates with improved patient outcomes and reduced environmental impacts associated with traditional healthcare models (Alahmari et al., 2022; Murphy et al., 2021).

Recent advancements in AI are rapidly transforming the landscape of sustainable healthcare. Generative AI, for instance, is revolutionizing drug discovery by accelerating the identification of potential therapeutic compounds and optimizing clinical trial designs. Federated learning is another cutting-edge development that enhances data privacy by enabling collaborative model training without the need to centralize sensitive patient information. These advancements not only improve the efficiency and effectiveness of healthcare but also contribute to sustainability by reducing resource consumption and minimizing adverse impacts (Lee & Yoon, 2021; Choudhury & Asan, 2020).

4.1. Advancements in AI Technologies

The advancements in artificial intelligence (AI) technologies are reshaping the landscape of sustainable healthcare, offering innovative solutions that enhance patient care, optimize resource utilization, and improve overall healthcare outcomes. The integration of machine learning, natural language processing, and computer vision into healthcare practices has led to significant breakthroughs in diagnostics, treatment personalization, and operational efficiency (Huang et al., 2022). These technologies are not only augmenting the capabilities of healthcare professionals but are also paving the way for more sustainable healthcare systems that can respond effectively to the growing demands of patient care. Machine learning, a subset of AI, has demonstrated remarkable potential in analyzing complex medical data, enabling healthcare providers to make informed decisions based on predictive analytics (Huang et al., 2022). For instance, recent studies have highlighted the development of specialized deep learning architectures, such as the Bidirectional Long Short-Term Memory (BiLSTM) model, which has achieved superior accuracy in diagnosing conditions like acute ST-elevation myocardial infarction (STEMI) from electrocardiograms (ECGs) (Huang et al., 2022). This level of diagnostic precision not only enhances patient outcomes but also reduces the burden on healthcare systems by minimizing unnecessary procedures and hospitalizations, thereby contributing to sustainability (Pedro et al., 2023). Natural language processing (NLP) is another critical advancement that is transforming healthcare communication and documentation. NLP algorithms can analyze unstructured data from clinical notes, patient records, and research articles, facilitating the extraction of valuable insights that can inform clinical decision-making (Quazi, Mohammad, & Gorrepati, 2024). By streamlining the documentation process and enhancing the accessibility of patient information, NLP technologies help healthcare providers focus more on patient care rather than administrative tasks, ultimately leading to improved efficiency and resource allocation (Lee & Yoon, 2021). Furthermore, AI-driven chatbots and virtual assistants are emerging as tools for patient engagement, providing instant access to medical information and support, which empowers patients to take an active role in their healthcare (Ahanin, Sade, & Tat, 2022). Computer vision, another significant AI technology, is revolutionizing medical imaging by enabling faster and more accurate interpretations of diagnostic images. AI algorithms can detect anomalies in radiographs, MRIs, and CT scans with a level of precision that often surpasses human capabilities (Ahanin, Sade, & Tat, 2022). This capability not only accelerates the diagnostic process but also enhances the accuracy of disease detection, which is crucial for timely interventions. The integration of AI in imaging technologies is particularly beneficial in resource-limited settings, where access to specialized radiologists may be scarce, thus promoting equity in healthcare delivery (Ying et al., 2024). Moreover, the application of AI technologies extends beyond diagnostics to encompass personalized treatment plans tailored to individual patient needs. By analyzing vast datasets that include genomic information, lifestyle factors, and previous treatment outcomes, AI can identify the most effective therapeutic strategies for patients (Naqvi et al., 2023). This personalized approach not only improves treatment efficacy but also reduces the likelihood of adverse effects, thereby enhancing patient safety and satisfaction. The ability to tailor treatments based on individual characteristics is a significant step toward achieving sustainable healthcare, as it optimizes resource use and minimizes waste associated with ineffective treatments (Familoni, 2024). The advancements in AI technologies also facilitate the integration of wearable health devices, which are becoming increasingly prevalent in monitoring patient health in real-time. These devices collect continuous data on various health parameters, such as heart rate, blood pressure, and physical activity levels, which AI algorithms can analyze to provide actionable insights for both patients and healthcare providers (Secara & Hordiiuk,

2024). The convergence of AI and wearable technology enables proactive health management, allowing for early detection of potential health issues and timely interventions, which are essential for reducing healthcare costs and improving population health outcomes (Naqvi et al., 2023). Despite the promising advancements in AI technologies, there are challenges that must be addressed to fully realize their potential in sustainable healthcare. Issues related to data privacy, algorithmic bias, and the need for robust regulatory frameworks are critical considerations that healthcare stakeholders must navigate (Petersson et al., 2022; Arigbabu et al., 2024). Ensuring that AI systems are developed and implemented ethically is paramount to building trust among healthcare professionals and patients alike. Furthermore, continuous education and training for healthcare providers on the use of AI technologies will be essential to maximize their benefits while minimizing potential risks (O'Connor et al., 2023). The advancements in AI technologies are fundamentally transforming the healthcare landscape, offering innovative solutions that enhance patient care, optimize resource utilization, and promote sustainability. As AI continues to evolve, its integration into healthcare practices will likely lead to more efficient, personalized, and equitable healthcare systems. However, addressing the associated challenges and fostering a collaborative approach among stakeholders will be crucial to ensuring that the benefits of AI are realized in a responsible and sustainable manner.

4.2. Integration with Other Emerging Technologies

The integration of artificial intelligence (AI) with other emerging technologies is a pivotal aspect of advancing sustainable healthcare systems. This convergence not only enhances the capabilities of AI but also addresses critical challenges within the healthcare sector, such as data security, interoperability, and patient engagement. Among the most promising integrations are those involving blockchain technology, the Internet of Things (IoT), and big data analytics, each contributing uniquely to the optimization of healthcare delivery and management. Blockchain technology, in particular, has emerged as a powerful ally for AI in healthcare. By providing a decentralized and secure framework for data sharing, blockchain enhances the integrity and privacy of health information. The combination of AI and blockchain can facilitate the development of more robust electronic health record (EHR) systems that ensure patient data is securely stored and accessible only to authorized personnel (Rao & Manvi, 2023; Biswas & Singh, 2024). This integration addresses significant concerns regarding data breaches and unauthorized access, which are prevalent in traditional healthcare systems. Moreover, the use of blockchain can streamline the process of data verification, enabling AI algorithms to access high-quality, reliable data for analysis and decision-making (Tagde et al., 2021). As a result, healthcare providers can leverage AI-driven insights while maintaining patient confidentiality and trust. The Internet of Things (IoT) also plays a crucial role in the integration of AI technologies within healthcare. IoT devices, such as wearable health monitors and smart medical devices, continuously collect real-time data on patients' health metrics. When combined with AI, this data can be analyzed to provide personalized health insights and predictive analytics that inform clinical decisions (Yu et al., 2024; Venkatraman et al., 2023). For instance, AI algorithms can process data from IoT devices to detect early signs of health deterioration, enabling timely interventions that can prevent hospitalizations and reduce healthcare costs (Ara & Mifa, 2024). Furthermore, the integration of AI with IoT enhances remote patient monitoring capabilities, allowing healthcare providers to manage chronic conditions more effectively and improve patient outcomes (Gunasekeran et al., 2021). This synergy not only optimizes resource utilization but also promotes a more proactive approach to healthcare, aligning with the principles of sustainability. Big data analytics is another critical component that complements AI in the healthcare domain. The vast amounts of data generated from various sources, including EHRs, clinical trials, and patient interactions, present both opportunities and challenges for healthcare systems (Muhunzi, 2024; Subrahmanya et al., 2021). By integrating big data analytics with AI, healthcare organizations can harness the power of advanced analytical techniques to extract meaningful insights from complex datasets. This integration enables healthcare providers to identify trends, predict disease outbreaks, and tailor interventions to specific populations (Badawy, 2023; Thakur et al., 2023). For example, AI-driven big data analytics can facilitate the identification of at-risk populations, allowing for targeted public health initiatives that can mitigate the spread of diseases and improve overall community health (Muhunzi, Kitambala, & Mashauri, 2024; Badawy, 2023). The ability to analyze large datasets in real-time enhances decision-making processes and fosters a more efficient allocation of healthcare resources. Moreover, the integration of AI with big data analytics and IoT can lead to the development of intelligent health management systems that support personalized medicine. These systems can analyze individual patient data, including genetic information, lifestyle factors, and treatment responses, to recommend tailored treatment plans that optimize therapeutic outcomes (Yu et al., 2024; Parameshachari, Pelusi, & Goswami, 2025).This personalized approach not only improves patient satisfaction but also reduces the likelihood of adverse drug reactions and ineffective treatments, thereby enhancing the sustainability of healthcare practices (Ara & Mifa, 2024; Thakur et al., 2023). By leveraging the combined strengths of AI, big data, and IoT, healthcare providers can create a more responsive and patient-centered care model that aligns with the evolving needs of the population. Despite the promising potential of integrating AI with other emerging technologies, several challenges must be addressed to fully realize these benefits. Issues related to data interoperability, privacy, and ethical considerations remain significant barriers to the widespread adoption of these integrated systems (Petersson et al., 2022; Shittu et al., 2024). Ensuring that different technologies can communicate effectively and share data securely is essential for creating a seamless healthcare experience. Additionally, healthcare organizations must prioritize the development of regulatory frameworks that govern the use of AI and related technologies, ensuring that patient rights are protected while fostering innovation (Biswas & Singh, 2024; Jabarulla & Lee, 2021). The integration of AI with other emerging technologies such as blockchain, IoT, and big data analytics is transforming the healthcare landscape, offering innovative solutions that enhance patient care, optimize resource utilization, and promote sustainability. As these technologies continue to evolve, their synergistic effects will likely lead to more efficient, personalized, and equitable healthcare systems. However, addressing the associated challenges and fostering collaboration among stakeholders will be crucial to ensuring that the benefits of these integrated technologies are realized in a responsible and sustainable manner.

4.3. Role of Policy and Regulation

The effective integration of artificial intelligence (AI) in sustainable healthcare systems is heavily influenced by the establishment of robust policy frameworks and regulatory measures. As AI technologies continue to evolve and permeate various aspects of healthcare, it is imperative that governments, regulatory bodies, and healthcare organizations collaborate to create guidelines that ensure the ethical, safe, and effective use of AI. This section discusses the critical role of policy and regulation in shaping the future of AI in healthcare, addressing ethical considerations, data privacy, and the need for continuous oversight. One of the primary challenges in the implementation of AI in healthcare is the lack of comprehensive regulatory frameworks that can adapt to the rapid advancements in technology.

Current regulations often lag behind technological innovations, creating a gap that can hinder the safe deployment of AI applications (Hasan et al., 2024; Krishnan Ganapathy, 2021). For instance, the European Union has made strides with the General Data Protection Regulation (GDPR), which provides a framework for data protection and privacy; however, there remains a need for specific regulations tailored to the unique challenges posed by AI technologies in healthcare (Sung et al., 2023; Meszaros, Minari, & Huys, 2022). Policymakers must prioritize the development of clear guidelines that address the ethical implications of AI, including issues related to algorithmic bias, transparency, and accountability (Zhang & Zhang, 2023; Aluthge Don, 2024). Moreover, the ethical considerations surrounding AI in healthcare are paramount. As AI systems are increasingly utilized for decision-making in clinical settings, concerns regarding bias and fairness in algorithmic outcomes have come to the forefront (Liu & Wu, 2022; Aquino et al., 2023). Regulatory bodies must establish standards that ensure AI algorithms are developed and tested in ways that minimize bias and promote equitable healthcare delivery. This includes implementing "privacy by design" principles, which advocate for the incorporation of privacy measures throughout the AI development process (Pedro et al., 2023). By prioritizing ethical considerations, policymakers can foster trust among healthcare professionals and patients, which is essential for the successful adoption of AI technologies. The role of healthcare professionals in the regulatory landscape cannot be overstated. Physicians and other healthcare providers express a strong desire for regulatory oversight to ensure patient safety and confidentiality when utilizing AI tools (Richardson et al., 2021). Engaging healthcare professionals in the regulatory process is crucial, as their insights can inform the development of guidelines that reflect the realities of clinical practice. Collaborative efforts between policymakers, healthcare providers, ethicists, and AI developers can lead to the creation of comprehensive regulations that address the multifaceted challenges associated with AI in (Hasan et al., 2024; Krishnan Ganapathy, 2021). Such collaboration is vital for ensuring that AI technologies are implemented in ways that enhance patient care while safeguarding their rights. Continuous monitoring and evaluation of AI systems post-implementation are also critical components of effective regulation. As AI algorithms are updated and refined over time, regulatory agencies must develop mechanisms for ongoing oversight to ensure that these systems continue to operate safely and effectively (Meszaros, Minari, & Huys, 2022; Zhang & Zhang, 2023). This includes establishing protocols for post-market surveillance that allow for the assessment of AI performance in real-world settings, enabling timely interventions when issues arise. By implementing robust monitoring frameworks, regulatory bodies can ensure that AI technologies remain aligned with ethical standards and continue to serve the best interests of patients and healthcare providers alike. Furthermore, public engagement and education are essential for fostering a supportive environment for AI in healthcare. Patients and the general public must be informed about the benefits and risks associated with AI technologies to build trust and acceptance (Richardson et al., 2021; Warrington & Holm, 2024). Policymakers should prioritize initiatives that promote transparency in AI applications, ensuring that patients understand how their data is used and the implications of AI-driven decisions in their care. By fostering an informed public dialogue, stakeholders can address concerns and misconceptions surrounding AI, ultimately leading to greater acceptance and utilization of these technologies in healthcare. In conclusion, the role of policy and regulation in the integration of AI into sustainable healthcare systems is critical. As AI technologies continue to advance, it is essential for regulatory bodies to establish comprehensive frameworks that address ethical considerations, promote transparency, and ensure patient safety. Collaborative efforts among policymakers, healthcare professionals, and AI developers will be vital in shaping regulations that support the responsible use of AI in healthcare. By prioritizing continuous oversight and public engagement, stakeholders can create an environment conducive to the successful implementation of AI technologies, ultimately enhancing the sustainability and effectiveness of healthcare systems.

4.4. Global Collaboration and Knowledge Sharing

The advancement of artificial intelligence (AI) in sustainable healthcare is significantly enhanced through global collaboration and knowledge sharing. As healthcare challenges transcend national borders, the need for international partnerships and cooperative frameworks becomes increasingly critical. Collaborative efforts among governments, healthcare organizations, academic institutions, and technology developers can facilitate the sharing of best practices, resources, and innovations, ultimately leading to improved health outcomes worldwide. One of the primary benefits of global collaboration is the ability to leverage diverse expertise and experiences in AI implementation across different healthcare systems. For instance, low- and middle-income countries (LMICs) face unique challenges in healthcare delivery, and insights gained from AI applications in these contexts can inform strategies for sustainable development (Alami et al., 2020). By fostering partnerships that prioritize knowledge sharing, stakeholders can identify contextual facilitators and obstacles, enabling the development of AI solutions that are tailored to specific regional needs. This approach aligns with the Sustainable Development Goals (SDGs), particularly Goal 17, which emphasizes the importance of partnerships for achieving sustainable development (Alami et al., 2020). Furthermore, the ethical use of AI in healthcare necessitates a collaborative approach to data sharing and governance. The sharing of clinical imaging data, for example, is essential for training robust AI models that can enhance diagnostic accuracy and patient care (Larson et al., 2020). However, ethical considerations surrounding data privacy and security must be addressed to build trust among stakeholders. Establishing a framework that promotes responsible data sharing while ensuring patient confidentiality is crucial. This framework should involve all parties that utilize clinical data, including for-profit entities, thereby embedding trustworthiness into data-sharing efforts (Larson et al., 2020). By creating a culture of transparency and accountability, stakeholders can foster an environment conducive to innovation and collaboration. The bibliometric analysis of AI research in healthcare highlights the increasing collaboration among researchers from different countries and disciplines (Guo et al., 2020; Aldousari & Kithinji, 2024). This trend underscores the importance of interdisciplinary partnerships in advancing AI technologies. By bringing together computer scientists, data scientists, clinicians, and medical informaticians, collaborative research efforts can lead to the development of innovative AI applications that address pressing healthcare challenges. Such collaborations not only enhance the quality of research but also facilitate the dissemination of knowledge and best practices across borders, ultimately benefiting global health outcomes (Guo et al., 2020; Aldousari & Kithinji, 2024). Moreover, global collaboration can play a pivotal role in addressing disparities in AI adoption and implementation. As highlighted in various studies, there are significant disparities in access to AI technologies between high-income and low-income countries (Soladzha, 2024; Aderibigbe et al., 2023). Collaborative initiatives that focus on capacity building, education, and training can help bridge these gaps. For instance, partnerships between developed and developing countries can facilitate knowledge transfer and skill development, empowering healthcare professionals in LMICs to effectively utilize AI technologies in their practice (Aderibigbe et al., 2023; Folorunso et al., 2024). This approach not only promotes equity in healthcare access but also fosters sustainable advancements in AI applications. In addition to fostering partnerships, the establishment of international standards and guidelines for AI in healthcare is essential for promoting responsible innovation. The development of global ethical frameworks for AI technologies can provide a foundation for consistent practices across different regions (Hoseini, 2023; Jobin, Ienca, & Vayena, 2019). Such frameworks should prioritize transparency, accountability, and fairness, ensuring that AI applications are developed and deployed in ways that respect human rights and promote social good. By aligning local policies with global standards, stakeholders can facilitate cross-border data sharing and collaboration, ultimately enhancing the effectiveness of AI in healthcare (Folorunso et al., 2024; Hoseini, 2023). The ongoing COVID-19 pandemic has further underscored the importance of global collaboration in healthcare. The crisis has prompted unprecedented levels of cooperation among countries, organizations, and researchers to leverage AI and digital technologies for pandemic response and management This collaborative spirit can serve as a model for future initiatives aimed at addressing global health challenges. By harnessing the collective expertise and resources of the international community, stakeholders can develop innovative AI solutions that enhance healthcare delivery and resilience in the face of future crises (Puaschunder, 2020; Tidjon & Khomh, 2022). In conclusion, global collaboration and knowledge sharing are essential components of advancing AI in sustainable healthcare. By fostering partnerships that prioritize ethical data sharing, interdisciplinary research, and capacity building, stakeholders can enhance the effectiveness and equity of AI applications in healthcare. The establishment of international standards and guidelines will further support responsible innovation, ensuring that AI technologies are developed and deployed in ways that benefit all members of society. As the global community continues to navigate the complexities of healthcare challenges, collaborative efforts will be crucial in realizing the full potential of AI in promoting sustainable health outcomes.

4.5. Patient-Centric Approaches

In the evolving landscape of healthcare, patient-centric approaches are becoming increasingly vital, particularly in the context of integrating artificial intelligence (AI) technologies. These approaches prioritize the needs, preferences, and values of patients, ensuring that they are actively involved in their own care processes. By leveraging AI, healthcare systems can enhance patient engagement, improve health outcomes, and promote sustainability within healthcare delivery. The significance of patient-centric approaches in sustainable healthcare highlights the role of AI in facilitating these strategies. One of the primary benefits of patient-centric care is the empowerment of patients through information and education. Patients who are well-informed about their health conditions and treatment options are more likely to engage actively in their care, leading to better health outcomes (Wong & Leland, 2018; Witkowski, Okhai, & Neely, 2024). AI technologies can play a crucial role in this regard by providing personalized health information and recommendations tailored to individual patient needs. For instance, AI-driven applications can analyze patient data and generate insights that help patients understand their conditions and treatment options, thereby reducing anxiety and uncertainty (Awuah et al., 2024). This empowerment fosters a collaborative relationship between patients and healthcare providers, enhancing the overall quality of care. Moreover, AI can facilitate shared decision-making, a cornerstone of patient-centered care. By providing healthcare professionals with advanced analytics and predictive modeling, AI tools can support clinicians in discussing treatment options with patients based on their unique circumstances and preferences (Al Kuwaiti et al., 2023). This collaborative approach not only respects patient autonomy but also aligns treatment plans with patients' values and goals, ultimately leading to improved adherence and satisfaction with care (Liang et al., 2020). The integration of AI in shared decision-making processes can thus enhance the effectiveness of interventions and promote a more sustainable healthcare model. The COVID-19 pandemic has underscored the importance of patient engagement and the potential of virtual technologies in facilitating this engagement. During the pandemic, many healthcare organizations adapted their patient engagement strategies to leverage telehealth and digital communication tools, allowing patients to participate in their care remotely (Marcinow et al., 2023; Tripp et al., 2022). These virtual platforms have proven effective in maintaining patient connections and ensuring that the patient voice remains central to care delivery. As healthcare systems continue to embrace digital solutions, the integration of AI can further enhance these virtual engagement strategies by providing real-time feedback and personalized support to patients Tripp et al., 2022). Additionally, patient-centric approaches can contribute to the sustainability of healthcare systems by improving care coordination and reducing unnecessary healthcare utilization. Research has shown that patient-centered care can lead to better coordination of services, particularly in complex cases such as oncology, where timely access to care is crucial (Liang et al., 2020; Saviano et al., 2018). By utilizing AI to streamline care pathways and facilitate communication among healthcare providers, patient-centric approaches can help prevent avoidable hospitalizations and reduce the overall burden on healthcare resources. This not only enhances patient outcomes but also contributes to the sustainability of healthcare systems by optimizing resource utilization (Saviano et al., 2018). Furthermore, the incorporation of patient feedback into the design and implementation of AI technologies is essential for ensuring that these tools meet the needs of diverse patient populations. Engaging patients in the co-creation of AI solutions can lead to more relevant and effective applications that address specific health challenges (Toncinic, de Wildt-Liesveld, & Vrijhoef, 2020; Nelson et al., 2020). For example, understanding patient perspectives on the use of AI in skin cancer screening has highlighted the importance of addressing concerns related to equity and access, particularly among underrepresented groups (Nelson et al., 2020). By prioritizing patient input, healthcare organizations can develop AI technologies that are not only effective but also equitable and inclusive. Despite the numerous benefits of patient-centric approaches, challenges remain in their implementation. Barriers such as health literacy disparities, technological access, and resistance to change among healthcare providers can hinder the successful adoption of these strategies (Kwame & Petrucka, 2021; Clery et al., 2021). To overcome these challenges, healthcare organizations must invest in training and education programs that equip both patients and providers with the necessary skills to engage effectively with AI technologies (Kwame & Petrucka, 2021). Additionally, fostering a culture of collaboration and openness within healthcare organizations can facilitate the integration of patient-centric approaches into routine practice. In conclusion, patient-centric approaches are essential for promoting sustainable healthcare, particularly in the context of AI integration. By empowering patients, facilitating shared decision-making, and leveraging virtual technologies, healthcare systems can enhance patient engagement and improve health outcomes. The incorporation of patient feedback in the development of AI solutions further ensures that these technologies are relevant and effective. As healthcare continues to evolve, prioritizing patient-centric strategies will be crucial for achieving a more sustainable and equitable healthcare system.

5. CONCLUSION

AI algorithms represent a transformative force in the quest for sustainable healthcare. By optimizing resource use, enhancing preventive care, facilitating telemedicine, accelerating drug discovery, and enabling personalized treatment, these technologies can significantly improve both patient outcomes and the overall sustainability of healthcare systems. This chapter has illustrated AI's transformative impact on sustainable healthcare, showcasing advancements in diagnostics, personalized treatment, and operational efficiency. Key takeaways highlight AI's ability to enhance precision and accessibility through early disease detection via medical imaging and telemedicine solutions that broaden care delivery. Sustainability gains are realized through optimized resource utilization, waste reduction, and the development of energy-efficient AI models. However, significant challenges persist, including ethical considerations such as bias and accountability, regulatory hurdles related to global standards, and the need for equitable adoption across diverse healthcare systems.

Looking ahead, the future of AI in sustainable healthcare depends on collaborative frameworks that integrate policymakers, clinicians, and technologists to address existing ethical and regulatory gaps. Green AI initiatives will be crucial, demanding a balance between performance and environmental costs, such as the development of lower-carbon algorithms. Moreover, the development of patient-centered AI tools, designed with inclusivity and transparency, will be essential for driving trust and scalability. The path forward necessitates not only technological advancements but also a steadfast commitment to equity and sustainability, ensuring that AI benefits all patients and the planet, especially in consideration of global AI equity.

REFERENCES

Abou Ghayda, R.. (2024). Artificial intelligence in andrology: From semen analysis to image diagnostics. *The World Journal of Men's Health*, *42*(1), 39. DOI: 10.5534/wjmh.230050 PMID: 37382282

Aderibigbe, A. O.Adebayo Olusegun AderibigbePeter Efosa OhenhenNwabueze Kelvin NwaobiaJoachim Osheyor GidiagbaEmmanuel Chigozie Ani. (2023). Artificial intelligence in developing countries: Bridging the gap between potential and implementation. *Computer Science & IT Research Journal*, *4*(3), 185–199. DOI: 10.51594/csitrj.v4i3.629

Ahanin, E., Sade, A. B., & Tat, H. H. (2022). Applications of artificial intelligence and voice assistant in healthcare. *International Journal of Academic Research in Business & Social Sciences*, *12*(12), 2545–2554. DOI: 10.6007/IJARBSS/v12-i12/16048

Ahmed, A., & Adil, K. (2023). *Transforming Healthcare Systems with Artificial Intelligence: Revolutionizing Efficiency*. Quality, and Patient Care.

Al-Karawi, D., Al-Zaidi, S., Helael, K. A., Obeidat, N., Mouhsen, A. M., Ajam, T., Alshalabi, B. A., Salman, M., & Ahmed, M. H. (2024). A Review of Artificial Intelligence in Breast Imaging. *Tomography : a Journal for Imaging Research*, *10*(5), 705–726. DOI: 10.3390/tomography10050055 PMID: 38787015

Al Kuwaiti, A., Nazer, K., Al-Reedy, A., Al-Shehri, S., Al-Muhanna, A., Subbarayalu, A. V., Al Muhanna, D., & Al-Muhanna, F. A. (2023). A review of the role of artificial intelligence in healthcare. *Journal of Personalized Medicine*, *13*(6), 951. DOI: 10.3390/jpm13060951 PMID: 37373940

Alahmari, N., Alswedani, S., Alzahrani, A., Katib, I., Albeshri, A., & Mehmood, R. (2022). Musawah: A data-driven ai approach and tool to co-create healthcare services with a case study on cancer disease in Saudi Arabia. *Sustainability (Basel)*, *14*(6), 3313. DOI: 10.3390/su14063313

Alami, H., Rivard, L., Lehoux, P., Hoffman, S. J., Cadeddu, S. B. M., Savoldelli, M., Samri, M. A., Ag Ahmed, M. A., Fleet, R., & Fortin, J.-P. (2020). Artificial intelligence in health care: Laying the Foundation for Responsible, sustainable, and inclusive innovation in low-and middle-income countries. *Globalization and Health*, *16*(1), 1–6. DOI: 10.1186/s12992-020-00584-1 PMID: 32580741

Alasasfeh, H. O., Alomari, T., & Ibbini, M. S. (2021, March). Deep Learning Approach for COVID-19 Detection Based on X-Ray Images. In 2021 18th International Multi-Conference on Systems, Signals & Devices (SSD) (pp. 1-6). IEEE.

Aldousari, E., & Kithinji, D. (2024). Artificial intelligence and health information: A bibliometric analysis of three decades of research. *Health Informatics Journal*, *30*(3), 14604582241283969. DOI: 10.1177/14604582241283969 PMID: 39262107

Alnasser, B. (2023). A Review of Literature on the Economic Implications of Implementing Artificial Intelligence in Healthcare. *E-Health Telecommunication Systems and Networks*, *12*(3), 35–48. DOI: 10.4236/etsn.2023.123003

Alowais, S. A., Alghamdi, S. S., Alsuhebany, N., Alqahtani, T., Alshaya, A. I., Almohareb, S. N., Aldairem, A., Alrashed, M., Bin Saleh, K., Badreldin, H. A., Al Yami, M. S., Al Harbi, S., & Albekairy, A. M. (2023). Revolutionizing healthcare: The role of artificial intelligence in clinical practice. *BMC Medical Education, 23*(1), 689. DOI: 10.1186/s12909-023-04698-z PMID: 37740191

Aluthge Don, Y., *Regulatory Perspectives of AI as Medical Device: a scoping review.* 2024.

Anyanwu, E. C.. (2024). Artificial intelligence in healthcare: A review of ethical dilemmas and practical applications. *International Medical Science Research Journal, 4*(2), 126–140. DOI: 10.51594/imsrj.v4i2.755

Aquino, Y. S. J., Carter, S. M., Houssami, N., Braunack-Mayer, A., Win, K. T., Degeling, C., Wang, L., & Rogers, W. A. (2023). Practical, epistemic and normative implications of algorithmic bias in healthcare artificial intelligence: A qualitative study of multidisciplinary expert perspectives. *Journal of Medical Ethics*, jme-2022-108850. DOI: 10.1136/jme-2022-108850 PMID: 36823101

Aquino, Y. S. J., Rogers, W. A., Braunack-Mayer, A., Frazer, H., Win, K. T., Houssami, N., Degeling, C., Semsarian, C., & Carter, S. M. (2023). Utopia versus dystopia: Professional perspectives on the impact of healthcare artificial intelligence on clinical roles and skills. *International Journal of Medical Informatics, 169*, 104903. DOI: 10.1016/j.ijmedinf.2022.104903 PMID: 36343512

Ara, A., & Mifa, A. F. (2024). Integrating artificial intelligence and big data in mobile health: A systematic review of innovations and challenges in healthcare systems. Global Mainstream Journal of Business, Economics, Development & Project Management, 3(01), 01-16.

Arigbabu, A. T., Olaniyi, O. O., Adigwe, C. S., Adebiyi, O. O., & Ajayi, S. A. (2024). Data governance in AI-enabled healthcare systems: A case of the project nightingale. *Asian Journal of Research in Computer Science, 17*(5), 85–107. DOI: 10.9734/ajrcos/2024/v17i5441

Arnar, D. O., Oddsson, S. J., Gunnarsdottir, T., Gudlaugsdottir, G. J., Gudmundsson, E. F., Ketilsdóttir, A., Halldorsdottir, H., Hrafnkelsdottir, T. J., Hallsson, H., Amundadottir, M. L., & Thorgeirsson, T. (2022). Improving outpatient care for heart failure through digital innovation: A feasibility study. *Pilot and Feasibility Studies, 8*(1), 242. DOI: 10.1186/s40814-022-01206-w PMID: 36451212

Awuah, W. A., Aderinto, N., Poornaselvan, J., Tan, J. K., Shah, M. H., Ashinze, P., Pujari, A. G., Bharadwaj, H. R., Abdul-Rahman, T., & Atallah, O. (2024). Empowering health care consumers & understanding patients' perspectives on AI integration in oncology and surgery: A perspective. *Health Science Reports, 7*(7), e2268. DOI: 10.1002/hsr2.2268 PMID: 39050906

Babarinde, A. O.. (2023). Review of AI applications in Healthcare: Comparative insights from the USA and Africa. *International Medical Science Research Journal, 3*(3), 92–107. DOI: 10.51594/imsrj.v3i3.641

Badawy, M. (2023). *Integrating Artificial Intelligence and Big Data into Smart Healthcare Systems: A Comprehensive Review of Current Practices and Future Directions.* Artificial Intelligence Evolution.

Barriga, A., Rutle, A., & Heldal, R. (2020). Improving Model Repair through Experience Sharing. *Journal of Object Technology, 19*(2), 13–1.

Batra, A. M., & Reche, A. (2023). A new era of dental care: Harnessing artificial intelligence for better diagnosis and treatment. *Cureus*, *15*(11). PMID: 38143639

Biswas, I., & Singh, R. (2024). "Application Of AI And Blockchain In Healthcare Industry"–A Review. *Journal of Advanced Zoology*, *45*(2). Advance online publication. DOI: 10.53555/jaz.v45i2.3983

Botwe, B. O., Antwi, W. K., Arkoh, S., & Akudjedu, T. N. (2021). Radiographers' perspectives on the emerging integration of artificial intelligence into diagnostic imaging: The Ghana study. *Journal of Medical Radiation Sciences*, *68*(3), 260–268. DOI: 10.1002/jmrs.460 PMID: 33586361

Brown, N., Ertl, P., Lewis, R., Luksch, T., Reker, D., & Schneider, N. (2020). Artificial intelligence in chemistry and drug design. *Journal of Computer-Aided Molecular Design*, *34*(7), 709–715. DOI: 10.1007/s10822-020-00317-x PMID: 32468207

Cai, C., Wang, S., Xu, Y., Zhang, W., Tang, K., Ouyang, Q., Lai, L., & Pei, J. (2020). Transfer learning for drug discovery. *Journal of Medicinal Chemistry*, *63*(16), 8683–8694. DOI: 10.1021/acs.jmedchem.9b02147 PMID: 32672961

Chew, H. S. J., & Achananuparp, P. (2022). Perceptions and needs of artificial intelligence in health care to increase adoption: Scoping review. *Journal of Medical Internet Research*, *24*(1), e32939. DOI: 10.2196/32939 PMID: 35029538

Chokshi, S. K., & Mann, D. M. (2018). Innovating from within: A process model for user-centered digital development in academic medical centers. *JMIR Human Factors*, *5*(4), e11048. DOI: 10.2196/11048 PMID: 30567688

Chomutare, T., Tejedor, M., Svenning, T. O., Marco-Ruiz, L., Tayefi, M., Lind, K., Godtliebsen, F., Moen, A., Ismail, L., Makhlysheva, A., & Ngo, P. D. (2022). Artificial intelligence implementation in healthcare: A theory-based scoping review of barriers and facilitators. *International Journal of Environmental Research and Public Health*, *19*(23), 16359. DOI: 10.3390/ijerph192316359 PMID: 36498432

Choudhury, A., & Asan, O. (2020). Role of artificial intelligence in patient safety outcomes: Systematic literature review. *JMIR Medical Informatics*, *8*(7), e18599. DOI: 10.2196/18599 PMID: 32706688

Claudy, M. C., Aquino, K., & Graso, M. (2022). Artificial intelligence can't be charmed: The effects of impartiality on laypeople's algorithmic preferences. *Frontiers in Psychology*, *13*, 898027. DOI: 10.3389/fpsyg.2022.898027 PMID: 35846643

Clery, P., d'Arch Smith, S., Marsden, O., & Leedham-Green, K. (2021). Sustainability in quality improvement (SusQI): A case-study in undergraduate medical education. *BMC Medical Education*, *21*(1), 425. DOI: 10.1186/s12909-021-02817-2 PMID: 34384400

Coeckelbergh, M. (2021). AI for climate: Freedom, justice, and other ethical and political challenges. *AI and Ethics*, *1*(1), 67–72. DOI: 10.1007/s43681-020-00007-2

Cripps, M., & Scarbrough, H. (2022). Making digital health "solutions" sustainable in healthcare systems: A practitioner perspective. *Frontiers in Digital Health*, *4*, 727421. DOI: 10.3389/fdgth.2022.727421 PMID: 35434699

Dara, S., Dhamercherla, S., Jadav, S. S., Babu, C. H. M., & Ahsan, M. J. (2022). Machine learning in drug discovery: A review. *Artificial Intelligence Review*, *55*(3), 1947–1999. DOI: 10.1007/s10462-021-10058-4 PMID: 34393317

Ding, H., Wu, J., Zhao, W., Matinlinna, J. P., Burrow, M. F., & Tsoi, J. K. H. (2023). Artificial intelligence in dentistry—A review. *Frontiers in Dental Medicine*, *4*, 1085251. DOI: 10.3389/fdmed.2023.1085251 PMID: 39935549

El Morr, C., & Ali-Hassan, H. (2019). *Analytics in healthcare: a practical introduction*. Springer. DOI: 10.1007/978-3-030-04506-7

Ergün, O., Serel, T. A., Öztürk, S. A., Serel, H. B., Soyupek, S., & Hoşcan, B. (2024). Deep-learning-based diagnosis and grading of vesicoureteral reflux: A novel approach for improved clinical decision-making: Vesicoureteral reflux and deep learning. *Journal of Surgery and Medicine*, *8*(1), 12–16. DOI: 10.28982/josam.8020

Eshwar, M. (2023). Exploring the potential of artificial intelligence in healthcare: Possibilities and challenges. *International Scientific Journal of Engineering and Management*, *2*(04). Advance online publication. DOI: 10.55041/ISJEM00408

Familoni, B.Babajide Tolulope Familoni. (2024). Ethical frameworks for AI in healthcare entrepreneurship: A theoretical examination of challenges and approaches. *International Journal of Frontiers in Biology and Pharmacy Research*, *5*(1), 57–65. DOI: 10.53294/ijfbpr.2024.5.1.0032

Folorunso, A.. (2024). A policy framework on AI usage in developing countries and its impact. *Global Journal of Engineering and Technology Advances*, *21*(01), 154–166. DOI: 10.30574/gjeta.2024.21.1.0192

Gama, F., Tyskbo, D., Nygren, J., Barlow, J., Reed, J., & Svedberg, P. (2022). Implementation frameworks for artificial intelligence translation into health care practice: Scoping review. *Journal of Medical Internet Research*, *24*(1), e32215. DOI: 10.2196/32215 PMID: 35084349

Gawriljuk, V. O., Foil, D. H., Puhl, A. C., Zorn, K. M., Lane, T. R., Riabova, O., Makarov, V., Godoy, A. S., Oliva, G., & Ekins, S. (2021). Development of machine learning models and the discovery of a new antiviral compound against yellow fever virus. *Journal of Chemical Information and Modeling*, *61*(8), 3804–3813. DOI: 10.1021/acs.jcim.1c00460 PMID: 34286575

Gou, F., Liu, J., Xiao, C., & Wu, J. (2024). Research on artificial-intelligence-assisted medicine: A survey on medical artificial intelligence. *Diagnostics (Basel)*, *14*(14), 1472. DOI: 10.3390/diagnostics14141472 PMID: 39061610

Guerra, R. (2024). Enhancing risk management in hospitals: Leveraging artificial intelligence for improved outcomes. *Italian Journal of Medicine*, *18*(2). Advance online publication. DOI: 10.4081/itjm.2024.1721

Gunasekeran, D. V., Tseng, R. M. W. W., Tham, Y.-C., & Wong, T. Y. (2021). Applications of digital health for public health responses to COVID-19: A systematic scoping review of artificial intelligence, telehealth and related technologies. *NPJ Digital Medicine*, *4*(1), 40. DOI: 10.1038/s41746-021-00412-9 PMID: 33637833

Guo, Y., Hao, Z., Zhao, S., Gong, J., & Yang, F. (2020). Artificial intelligence in health care: Bibliometric analysis. *Journal of Medical Internet Research, 22*(7), e18228. DOI: 10.2196/18228 PMID: 32723713

Hasan, H. E., Jaber, D., Khabour, O. F., & Alzoubi, K. H. (2024). Ethical considerations and concerns in the implementation of AI in pharmacy practice: A cross-sectional study. *BMC Medical Ethics, 25*(1), 55. DOI: 10.1186/s12910-024-01062-8 PMID: 38750441

Hassanien, A. E., & Mononteliza, J. (2020). Autonomous driving path planning based on sarsa-dyna algorithm. *Asia-pacific J Convergent Res Interchange, 6*(7), 59–70. DOI: 10.47116/apjcri.2020.07.06

Hessel, M., Soyer, H., Espeholt, L., Czarnecki, W., Schmitt, S., & Van Hasselt, H. (2019, July). Multi-task deep reinforcement learning with popart. *Proceedings of the AAAI Conference on Artificial Intelligence, 33*(01), 3796–3803.

Hoseini, F. (2023). AI Ethics: A Call for Global Standards in Technology Development. *AI and Tech in Behavioral and Social Sciences, 1*(4), 1–3. DOI: 10.61838/kman.aitech.1.4.1

Hoseini, M. (2023). Patient Experiences with AI in Healthcare Settings. *AI and Tech in Behavioral and Social Sciences, 1*(3), 12–18. DOI: 10.61838/kman.aitech.1.3.3

Hosny, A., Parmar, C., Quackenbush, J., Schwartz, L. H., & Aerts, H. J. W. L. (2018). Artificial intelligence in radiology. *Nature Reviews. Cancer, 18*(8), 500–510. DOI: 10.1038/s41568-018-0016-5 PMID: 29777175

Huang, J.-D., Wang, J., Ramsey, E., Leavey, G., Chico, T. J. A., & Condell, J. (2022). Applying artificial intelligence to wearable sensor data to diagnose and predict cardiovascular disease: A review. *Sensors (Basel), 22*(20), 8002. DOI: 10.3390/s22208002 PMID: 36298352

Huang, X., Wang, H., She, C., Feng, J., Liu, X., Hu, X., Chen, L., & Tao, Y. (2022). Artificial intelligence promotes the diagnosis and screening of diabetic retinopathy. *Frontiers in Endocrinology, 13*, 946915. DOI: 10.3389/fendo.2022.946915 PMID: 36246896

Hwang, D.-K., Hsu, C.-C., Chang, K.-J., Chao, D., Sun, C.-H., Jheng, Y.-C., Yarmishyn, A. A., Wu, J.-C., Tsai, C.-Y., Wang, M.-L., Peng, C.-H., Chien, K.-H., Kao, C.-L., Lin, T.-C., Woung, L.-C., Chen, S.-J., & Chiou, S.-H. (2019). Artificial intelligence-based decision-making for age-related macular degeneration. *Theranostics, 9*(1), 232–245. DOI: 10.7150/thno.28447 PMID: 30662564

Iovino, L., Barriga Rodriguez, A., Rutle, A., & Heldal, R. (2020). Model repair with quality-based reinforcement learning.

Ismail, A. F. M. F., Sam, M. F. M., Bakar, K. A., Ahamat, A., Adam, S., & Qureshi, M. I. (2022). Artificial intelligence in healthcare business ecosystem: a bibliometric study. International journal of online and biomedical engineering, 18(9), 100-114.

Issa, W. B., Shorbagi, A., Al-Sharman, A., Rababa, M., Al-Majeed, K., Radwan, H., Refaat Ahmed, F., Al-Yateem, N., Mottershead, R., Abdelrahim, D. N., Hijazi, H., Khasawneh, W., Ali, I., Abbas, N., & Fakhry, R. (2024). Shaping the future: perspectives on the Integration of Artificial Intelligence in health profession education: a multi-country survey. *BMC Medical Education, 24*(1), 1166. DOI: 10.1186/s12909-024-06076-9 PMID: 39425151

Jabarulla, M. Y., & Lee, H.-N. (2021). A blockchain and artificial intelligence-based, patient-centric healthcare system for combating the COVID-19 pandemic: Opportunities and applications. In *Healthcare*. Mdpi.

Jansson, M., Ohtonen, P., Alalääkkölä, T., Heikkinen, J., Mäkiniemi, M., Lahtinen, S., Lahtela, R., Ahonen, M., Jämsä, S., & Liisantti, J. (2022). Artificial intelligence-enhanced care pathway planning and scheduling system: Content validity assessment of required functionalities. *BMC Health Services Research*, *22*(1), 1513. DOI: 10.1186/s12913-022-08780-y PMID: 36510176

Jobin, A., Ienca, M., & Vayena, E. (2019). The global landscape of AI ethics guidelines. *Nature Machine Intelligence*, *1*(9), 389–399. DOI: 10.1038/s42256-019-0088-2

Kale, G. A. (2019). Artificial Intelligence in Healthcare-Opportunities and Challenges.

Katirai, A. (2023). The ethics of advancing artificial intelligence in healthcare: Analyzing ethical considerations for Japan's innovative AI hospital system. *Frontiers in Public Health*, *11*, 1142062. DOI: 10.3389/fpubh.2023.1142062 PMID: 37529426

Krishnan Ganapathy, M. N. (2021). Artificial intelligence and healthcare regulatory and legal concerns. *Telehealth and Medicine Today*, *6*(2).

Kumar, K.. (2023). Artificial intelligence and machine learning based intervention in medical infrastructure: a review and future trends. In *Healthcare*. MDPI.

Kwame, A., & Petrucka, P. M. (2021). A literature-based study of patient-centered care and communication in nurse-patient interactions: Barriers, facilitators, and the way forward. *BMC Nursing*, *20*(1), 158. DOI: 10.1186/s12912-021-00684-2 PMID: 34479560

Laï, M.-C., Brian, M., & Mamzer, M.-F. (2020). Perceptions of artificial intelligence in healthcare: Findings from a qualitative survey study among actors in France. *Journal of Translational Medicine*, *18*(1), 1–13. DOI: 10.1186/s12967-019-02204-y PMID: 31918710

Larson, D. B., Magnus, D. C., Lungren, M. P., Shah, N. H., & Langlotz, C. P. (2020). Ethics of using and sharing clinical imaging data for artificial intelligence: A proposed framework. *Radiology*, *295*(3), 675–682. DOI: 10.1148/radiol.2020192536 PMID: 32208097

Lee, D., & Yoon, S. N. (2021). Application of artificial intelligence-based technologies in the healthcare industry: Opportunities and challenges. *International Journal of Environmental Research and Public Health*, *18*(1), 271. DOI: 10.3390/ijerph18010271 PMID: 33401373

Li, H., Zheng, Y., Xie, P., Ng, T. K., Qiu, K., & Zhang, G. (2023). Cost-effectiveness analysis of telemedicine and artificial intelligence-based diabetic retinopathy screening in urban and rural China.

Li, R., Yang, Z., Zhang, Y., Bai, W., Du, Y., Sun, R., Tang, J., Wang, N., & Liu, H. (2022). Cost-effectiveness and cost-utility of traditional and telemedicine combined population-based age-related macular degeneration and diabetic retinopathy screening in rural and urban China. *The Lancet Regional Health. Western Pacific*, *23*, 23. DOI: 10.1016/j.lanwpc.2022.100435 PMID: 35355615

Liang, H., Tao, L., Ford, E. W., Beydoun, M. A., & Eid, S. M. (2020). The patient-centered oncology care on health care utilization and cost: A systematic review and meta-analysis. *Health Care Management Review*, *45*(4), 364–376. DOI: 10.1097/HMR.0000000000000226 PMID: 30335617

Liu, T. A., & Wu, J.-H. (2022). The ethical and societal considerations for the rise of artificial intelligence and big data in ophthalmology. *Frontiers in Medicine*, *9*, 845522. DOI: 10.3389/fmed.2022.845522 PMID: 35836952

Marcinow, M., Sandercock, J., Cadel, L., Singh, H., Guilcher, S. J. T., Dowedoff, P., Maybee, A., Law, S., Fancott, C., & Kuluski, K. (2023). A qualitative study exploring how patient engagement activities were sustained or adapted in Canadian healthcare organizations during the COVID-19 pandemic. *PLoS One*, *18*(3), e0282890. DOI: 10.1371/journal.pone.0282890 PMID: 36928262

Mather, C., & Almond, H. (2022). Using COMPASS (Context Optimisation Model for Person-Centred Analysis and Systematic Solutions) theory to augment implementation of digital health solutions. *International Journal of Environmental Research and Public Health*, *19*(12), 7111. DOI: 10.3390/ijerph19127111 PMID: 35742360

Mayr, A., Klambauer, G., Unterthiner, T., Steijaert, M., Wegner, J. K., Ceulemans, H., Clevert, D.-A., & Hochreiter, S. (2018). Large-scale comparison of machine learning methods for drug target prediction on ChEMBL. *Chemical Science (Cambridge)*, *9*(24), 5441–5451. DOI: 10.1039/C8SC00148K PMID: 30155234

Meszaros, J., Minari, J., & Huys, I. (2022). The future regulation of artificial intelligence systems in healthcare services and medical research in the European Union. *Frontiers in Genetics*, *13*, 927721. DOI: 10.3389/fgene.2022.927721 PMID: 36267404

Mikava, N., & Mamulaidze, T. (2023). Implications Of Artificial Intelligence In Healthcare In Developing Countries: Perspectives And Challenges. *Agora International Journal of Economical Sciences*, *17*(2), 110–120. DOI: 10.15837/aijes.v17i2.6448

Movahed, M., & Bilderback, S. (2024). Evaluating the readiness of healthcare administration students to utilize AI for sustainable leadership: A survey study. *Journal of Health Organization and Management*, *38*(4), 567–582. DOI: 10.1108/JHOM-12-2023-0385 PMID: 38858220

Muhunzi, D., Kitambala, L., & Mashauri, H. L. (2024). Big data analytics in the healthcare sector: Opportunities and challenges in developing countries. A literature review. *Health Informatics Journal*, *30*(4), 14604582241294217. DOI: 10.1177/14604582241294217 PMID: 39434249

Muley, A., Muzumdar, P., Kurian, G., & Basyal, G. P. (2023). Risk of AI in Healthcare: A comprehensive literature review and study framework. arXiv preprint arXiv:2309.14530.

Murphy, K., Di Ruggiero, E., Upshur, R., Willison, D. J., Malhotra, N., Cai, J. C., Malhotra, N., Lui, V., & Gibson, J. (2021). Artificial intelligence for good health: A scoping review of the ethics literature. *BMC Medical Ethics*, *22*(1), 1–17. DOI: 10.1186/s12910-021-00577-8 PMID: 33588803

Nadarzynski, T., Miles, O., Cowie, A., & Ridge, D. (2019). Acceptability of artificial intelligence (AI)-led chatbot services in healthcare: A mixed-methods study. *Digital Health*, *5*, 2055207619871808. DOI: 10.1177/2055207619871808 PMID: 31467682

Naqvi, S. G., Nasir, T., Azam, H., & Zafar, L. (2023). Artificial intelligence in healthcare. *Pakistan Journal of Humanities and Social Sciences*, *11*(2), 1361–1367.

Nelson, C. A., Pérez-Chada, L. M., Creadore, A., Li, S. J., Lo, K., Manjaly, P., Pournamdari, A. B., Tkachenko, E., Barbieri, J. S., Ko, J. M., Menon, A. V., Hartman, R. I., & Mostaghimi, A. (2020). Patient perspectives on the use of artificial intelligence for skin cancer screening: A qualitative study. *JAMA Dermatology*, *156*(5), 501–512. DOI: 10.1001/jamadermatol.2019.5014 PMID: 32159733

Neto, L. M., & Endo, P. T. (2023). The use of Convolutional Neural Network to classify Congenital Syphilis with image representations of tabular data.

Nor, N. A. M., Mohamed, A., & Mutalib, S. (2020). Prevalence of hypertension: Predictive analytics review. *IAES International Journal of Artificial Intelligence*, *9*(4), 576. DOI: 10.11591/ijai.v9.i4.pp576-583

O'Connor, S., Yan, Y., Thilo, F. J. S., Felzmann, H., Dowding, D., & Lee, J. J. (2023). Artificial intelligence in nursing and midwifery: A systematic review. *Journal of Clinical Nursing*, *32*(13-14), 2951–2968. DOI: 10.1111/jocn.16478 PMID: 35908207

Ogaga, D., & Zhao, H. (2023). The Rise of Artificial Intelligence and Machine Learning in HealthCare Industry. International Journal of Research and Innovation in Applied Science.

Oh, S. H., Lee, S. J., & Park, J. (2022). Precision medicine for hypertension patients with type 2 diabetes via reinforcement learning. *Journal of Personalized Medicine*, *12*(1), 87. DOI: 10.3390/jpm12010087 PMID: 35055402

Okolo, C. A., Olorunsogo, T., & Babawarun, O. (2024). A comprehensive review of AI applications in personalized medicine. *International Journal of Science and Research Archive*, *11*(1), 2544–2549. DOI: 10.30574/ijsra.2024.11.1.0338

Olorunsogo, T.. (2024). Ethical considerations in AI-enhanced medical decision support systems: A review. *World Journal of Advanced Engineering Technology and Sciences*, *11*(1), 329–336. DOI: 10.30574/wjaets.2024.11.1.0061

Parameshachari, B., Pelusi, D., & Goswami, B. (2025). *AI-Driven Big Data Analytics for Mobile Healthcare*. Wiley Online Library.

Parekh, V. S., & Jacobs, M. A. (2019). Deep learning and radiomics in precision medicine. *Expert Review of Precision Medicine and Drug Development*, *4*(2), 59–72. DOI: 10.1080/23808993.2019.1585805 PMID: 31080889

Pedro, A. R., Dias, M. B., Laranjo, L., Cunha, A. S., & Cordeiro, J. V. (2023). Artificial intelligence in medicine: A comprehensive survey of medical doctor's perspectives in Portugal. *PLoS One*, *18*(9), e0290613. DOI: 10.1371/journal.pone.0290613 PMID: 37676884

Pereira, T.. (2021). Sharing biomedical data: Strengthening ai development in healthcare. In *Healthcare*. MDPI.

Petersson, L., Larsson, I., Nygren, J. M., Nilsen, P., Neher, M., Reed, J. E., Tyskbo, D., & Svedberg, P. (2022). Challenges to implementing artificial intelligence in healthcare: A qualitative interview study with healthcare leaders in Sweden. *BMC Health Services Research*, *22*(1), 850. DOI: 10.1186/s12913-022-08215-8 PMID: 35778736

Poalelungi, D. G., Musat, C. L., Fulga, A., Neagu, M., Neagu, A. I., Piraianu, A. I., & Fulga, I. (2023). Advancing patient care: How artificial intelligence is transforming healthcare. *Journal of Personalized Medicine*, *13*(8), 1214. DOI: 10.3390/jpm13081214 PMID: 37623465

Puaschunder, J. M. (2020). *The future of Artificial Intelligence in international healthcare: An index.* in *Proceedings of the 17th international RAIS conference on social sciences and humanities*. Scientia Moralitas Research Institute. DOI: 10.2139/ssrn.3623530

Quazi, F., Mohammad, A. S., & Gorrepati, N. (2024). Transforming Treatment and Diagnostics in Healthcare using AI. *Available atSSRN* 4942334.

Rahmani, A. M., Yousefpoor, E., Yousefpoor, M. S., Mehmood, Z., Haider, A., Hosseinzadeh, M., & Ali Naqvi, R. (2021). Machine learning (ML) in medicine: Review, applications, and challenges. *Mathematics*, *9*(22), 2970.

Rajalakshmi, R., Prathiba, V., Arulmalar, S., & Usha, M. (2021). Review of retinal cameras for global coverage of diabetic retinopathy screening. *Eye (London, England)*, *35*(1), 162–172. DOI: 10.1038/s41433-020-01262-7 PMID: 33168977

Rao, K. P. N., & Manvi, S. (2023). Survey on electronic health record management using amalgamation of artificial intelligence and blockchain technologies. *Acta Informatica Pragensia*, *12*(1), 179–199. DOI: 10.18267/j.aip.194

Rathore, F. A., & Rathore, M. A. (2023). The emerging role of artificial intelligence in healthcare. *JPMA. The Journal of the Pakistan Medical Association*, *73*(7), 1368–1369. DOI: 10.47391/JPMA.23-48 PMID: 37469045

Reker, D. (2019). Practical considerations for active machine learning in drug discovery. *Drug Discovery Today. Technologies*, *32*, 73–79. DOI: 10.1016/j.ddtec.2020.06.001 PMID: 33386097

Richardson, J. P., Smith, C., Curtis, S., Watson, S., Zhu, X., Barry, B., & Sharp, R. R. (2021). Patient apprehensions about the use of artificial intelligence in healthcare. *NPJ Digital Medicine*, *4*(1), 140. DOI: 10.1038/s41746-021-00509-1 PMID: 34548621

Saviano, M., Bassano, C., Piciocchi, P., Di Nauta, P., & Lettieri, M. (2018). Monitoring viability and sustainability in healthcare organizations. *Sustainability (Basel)*, *10*(10), 3548. DOI: 10.3390/su10103548

Secara, I.-A., & Hordiiuk, D. (2024). Personalized Health Monitoring Systems: Integrating Wearable and AI. *Journal of Intelligent Learning Systems and Applications*, *16*(02), 44–52. DOI: 10.4236/jilsa.2024.162004

Secinaro, S., Calandra, D., Secinaro, A., Muthurangu, V., & Biancone, P. (2021). The role of artificial intelligence in healthcare: A structured literature review. *BMC Medical Informatics and Decision Making*, *21*(1), 1–23. DOI: 10.1186/s12911-021-01488-9 PMID: 33836752

Shameer, K., Johnson, K. W., Glicksberg, B. S., Dudley, J. T., & Sengupta, P. P. (2018). Machine learning in cardiovascular medicine: Are we there yet? *Heart (British Cardiac Society), 104*(14), 1156–1164. DOI: 10.1136/heartjnl-2017-311198 PMID: 29352006

Shittu, R. A.. (2024). The role of business intelligence tools in improving healthcare patient outcomes and operations. *World Journal of Advanced Research and Reviews, 24*(2), 1039–1060. DOI: 10.30574/wjarr.2024.24.2.3414

Shorten, C., & Khoshgoftaar, T. M. (2019). A survey on image data augmentation for deep learning. *Journal of Big Data, 6*(1), 1–48. DOI: 10.1186/s40537-019-0197-0

Singi, S. R., Sathe, S., Reche, A. R., Sibal, A., & Mantri, N. (2022). Extended arm of precision in prosthodontics: Artificial intelligence. *Cureus, 14*(11). Advance online publication. DOI: 10.7759/cureus.30962 PMID: 36465202

Soladzha, O. (2024). Using Artificial Intelligence To Protect Human Rights: Development Of Sustainable Plastic Waste Recycling In Nigeria. Bulletin of the V.N. Karazin Kharkiv National University. Series. Law

Steerling, E., Siira, E., Nilsen, P., Svedberg, P., & Nygren, J. (2023). Implementing AI in healthcare—the relevance of trust: A scoping review. *Frontiers in Health Services, 3*, 1211150. DOI: 10.3389/frhs.2023.1211150 PMID: 37693234

Stewart, J., Lu, J., Gahungu, N., Goudie, A., Fegan, P. G., Bennamoun, M., Sprivulis, P., & Dwivedi, G. (2023). Western Australian medical students' attitudes towards artificial intelligence in healthcare. *PLoS One, 18*(8), e0290642. DOI: 10.1371/journal.pone.0290642 PMID: 37651380

Sung, J. J., Savulescu, J., Ngiam, K. Y., An, B., Ang, T. L., Yeoh, K. G., Cham, T.-J., Tsao, S., & Chua, T. S. (2023). Artificial intelligence for gastroenterology: Singapore artificial intelligence for Gastroenterology Working Group Position Statement. *Journal of Gastroenterology and Hepatology, 38*(10), 1669–1676. DOI: 10.1111/jgh.16241 PMID: 37277693

Tagde, P., Tagde, S., Bhattacharya, T., Tagde, P., Chopra, H., Akter, R., Kaushik, D., & Rahman, M. H. (2021). Blockchain and artificial intelligence technology in e-Health. *Environmental Science and Pollution Research International, 28*(38), 52810–52831. DOI: 10.1007/s11356-021-16223-0 PMID: 34476701

Temsah, M.-H., Alhuzaimi, A. N., Almansour, M., Aljamaan, F., Alhasan, K., Batarfi, M. A., Altamimi, I., Alharbi, A., Alsuhaibani, A. A., Alwakeel, L., Alzahrani, A. A., Alsulaim, K. B., Jamal, A., Khayat, A., Alghamdi, M. H., Halwani, R., Khan, M. K., Al-Eyadhy, A., & Nazer, R. (2024). Art or artifact: Evaluating the accuracy, appeal, and educational value of AI-generated imagery in DALL· E 3 for illustrating congenital heart diseases. *Journal of Medical Systems, 48*(1), 54. DOI: 10.1007/s10916-024-02072-0 PMID: 38780839

Thakur, S.. (2023). *Big data and artificial intelligence in ophthalmology.*

Tidjon, L. N., & Khomh, F. (2022). The different faces of ai ethics across the world: a principle-implementation gap analysis. arXiv preprint arXiv:2206.03225.

Toncinic, S., de Wildt-Liesveld, R., & Vrijhoef, H. (2020). Evaluation of a digital platform that engages stakeholders in the co-creation of healthcare innovations: A mixed-methods study. *International Journal of Care Coordination*, *23*(1), 33–42. DOI: 10.1177/2053434520913578

Tripp, L., Vanstone, M., Canfield, C., Leslie, M., Levasseur, M. A., Panday, J., Rowland, P., Wilson, G., You, J., & Abelson, J. (2022). The impact of COVID-19 on patient engagement in the health system: Results from a Pan-Canadian survey of patient, family and caregiver partners. *Health Expectations*, *25*(2), 744–753. DOI: 10.1111/hex.13421 PMID: 35023267

Tsiakas, K., Abujelala, M., & Makedon, F. (2018). Task engagement as personalization feedback for socially-assistive robots and cognitive training. *Technologies*, *6*(2), 49. DOI: 10.3390/technologies6020049

Udegbe, F. C.Francisca Chibugo UdegbeOgochukwu Roseline EbulueCharles Chukwudalu EbulueC-hukwunonso Sylvester Ekesiobi. (2024). AI's impact on personalized medicine: Tailoring treatments for improved health outcomes. *Engineering Science & Technology Journal*, *5*(4), 1386–1394. DOI: 10.51594/estj.v5i4.1040

Vamathevan, J., Clark, D., Czodrowski, P., Dunham, I., Ferran, E., Lee, G., Li, B., Madabhushi, A., Shah, P., Spitzer, M., & Zhao, S. (2019). Applications of machine learning in drug discovery and development. *Nature Reviews. Drug Discovery*, *18*(6), 463–477. DOI: 10.1038/s41573-019-0024-5 PMID: 30976107

Vatansever, S., Schlessinger, A., Wacker, D., Kaniskan, H. Ü., Jin, J., Zhou, M.-M., & Zhang, B. (2021). Artificial intelligence and machine learning-aided drug discovery in central nervous system diseases: State-of-the-arts and future directions. *Medicinal Research Reviews*, *41*(3), 1427–1473. DOI: 10.1002/med.21764 PMID: 33295676

Vella, D., & Ebejer, J.-P. (2022). Few-shot learning for low-data drug discovery. *Journal of Chemical Information and Modeling*, *63*(1), 27–42. DOI: 10.1021/acs.jcim.2c00779 PMID: 36410391

Venkatraman, S., Parvin, S., Mansoor, W., & Gawanmeh, A. (2023). Big data analytics and internet of things for personalised healthcare: opportunities and challenges. International Journal of Electrical & Computer Engineering (2088-8708), 13(4).

Victor, N. O. C. (2023). An experimental case study on how AI may improve communi-cation and re-source allocation. *International Journal of Artificial Intelligence and Machine Learning*, *3*(1), 10–18.

Vishwakarma, L. P.. (2023). Application of artificial intelligence for resilient and sustainable healthcare system: Systematic literature review and future research directions. *International Journal of Production Research*, •••, 1–23.

Wang, L., Zhang, W., He, X., & Zha, H. (2018, July). Supervised reinforcement learning with recurrent neural network for dynamic treatment recommendation. In Proceedings of the 24th ACM SIGKDD international conference on knowledge discovery & data mining (pp. 2447-2456).

Warrington, D. J., & Holm, S. (2024). Healthcare ethics and artificial intelligence: A UK doctor survey. *BMJ Open*, *14*(12), e089090. DOI: 10.1136/bmjopen-2024-089090 PMID: 39806591

Williamson, S. M., & Prybutok, V. (2024). Balancing privacy and progress: A review of privacy challenges, systemic oversight, and patient perceptions in AI-driven healthcare. *Applied Sciences (Basel, Switzerland), 14*(2), 675. DOI: 10.3390/app14020675

1. Witkowski, K., Okhai, R., & Neely, S. R. (2024). Public perceptions of artificial intelligence in healthcare: Ethical concerns and opportunities for patient-centered care. *BMC Medical Ethics, 25*(1), 1–11. DOI: 10.1186/s12910-024-01066-4 PMID: 38909180

Wong, C., & Leland, N. E. (2018). Clinicians' perspectives of patient engagement in post-acute care: A social ecological approach. *Physical & Occupational Therapy in Geriatrics, 36*(1), 29–42. DOI: 10.1080/02703181.2017.1407859 PMID: 29805191

Yelne, S., Chaudhary, M., Dod, K., Sayyad, A., & Sharma, R. (2023). Harnessing the power of AI: A comprehensive review of its impact and challenges in nursing science and healthcare. *Cureus, 15*(11). Advance online publication. DOI: 10.7759/cureus.49252 PMID: 38143615

Yin, J., Ngiam, K. Y., & Teo, H. H. (2021). Role of artificial intelligence applications in real-life clinical practice: Systematic review. *Journal of Medical Internet Research, 23*(4), e25759. DOI: 10.2196/25759 PMID: 33885365

Ying, L., Li, S., Chen, C., Yang, F., Li, X., Chen, Y., Ding, Y., Chang, G., Li, J., & Wang, X. (2024). Screening/diagnosis of pediatric endocrine disorders through the artificial intelligence model in different language settings. *European Journal of Pediatrics, 183*(6), 2655–2661. DOI: 10.1007/s00431-024-05527-1 PMID: 38502320

Young, A. T., Amara, D., Bhattacharya, A., & Wei, M. L. (2021). Patient and general public attitudes towards clinical artificial intelligence: A mixed methods systematic review. *The Lancet. Digital Health, 3*(9), e599–e611. DOI: 10.1016/S2589-7500(21)00132-1 PMID: 34446266

Yousefi, Z., Saadati, N., & Saadati, S. A. (2023). AI in Elderly Care: Understanding the Implications for Independence and Social Interaction. *AI and Tech in Behavioral and Social Sciences, 1*(4), 26–32. DOI: 10.61838/kman.aitech.1.4.5

Yu, S., Jeon, B. R., Liu, C., Kim, D., Park, H.-I., Park, H. D., Shin, J. H., Lee, J. H., Choi, Q., Kim, S., Yun, Y. M., & Cho, E.-J. (2024). Laboratory preparation for digital medicine in healthcare 4.0: An investigation into the awareness and applications of big data and artificial intelligence. *Annals of Laboratory Medicine, 44*(6), 562–571. DOI: 10.3343/alm.2024.0111 PMID: 38953115

Yu, Y., Niu, J., Yu, Y., Xia, S., & Sun, S. (2024). AI predictive modeling of survival outcomes for renal cancer patients undergoing targeted therapy. *Scientific Reports, 14*(1), 26156. DOI: 10.1038/s41598-024-77638-6 PMID: 39478092

Zhang, J., & Zhang, Z. (2023). Ethics and governance of trustworthy medical artificial intelligence. *BMC Medical Informatics and Decision Making, 23*(1), 7. DOI: 10.1186/s12911-023-02103-9 PMID: 36639799

KEY TERMS AND DEFINITIONS

Artificial Intelligence (AI): Computer systems designed to perform tasks that typically require human intelligence, such as diagnosing diseases or analyzing medical images.

Machine Learning (ML): A type of AI where systems learn from data to improve their performance without being explicitly programmed.

Natural Language Processing (NLP): AI technology that helps computers understand, interpret, and respond to human language (e.g., analyzing doctor's notes or patient conversations).

Predictive Analytics: Using AI to forecast future health events (e.g., predicting patient readmissions) based on historical data.

Convolutional Neural Network (CNN): An AI model specialized in analyzing visual data like X-rays or MRIs by detecting patterns in images.

Reinforcement Learning (RL): AI that learns by trial and error, refining actions based on rewards (e.g., optimizing treatment plans over time).

Telemedicine: Remote healthcare delivery using digital tools, often enhanced by AI for diagnostics or monitoring.

Algorithmic Bias: When AI systems produce unfair outcomes due to skewed or unrepresentative training data.

Electronic Health Records (EHRs): Digital versions of patient medical histories used by AI for analysis and decision-making.

Sustainability in Healthcare: Practices that reduce environmental impact while maintaining care quality—AI helps by optimizing resources and minimizing waste.

Chapter 2
AI Tools and Applications in Managing Immunological Disorders

Sangjin Kim
https://orcid.org/0009-0008-5882-3778
Korea University, South Korea

Seunggyu Lee
Korea University, South Korea

Seohoon Jin
https://orcid.org/0000-0001-9310-9504
Korea University, South Korea

Jai Woo Lee
https://orcid.org/0000-0002-4385-2831
Korea University, South Korea

ABSTRACT

The goals of this chapter are to review artificial intelligence and big data techniques in precision medicine and corroborate applications of artificial intelligence techniques to solve challenges in immunological disorders. The integration of artificial intelligence in precision medicine has strengthened immunology in biomedical sciences. Precision medicine detects the health outcomes of specific patients. Biomedical studies have shown that clinical research defining the integration of artificial intelligence and precision medicine will present solutions for the challenging issues in precision medicine. This chapter covers various features of artificial intelligence in precision medicine that may nourish biomedical science research. We discuss how artificial intelligence solidifies the technical environment of precision medicine and the application of artificial intelligence methods to analyze biomedical big data of immunological disorders.

DOI: 10.4018/979-8-3693-9725-1.ch002

1. INTRODUCTION

The goals of this chapter were to: (1) review artificial intelligence and big data techniques in precision medicine, and 2) corroborate applications of artificial intelligence techniques to solve challenges in immunological disorders. The integration of artificial intelligence in precision medicine has strengthened immunology in biomedical sciences (Filipp, 2019). Precision medicine detects the health outcomes of specific patients (Johnson et al., 2021).

Biomedical studies have shown that clinical research defining the integration of artificial intelligence and precision medicine will present solutions for the challenging issues in precision medicine (Quazi, 2022). This chapter covers various features of artificial intelligence in precision medicine that may nourish biomedical science research. It is crucial to note how artificial intelligence solidifies the technical environment of precision medicine and the application of artificial intelligence methods to analyze biomedical big data in precision medicine (Yang et al., 2024). Genetic and environmental factors may affect immune responses (Mangino et al., 2017). The development of the disease is often associated with the activation of T and B lymphocytes, the production of autoantibodies, and the release of various proinflammatory cytokines and chemokines (Bhol et al., 2024). Options for treatment involve symptom management, disease progression prevention using immunosuppressive agents, antiproliferative drugs like mycophenolate mofetil, and corticosteroids along with other anti-inflammatory drugs known for the side effects (Moingeon, 2023). Over the last ten years, there have been advancements in developing monoclonal antibodies and other biological drugs that target cytokines, or components of proinflammatory pathways, leading to improved treatment outcomes because of the higher specificity and lower toxicity compared to broadly acting immunomodulatory agents (Donnelly et al., 2009).

A wide range of disorders can be defined by the dysregulation of the immune system over abnormal or modified immune reactions (Long et al., 2023). The immune system targets its tissues and inflammatory conditions where the immune system is constantly overactive, due to bacteria living harmoniously on the body (Chaplin, 2010). The immune system reacts to harmless substances, primary immunodeficiencies caused by genetic defects at birth, and blood cancers like leukemias and lymphomas that impact the immune system (Achilles et al., 2014). Many infectious diseases can cause critical disruptions to the immune system (Zheng et al., 2020). Despite the distinct pathophysiological mechanisms, the distinct conditions have led to high levels of similarities (Kuruvilla et al., 2019). Modeling artificial intelligence in precision medicine is beneficial for illustrating the diversity among patients related to a particular disease, including the immune system imbalances, organs, overall symptoms, and reactions to current therapies (Danieli et al., 2024).

Precision medicine involving computational methods requires sophisticated computing systems to observe and analyze complex data (Thirunavukarasu et al., 2022). Advancements in precision medicine may depend on accurate and reliable predictive models that incorporate databases for multi-omics data, high-resolution imaging data, and environmental data (Pammi et al., 2023). These advancements will enable the development of more complex patient models, and complete digital replicas of the human body (Zhang et al., 2024). More sophisticated models may follow normal immune reactions after handling disease-causing agents or receiving a vaccine, serving as a standard to accurately detect abnormal regulation (Laupèze et al., 2021). While causal disease models from systems biology are currently employed for assessing drug effectiveness, they can be useful in evaluating the safety risks of drug candidates that target components of adverse outcome pathways (Boland et al., 2016). Improved computational techniques may evaluate the importance of combination therapies because it is impossible to test all potential combinations in clinical trials. The validation of complex models may require higher computing power for the big data analytics of various biomedical datasets. Multiple recommendations have been set up regarding data management, curation, pre-processing, and simulation (Güvenç Paltun et al., 2021). Current models based on artificial intelligence provide innovative methods to accelerate the creation and advancement of effective treatments, with many current uses in managing immune disorders (Wiljer et al., 2021). Artificial intelligence plays a crucial role in analyzing and predicting the complex systems of immunology through its machine learning and data analysis techniques. Artificial intelligence contributes to efficiently analyzing complex immunological data using dimensionality reduction techniques (Amir et al., 2013). By compressing vast amounts of data and extracting essential elements, it helps to more accurately predict human immune responses (Saeys et al., 2016). These technologies significantly contribute to modeling interactions between immune cells, advancing cancer immunology research, and developing diagnostics and treatment methods (Efremova et al., 2020). Artificial intelligence is utilized as a valuable tool in immunological research to analyze nonlinear relationships and predict immune responses (Libbrecht & Noble, 2015). In the process of modeling interactions among various immune cell types and understanding the complex relationships between genes and pathways, Artificial intelligence can aid in the prevention and treatment of diseases such as autoimmune disorders, infections, and cancer (Sachs et al., 2005). In immunological research, Artificial intelligence is evolving beyond simple pattern recognition to model causal relationships between disease progression and immune responses, presenting new possibilities for the development and application of immunotherapies.

It is significant to assess how artificial intelligence methods can impact precision medicine and check future opportunities, focusing on precision medicine related to individual patient needs (Ahmed et al., 2020). The application of artificial intelligence in precision medicine can design intelligent machines by using machine learning techniques, inspired by the physiology of primate brains (Vatansever et al., 2021). Artificial intelligence combines various technologies that include different aspects of human intelligence seen in generative artificial intelligence like ChatGPT (Rodriguez et al., 2024). Artificial intelligence, when combined with human intelligence, enables the identification of patterns in patient data to develop predictive models that can guide significant decision-making (Lv et al., 2024). In the realm of immune diseases, the application of artificial intelligence may generate models that are employed to classify patients, select appropriate treatment objectives, pinpoint and enhance promising drug discovery possibilities, and determine individuals who may respond positively to the medication (Alhasan & Hasaneen, 2021). The medical community must evaluate the value and potential opportunities of artificial intelligence in healthcare and recognize its limitations in treating various diseases for it to be beneficial (Rahman et al., 2024). Anticipating how inhibitors will be responded to remains a healthcare requirement that has not yet been fulfilled. It is necessary to identify artificial intelligence predictive biomarkers to classify inhibitor-treated patients into responders and non-responders (Yao et al., 2024).

2. PRECISION MEDICINE

Using extensive multidimensional biological datasets that include individual heterogeneity in genes, and environment, precision medicine aims to develop and optimize diagnostic and therapeutic solutions (Uddin et al., 2019). Medical professionals can obtain the chance to more precisely customize early interventions for every patient and artificial intelligence systems can reasonably estimate the risk of disease using multidimensional clinical and biological data by utilizing high performance computer capabilities

(X. Sun et al., 2023). Conversely, there has been less advancement in the field of neurodevelopmental disorders, such as epilepsy, autism spectrum disorder, intellectual disability, etc. Phenotypic and etiological heterogeneity, as well as the uncommon and penetrant nature of the underlying risk variants, complicate the quantification of risk from the patterns of genomic variation, including the functional characterization of genes and variants (Uffelmann et al., 2021). Although genes and variants may offer additional sufficient clues, structural and functional brain imaging as well as neuropsychological and neurophysiological markers frequently need further research to reach diagnostic sensitivity (Roalf & Gur, 2017). The question of whether artificial intelligence can provide a breakthrough in forecasting the prognosis and dangers of diseases is thus at the heart of the precision medicine dilemma (Abdallah et al., 2023).

The ideas behind precision medicine indicate that subpopulations with varying disease risk, prognosis, and responsiveness to treatment can be recognized due to variations in underlying biology and other factors (Krzyszczyk et al., 2018). The phenotypic or genotypic structures can be found using deep learning algorithms to train multidimensional datasets that capture variations in biological mechanisms (Crossa et al., 2024). Based on the biomedical and demographic characteristics of each patient, datasets can then be used to predict prognosis, treatment response, disease risk, and other outcomes (Ghofrani & Taherdoost, 2024). Precision medicine will provide clinicians with the opportunity to more precisely tailor interventions regarding disease-modifying or preventative unlike the current inductive process of symptom classification and occasionally imprecise process of treatment decisions (Seyhan & Carini, 2019). Large multidimensional biological and clinical datasets are now accessible with the collaborative efforts of the global scientific community and the exponential growth in computer capabilities in recent years. Processing multidimensional datasets requires high-performance computing, one of challenges in the field of precision medicine (Prosperi et al., 2018). Artificial intelligence-based prediction systems for cardiovascular disease and cancer have recently demonstrated encouraging outcomes, accurately predicting the risk and onset of disease (Singh et al., 2024). The available precise biological measures, sufficient quantification of pertinent environmental factors, and the identification of variations of known penetrance are all necessary for the success of precision medicine (Bagger et al., 2024). There are several barriers to adopting a comparable strategy to the category of immunological disorders. A collection of conditions with early infancy onset that affect many areas of immune development, and higher physiological processes. The immunological disorders in the field of precision medicine include severe disease that affect several areas of physiological and even cognitive functioning, as well as severe and widespread disorders (Khosravi-Maharlooei et al., 2022). Certain immunological disorders are extremely uncommon, especially single gene disorders with more serious physiological health effects. Due in part to the high rates of co-morbidity, immunological disorders may cause significant functional impairment (Rosenblum et al., 2012).

AI-based technologies come with many advantages and some drawbacks in the medical field. One of the biggest advantages is enhanced diagnostic capabilities (Topol, 2019). AI can analyze vast amounts of medical data to detect diseases more accurately and quickly (Rajkomar, Oren, et al., 2018). For example, it helps classify diseases by utilizing patient records, imaging results, and genetic information, which supports doctors' decision-making and improves the accuracy of treatments (Gurovich et al., 2019; Najjar, 2023). AI can play a significant role in cancer diagnosis, as combining traditional blood tests or liquid biopsies with AI analysis can lead to more accurate early detection of cancer (Ardila et al., 2019; Campanella et al., 2019; Esteva et al., 2017; McKinney et al., 2020). Furthermore, AI can develop personalized treatment plans by considering a patient's genetic makeup, lifestyle, and medical history, maximizing the effectiveness of treatments (Chen et al., 2025; Parekh et al., 2023; Schork, 2019).

Through predictive analytics, AI analyzes a patient's health status and helps predict potential future issues, enabling preventive measures (Dong et al., 2025; Tomašev et al., 2019). This type of prediction can play a crucial role, particularly in chronic diseases and cancers (Attia et al., 2019; Weng et al., 2017). In drug development, AI is also important for quickly identifying drug candidates and predicting their efficacy, providing a much faster and more efficient method than traditional research and development processes (Chen et al., 2018; Jumper et al., 2021; Seo, S., & Lee, J. W., 2024; Stokes et al., 2020; Wu et al., 2024). Additionally, AI facilitates remote patient monitoring, allowing healthcare providers to track patients' health indicators in real time and intervene immediately when issues arise.

The fusion of AI and precision medicine is an ongoing innovative change. Recently, efforts to build data repositories have been actively undertaken in various countries, including the United States, which serves as a critical stepping stone for the adoption of precision medicine (Wahl et al., 2018). For instance, examples like the UK Biobank, Japan Biobank, and the Australian Genomics Health Alliance illustrate the rapidly changing attitudes towards precision medicine on a global scale (Khan et al., 2024). These advancements suggest that the combination of AI and precision medicine is not merely theoretical but can indeed establish itself as a practical medical innovation.

3. DEFINITIONS AND ROLES OF ARTIFICIAL INTELLIGENCE

Artificial intelligence refers to the capability of computers to simulate and model human cognitive functions (Xu et al., 2021). Artificial intelligence employs technologies to allow computers or machines to possess capabilities in areas such as planning, learning and sensing (Datta et al., 2024). Artificial intelligence systems identify surroundings, make decisions, and gain knowledge by repeating experiments. Artificial intelligence can be explained as a model that unifies learning theories to examine and implement the functions in optimizing learning processes (Prasetyo et al., 2024). The model related to cognitive psychology, bioinformatics, and computation, follows a causal learning mechanism that illustrates how learning processes can be conducted. The model describes how knowledge acquired through learning processes is collected, combined, or shared in the various research fields (Gorriz Sáez et al., 2023). Practice implications, evaluation standards, and a discussion of limitations are incorporated to understand learning processes in the field of artificial intelligence. Equipped with the suggested model, artificial intelligence developers can collaborate with learning designers, researchers, and practitioners to utilize the theoretical or practical roles to enhance personal learning, team efficiency, and the creation of knowledge communities (Gibson et al., 2023).

3.1 What Makes an Artificial Intelligence Model?

Reevaluating learning theories in the era of artificial intelligence and big data is required for the following reasons. The insights from evolution and complexity for an ongoing adaptation of theories to actual circumstances should be considered. Enhanced computational models of learning may enrich the comprehension of existing theories and broaden the scope and impact of both symbolic and literal humanities (Vossoughi et al., 2023). The circumstances related to artificial intelligence bring broader ideas and unify concepts with the advancements in the field of learning sciences. Evolution and development in complexity theory highlight the inherent function of learning as a component of exploration and investigating niches in a broader environment through gradual steps and advances (Colther & Doussoulin, 2024). The great advancements in artificial intelligence and big data have arrived at a point where the societal roles of artificial intelligence are more crucial than ever. Utilizing artificial intelligence methods can provide a summary that demonstrates connections and shared processes within learning processes (Akgun & Greenhow, 2022). This unification provides a new perspective on the promising functions of artificial intelligence in biomedical sciences (Ali et al., 2023; Kulikowski, 2019).

A steady trend in the development of artificial intelligence is illustrated for the understanding of advanced human intelligence (Dong et al., 2020). As the artificial intelligence effect, when a computer accomplishes a task, the difficulties in defining artificial intelligence arise not from mistakes or carelessness, but from the continuous endeavor to precisely pinpoint the intelligence. With the various definitions examined in this context and beyond, a wide-ranging definition of artificial intelligence has been adopted (Guan et al., 2023). Focusing exclusively on deep learning would overlook how numerous current challenges impact various elements of artificial intelligence, including logical systems (Collins et al., 2021). One challenge regarding artificial intelligence is the black box inquiry. Many artificial intelligence applications utilized by governments do not implement advanced methods such as deep learning and exhibit several significant problems that require attention in research and development (Marey et al., 2024).

3.2 How Can We Translate Insights from Artificial Intelligence Models to Precision Medicine?

The traits of the scientific domain suggest that the comprehension of artificial intelligence will progress over time (Bianchini et al., 2022). Instead of considering artificial intelligence as a clearly defined field with simplified definitions and methods, it is more advantageous to examine a complex and diverse area focusing on a specific target. The spot on that horizon symbolizes the understanding and emulation of all human mental capabilities (Strachan et al., 2024). Numerous specialists believe that artificial intelligence plays a major role in daily life, and a comprehensive grasp of artificial intelligence as well as computer science fundamentals will be essential for upcoming careers in science and engineering (Huang & Rust, 2018). Expertise in artificial intelligence and computer science will be as important as traditional fields of studies. By drawing an analogy with the learning processes, artificial intelligence concepts may be developed to encompass modules designed for different age ranges throughout multiple demographic levels (Padovano & Cardamone, 2024). Key artificial intelligence topics are linked to search-related problem solving, sorting algorithms, graphs, and data structures. Progress in artificial intelligence prompts inquiries regarding not only the current nature of scientific practices but also regarding technical elements within the practices (Hosny et al., 2018). The inquiry into science practices can be examined regarding scientific activities performed exclusively by people. As artificial intelligence tools become more essential to scientific practices, the concept of cutting-edge elements affects science education since learning environments must adjust to artificial intelligence as a partner in scientific endeavors, where researchers and practitioners collaboratively utilize the tools to tackle scientific challenges (Wang et al., 2024). The role and influence of artificial intelligence on scientific practices will create additional requirements for the research and development sector. The demands are like any new initiative aimed at revising or enhancing educational goals and outcomes, potentially necessitating a shift in the curriculum's content and structure, along with various reforms in assessment, teaching methods, and educator training (Chen et al., 2020).

Therefore, integrating artificial intelligence into science education presents a significant challenge that necessitates substantial systemic changes by creating intelligent machines that can perform activities typically requiring human intelligence, such as understanding speech, evaluating images, interpreting natural language, playing games, and operating vehicles (Chen & Zhu, 2023).

Statistics is a branch of mathematics centered on gathering, analyzing, interpreting, presenting, and organizing data and statistical methods are utilized to evaluate and comprehend data to make inferences about populations derived from samples (Omone et al., 2021). Artificial intelligence relies heavily on statistical methods to extract knowledge from biomedical data and produce estimation in healthcare (Davenport & Kalakota, 2019). Statistical methods enable artificial intelligence systems to identify patterns, uncover associations, and make inferences from biomedical data (Jamialahmadi et al., 2024). Pattern recognition usually involves the classification of patterns in supervised learning and clustering of patterns in unsupervised learning (Schwenker & Trentin, 2014). The recent advancement in available large-scale datasets has resulted in the integration of machines and deep learning in modern pattern recognition techniques. Regression analysis is a statistical method used in artificial intelligence to identify the relationship between a dependent variable and one or more independent variables (Vetter & Schober, 2018). Bayesian Statistics is a statistical method used in artificial intelligence to determine the probability of an event by merging prior knowledge with new data by generating prediction and optimizing decision making processes (Goligher et al., 2024). Statistical methods utilized in artificial intelligence to extract insights from data without explicit programming are known as algorithms for machine learning (Sarker). Neural networks represent a class of machine learning algorithms employed in artificial intelligence to examine the structure and function of the human brain (Abiodun et al., 2018).

The rapid advancement of artificial intelligence technology gives analysis tools in clinical settings, potentially transforming healthcare services (Alhejaily, 2024). It is crucial to record and share information about the role of artificial intelligence in clinical practice, to prepare healthcare professionals with the understanding of resources needed for successful application in patient care. The understanding of the function of artificial intelligence in healthcare can be enhanced by examining biomedical data essential for recognizing irregularities in the biological mechanisms (Khalifa & Albadawy, 2024). A reliable monitoring system can be utilized to identify patterns in data. Machine learning methods provide the automation of biomedical research processes, allowing for the categorization of normal and abnormal patterns through the establishment of decision boundaries (Sirocchi et al., 2024). Artificial intelligence methods include the support vector machine, random forest, neural network, etc. These models can be classified as supervised learning, unsupervised learning, semi-supervised learning, reinforcement learning, etc (Barragán-Montero et al., 2021).

However, the use of AI-based technologies in the medical field also comes with several drawbacks. The first disadvantage is the lack of sufficient and well-annotated data for training AI. The scarcity of extensive datasets that reflect diverse patient populations and varying cancer burdens can hinder the effective use of AI. Additionally, concerns about data privacy and security arise when handling patient data (Kaissis et al., 2020). AI systems must collect and store large amounts of sensitive patient information, making it crucial to manage this data securely (Rieke et al., 2020).

While AI can enhance efficiency, it cannot replace human contact. Some patients may prefer emotional support from humans over mechanical responses, which is a challenge for AI systems to provide. There is also the issue of algorithmic bias (Obermeyer et al., 2019). Since AI systems rely on the data they are trained on, biased data can lead to biased decisions by the algorithms (Vyas et al., 2020). This poses a risk of exacerbating healthcare inequality (Rajkomar, Hardt, et al., 2018). Furthermore, an over-reliance on AI technology may weaken the ability of healthcare professionals to make critical decisions.

A key consideration at the intersection of AI and precision medicine is data protection (Morley et al., 2020). It is essential to establish rigorous regulations to ensure that patient privacy is safeguarded during the process of collecting and integrating various types of data. To address this, a secure and well-regulated ecosystem for data storage, management, and sharing must be developed (Gerke et al., 2020).

4. IMMUNOLOGICAL DISORDERS

Autoimmune diseases occur due to a failure of immunologic tolerance, resulting in an immune reaction. In many cases, the triggers that start the immune response to self-molecules remain unclear, but several studies indicate links to environmental and genetic factors, as well as specific types of infections (Cooper et al., 1999; Ercolini & Miller, 2009; Jörg et al., 2016). The populations are affected by autoimmune diseases, often displaying symptoms of various disorders (Miller, 2023). It has been shown that several prevalent health issues like atherosclerosis and inflammatory bowel disease could involve an autoimmune problem (Weissman et al., 2020). While the fundamental mechanisms behind this predisposition have been studied, it is recognized that a significant portion of the evidence demonstrating the onset of autoimmune diseases is derived from animal models and human research (Rosenblum et al., 2015).

A limited quantity of autoreactive B and T cells is a typical component of the immune cell population, as the generation of autoantibodies is seen in healthy individuals in the mechanisms of autoimmune disease (Pisetsky, 2023). Tolerance is upheld through the regulatory interactions among different cell types and soluble mediators. Under specific circumstances, tolerance may be disrupted, leading to the development of an autoimmune condition (Pelanda & Piccirillo, 2008). The onset of autoimmune diseases may rely on a favorable genetic predisposition, but triggering agents like viral, bacterial, or chemical exposures result in changed self-reactivity. There exist various hypotheses concerning how genetics and environmental influences might contribute to overcoming the resistance to reactivity with self-antigens. Immune effector mechanisms that enhance or support the specific responses of T- and B-lymphocytes are crucial in the immune response as well (Molina & Shoenfeld, 2005). These nonspecific entities act as an initial defense against possible pathogens and comprise various leukocytes like macrophages, natural killer cells, and polymorphonuclear leukocytes, along with soluble mediators such as complement and cytokines (Lodoen & Lanier, 2006). Several autoimmune disorders exhibit distinct irregularities in cytokine production, indicating that these soluble agents might be involved in both the onset and development of the disease (Kunz & Ibrahim, 2009).

Autoimmunity involves self-reactive immune elements, while autoimmune disease consists of autoimmunity along with pathological changes (Castro & Gourley, 2010). Autoimmunity and autoimmune diseases are significantly rising in various regions globally, probably due to alterations in the interactions with environmental factors (Wang et al., 2015). The findings suggest that significant changes in diet, exposure to xenobiotics, air pollution, infections, individual lifestyles, stress levels, and climate change are responsible for these increases (Miller, 2025). Enhancing the diagnostic, therapeutic, and preventive methods can provide novel and sufficient approaches to overcome autoimmune diseases.

5. AI APPLICATIONS IN IMMUNOLOGICAL DISORDERS

Precision medicine is a healthcare strategy that employs different technologies to enable tailored diagnosis and treatment for individuals (Ho et al., 2020). The availability of technologies such as high-performance computing and vast biological datasets is crucial for developing a precision medicine strategy that can greatly influence healthcare (Quazi, 2022). A collection of computer algorithms can identify patterns in multidimensional datasets subsequently used to predict or improve results based on information about individual patients (Fountzilas et al., 2025). Algorithms in artificial intelligence employ learning methods based on classification or pattern recognition to examine input data, allowing for predictions from cumulative datasets. In clinical medicine, using results from pathological samples enables the prediction of diagnosis for the pathological samples acquired from new patients (Kumar et al., 2023). Multifaceted biological data and artificial intelligence methods will be necessary to unravel the pathogenicity (Shao et al., 2024). Numerous penetrant variants are recognized to exhibit multiple clinical manifestations, and a variety of conditions are built by diverse presentations associated with phenotypic heterogeneity (Y. H. Sun et al., 2023).

Artificial intelligence transforms allergy and immunology by incorporating advanced technology to improve patient results and revolutionize clinical practices and research (Goktas & Damadoglu). Artificial intelligence can improve diagnostic methods, including models that forecast allergen sensitivity and refined immunotherapy approaches. Large-scale datasets can be used to facilitate a better comprehension of allergic conditions and immune system reactions, resulting in more precise, efficient, and effective therapies (MacMath et al., 2023). The application of artificial intelligence enables care via allergen mapping, automated patient tracking, and targeted immunotherapy. The incorporation of artificial intelligence techniques into clinical settings provides allergy and immunology features for health care services (Carini & Seyhan, 2024).

Research in artificial intelligence in the medical field has grown tremendously in the past ten years, with studies demonstrating the capability of artificial intelligence algorithms to optimize clinical practices and services (Alowais et al., 2023). Research and development which can develop artificial intelligence models have grown to assist in recognizing inherited immunity disorders. Utilizing more extensive electronic health record data sets can greatly enhance the early detection of inherited immunity disorders with improvements in phenotyping accuracy and advancements in artificial intelligence methods. The use of artificial intelligence techniques in identifying immunological disorders encounters obstacles with substantial data backup (C. Zhang et al., 2023). The utilization of artificial intelligence techniques enables substantial data support for model training in big data analytics (Barja-Martinez et al., 2021). Although artificial intelligence techniques provide optimal prediction and diagnosis outcomes, the interpretability of big data analytics is limited. The algorithms and technologies of artificial intelligence have been advanced, and the outcomes depend on the specific technologies and algorithms, influencing the precision of acquiring disease-related information. Artificial intelligence algorithms are effective for healthcare information, the algorithms can be used to manage various data types, and the predictive performance has been gradually improved as the volume of input data increases (Bohr & Memarzadeh, 2020). A solution to facilitate effective information extraction for healthcare analytics is to collaborate data science teams, clinical practitioners, and laboratory scientists. In this manner, the technical expertise of data scientists can enhance the knowledge of clinical and scientific domain experts to improve data extraction, dataset creation, and analysis throughout a thorough and pertinent process.

Building on these general applications, the following sections explore specialized AI tools such as those for analyzing the tumor immune microenvironment, predicting T cell antigens, and developing personalized cancer vaccines which effectively illustrate the transformative impact of AI on precision immunotherapy.

5.1 AI Tools for Tumor Immune Microenvironment Analysis

To analyze the immunological characteristics of the tumor microenvironment, artificial intelligence-based tools have been widely employed. A notable example is IOBR (Immuno-Oncology Biological Research), an R package designed to integrate multi-omics data to compute various indicators related to the tumor immune microenvironment (TME) (Zeng et al., 2021). IOBR consolidates several algorithms—including CIBERSORT, TIMER, and others—to quantitatively assess the composition of immune cells and molecular signatures within tumor tissues (Newman et al., 2015). It further correlates these immunological metrics with clinical data, thus enhancing the understanding of patient prognosis. For instance, transcriptome analysis from the IMvigor210 cohort (involving patients treated with anti-PD-L1 inhibitors) revealed that the infiltration of M1 macrophages could serve as a significant biomarker predicting treatment response .

5.2 Application of AI in Antigen Prediction and Vaccine Design

In the fields of immunological research and vaccine development, AI-driven software plays a crucial role in the efficient prediction of T cell antigens. An exemplary tool, MHCflurry, predicts the binding affinity of peptides to MHC class I molecules, thereby aiding in the identification of immunogenic epitopes for vaccine target selection in both cancer and infectious disease research (O'Donnell et al., 2020). Utilizing deep learning models trained on extensive experimental datasets, MHCflurry achieves superior accuracy compared to conventional methods. Its high-throughput capability—processing over 7,000 peptide predictions per second—enables rapid screening of potential antigens. This efficiency significantly streamlines the selection process, allowing researchers to focus on the most promising candidates for experimental validation and subsequent vaccine design.

5.3 Case Study of Personalized Cancer Vaccine Development

AI techniques are also integral to personalized cancer vaccine development, where the objective is to tailor immunotherapeutic targets based on individual tumor genomic profiles (Kumar et al., 2024). In the PGV-001 clinical trial, for instance, a pipeline was implemented that integrated exome sequencing with transcriptomic analysis to identify patient-specific mutations and predict corresponding neoantigen candidates (Rubinsteyn et al., 2018). This personalized vaccine design pipeline comprises several AI modules, including Isovar and Vaxrank. Isovar analyzes tumor mutation data in conjunction with RNA expression profiles to derive mutant protein sequences that serve as potential neoantigens . Subsequently, Vaxrank evaluates these mutant peptides by predicting their binding affinities to MHC molecules and ranking them based on both binding strength and expression levels. This prioritization process enables the selection of neoantigens most likely to elicit a robust immune response, thereby underscoring the feasibility and effectiveness of individualized immunotherapy strategies .

6. CONCLUSIONS

Electronic health records and research data are growing rapidly, while patients are experiencing longer lifespans with increasing complexity (Casey et al., 2016). Well-designed computational tools can aid in understanding clinical and scientific data, minimize medical mistakes, and reduce morbidity. Due to these factors, artificial intelligence and machine learning have sparked curiosity in the healthcare field and are progressing applications across diagnostic, quality-care, and research areas. By aiding disease diagnosis, computation techniques can identify patients who are at risk for primary immunodeficiency diseases. For instance, a risk-assessment algorithm can be integrated into a health plan data pipeline to detect patients with health issues, risks, or clinical paths to promote early intervention. Analyzing structured laboratory data based on rules can facilitate population-wide evaluation of the disease risk (Wen et al., 2022). However, these methods ought to be regarded as the beginning of the possibilities in clinical immunology, which extend from discovering new disease genes to choosing subjects for participation in clinical trials. According to every standard of the definition, healthcare data qualifies as big data. In general, big data pertains to data that is of enormous size, collected at high speed, and exhibits considerable diversity. This dual nature of big data requires attention for both its effective utilization and the management of complexity. Distinct big data characteristics also necessitate tools to perform data inference. Conventional artificial intelligence algorithms are crafted to process vast quantities of data and identify patterns (Elhaddad & Hamam, 2024). Data can be gathered from regular clinical, lab, and claims information to create examples examined by the model according to a specified task. Artificial intelligence algorithms assign greater importance to specific features that are linked to predicting a labeled class outcome based on the method schema selected. Artificial intelligence algorithms are capable of processing substantial volumes of diverse and intricate data, evaluated based on features acquired during training, resulting in a prediction that can be utilized effectively (B. Zhang et al., 2023).

In the future, the convergence of AI and precision medicine is likely to continue evolving healthcare innovations. To facilitate this, several solutions are necessary. First, standardization and sharing of data must be implemented (Wilkinson et al., 2016). It is essential to standardize the data collected from various sources to ensure consistent processing, allowing AI to produce more accurate and reliable results. Additionally, to enhance applicability in diverse environments, various infrastructures need to be established (Wahl et al., 2018). Collaboration and investment between the government and the private sector are crucial, especially in low-income countries where subsidies or support programs are needed to increase access to AI technology. For AI and precision medicine technologies to be successfully integrated into the medical field, ethical standards must be established alongside transparent and accountable regulatory and legal frameworks (Morley et al., 2020). AI must be ensured to operate fairly in healthcare, serving to complement rather than replace human intuition. Furthermore, training and education on AI technology for healthcare professionals are essential. This will enable doctors to effectively use AI as an assistive tool. Lastly, building trust with patients and the public is crucial. Providing clear information about how AI technology operates and how data is processed, along with rigorous management of privacy and security, is necessary to gain that trust.

REFERENCES

Abdallah, S., Sharifa, M., Almadhoun, M. K. I. K., Khawar, M. M.Sr, Shaikh, U., Balabel, K. M., Saleh, I., Manzoor, A., Mandal, A. K., & Ekomwereren, O. (2023). The impact of artificial intelligence on optimizing diagnosis and treatment plans for rare genetic disorders. *Cureus*, *15*(10). Advance online publication. DOI: 10.7759/cureus.46860 PMID: 37954711

Abiodun, O. I., Jantan, A., Omolara, A. E., Dada, K. V., Mohamed, N. A., & Arshad, H. (2018). State-of-the-art in artificial neural network applications: A survey. *Heliyon*, *4*(11), e00938. DOI: 10.1016/j.heliyon.2018.e00938 PMID: 30519653

Achilles, S. L., Creinin, M. D., Stoner, K. A., Chen, B. A., Meyn, L., & Hillier, S. L. (2014). Changes in genital tract immune cell populations after initiation of intrauterine contraception. *American journal of obstetrics and gynecology, 211*(5), 489. e481-489. e489.

Ahmed, Z., Mohamed, K., Zeeshan, S., & Dong, X. (2020). Artificial intelligence with multi-functional machine learning platform development for better healthcare and precision medicine. *Database : The Journal of Biological Databases and Curation*, *2020*, baaa010. DOI: 10.1093/database/baaa010 PMID: 32185396

Akgun, S., & Greenhow, C. (2022). Artificial intelligence in education: Addressing ethical challenges in K-12 settings. *AI and Ethics*, *2*(3), 431–440. DOI: 10.1007/s43681-021-00096-7 PMID: 34790956

Alhasan, M., & Hasaneen, M. (2021). Digital imaging, technologies and artificial intelligence applications during COVID-19 pandemic. *Computerized Medical Imaging and Graphics*, *91*, 101933. DOI: 10.1016/j.compmedimag.2021.101933 PMID: 34082281

Alhejaily, A.-M. G. (2024). Artificial intelligence in healthcare. *Biomedical Reports*, *22*(1), 11. DOI: 10.3892/br.2024.1889 PMID: 39583770

Ali, S., Akhlaq, F., Imran, A. S., Kastrati, Z., Daudpota, S. M., & Moosa, M. (2023). The enlightening role of explainable artificial intelligence in medical & healthcare domains: A systematic literature review. *Computers in Biology and Medicine*, *166*, 107555. DOI: 10.1016/j.compbiomed.2023.107555 PMID: 37806061

Alowais, S. A., Alghamdi, S. S., Alsuhebany, N., Alqahtani, T., Alshaya, A. I., Almohareb, S. N., Aldairem, A., Alrashed, M., Bin Saleh, K., Badreldin, H. A., Al Yami, M. S., Al Harbi, S., & Albekairy, A. M. (2023). Revolutionizing healthcare: The role of artificial intelligence in clinical practice. *BMC Medical Education*, *23*(1), 689. DOI: 10.1186/s12909-023-04698-z PMID: 37740191

Amir, E.-D., Davis, K. L., Tadmor, M. D., Simonds, E. F., Levine, J. H., Bendall, S. C., Shenfeld, D. K., Krishnaswamy, S., Nolan, G. P., & Pe'er, D. (2013). viSNE enables visualization of high dimensional single-cell data and reveals phenotypic heterogeneity of leukemia. *Nature Biotechnology*, *31*(6), 545–552. DOI: 10.1038/nbt.2594 PMID: 23685480

Ardila, D., Kiraly, A. P., Bharadwaj, S., Choi, B., Reicher, J. J., Peng, L., Tse, D., Etemadi, M., Ye, W., Corrado, G., Naidich, D. P., & Shetty, S. (2019). End-to-end lung cancer screening with three-dimensional deep learning on low-dose chest computed tomography. *Nature Medicine*, *25*(6), 954–961. DOI: 10.1038/s41591-019-0447-x PMID: 31110349

Attia, Z. I., Noseworthy, P. A., Lopez-Jimenez, F., Asirvatham, S. J., Deshmukh, A. J., Gersh, B. J., Carter, R. E., Yao, X., Rabinstein, A. A., Erickson, B. J., Kapa, S., & Friedman, P. A. (2019). An artificial intelligence-enabled ECG algorithm for the identification of patients with atrial fibrillation during sinus rhythm: A retrospective analysis of outcome prediction. *Lancet*, *394*(10201), 861–867. DOI: 10.1016/S0140-6736(19)31721-0 PMID: 31378392

Bagger, F. O., Borgwardt, L., Jespersen, A. S., Hansen, A. R., Bertelsen, B., Kodama, M., & Nielsen, F. C. (2024). Whole genome sequencing in clinical practice. *BMC Medical Genomics*, *17*(1), 39. DOI: 10.1186/s12920-024-01795-w PMID: 38287327

Barja-Martinez, S., Aragüés-Peñalba, M., Munné-Collado, Í., Lloret-Gallego, P., Bullich-Massagué, E., & Villafafila-Robles, R. (2021). Artificial intelligence techniques for enabling Big Data services in distribution networks: A review. *Renewable & Sustainable Energy Reviews*, *150*, 111459. DOI: 10.1016/j.rser.2021.111459

Barragán-Montero, A., Javaid, U., Valdés, G., Nguyen, D., Desbordes, P., Macq, B., Willems, S., Vandewinckele, L., Holmström, M., Löfman, F., Michiels, S., Souris, K., Sterpin, E., & Lee, J. A. (2021). Artificial intelligence and machine learning for medical imaging: A technology review. *Physica Medica*, *83*, 242–256. DOI: 10.1016/j.ejmp.2021.04.016 PMID: 33979715

Bhol, N. K., Bhanjadeo, M. M., Singh, A. K., Dash, U. C., Ojha, R. R., Majhi, S., Duttaroy, A. K., & Jena, A. B. (2024). The interplay between cytokines, inflammation, and antioxidants: Mechanistic insights and therapeutic potentials of various antioxidants and anti-cytokine compounds. *Biomedicine and Pharmacotherapy*, *178*, 117177. DOI: 10.1016/j.biopha.2024.117177 PMID: 39053423

Bianchini, S., Müller, M., & Pelletier, P. (2022). Artificial intelligence in science: An emerging general method of invention. *Research Policy*, *51*(10), 104604. DOI: 10.1016/j.respol.2022.104604

Bohr, A., & Memarzadeh, K. (2020). The rise of artificial intelligence in healthcare applications. In *Artificial Intelligence in healthcare* (pp. 25–60). Elsevier. DOI: 10.1016/B978-0-12-818438-7.00002-2

Boland, M. R., Jacunski, A., Lorberbaum, T., Romano, J. D., Moskovitch, R., & Tatonetti, N. P. (2016). Systems biology approaches for identifying adverse drug reactions and elucidating their underlying biological mechanisms. *Wiley Interdisciplinary Reviews. Systems Biology and Medicine*, *8*(2), 104–122. DOI: 10.1002/wsbm.1323 PMID: 26559926

Campanella, G., Hanna, M. G., Geneslaw, L., Miraflor, A., Werneck Krauss Silva, V., Busam, K. J., Brogi, E., Reuter, V. E., Klimstra, D. S., & Fuchs, T. J. (2019). Clinical-grade computational pathology using weakly supervised deep learning on whole slide images. *Nature Medicine*, *25*(8), 1301–1309. DOI: 10.1038/s41591-019-0508-1 PMID: 31308507

Carini, C., & Seyhan, A. A. (2024). Tribulations and future opportunities for artificial intelligence in precision medicine. *Journal of Translational Medicine*, *22*(1), 411. DOI: 10.1186/s12967-024-05067-0 PMID: 38702711

Casey, J. A., Schwartz, B. S., Stewart, W. F., & Adler, N. E. (2016). Using electronic health records for population health research: A review of methods and applications. *Annual Review of Public Health*, *37*(1), 61–81. DOI: 10.1146/annurev-publhealth-032315-021353 PMID: 26667605

Castro, C., & Gourley, M. (2010). Diagnostic testing and interpretation of tests for autoimmunity. *The Journal of Allergy and Clinical Immunology*, *125*(2), S238–S247. DOI: 10.1016/j.jaci.2009.09.041 PMID: 20061009

Chaplin, D. D. (2010). Overview of the immune response. *The Journal of Allergy and Clinical Immunology*, *125*(2), S3–S23. DOI: 10.1016/j.jaci.2009.12.980 PMID: 20176265

Chen, B., & Zhu, X. (2023). Integrating generative AI in knowledge building. *Computers and Education: Artificial Intelligence*, *5*, 100184.

Chen, H., Engkvist, O., Wang, Y., Olivecrona, M., & Blaschke, T. (2018). The rise of deep learning in drug discovery. *Drug Discovery Today*, *23*(6), 1241–1250. DOI: 10.1016/j.drudis.2018.01.039 PMID: 29366762

Chen, L., Chen, P., & Lin, Z. (2020). Artificial intelligence in education: A review. *IEEE Access : Practical Innovations, Open Solutions*, *8*, 75264–75278. DOI: 10.1109/ACCESS.2020.2988510

Chen, Y.-M., Hsiao, T.-H., Lin, C.-H., & Fann, Y. C. (2025). Unlocking precision medicine: Clinical applications of integrating health records, genetics, and immunology through artificial intelligence. *Journal of Biomedical Science*, *32*(1), 16. DOI: 10.1186/s12929-024-01110-w PMID: 39915780

Collins, C., Dennehy, D., Conboy, K., & Mikalef, P. (2021). Artificial intelligence in information systems research: A systematic literature review and research agenda. *International Journal of Information Management*, *60*, 102383. DOI: 10.1016/j.ijinfomgt.2021.102383

Colther, C., & Doussoulin, J. P. (2024). Artificial intelligence: Driving force in the evolution of human knowledge. *Journal of Innovation & Knowledge*, *9*(4), 100625. DOI: 10.1016/j.jik.2024.100625

Cooper, G. S., Miller, F. W., & Pandey, J. P. (1999). The role of genetic factors in autoimmune disease: Implications for environmental research. *Environmental Health Perspectives*, *107*(suppl 5), 693–700. PMID: 10502533

Crossa, J., Montesinos-Lopez, O. A., Costa-Neto, G., Vitale, P., Martini, J. W., Runcie, D., Fritsche-Neto, R., Montesinos-Lopez, A., Pérez-Rodríguez, P., & Gerard, G. (2024). Machine learning algorithms translate big data into predictive breeding accuracy. *Trends in Plant Science*. PMID: 39462718

Danieli, M. G., Brunetto, S., Gammeri, L., Palmeri, D., Claudi, I., Shoenfeld, Y., & Gangemi, S. (2024). Machine learning application in autoimmune diseases: State of art and future prospectives. *Autoimmunity Reviews*, *23*(2), 103496. DOI: 10.1016/j.autrev.2023.103496 PMID: 38081493

Datta, S. D., Islam, M., Sobuz, M. H. R., Ahmed, S., & Kar, M. (2024). Artificial intelligence and machine learning applications in the project lifecycle of the construction industry: A comprehensive review. *Heliyon*, *10*(5), e26888. DOI: 10.1016/j.heliyon.2024.e26888 PMID: 38444479

Davenport, T., & Kalakota, R. (2019). The potential for artificial intelligence in healthcare. *Future Healthcare Journal*, *6*(2), 94–98. DOI: 10.7861/futurehosp.6-2-94 PMID: 31363513

Dong, C., Ji, Y., Fu, Z., Qi, Y., Yi, T., Yang, Y., Sun, Y., & Sun, H. (2025). Precision management in chronic disease: An AI empowered perspective on medicine-engineering crossover. *iScience*, *28*(3), 112044. DOI: 10.1016/j.isci.2025.112044 PMID: 40104052

Dong, Y., Hou, J., Zhang, N., & Zhang, M. (2020). Research on how human intelligence, consciousness, and cognitive computing affect the development of artificial intelligence. *Complexity*, *2020*(1), 1680845. DOI: 10.1155/2020/1680845

Donnelly, R. P., Young, H. A., & Rosenberg, A. S. (2009). An overview of cytokines and cytokine antagonists as therapeutic agents. *Annals of the New York Academy of Sciences*, *1182*(1), 1–13. DOI: 10.1111/j.1749-6632.2009.05382.x PMID: 20074270

Efremova, M., Vento-Tormo, M., Teichmann, S. A., & Vento-Tormo, R. (2020). CellPhoneDB: Inferring cell–cell communication from combined expression of multi-subunit ligand–receptor complexes. *Nature Protocols*, *15*(4), 1484–1506. DOI: 10.1038/s41596-020-0292-x PMID: 32103204

Elhaddad, M., & Hamam, S. (2024). AI-driven clinical decision support systems: An ongoing pursuit of potential. *Cureus*, *16*(4). Advance online publication. DOI: 10.7759/cureus.57728 PMID: 38711724

Ercolini, A., & Miller, S. (2009). The role of infections in autoimmune disease. *Clinical and Experimental Immunology*, *155*(1), 1–15. DOI: 10.1111/j.1365-2249.2008.03834.x PMID: 19076824

Esteva, A., Kuprel, B., Novoa, R. A., Ko, J., Swetter, S. M., Blau, H. M., & Thrun, S. (2017). Dermatologist-level classification of skin cancer with deep neural networks. *Nature*, *542*(7639), 115–118. DOI: 10.1038/nature21056 PMID: 28117445

Filipp, F. V. (2019). Opportunities for artificial intelligence in advancing precision medicine. *Current Genetic Medicine Reports*, *7*(4), 208–213. DOI: 10.1007/s40142-019-00177-4 PMID: 31871830

Fountzilas, E., Pearce, T., Baysal, M. A., Chakraborty, A., & Tsimberidou, A. M. (2025). Convergence of evolving artificial intelligence and machine learning techniques in precision oncology. *npj. Digital Medicine*, *8*(1), 75. PMID: 39890986

Gerke, S., Minssen, T., & Cohen, G. (2020). Ethical and legal challenges of artificial intelligence-driven healthcare. In *Artificial intelligence in healthcare* (pp. 295–336). Elsevier. DOI: 10.1016/B978-0-12-818438-7.00012-5

Ghofrani, A., & Taherdoost, H. (2024). Biomedical data analytics for better patient outcomes. *Drug Discovery Today*, •••, 104280. PMID: 39732322

Gibson, D., Kovanovic, V., Ifenthaler, D., Dexter, S., & Feng, S. (2023). Learning theories for artificial intelligence promoting learning processes. *British Journal of Educational Technology*, *54*(5), 1125–1146. DOI: 10.1111/bjet.13341

Goktas, P., & Damadoglu, E. (2025). Future of allergy and immunology: Is artificial intelligence the key in the digital era? *Annals of Allergy, Asthma & Immunology, 134*(4), 396–407.

Goligher, E. C., Heath, A., & Harhay, M. O. (2024). Bayesian statistics for clinical research. *Lancet, 404*(10457), 1067–1076. DOI: 10.1016/S0140-6736(24)01295-9 PMID: 39277290

Gorriz Sáez, J. M., Álvarez Illán, I., Arco Martín, J. E., Castillo Barnes, D., Formoso, M. A., Gallego Molina, N. J., Jiménez Mesa, C., Martínez Murcia, F. J., Ortiz García, A., & Ramírez Pérez De Inestrosa, J. (2023). Computational approaches to Explainable Artificial Intelligence: Advances in theory, applications and trends.

Guan, Z., Li, H., Liu, R., Cai, C., Liu, Y., Li, J., Wang, X., Huang, S., Wu, L., Liu, D., Yu, S., Wang, Z., Shu, J., Hou, X., Yang, X., Jia, W., & Sheng, B. (2023). Artificial intelligence in diabetes management: Advancements, opportunities, and challenges. *Cell Reports Medicine, 4*(10), 101213. DOI: 10.1016/j.xcrm.2023.101213 PMID: 37788667

Gurovich, Y., Hanani, Y., Bar, O., Nadav, G., Fleischer, N., Gelbman, D., Basel-Salmon, L., Krawitz, P. M., Kamphausen, S. B., Zenker, M., Bird, L. M., & Gripp, K. W. (2019). Identifying facial phenotypes of genetic disorders using deep learning. *Nature Medicine, 25*(1), 60–64. DOI: 10.1038/s41591-018-0279-0 PMID: 30617323

Güvenç Paltun, B., Kaski, S., & Mamitsuka, H. (2021). Machine learning approaches for drug combination therapies. *Briefings in Bioinformatics, 22*(6), bbab293. DOI: 10.1093/bib/bbab293 PMID: 34368832

Ho, D., Quake, S. R., McCabe, E. R., Chng, W. J., Chow, E. K., Ding, X., Gelb, B. D., Ginsburg, G. S., Hassenstab, J., Ho, C.-M., Mobley, W. C., Nolan, G. P., Rosen, S. T., Tan, P., Yen, Y., & Zarrinpar, A. (2020). Enabling technologies for personalized and precision medicine. *Trends in Biotechnology, 38*(5), 497–518. DOI: 10.1016/j.tibtech.2019.12.021 PMID: 31980301

Hosny, A., Parmar, C., Quackenbush, J., Schwartz, L. H., & Aerts, H. J. (2018). Artificial intelligence in radiology. *Nature Reviews. Cancer, 18*(8), 500–510. DOI: 10.1038/s41568-018-0016-5 PMID: 29777175

Huang, M.-H., & Rust, R. T. (2018). Artificial intelligence in service. *Journal of Service Research, 21*(2), 155–172. DOI: 10.1177/1094670517752459

Jamialahmadi, H., Khalili-Tanha, G., Nazari, E., & Rezaei-Tavirani, M. (2024). Artificial intelligence and bioinformatics: A journey from traditional techniques to smart approaches. *Gastroenterology and Hepatology from Bed To Bench, 17*(3), 241. PMID: 39308539

Johnson, K. B., Wei, W. Q., Weeraratne, D., Frisse, M. E., Misulis, K., Rhee, K., Zhao, J., & Snowdon, J. L. (2021). Precision medicine, AI, and the future of personalized health care. *Clinical and Translational Science, 14*(1), 86–93. DOI: 10.1111/cts.12884 PMID: 32961010

Jörg, S., Grohme, D. A., Erzler, M., Binsfeld, M., Haghikia, A., Müller, D. N., Linker, R. A., & Kleinewietfeld, M. (2016). Environmental factors in autoimmune diseases and their role in multiple sclerosis. *Cellular and Molecular Life Sciences : CMLS, 73*(24), 4611–4622. DOI: 10.1007/s00018-016-2311-1 PMID: 27491297

Jumper, J., Evans, R., Pritzel, A., Green, T., Figurnov, M., Ronneberger, O., Tunyasuvunakool, K., Bates, R., Žídek, A., Potapenko, A., Bridgland, A., Meyer, C., Kohl, S. A. A., Ballard, A. J., Cowie, A., Romera-Paredes, B., Nikolov, S., Jain, R., Adler, J., & Hassabis, D. (2021). Highly accurate protein structure prediction with AlphaFold. *Nature, 596*(7873), 583–589. DOI: 10.1038/s41586-021-03819-2 PMID: 34265844

Kaissis, G. A., Makowski, M. R., Rückert, D., & Braren, R. F. (2020). Secure, privacy-preserving and federated machine learning in medical imaging. *Nature Machine Intelligence, 2*(6), 305–311. DOI: 10.1038/s42256-020-0186-1

Khalifa, M., & Albadawy, M. (2024). Artificial intelligence for clinical prediction: Exploring key domains and essential functions. *Computer Methods and Programs in Biomedicine Update, 5*, 100148. DOI: 10.1016/j.cmpbup.2024.100148

Khan, M. S., Umer, H., & Faruqe, F. (2024). Artificial intelligence for low income countries. *Humanities & Social Sciences Communications, 11*(1), 1–13. DOI: 10.1057/s41599-024-03947-w

Khosravi-Maharlooei, M., Madley, R., Borsotti, C., Ferreira, L. M., Sharp, R. C., Brehm, M. A., Greiner, D. L., Parent, A. V., Anderson, M. S., Sykes, M., & Creusot, R. J. (2022). Modeling human T1D-associated autoimmune processes. *Molecular Metabolism, 56*, 101417. DOI: 10.1016/j.molmet.2021.101417 PMID: 34902607

Krzyszczyk, P., Acevedo, A., Davidoff, E. J., Timmins, L. M., Marrero-Berrios, I., Patel, M., White, C., Lowe, C., Sherba, J. J., & Hartmanshenn, C. (2018). The growing role of precision and personalized medicine for cancer treatment. *Technology, 6*(03n04), 79-100.

Kulikowski, C. A. (2019). Beginnings of artificial intelligence in medicine (AIM): Computational artifice assisting scientific inquiry and clinical art–with reflections on present aim challenges. *Yearbook of Medical Informatics, 28*(01), 249–256. DOI: 10.1055/s-0039-1677895 PMID: 31022744

Kumar, A., Dixit, S., Srinivasan, K., & Vincent, P. D. R. (2024). Personalized cancer vaccine design using AI-powered technologies. *Frontiers in Immunology, 15*, 1357217. DOI: 10.3389/fimmu.2024.1357217 PMID: 39582860

Kumar, Y., Koul, A., Singla, R., & Ijaz, M. F. (2023). Artificial intelligence in disease diagnosis: A systematic literature review, synthesizing framework and future research agenda. *Journal of Ambient Intelligence and Humanized Computing, 14*(7), 8459–8486. DOI: 10.1007/s12652-021-03612-z PMID: 35039756

Kunz, M., & Ibrahim, S. M. (2009). Cytokines and cytokine profiles in human autoimmune diseases and animal models of autoimmunity. *Mediators of Inflammation, 2009*(1), 979258. DOI: 10.1155/2009/979258 PMID: 19884985

Kuruvilla, M. E., Lee, F. E.-H., & Lee, G. B. (2019). Understanding asthma phenotypes, endotypes, and mechanisms of disease. *Clinical Reviews in Allergy & Immunology, 56*(2), 219–233. DOI: 10.1007/s12016-018-8712-1 PMID: 30206782

Laupèze, B., Del Giudice, G., Doherty, M. T., & Van der Most, R. (2021). Vaccination as a preventative measure contributing to immune fitness. *npj. Vaccines, 6*(1), 93. PMID: 34315886

Libbrecht, M. W., & Noble, W. S. (2015). Machine learning applications in genetics and genomics. *Nature Reviews. Genetics*, *16*(6), 321–332. DOI: 10.1038/nrg3920 PMID: 25948244

Lodoen, M. B., & Lanier, L. L. (2006). Natural killer cells as an initial defense against pathogens. *Current Opinion in Immunology*, *18*(4), 391–398. DOI: 10.1016/j.coi.2006.05.002 PMID: 16765573

Long, A., Kleiner, A., & Looney, R. J. (2023). Immune dysregulation. *The Journal of Allergy and Clinical Immunology*, *151*(1), 70–80. DOI: 10.1016/j.jaci.2022.11.001 PMID: 36608984

Lv, C., Guo, W., Yin, X., Liu, L., Huang, X., Li, S., & Zhang, L. (2024). Innovative applications of artificial intelligence during the COVID-19 pandemic. *Infectious Medicine*, *3*(1), 100095. DOI: 10.1016/j.imj.2024.100095 PMID: 38586543

MacMath, D., Chen, M., & Khoury, P. (2023). Artificial intelligence: Exploring the future of innovation in allergy immunology. *Current Allergy and Asthma Reports*, *23*(6), 351–362. DOI: 10.1007/s11882-023-01084-z PMID: 37160554

Mangino, M., Roederer, M., Beddall, M. H., Nestle, F. O., & Spector, T. D. (2017). Innate and adaptive immune traits are differentially affected by genetic and environmental factors. *Nature Communications*, *8*(1), 13850. DOI: 10.1038/ncomms13850 PMID: 28054551

Marey, A., Arjmand, P., Alerab, A. D. S., Eslami, M. J., Saad, A. M., Sanchez, N., & Umair, M. (2024). Explainability, transparency and black box challenges of AI in radiology: Impact on patient care in cardiovascular radiology. *The Egyptian Journal of Radiology and Nuclear Medicine*, *55*(1), 183. DOI: 10.1186/s43055-024-01356-2

McKinney, S. M., Sieniek, M., Godbole, V., Godwin, J., Antropova, N., Ashrafian, H., Back, T., Chesus, M., Corrado, G. S., Darzi, A., Etemadi, M., Garcia-Vicente, F., Gilbert, F. J., Halling-Brown, M., Hassabis, D., Jansen, S., Karthikesalingam, A., Kelly, C. J., King, D., & Shetty, S. (2020). International evaluation of an AI system for breast cancer screening. *Nature*, *577*(7788), 89–94. DOI: 10.1038/s41586-019-1799-6 PMID: 31894144

Miller, F. W. (2023). The increasing prevalence of autoimmunity and autoimmune diseases: An urgent call to action for improved understanding, diagnosis, treatment, and prevention. *Current Opinion in Immunology*, *80*, 102266. DOI: 10.1016/j.coi.2022.102266 PMID: 36446151

Miller, F. W. (2025). Environment, Lifestyles, and Climate Change: The Many Nongenetic Contributors to The Long and Winding Road to Autoimmune Diseases. *Arthritis Care and Research*, *77*(1), 3–11. DOI: 10.1002/acr.25423 PMID: 39228044

Moingeon, P. (2023). Artificial intelligence-driven drug development against autoimmune diseases. *Trends in Pharmacological Sciences*, *44*(7), 411–424. DOI: 10.1016/j.tips.2023.04.005 PMID: 37268540

Molina, V., & Shoenfeld, Y. (2005). Infection, vaccines and other environmental triggers of autoimmunity. *Autoimmunity*, *38*(3), 235–245. DOI: 10.1080/08916930500050277 PMID: 16126512

Morley, J., Machado, C. C., Burr, C., Cowls, J., Joshi, I., Taddeo, M., & Floridi, L. (2020). The ethics of AI in health care: A mapping review. *Social Science & Medicine*, *260*, 113172. DOI: 10.1016/j.socscimed.2020.113172 PMID: 32702587

Najjar, R. (2023). Redefining radiology: A review of artificial intelligence integration in medical imaging. *Diagnostics (Basel), 13*(17), 2760. DOI: 10.3390/diagnostics13172760 PMID: 37685300

Newman, A. M., Liu, C. L., Green, M. R., Gentles, A. J., Feng, W., Xu, Y., Hoang, C. D., Diehn, M., & Alizadeh, A. A. (2015). Robust enumeration of cell subsets from tissue expression profiles. *Nature Methods*, *12*(5), 453–457. DOI: 10.1038/nmeth.3337 PMID: 25822800

O'Donnell, T. J., Rubinsteyn, A., & Laserson, U. (2020). MHCflurry 2.0: improved pan-allele prediction of MHC class I-presented peptides by incorporating antigen processing. *Cell systems, 11*(1), 42-48. e47.

Obermeyer, Z., Powers, B., Vogeli, C., & Mullainathan, S. (2019). Dissecting racial bias in an algorithm used to manage the health of populations. *Science*, *366*(6464), 447–453. DOI: 10.1126/science.aax2342 PMID: 31649194

Omone, O. M., Kovács, L., & Kozlovszky, M. (2021). The Basic Application of Biostatistics to Biomedical Science Using R Programming. 2021 IEEE 19th World Symposium on Applied Machine Intelligence and Informatics (SAMI).

Padovano, A., & Cardamone, M. (2024). Towards human-AI collaboration in the competency-based curriculum development process: The case of industrial engineering and management education. *Computers and Education: Artificial Intelligence*, *7*, 100256.

Pammi, M., Aghaeepour, N., & Neu, J. (2023). Multiomics, artificial intelligence, and precision medicine in perinatology. *Pediatric Research*, *93*(2), 308–315. DOI: 10.1038/s41390-022-02181-x PMID: 35804156

Parekh, A.-D. E., Shaikh, O. A., Manan, S., & Al Hasibuzzaman, M. (2023). Artificial intelligence (AI) in personalized medicine: AI-generated personalized therapy regimens based on genetic and medical history. *Annals of Medicine and Surgery (London)*, *85*(11), 5831–5833. DOI: 10.1097/MS9.0000000000001320 PMID: 37915639

Pelanda, R., & Piccirillo, C. A. (2008). Tolerance, immune regulation, and autoimmunity: Cells and cytokines that make a difference. *Current Opinion in Immunology*, *20*(6), 629–631. DOI: 10.1016/j.coi.2008.10.005 PMID: 18977298

Pisetsky, D. S. (2023). Pathogenesis of autoimmune disease. *Nature Reviews. Nephrology*, *19*(8), 509–524. DOI: 10.1038/s41581-023-00720-1 PMID: 37165096

Prasetyo, M. L., Peranginangin, R. A., Martinovic, N., Ichsan, M., & Wicaksono, H. (2024). Artificial intelligence in open innovation project management: A systematic literature review on technologies, applications, and integration requirements. *Journal of Open Innovation*, •••, 100445.

Prosperi, M., Min, J. S., Bian, J., & Modave, F. (2018). Big data hurdles in precision medicine and precision public health. *BMC Medical Informatics and Decision Making*, *18*(1), 1–15. DOI: 10.1186/s12911-018-0719-2 PMID: 30594159

Quazi, S. (2022). Artificial intelligence and machine learning in precision and genomic medicine. *Medical Oncology (Northwood, London, England)*, *39*(8), 120. DOI: 10.1007/s12032-022-01711-1 PMID: 35704152

Rahman, A., Debnath, T., Kundu, D., Khan, M. S. I., Aishi, A. A., Sazzad, S., Sayduzzaman, M., & Band, S. S. (2024). Machine learning and deep learning-based approach in smart healthcare: Recent advances, applications, challenges and opportunities. *AIMS Public Health*, *11*(1), 58–109. DOI: 10.3934/publichealth.2024004 PMID: 38617415

Rajkomar, A., Hardt, M., Howell, M. D., Corrado, G., & Chin, M. H. (2018). Ensuring fairness in machine learning to advance health equity. *Annals of Internal Medicine*, *169*(12), 866–872. DOI: 10.7326/M18-1990 PMID: 30508424

Rajkomar, A., Oren, E., Chen, K., Dai, A. M., Hajaj, N., Hardt, M., Liu, P. J., Liu, X., Marcus, J., & Sun, M. (2018). Scalable and accurate deep learning with electronic health records. *npj. Digital Medicine*, *1*(1), 18. PMID: 31304302

Rieke, N., Hancox, J., Li, W., Milletari, F., Roth, H. R., Albarqouni, S., Bakas, S., Galtier, M. N., Landman, B. A., & Maier-Hein, K. (2020). The future of digital health with federated learning. *npj. Digital Medicine*, *3*(1), 119. PMID: 33015372

Roalf, D. R., & Gur, R. C. (2017). Functional brain imaging in neuropsychology over the past 25 years. *Neuropsychology*, *31*(8), 954–971. DOI: 10.1037/neu0000426 PMID: 29376672

Rodriguez, D. V., Lawrence, K., Gonzalez, J., Brandfield-Harvey, B., Xu, L., Tasneem, S., Levine, D. L., & Mann, D. (2024). Leveraging generative AI tools to support the development of digital solutions in health care research: Case study. *JMIR Human Factors*, *11*(1), e52885. DOI: 10.2196/52885 PMID: 38446539

Rosenblum, M. D., Gratz, I. K., Paw, J. S., & Abbas, A. K. (2012). Treating human autoimmunity: current practice and future prospects. *Science translational medicine, 4*(125), 125sr121-125sr121.

Rosenblum, M. D., Remedios, K. A., & Abbas, A. K. (2015). Mechanisms of human autoimmunity. *The Journal of Clinical Investigation*, *125*(6), 2228–2233. DOI: 10.1172/JCI78088 PMID: 25893595

Rubinsteyn, A., Kodysh, J., Hodes, I., Mondet, S., Aksoy, B. A., Finnigan, J. P., Bhardwaj, N., & Hammerbacher, J. (2018). Computational pipeline for the PGV-001 neoantigen vaccine trial. *Frontiers in Immunology*, *8*, 1807. DOI: 10.3389/fimmu.2017.01807 PMID: 29403468

Sachs, K., Perez, O., Pe'er, D., Lauffenburger, D. A., & Nolan, G. P. (2005). Causal protein-signaling networks derived from multiparameter single-cell data. *Science*, *308*(5721), 523–529. DOI: 10.1126/science.1105809 PMID: 15845847

Saeys, Y., Van Gassen, S., & Lambrecht, B. N. (2016). Computational flow cytometry: Helping to make sense of high-dimensional immunology data. *Nature Reviews. Immunology*, *16*(7), 449–462. DOI: 10.1038/nri.2016.56 PMID: 27320317

Sarker, I. H. (•••). Investigating undergraduate students' intention to engage in artificial intelligence learning. *SN Computer Science*, *3*(2), 158–158. DOI: 10.1007/s42979-022-01043-x PMID: 35194580

Schork, N. J. (2019). Artificial intelligence and personalized medicine. *Precision medicine in Cancer therapy*, 265-283.

Schwenker, F., & Trentin, E. (2014). Pattern classification and clustering: A review of partially supervised learning approaches. *Pattern Recognition Letters*, *37*, 4–14. DOI: 10.1016/j.patrec.2013.10.017

Seo, S., & Lee, J. W. (2024). Applications of Big Data and AI-Driven Technologies in CADD (Computer-Aided Drug Design). In Gore, M., & Jagtap, U. B. (Eds.), *Computational Drug Discovery and Design* (pp. 295–305)., DOI: 10.1007/978-1-0716-3441-7_16

Seyhan, A. A., & Carini, C. (2019). Are innovation and new technologies in precision medicine paving a new era in patients centric care? *Journal of Translational Medicine*, *17*(1), 114. DOI: 10.1186/s12967-019-1864-9 PMID: 30953518

Shao, J., Ma, J., Yu, Y., Zhang, S., Wang, W., Li, W., & Wang, C. (2024). A multimodal integration pipeline for accurate diagnosis, pathogen identification, and prognosis prediction of pulmonary infections. *Innovation (Cambridge (Mass.))*, *5*(4), 100648. DOI: 10.1016/j.xinn.2024.100648 PMID: 39021525

Singh, M., Kumar, A., Khanna, N. N., Laird, J. R., Nicolaides, A., Faa, G., Johri, A. M., Mantella, L. E., Fernandes, J. F. E., Teji, J. S., Singh, N., Fouda, M. M., Singh, R., Sharma, A., Kitas, G., Rathore, V., Singh, I. M., Tadepalli, K., Al-Maini, M., & Suri, J. S. (2024). Artificial intelligence for cardiovascular disease risk assessment in personalised framework: A scoping review. *EClinicalMedicine*, *73*, 73. DOI: 10.1016/j.eclinm.2024.102660 PMID: 38846068

Sirocchi, C., Bogliolo, A., & Montagna, S. (2024). Medical-informed machine learning: Integrating prior knowledge into medical decision systems. *BMC Medical Informatics and Decision Making*, *24*(S4, Suppl 4), 186. DOI: 10.1186/s12911-024-02582-4 PMID: 38943085

Stokes, J. M., Yang, K., Swanson, K., Jin, W., Cubillos-Ruiz, A., Donghia, N. M., MacNair, C. R., French, S., Carfrae, L. A., & Bloom-Ackermann, Z. (2020). A deep learning approach to antibiotic discovery. *Cell, 180*(4), 688-702. e613.

Strachan, J. W., Albergo, D., Borghini, G., Pansardi, O., Scaliti, E., Gupta, S., Saxena, K., Rufo, A., Panzeri, S., Manzi, G., Graziano, M. S. A., & Becchio, C. (2024). Testing theory of mind in large language models and humans. *Nature Human Behaviour*, *8*(7), 1285–1295. DOI: 10.1038/s41562-024-01882-z PMID: 38769463

Sun, X., Yin, Y., Yang, Q., & Huo, T. (2023). Artificial intelligence in cardiovascular diseases: Diagnostic and therapeutic perspectives. *European Journal of Medical Research*, *28*(1), 242. DOI: 10.1186/s40001-023-01065-y PMID: 37475050

Sun, Y. H., Wu, Y.-L., & Liao, B.-Y. (2023). Phenotypic heterogeneity in human genetic diseases: Ultrasensitivity-mediated threshold effects as a unifying molecular mechanism. *Journal of Biomedical Science*, *30*(1), 58. DOI: 10.1186/s12929-023-00959-7 PMID: 37525275

Thirunavukarasu, R., Gnanasambandan, R., Gopikrishnan, M., & Palanisamy, V. (2022). Towards computational solutions for precision medicine based big data healthcare system using deep learning models: A review. *Computers in Biology and Medicine*, *149*, 106020. DOI: 10.1016/j.compbiomed.2022.106020 PMID: 36088715

Tomašev, N., Glorot, X., Rae, J. W., Zielinski, M., Askham, H., Saraiva, A., Mottram, A., Meyer, C., Ravuri, S., Protsyuk, I., Connell, A., Hughes, C. O., Karthikesalingam, A., Cornebise, J., Montgomery, H., Rees, G., Laing, C., Baker, C. R., Peterson, K., & Mohamed, S. (2019). A clinically applicable approach to continuous prediction of future acute kidney injury. *Nature*, *572*(7767), 116–119. DOI: 10.1038/s41586-019-1390-1 PMID: 31367026

Topol, E. J. (2019). High-performance medicine: The convergence of human and artificial intelligence. *Nature Medicine*, *25*(1), 44–56. DOI: 10.1038/s41591-018-0300-7 PMID: 30617339

Uddin, M., Wang, Y., & Woodbury-Smith, M. (2019). Artificial intelligence for precision medicine in neurodevelopmental disorders. *npj. Digital Medicine*, *2*(1), 112. PMID: 31799421

Uffelmann, E., Huang, Q. Q., Munung, N. S., De Vries, J., Okada, Y., Martin, A. R., Martin, H. C., Lappalainen, T., & Posthuma, D. (2021). Genome-wide association studies. *Nature Reviews. Methods Primers*, *1*(1), 59. DOI: 10.1038/s43586-021-00056-9

Vatansever, S., Schlessinger, A., Wacker, D., Kaniskan, H. Ü., Jin, J., Zhou, M. M., & Zhang, B. (2021). Artificial intelligence and machine learning-aided drug discovery in central nervous system diseases: State-of-the-arts and future directions. *Medicinal Research Reviews*, *41*(3), 1427–1473. DOI: 10.1002/med.21764 PMID: 33295676

Vetter, T. R., & Schober, P. (2018). Regression: The apple does not fall far from the tree. *Anesthesia and Analgesia*, *127*(1), 277–283. DOI: 10.1213/ANE.0000000000003424 PMID: 29771712

Vossoughi, S., Marin, A., & Bang, M. (2023). Toward Just and Sustainable Futures: Human Learning and Relationality Within Socio-Ecological Systems. *Review of Research in Education*, *47*(1), 218–273. DOI: 10.3102/0091732X231223505

Vyas, D. A., Eisenstein, L. G., & Jones, D. S. (2020). *Hidden in plain sight—reconsidering the use of race correction in clinical algorithms* (Vol. 383). Mass Medical Soc.

Wahl, B., Cossy-Gantner, A., Germann, S., & Schwalbe, N. R. (2018). Artificial intelligence (AI) and global health: How can AI contribute to health in resource-poor settings? *BMJ Global Health*, *3*(4), e000798. DOI: 10.1136/bmjgh-2018-000798 PMID: 30233828

Wang, L., Wang, F. S., & Gershwin, M. E. (2015). Human autoimmune diseases: A comprehensive update. *Journal of Internal Medicine*, *278*(4), 369–395. DOI: 10.1111/joim.12395 PMID: 26212387

Wang, S., Wang, F., Zhu, Z., Wang, J., Tran, T., & Du, Z. (2024). Artificial intelligence in education: A systematic literature review. *Expert Systems with Applications*, *252*, 124167. DOI: 10.1016/j.eswa.2024.124167

Weissman, S., Sinh, P., Mehta, T. I., Thaker, R. K., Derman, A., Heiberger, C., Qureshi, N., Amrutiya, V., Atoot, A., Dave, M., & Tabibian, J. H. (2020). Atherosclerotic cardiovascular disease in inflammatory bowel disease: The role of chronic inflammation. *World Journal of Gastrointestinal Pathophysiology*, *11*(5), 104–113. DOI: 10.4291/wjgp.v11.i5.104 PMID: 32832194

Wen, X., Leng, P., Wang, J., Yang, G., Zu, R., Jia, X., Zhang, K., Mengesha, B. A., Huang, J., Wang, D., & Luo, H. (2022). Clinlabomics: Leveraging clinical laboratory data by data mining strategies. *BMC Bioinformatics*, *23*(1), 387. DOI: 10.1186/s12859-022-04926-1 PMID: 36153474

Weng, S. F., Reps, J., Kai, J., Garibaldi, J. M., & Qureshi, N. (2017). Can machine-learning improve cardiovascular risk prediction using routine clinical data? *PLoS One*, *12*(4), e0174944. DOI: 10.1371/journal.pone.0174944 PMID: 28376093

Wiljer, D., Salhia, M., Dolatabadi, E., Dhalla, A., Gillan, C., Al-Mouaswas, D., Jackson, E., Waldorf, J., Mattson, J., Clare, M., Lalani, N., Charow, R., Balakumar, S., Younus, S., Jeyakumar, T., Peteanu, W., & Tavares, W. (2021). Accelerating the appropriate adoption of artificial intelligence in health care: Protocol for a multistepped approach. *JMIR Research Protocols*, *10*(10), e30940. DOI: 10.2196/30940 PMID: 34612839

Wilkinson, M. D., Dumontier, M., Aalbersberg, I. J., Appleton, G., Axton, M., Baak, A., Blomberg, N., Boiten, J.-W., da Silva Santos, L. B., Bourne, P. E., Bouwman, J., Brookes, A. J., Clark, T., Crosas, M., Dillo, I., Dumon, O., Edmunds, S., Evelo, C. T., Finkers, R., & Mons, B. (2016). The FAIR Guiding Principles for scientific data management and stewardship. *Scientific Data*, *3*(1), 1–9. DOI: 10.1038/sdata.2016.18 PMID: 26978244

Wu, Y., Ma, L., Li, X., Yang, J., Rao, X., Hu, Y., Xi, J., Tao, L., Wang, J., Du, L., Chen, G., & Liu, S. (2024). The role of artificial intelligence in drug screening, drug design, and clinical trials. *Frontiers in Pharmacology*, *15*, 1459954. DOI: 10.3389/fphar.2024.1459954 PMID: 39679365

Xu, Y., Liu, X., Cao, X., Huang, C., Liu, E., Qian, S., Liu, X., Wu, Y., Dong, F., Qiu, C.-W., Qiu, J., Hua, K., Su, W., Wu, J., Xu, H., Han, Y., Fu, C., Yin, Z., Liu, M., & Zhang, J. (2021). Artificial intelligence: A powerful paradigm for scientific research. *Innovation (Cambridge (Mass.))*, *2*(4), 100179. DOI: 10.1016/j.xinn.2021.100179 PMID: 34877560

Yang, X., Huang, K., Yang, D., Zhao, W., & Zhou, X. (2024). Biomedical big data technologies, applications, and challenges for precision medicine: A review. *Global Challenges (Hoboken, NJ)*, *8*(1), 2300163. DOI: 10.1002/gch2.202300163 PMID: 38223896

Yao, J., Lin, X., Zhang, X., Xie, M., Ma, X., Bao, X., Song, J., Liang, Y., Wang, Q., & Xue, X. (2024). Predictive biomarkers for immune checkpoint inhibitors therapy in lung cancer. *Human Vaccines & Immunotherapeutics*, *20*(1), 2406063. DOI: 10.1080/21645515.2024.2406063 PMID: 39415535

Zeng, D., Ye, Z., Shen, R., Yu, G., Wu, J., Xiong, Y., Zhou, R., Qiu, W., Huang, N., Sun, L., Li, X., Bin, J., Liao, Y., Shi, M., & Liao, W. (2021). IOBR: Multi-omics immuno-oncology biological research to decode tumor microenvironment and signatures. *Frontiers in Immunology*, *12*, 687975. DOI: 10.3389/fimmu.2021.687975 PMID: 34276676

Zhang, B., Shi, H., & Wang, H. (2023). Machine learning and AI in cancer prognosis, prediction, and treatment selection: A critical approach. *Journal of Multidisciplinary Healthcare*, *16*, 1779–1791. DOI: 10.2147/JMDH.S410301 PMID: 37398894

Zhang, C., Xu, J., Tang, R., Yang, J., Wang, W., Yu, X., & Shi, S. (2023). Novel research and future prospects of artificial intelligence in cancer diagnosis and treatment. *Journal of Hematology & Oncology*, *16*(1), 114. DOI: 10.1186/s13045-023-01514-5 PMID: 38012673

Zhang, K., Zhou, H.-Y., Baptista-Hon, D. T., Gao, Y., Liu, X., Oermann, E., Xu, S., Jin, S., Zhang, J., Sun, Z., Yin, Y., Razmi, R. M., Loupy, A., Beck, S., Qu, J., & Wu, J. (2024). Concepts and applications of digital twins in healthcare and medicine. *Patterns (New York, N.Y.)*, *5*(8), 101028. DOI: 10.1016/j.patter.2024.101028 PMID: 39233690

Zheng, D., Liwinski, T., & Elinav, E. (2020). Interaction between microbiota and immunity in health and disease. *Cell Research*, *30*(6), 492–506. DOI: 10.1038/s41422-020-0332-7 PMID: 32433595

Chapter 3
AI-Enhanced Diagnosis for Immunological Disorders

Irina Negut
https://orcid.org/0000-0003-4038-7548
National Institute for Lasers, Plasma, and Radiation Physics, Romania

Anita Visan
https://orcid.org/0000-0003-0539-4160
National Institute for Lasers, Plasma, and Radiation Physics, Romania

ABSTRACT

The integration of Artificial Intelligence (AI) in immunological disorder diagnosis is transforming medical diagnostics by enabling rapid and accurate decision-making. This chapter explores AI-enhanced techniques, including machine learning, deep learning, and natural language processing, in identifying disease biomarkers, predicting progression, and optimizing personalized treatments. Key methodologies such as convolutional neural networks for imaging, support vector machines for classification, and AI-assisted genomic analysis are discussed. Additionally, the role of big data, electronic health records, and federated learning in improving diagnostic accuracy is examined. While AI offers significant advancements, challenges like data heterogeneity, bias, and regulatory compliance remain. The chapter highlights AI's future potential in precision medicine, enhancing early disease detection and improving patient outcomes.

1 INTRODUCTION

Immunological disorders, including autoimmune diseases, immunodeficiencies, and hypersensitivity reactions, pose diagnostic challenges due to complex pathophysiology and diverse symptoms. These conditions involve dysregulated immune responses, leading to inflammation, tissue damage, or impaired immunity. Traditional diagnostics, like serological tests and genetic assays, are time-intensive and often imprecise in overlapping cases. AI integration enhances accuracy, predictive analytics, and personalized care, transforming diagnosis and treatment.

This chapter explores the groundbreaking impact of AI on the diagnosis and management of immunological disorders, a domain characterized by complexity, heterogeneity, and evolving challenges.

DOI: 10.4018/979-8-3693-9725-1.ch003

AI encompasses a suite of technologies such as machine learning (ML), deep learning (DL), and natural language processing (NLP) that enable the analysis of vast and complex datasets (Ahmed et al. 2020), (Hanna et al. 2025), (Rashidi et al. 2025). These technologies have been transformative in uncovering novel biomarkers, improving diagnostic workflows, and predicting disease progression. For example, AI models trained on multi-omics datasets, including genomic, transcriptomic, and proteomic data, have identified previously unrecognized biomarkers for systemic lupus erythematosus (SLE) and rheumatoid arthritis (RA), thereby enabling earlier and more accurate diagnoses (Adamichou et al. 2021), (Dudek et al. 2024).

In imaging diagnostics, AI-powered tools have proven instrumental in enhancing the interpretation of radiographic and histopathological data. Convolutional neural networks (CNNs), a subset of DL, have been used to detect subtle inflammatory changes in tissue scans and joint erosions in conditions like RA, with greater precision than traditional methods (Rigamonti et al. 2023), (Zarubin et al. 2022), (C. Zhao et al. 2020). In systemic autoimmune diseases, AI-enhanced imaging has facilitated the early detection of disease-specific morphological patterns, offering clinicians valuable insights for timely interventions.

AI excels in integrating multi-omics data to uncover disease mechanisms and stratify patients. In primary immunodeficiencies (PIDs), AI accelerates the identification of genetic mutations and immune dysfunction markers, enabling early diagnosis and personalized treatment (Westermann-Clark et al. 2021), (Simon et al. 2020). Similarly, AI tools combining transcriptomic and proteomic data have been used to delineate disease endotypes in asthma and atopic dermatitis, advancing precision medicine approaches (Guida et al. 2022), (Almuhanna et al. 2024), (Yuemeng Wu et al. 2023).

AI has also shown promise in predictive modeling for disease progression and treatment outcomes. ML models that integrate genetic predisposition, environmental exposures, and patient history can forecast disease flares and treatment responses with high accuracy. In multiple sclerosis (MS), for example, predictive algorithms using neuroimaging and cerebrospinal fluid biomarkers have enabled clinicians to anticipate disease activity and optimize therapeutic regimens (PRIETL et al. 2023), (Yijun Zhao et al. 2017).

In hypersensitivity disorders such as asthma, AI tools analyzing environmental and physiological data have demonstrated the ability to predict exacerbations, aiding in proactive disease management (Guida et al. 2022).

AI-driven predictive modeling helps clinicians anticipate disease flares and treatment responses by integrating genetic, environmental, and clinical data. Wearable technologies, powered by AI, revolutionize real-time monitoring in diseases like asthma, enabling proactive care and personalized management (Almuhanna et al. 2024).

Despite AI's potential in immunological diagnostics, challenges persist. Data scarcity and quality issues impact model reliability, particularly in rare disorders. Ethical concerns, including data privacy and bias, require compliance with HIPAA (Health Insurance Portability and Accountability Act) and GDPR (General Data Protection Regulation). The interpretability of AI outputs remains crucial for clinical adoption, highlighting the need for user-friendly interfaces and transparent algorithms to ensure equitable healthcare outcomes (Bakare et al. 2024).

In conclusion, AI-enhanced diagnostics are revolutionizing immunological disorder management, enabling earlier detection, precise treatments, and improved patient outcomes through data integration, predictive modeling, and imaging analysis. However, challenges in data quality, interpretability, and ethics must be addressed for widespread adoption. Ongoing research and interdisciplinary collaboration are key to unlocking AI's full potential in immunological healthcare.

2 AI APPLICATIONS IN IMMUNOLOGICAL DIAGNOSIS

2.1 Introduction to AI in Healthcare Diagnostics

AI has emerged as a transformative force in modern healthcare, revolutionizing the landscape of medical diagnostics. Traditional diagnostic methods relied heavily on manual interpretation of medical images, laboratory tests, and clinical observations, often leading to time-consuming processes and potential human errors. The integration of AI into healthcare diagnostics has significantly enhanced efficiency, accuracy, and early disease detection, offering a paradigm shift toward precision medicine ("Application Research of Machine Learning Algorithms in Medical Diagnosis" 2024).

Historically, medical diagnostics relied heavily on human expertise, with clinicians manually analyzing medical images, interpreting laboratory test results, and correlating clinical symptoms to reach a diagnosis. These conventional methods, although effective, were often time-consuming, prone to human error, and limited by the availability of experienced specialists. The emergence of AI-powered diagnostic tools has significantly improved the accuracy, efficiency, and scalability of medical diagnostics, marking a crucial evolution in healthcare technology (Chakraborty et al. 2023). The historical trajectory of AI in diagnostics can be traced back to the 1950s and 1960s when early computational models were developed to assist in medical decision-making. One of the first AI applications in medicine was MYCIN, an expert system designed in the 1970s to aid in bacterial infection diagnosis and recommend antibiotic treatments. Despite its accuracy, MYCIN was never widely adopted due to computational limitations and resistance from the medical community (Frishberg 2025).

The shift from traditional diagnostic methods to AI-driven approaches has significantly improved the accuracy, efficiency, and accessibility of medical diagnostics. Traditional diagnostic methods largely depend on the expertise of healthcare professionals who interpret medical images, laboratory results, and clinical symptoms. While these approaches have been effective, they are often constrained by subjectivity, time limitations, human fatigue, and variability in diagnostic accuracy among practitioners.

One of the primary limitations of traditional diagnostic methods is variability in interpretation. Studies have shown that human radiologists may have differing interpretations of the same medical image, leading to inconsistencies in diagnosis. AI-based CNNs trained on large datasets can detect patterns in radiological images with greater consistency and reproducibility, thereby minimizing diagnostic errors (Deepa et al. 2023). Additionally, AI-powered tools can assist in decision support, offering second opinions to radiologists and reducing the chances of overlooking early-stage abnormalities.

Traditional methods also suffer from delays in diagnostic processes, particularly in regions with a shortage of specialized healthcare professionals. AI-driven chatbots and diagnostic assistants enable faster triaging by analyzing patient-reported symptoms and recommending appropriate testing or medical consultations. A study found that AI-driven chatbots significantly reduce waiting times in primary care settings by optimizing scheduling and initial assessments (Balakrishna and Solanki 2024).

Another key advantage of AI over traditional methods is early disease detection and predictive analytics. Traditional diagnostics often rely on disease symptoms becoming clinically evident, whereas AI models trained on longitudinal patient data can detect subtle biomarkers before symptoms manifest. AI algorithms have demonstrated significant success in predicting diabetes complications, neurodegenerative diseases, and cardiovascular events based on patient history and imaging data (Zeb et al. 2024).

The integration of NLP in AI further differentiates AI-driven diagnostics from traditional approaches. Traditional methods require healthcare providers to manually extract relevant data from electronic health records (EHRs), which can be time-consuming and error-prone. NLP automates this process by analyzing clinical notes, summarizing key patient information, and identifying risk factors, allowing for more informed clinical decision-making (Hasan and Farri 2019).

Despite these advancements, AI-driven diagnostic methods are not without challenges. The requirement for large, high-quality datasets remains a significant hurdle, as AI models need extensive training data to perform accurately across diverse populations. Moreover, concerns regarding AI bias, ethical considerations, and regulatory compliance must be addressed to ensure safe and effective deployment in clinical practice (Vasiliev et al. 2023). Nonetheless, ongoing advancements in explainable AI (XAI), federated learning, and ethical AI frameworks are helping to bridge these gaps and make AI-driven diagnostics more transparent and trustworthy.

In radiology, AI has played a pivotal role in enhancing image analysis and automated anomaly detection. DL algorithms, particularly CNNs, have demonstrated superior performance in detecting tumors, fractures, and pulmonary diseases from X-rays, CT scans, and MRIs, often surpassing human radiologists in terms of speed and accuracy. Studies indicate that AI-assisted radiology can reduce diagnostic errors by up to 30%, making it a valuable adjunct to human expertise (Vasiliev et al. 2023).

Pathology has also witnessed significant advancements through AI integration. Digital pathology systems, coupled with AI-powered image recognition software, enable rapid and precise identification of cancerous tissues, infectious diseases, and autoimmune disorders. AI algorithms trained on extensive histopathology datasets can efficiently classify tissue abnormalities and suggest differential diagnoses, reducing the burden on pathologists and accelerating the diagnostic workflow (Silva et al. 2023).

Beyond imaging and pathology, AI-driven clinical decision support systems (CDSSs) have emerged as powerful tools for disease prediction and personalized medicine. These systems utilize electronic health records (EHRs), genetic data, and real-time patient monitoring to detect early signs of diseases such as diabetes, cardiovascular conditions, and neurodegenerative disorders. By analyzing multimodal patient data, AI facilitates early intervention, reducing hospitalization rates and improving treatment outcomes (Artsi et al. 2024).

The transition from traditional diagnostics to AI-driven approaches is also evident in natural language processing (NLP) applications. AI-powered NLP models can extract clinically relevant insights from unstructured medical records, physician notes, and research literature, streamlining clinical workflows and reducing administrative burdens. These models enable automated diagnosis coding, medical summarization, and risk stratification, further optimizing healthcare delivery (Hasan and Farri 2019).

The role of AI in automated laboratory testing has significantly reduced the time required for disease diagnosis and prognosis. AI-driven automation in blood analysis, microbiology testing, and genetic screening enhances accuracy and minimizes human error. Machine learning algorithms analyze laboratory samples, identifying abnormalities in hematological and biochemical markers. Automated diagnostic systems powered by AI have shown promise in improving the detection of infectious diseases, endocrine disorders, and metabolic syndromes (Cyrielle et al. 2024).

Wearable health monitoring devices have further expanded AI applications in diagnostics, allowing real-time tracking of vital signs and early disease prediction. AI-integrated wearables utilize biosensors and IoT connectivity to collect and analyze physiological data such as heart rate, oxygen saturation, blood glucose levels, and body temperature. These devices support chronic disease management, remote patient monitoring, and early warning systems for critical health conditions. Recent advancements in

AI-powered wearables have enhanced their ability to detect cardiac arrhythmias, respiratory disorders, and neurological conditions, improving patient outcomes through proactive healthcare interventions (Haghayegh et al. 2024).

The continuous evolution of AI in medical diagnostics highlights its transformative potential in healthcare. By leveraging advanced AI frameworks, automated lab testing, and wearable health monitoring, AI-driven diagnostics offer unparalleled accuracy, efficiency, and scalability. Ongoing research and technological advancements will further refine these tools, ensuring their seamless integration into clinical practice and enhancing patient care worldwide (Gani et al. 2024).

As AI continues to evolve, its role in diagnostics will expand, incorporating advancements in explainable AI (XAI), federated learning, and multimodal deep learning. The seamless integration of AI into clinical practice will require ongoing validation studies, regulatory oversight, and interdisciplinary collaboration to ensure ethical implementation, data security, and unbiased decision-making. Despite the challenges, AI's potential to enhance diagnostic precision, expedite medical workflows, and improve patient outcomes underscores its critical role in the future of healthcare diagnostics (Singh et al. 2024).

2.2 Fundamentals of AI in Diagnostics

AI applications in diagnostics primarily rely on ML, DL, and NLP to analyze medical data, recognize patterns, and facilitate clinical decision-making. These technologies have been particularly instrumental in diagnosing immune-related disorders, where early detection and personalized treatment strategies are crucial (Singh et al. 2024).

ML models process vast amounts of structured clinical data, such as laboratory results, genetic markers, and imaging features, to develop predictive models for autoimmune diseases like rheumatoid arthritis, lupus, and multiple sclerosis. Algorithms such as support vector machines (SVMs) and random forests have demonstrated high accuracy in distinguishing autoimmune disorders from other inflammatory conditions (Deepa et al. 2023).

DL, a subset of ML, employs artificial neural networks to analyze complex medical images, such as CT scans, MRIs, and histopathology slides, aiding in the early detection of immune-related abnormalities. CNNs have been particularly effective in recognizing inflammatory patterns in lung scans for autoimmune-associated pulmonary diseases and detecting dermatological manifestations of immune disorders (Zeb et al. 2024).

NLP plays a crucial role in analyzing unstructured medical data, including electronic health records (EHRs), clinical notes, and biomedical literature. AI-driven NLP models can extract key clinical features from patient histories, improving the identification of early-stage immune diseases and enabling personalized treatment planning (Hasan and Farri 2019).

By integrating ML, DL, and NLP, AI-driven diagnostic systems have revolutionized the detection and management of immune-related disorders, enhancing diagnostic accuracy, reducing misdiagnoses, and enabling early therapeutic interventions. These advancements hold significant promise for precision medicine, improving patient outcomes in the field of immunology (Kwilinski et al. 2024).

AI-driven diagnostic methods leverage ML, DL, and NLP (**Table 1**) to provide automated, precise, and scalable solutions that improve healthcare outcomes (Dranove and Garthwaite 2022).

Table 1. Contributions of ML, DL, and NLP in medical diagnostics

AI technique	Application in medical diagnostics	Key benefits	References
ML	ML algorithms analyze structured patient data (e.g., lab results, imaging features, genetic markers) to detect patterns and create predictive models for disease diagnosis and prognosis. Decision trees and support vector machines (SVMs) aid in disease classification, while random forests improve diagnostic accuracy by aggregating multiple decision trees.	Enhances early diagnosis, improves predictive accuracy, and reduces human error in data analysis	("Application Research of Machine Learning Algorithms in Medical Diagnosis" 2024), (Muhsen et al. 2020)
DL	DL, a subset of ML, uses multi-layered artificial neural networks to extract hierarchical features from complex datasets. CNNs excel in medical imaging (CT scans, MRIs, histopathology) to identify disease patterns (e.g., autoimmune disorders). Recurrent Neural Networks (RNNs) and Transformer models analyze time-series clinical data for disease progression tracking.	Provides high accuracy in pattern recognition, aids in automated diagnosis, and enhances precision in medical imaging.	(Datta and Rohilla 2019), (Viswanathan et al. 1AD)
NLP	NLP automates the interpretation of unstructured medical text from electronic health records (EHRs), clinical notes, and biomedical literature. Named Entity Recognition (NER) and sentiment analysis extract clinically relevant insights such as symptom patterns and risk factors, supporting differential diagnosis.	Improves data extraction from clinical records, supports decision-making, and enhances medical text analysis.	(Mollaei et al. 2025)

2.3 Key AI Concepts and Tools Essential for Immunological Analysis

The integration of AI into immunological research and diagnostics has profoundly transformed our ability to detect, characterize, and treat immune-related disorders. AI-driven technologies enable the rapid and precise analysis of large-scale immunological datasets, significantly improving disease diagnosis, risk prediction, and personalized therapeutic strategies (Lu et al. 2024). These AI methodologies have revolutionized various aspects of immunology, including flow cytometry, immunohistochemistry (IHC), imaging mass cytometry, vaccine design, and antibody screening.

2.3.1 AI-Assisted Flow Cytometry in Immunological Diagnostics

One of the primary AI-driven tools in immunology is AI-assisted flow cytometry, which has significantly enhanced the classification and quantification of immune cells. Traditional flow cytometry relies on manual gating and expert evaluation, making it time-intensive and prone to variability between analysts. AI-powered platforms, such as DeepFlow™ and Cytopredict, automate this process using ML algorithms, which classify immune cell subtypes by analyzing multidimensional density–phenotype coupling. These AI models reduce the complexity and time required for analysis while maintaining or even improving diagnostic accuracy (Lu et al. 2024).

Flow cytometry plays a vital role in diagnosing primary immunodeficiencies, autoimmune diseases, and hematologic malignancies by identifying specific immune cell populations. AI-assisted gating has been particularly useful in detecting abnormal T-cell, B-cell, and natural killer (NK) cell populations, which are indicative of immune dysfunction. By leveraging unsupervised learning techniques, AI tools can uncover hidden immune dysregulation patterns, leading to more precise disease classifications (Poalelungi et al. 2024).

2.3.2 AI-Driven Immunohistochemistry and Digital Pathology

Immunohistochemistry (IHC) plays a crucial role in identifying biomarkers of immune-related diseases and cancers, but conventional interpretation methods often suffer from interobserver variability and subjective bias. AI-based digital pathology systems have emerged as powerful tools for improving IHC analysis by extracting quantitative immune markers and classifying disease phenotypes with high precision.

DL models trained on large datasets of histopathological images can recognize subtle patterns in immune cell infiltration, predict disease progression, and guide therapeutic decision-making. AI-based digital pathology has been particularly effective in hematologic malignancies, lupus nephritis, and rheumatoid arthritis, where immune infiltration plays a key role in disease pathology (Rigamonti et al. 2023).

In cancer immunotherapy, AI-assisted IHC staining analysis has improved patient stratification for immune checkpoint inhibitors (ICIs) by quantifying PD-L1, CD8+ T-cell infiltration, and other tumor immune markers. This precision-based approach has enhanced treatment efficacy, reduced unnecessary therapies, and provided deeper insights into the tumor microenvironment (Xu et al. 2021).

2.3.3 AI in Imaging Mass Cytometry and Spatial Immunoanalysis

AI-driven imaging mass cytometry has allowed researchers to study immune cell interactions within tissues, providing deeper insights into tumor immunology, autoimmunity, and infectious diseases. Unlike traditional histology, which provides only limited information on immune cell distributions, AI-assisted imaging mass cytometry can analyze dozens of immune markers simultaneously and visualize their spatial relationships within diseased tissues (J. Wu and Lin 2021).

For example, AI-based spatial transcriptomics has uncovered immune dysregulation patterns in multiple sclerosis (MS), lupus, and inflammatory bowel disease (IBD), enabling researchers to identify novel therapeutic targets. These models can predict immune cell migration, evaluate inflammatory cytokine gradients, and assess therapeutic responses to immunomodulatory drugs (Palm et al. 2022).

2.3.4. AI in Immunotherapy and Antibody Design

AI is revolutionizing immunotherapy by accelerating the development of monoclonal antibodies, checkpoint inhibitors, and personalized vaccines. DL models trained on antibody-protein interaction datasets have significantly enhanced the design and screening of therapeutic antibodies.

For instance, scifAI, an AI-powered antibody screening platform, predicts antibody affinity and specificity by analyzing their impact on immune cell activation. This AI-driven approach has expedited the discovery of immune checkpoint inhibitors, reducing drug development time and costs (Boushehri et al. 2023).

Furthermore, AI-assisted vaccine design platforms, such as DeepVacPred, predict antigenic peptide sequences capable of inducing protective immune responses. This technology has been instrumental in the development of COVID-19 vaccines and emerging cancer vaccines, facilitating the design of more effective and personalized immunization strategies (Qorri et al. 2024).

The integration of AI into immunological diagnostics, immunotherapy, and personalized medicine has unlocked unprecedented capabilities for early disease detection, immune response modeling, and biomarker discovery. AI-driven tools continue to enhance precision medicine approaches in immunology, leading to improved patient outcomes and groundbreaking advancements in immune-related disease management.

3 AI-POWERED BIOMARKER DISCOVERY

AI-assisted biomarker discovery is revolutionizing the diagnosis and treatment of immunological disorders by integrating multi-omics data, such as genomics, transcriptomics, and proteomics, to identify novel disease markers (**Figure 1**). The application of AI in biomarker discovery has enabled researchers to analyze vast datasets and extract meaningful insights, leading to more precise diagnostic and prognostic tools.

Figure 1. A multi-omics approach is essential for discovering and validating biomarkers that capture the multidimensional aspects of disease biology. This comprehensive effort requires integrating diverse 'omics' technologies, data types, databases, bioinformatics, and biostatistics to identify the most predictive biomarkers across DNA, RNA, protein, phenotype, and metabolite domains.

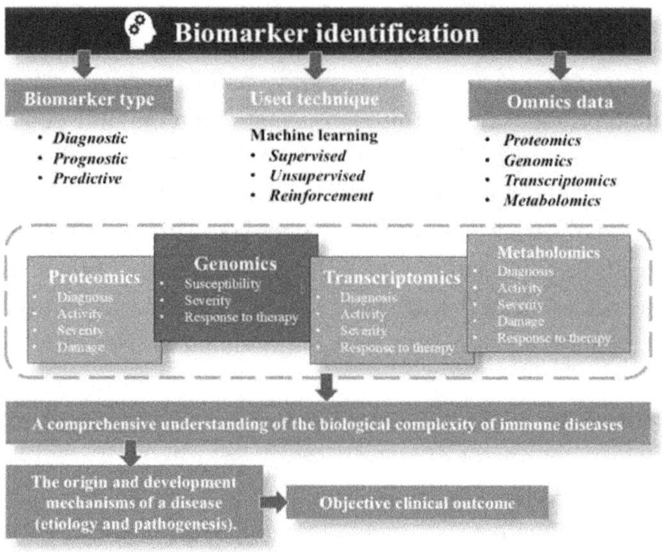

The integration of ML with high-dimensional "omics" data—such as genomics, proteomics, transcriptomics, and metabolomics—paired with clinical characteristics and "non-omics" data, offers a transformative opportunity to enhance precision and personalization in asthma care (Ray, Das, and Wenzel 2022).

AI-based computational models leverage ML algorithms to detect immune dysregulation patterns, improving differentiation between overlapping conditions. For example, AI has been instrumental in identifying biomarkers for autoimmune diseases such as SLE, RA, and primary immunodeficiencies, improving early detection and personalized treatment strategies (Laigle, Chadli, and Moingeon 2023).

A study showed AI can analyze angiogenesis and inflammatory markers to predict disease progression in autoimmune and cardiovascular disorders (Sundarraj et al. 2024). Such models rely on DL techniques to process high-throughput biological data, significantly improving the prediction of disease onset and patient stratification.

AI is transforming immunotherapy biomarker discovery through image analysis of histopathological slides, identifying tumor-infiltrating lymphocytes crucial in autoimmune and immunodeficiency disorders. By extracting meaningful data from complex images, AI enhances predictive modeling for treatment responses (Choi and Kim 2023). Also, AI has been instrumental in the discovery of novel immune complex biomarkers for lupus nephritis, demonstrating its potential for identifying circulating immune complexes that correlate with disease severity (Tang et al. 2022).

AI-driven flow cytometry enhances immune cell analysis, improving diagnostics for primary immunodeficiencies and autoimmune disorders. It enables rapid classification and enumeration of immune subsets, increasing efficiency, accuracy, and reducing human error, while accelerating detection of immune dysregulation patterns (Lu et al. 2024).

AI has also been applied to optimize digital pathology workflows, allowing for high-confidence biomarker profiling from hematoxylin and eosin (H&E) slides. By leveraging AI-driven computational pathology, researchers can identify molecular alterations in immune-related diseases, optimizing patient stratification for targeted therapies (Ofek et al. 2023). AI-driven pathology tools, combined with immunohistochemical biomarker scoring, contribute to more precise disease classification and improved treatment planning.

Furthermore, AI-powered immunosensors are emerging as effective tools for detecting autoimmune disease-related biomarkers, offering rapid and highly sensitive diagnostic solutions. These biosensors leverage AI to enhance specificity and improve real-time monitoring of immune response markers, significantly reducing the reliance on conventional laboratory-based diagnostics (Karachaliou and Livaniou 2023). By integrating AI with wearable biosensor technology, researchers are moving closer to real-time, point-of-care diagnostics that can improve patient outcomes through early disease detection.

Biomarker discovery leverages vast datasets from EHRs, sequencing, imaging, and biological samples. While traditional methods are time-intensive, AI-driven platforms automate feature selection, validation, and analysis, accelerating the process. AI models also predict biomarker-disease links, uncover patterns, and enhance diagnostic accuracy, crucial for complex disorders.

Several AI-powered platforms have emerged as indispensable resources for biomarker identification and validation. The following table (**Table 2**) presents some of the most recent and advanced AI-powered biomarker discovery databases and tools.

Table 2. Recent and advanced AI-powered biomarker discovery databases and tools for of immunological disorders

Database/tool	Description	Biomarker discovery	Reference
PandaOmics	AI-driven multi-omics data analysis platform for biomarker discovery	Identifies novel therapeutic targets and biomarkers using AI and bioinformatics	(Kamya et al. 2024)
IMPACT	Web server for immunotherapeutic predictive and prognostic biomarkers	Provides a comprehensive analysis of biomarkers associated with immune checkpoint inhibitors (ICI)	(Y. Liu et al. 2023)
BEST	AI-based biomarker discovery tool for solid tumors	Integrates gene expression data from over 50,000 tumor samples across multiple cancer types	(Z. Liu et al. 2023)
EDGE AI	AI-powered HLA-peptide analysis for immunotherapy and vaccine development	Predicts peptide-HLA interactions to guide T-cell-based vaccine development	(Klein et al. 2024, 904)
AI/ML-Derived Whole-Genome Biomarkers	AI-driven whole-genome biomarker discovery for neuroblastoma prognosis	Identifies survival-related biomarkers using ML on genomic data	(Alter et al. 2024)
TumorMapr™	AI-based spatial analytics for pathology and biomarker discovery	Uses explainable AI (xAI) to analyze fluorescence and mass spectrometry imaging datasets	(Newton et al. 2017)

AI-driven multi-omics analysis enhances biomarker discovery and disease stratification in SLE by integrating genomics, transcriptomics, and proteomics. ML-powered integration improves disease understanding, patient classification, and personalized treatments. Early, intermediate, and late integration methods optimize data consolidation, enabling robust analysis and precision medicine (Picard et al. 2021). DL models like DeepProg and DeFusion enhance survival prediction using multi-omics data. Initially applied to liver and breast cancers, these frameworks show promise for SLE, addressing data noise, improving accuracy, and capturing key disease patterns (Poirion et al. 2021), (W. Wang, Zhang, and Dai 2021).

Generative models for multi-omics integration have further expanded the scope of precision biomarker discovery by accommodating incomplete datasets while maintaining high classification performance (H.-S. Lee et al. 2024).

DL strategies like CustOmics allow for tailored treatment plans by providing interpretable and patient-specific results, thereby fostering personalized medicine in SLE biomarker discovery (Benkirane et al. 2023).

MOGAT, an innovative framework using graph attention networks, has shown promise in analyzing omics data to reveal disease pathways and enable precise patient categorization. This method has direct applications in unraveling the complexities of SLE (Tanvir et al. 2023). AI-driven causal modeling integrates genotype, environment, and phenotype to enhance SLE understanding. These models accurately predict disease mechanisms, aiding biomarker discovery and advancing personalized care (You Wu and Xie 2024).

Smartphone-based AI biosensors, equipped with advanced sensors like electrochemistry, fluorescence, and plasmon resonance, have become powerful tools for data processing and cloud integration (**Table 3**).

Table 3. Smartphone applications with insights and tools for the diagnosis, management, and tracking of immunological disorders, leveraging AI for enhanced accuracy and usability.

Application name	Description	Use in immunological disorders	Reference
Ada Health	Symptom assessment app using AI to provide health guidance.	Helps identify potential immunological conditions based on symptoms.	("Health. Powered by Ada.," n.d.)
SkinVision	AI-based app for analyzing skin conditions.	Monitors changes in skin lesions, aiding in detecting autoimmune-related skin changes.	("SkinVision I Skin Cancer Melanoma Detection App I SkinVision," n.d.)
Miiskin	Skin tracking app with AI-based lesion recognition.	Assists in tracking changes in skin conditions associated with immunological disorders.	("Online Dermatologist I Get a Virtual Dermatology Consultation," n.d.)
Symptomate	AI-powered symptom checker for various health conditions.	Suggests potential immunological conditions based on symptom analysis.	("Symptomate – Check Your Symptoms Online," n.d.)
Healthily	AI-based app for personal health checks.	Offers insights into potential immunological disorders based on health data.	("Healthily: Medically Verified Health Information You Need for Self-Care," n.d.)
MyTherapy	Medication tracker app with AI-driven adherence reminders.	Supports treatment adherence in patients with chronic immunological conditions.	("Medication Reminder and Pill Tracker App MyTherapy," n.d.)
KardiaMobile	AI-powered heart health app and device.	Detects heart irregularities that may be secondary to autoimmune diseases like lupus	("EKG Anywhere, Anytime I Kardia," n.d.)

4 AI IN ALLERGY AND HYPERSENSITIVITY DISORDERS

AI is revolutionizing the understanding and management of allergy and hypersensitivity disorders, including asthma, AD, and food allergies. By analyzing genetic, environmental, and immunological interactions, AI enhances biomarker discovery, early detection, and treatment optimization, advancing precision medicine in this field.

4.1 Food Allergies

Food allergies arise from an overactive immune response, where allergen-specific IgE antibodies trigger histamine release, causing reactions like hives to anaphylaxis (Schultes, Ernst, and Schmid 2021), (Shamji et al. 2021). Genetic factors, including IL-4, IL-13 (Namkung et al. 2011), and filaggrin mutations (Erdem et al. 2025), increase susceptibility., while environmental influences like diet and reduced microbial exposure contribute (K. H. Lee et al. 2020). A Th2-dominated immune response and epigenetic modifications further drive sensitization, with non-IgE mechanisms also playing a role in delayed immune reactions (Bellinghausen, Khatri, and Saloga 2022), (Cañas et al. 2021), (Bellanti 2024).

A pivotal study by Hardy et al. reviewed the role of biomarkers in allergen immunotherapy (AIT), highlighting the significance of allergen-specific IgE, IgG, and Tregs in assessing therapeutic responses. AI-based tools were employed to analyze trends in Th2 cytokine production, enabling the optimization of therapy protocols and paving the way for personalized treatment strategies (Hardy, Smeekens, and Kulis

2019). Alag et al. showed ML's ability to analyze DNA methylation data, identifying 13 genes linked to food allergies with high diagnostic accuracy. This highlights AI's potential in utilizing epigenetic insights for early and precise diagnosis (Alag 2019).

Innovative methodologies, such as bead-based epitope assays, have further enriched the biomarker discovery landscape. Suprun et al. introduced an assay capable of detecting allergenic IgE epitopes, enhancing sensitivity and providing a robust tool for phenotyping allergy severity (Suprun et al. 2019). Complementing this, van Bilsen et al. employed Bayesian networks and Topological Data Analysis (TDA) to uncover biomarkers linked to oral immunotherapy in food allergies, demonstrating the value of network-based approaches in clinical applications (van Bilsen et al. 2019).

Raikar et al. explored the application of ML in molecular profile analysis, demonstrating its potential in precision diagnostics and therapeutic interventions (Raikar, Raikar, and Somnache 2023). Similarly, Chen et al. developed an enzyme-linked immunosorbent assay-based microarray for detecting foodborne allergens, showing the utility of multiplexed immunological methods combined with AI analytics (Chen et al. 2023).

Emerging technologies like spatially resolved laser-activated cell sorting (SLACS) have also been integrated with AI to enhance biomarker identification and pathological analysis in allergy-related conditions (Jang et al. 2024). Additionally, Kamya et al. introduced PandaOmics, an AI platform designed for multi-omics integration, emphasizing its applicability in identifying novel biomarkers for various diseases, including allergies (Kamya et al. 2024).

4.2 Asthma

Asthma is a chronic airway disorder causing inflammation, obstruction, and bronchial hyperresponsiveness ("Global Initiative for Asthma," n.d.). It has allergic (Th2 high) and non-allergic (Th2 low) endotypes, with Th2-driven eosinophilic inflammation being most common (Nakagome and Nagata 2024). Genetic factors (e.g., IL33, IL4R, ORMDL3) (Sayers et al. 2024) and environmental triggers (allergens, pollution, infections) (Agache et al. 2024), (Aslam et al. 2024) influence susceptibility. Epigenetic modifications, like DNA methylation in FOXP3 and IL13, also impact disease severity (Mijač et al. 2024).

AI tools have shown promise in interpreting complex datasets, enabling clinicians to make informed decisions with higher precision (Kaplan et al. 2021). In respiratory medicine, the role of AI extends to diseases with overlapping symptoms such as asthma and chronic obstructive pulmonary disease (COPD). AI-powered models facilitate the interpretation of pulmonary function tests and assist in differential diagnosis, bridging a critical gap in the clinical workflow (Kaplan et al. 2021).

AI also enhances biomarker discovery, with omics technologies integrated to uncover asthma-specific markers. This integration supports better disease stratification and personalized treatment approaches. By using AI to analyze multi-omics data, researchers have identified critical biomarkers that contribute to asthma pathophysiology and treatment response (Guida et al. 2022).

Wearable technology represents another significant advancement in asthma care. A study on the AI Asthma Guard, a novel device that monitors environmental and physiological factors, demonstrates the potential for ML algorithms to predict asthma exacerbations, thereby enabling proactive management strategies (Almuhanna et al. 2024).

Non-invasive biomarkers, such as fractional exhaled nitric oxide, have been integrated with AI to monitor airway inflammation. This approach provides real-time insights into asthma control and predicts exacerbations with higher sensitivity than traditional methods (Menzies-Gow, Mansur, and Brightling 2020).

Another critical area of research involves phenotyping and disease progression modeling. AI-driven analytics have been employed to identify at-risk populations and monitor disease trajectory, particularly in overlapping conditions like asthma and COPD. These tools are critical for tailoring interventions to individual patient profiles (Feng et al. 2021).

4.3 Atopic Dermatitis

AD is a chronic inflammatory skin disorder causing itching, erythema, and recurrent lesions (Tian et al. 2024). It results from skin barrier defects (e.g., filaggrin mutations), Th2-driven immune dysregulation (IL-4, IL-13, IL-31) (Khatib et al. 2024)., and environmental triggers like allergens and pollutants(Asiniwasis et al. 2024) Th17 and Th22 pathways also contribute, particularly in certain AD subtypes (Laska et al. 2024), (Libon, Caron, and Nikkels 2024).

Advances in precision medicine are driving the development of biomarkers to guide therapy selection and predict disease outcomes. For instance, thymus and activation-regulated chemokine (TARC/CCL17) and serum IL-13 levels have emerged as potential biomarkers for disease severity and therapeutic response (Izuhara et al., n.d.).

A comprehensive study by Yu and Li provided an in-depth review of potential biomarkers for AD, including thymus and activation-regulated chemokine (TARC), CCL17, and IL-33. These biomarkers have proven effective in assessing disease severity and monitoring therapeutic outcomes, offering clinicians valuable tools for personalized patient management (Yu and Li 2022).

Bakker et al. leveraged Luminex technology to validate biomarker-based endotypes in AD, identifying key clusters linked to inflammatory pathways. This approach reinforced the significance of endotyping in tailoring interventions for diverse patient populations (Bakker et al. 2021).

Other studies have explored the utility of innovative techniques and methods for biomarker discovery. Wu et al. explored Th2-dominant serum biomarkers to predict the efficacy of dupilumab treatment in Chinese AD patients, further contributing to precision medicine approaches in this domain (Wu et al. 2023).

In pediatric populations, Meng et al. investigated plasma exosomal tRNA-derived fragments as biomarkers for AD, revealing their potential in understanding disease pathogenesis (L. Meng et al. 2021). Additionally, Li et al. utilized bioinformatics tools to identify diagnostic biomarkers for AD, linking them to immune cell infiltration and molecular pathways. This study demonstrated the power of AI in integrating genomic and molecular data to improve diagnostic accuracy and therapeutic decision-making (C. Li, Lu, and Han 2022).

5 AI IN IMMUNODEFICIENCY DISORDERS

PIDs are rare genetic disorders causing immune dysfunction and recurrent infections. AI-powered analytics improve genetic mutation and immune marker detection, enabling earlier, more accurate diagnoses and better therapeutic management for PIDs. ML models differentiate primary immunodeficiencies, supporting personalized treatment, while AI algorithms identify immune dysregulation patterns in rare disorders like anti-NMDAR encephalitis, providing key disease insights (Laigle, Chadli, and Moingeon 2023).

AI-driven systems enhance diagnostics by integrating genetic testing and immune profiling, aiding in identifying over 500 monogenic primary immunodeficiencies. These advancements enable earlier, more precise interventions, reducing disease-related morbidity (Klangkalya, Fleisher, and Rosenzweig 2024).

ML models are employed to distinguish between various PID subtypes. For instance, in autoimmune cytopenia, AI tools have guided semi-targeted therapies tailored to suspected pathogenic mechanisms. Such precision in therapy significantly improves clinical outcomes for chronic and refractory cases (Pacillo et al. 2022).

AI-assisted gene therapy, have opened new pathways for PID treatment. Autologous hematopoietic stem cell gene therapy has been applied to conditions like SCID (Severe Combined Immunodeficiency), with AI playing a pivotal role in optimizing genetic modification processes (Fox and Booth 2021).

Studies focusing on children with PID demonstrated how AI tools analyze immunoglobulin levels, vaccine titers, and lymphocyte subsets to distinguish between autoimmune cytopenias and other immune deficiencies. These findings suggest that integrating immune profiles into AI models can enhance early diagnosis and treatment personalization (Westermann-Clark et al. 2021).

Insights into PID and its predisposition to malignancies have been amplified using AI-based genomic analysis. For example, identifying genomic instability in B and T cells has provided critical data on the links between immune deficiencies and cancer predisposition (Mastio et al. 2020).

TREC (T-cell receptor excision circle) and KREC (kappa-deleting recombination excision circle) assays have been pivotal in detecting combined T and B cell immunodeficiencies. Research has demonstrated that AI integration into these testing frameworks can improve predictive accuracy, enabling early and precise detection of these conditions (Korsunskiy et al. 2020).

Whole-exome sequencing (WES) has enhanced PID diagnostics, especially in consanguineous populations with higher genetic predispositions. AI-assisted WES analysis achieved a 70% diagnostic success rate, highlighting AI's role in identifying genetic variants and enabling personalized treatment strategies (Simon et al. 2020).

Bayesian models have also played a critical role in PID diagnostics. These networks classify PID risk in patients presenting with recurrent infections by analyzing complex clinical and immunological data. Their high accuracy and ability to provide prescriptive analytics for targeted diagnostic evaluations underscore their clinical relevance (Rider et al. 2021).

For resource-limited settings, a customized genotyping approach using single nucleotide variants (SNVs) has demonstrated cost-effectiveness and diagnostic reliability. AI's role in identifying genetic mutations associated with immunodeficiencies has proven instrumental in these scenarios, offering equitable access to advanced diagnostics (Suratannon et al. 2020).

Causal Bayesian models offer key insights into phenotypic trajectories of PIDs like CVID and CID. By mapping relationships between clinical features and immunodeficiencies, these models enhance early detection and enable personalized care pathways (Papanastasiou et al. 2024).

5.1 AI-Driven Biomarker Discovery for Autoimmune Diseases

Autoimmune diseases arise from an abnormal immune response against self-antigens, leading to chronic inflammation and tissue damage. AI-based analysis of immune cell profiles, cytokine expression, and autoantibody patterns has improved diagnostic accuracy and disease stratification in autoimmune disorders.

5.1.1 Rheumatoid Arthritis

RA is an autoimmune condition characterized by chronic inflammation of the joints and systemic involvement (Khan et al. 2024). Traditional diagnostic methods often rely on serological markers, such as rheumatoid factor (RF) and anti-cyclic citrullinated peptide (anti-CCP) antibodies, which, although helpful, have limitations in sensitivity and specificity (Karami et al. 2024). Genetic factors such as HLA-DRB1 alleles and non-HLA genes (e.g., PTPN22, STAT4) play significant roles in disease susceptibility, while environmental factors like smoking and infections exacerbate disease onset by promoting citrullination and immune activation (Raheem and Alwandawi 2024), (Vetchinkina et al. 2021). RA's immunopathogenesis is driven by pro-inflammatory cytokines like TNF-α, IL-6, and IL-17, which lead to joint erosion, cartilage degradation, and chronic synovitis. Structural joint changes, including synovial hyperplasia and pannus formation, cause irreversible damage and functional impairment (Koper-Lenkiewicz et al. 2022).

Biomarkers like ACPAs and RF aid diagnosis and prognosis, while emerging tools like 14-3-3η protein and MBDA scores enhance personalized medicine, improving patient outcomes and quality of life (Rajdan, Srivastava, and Sharma 2024).

A study employing an isotope-labeling LC-MS-based metabolic profiling identified high-confidence RA biomarkers, including metabolites that differentiate RA patients from healthy controls. These metabolites were validated across multiple cohorts, demonstrating a high area under the curve (AUC) for diagnostic precision (Han et al. 2020).

Using transcriptomics datasets, a 16-gene biomarker panel was developed to differentiate RA from osteoarthritis with high accuracy. The model, validated with ML techniques like random forests and SVMs, achieved 96% classification accuracy (Long et al. 2019).

Advanced metabolomic studies identified a three-metabolite panel (L-cysteine, citric acid, and L-glutamine) predictive of RA. This panel was constructed using a random forest algorithm and validated through transcriptomics and targeted metabolomics, providing insights into the disease's biochemical pathways (He, Liu, and Gong 2021).

5.1.2 Systemic Lupus Erythematosus

Systemic lupus erythematosus (SLE) is a complex autoimmune disorder characterized by autoantibody production and multi-organ involvement. Genetic polymorphisms in HLA-DR2, HLA-DR3, IRF5, and complement deficiencies (C1q, C4) impair immune complex clearance, while environmental triggers like UV radiation, infections, and hormones contribute to disease onset (Ghodke-Puranik, Olferiev, and Crow 2024). ANAs and anti-dsDNA form immune complexes, leading to complement activation, inflammation, and organ damage, driven by type I interferons, TNF-α, and IL-6. Dysregulated apoptosis further perpetuates autoimmunity (Ghodke-Puranik, Olferiev, and Crow 2024), (Sutanto and Yuliasih 2023), (Elsayed, Kamaly, and Esmail 2022).

Proteomics and single-cell RNA sequencing have emerged as pivotal techniques for biomarker discovery in SLE. A study by Li et al. employed these methods to identify a six-protein combination that demonstrated excellent diagnostic performance and a nine-protein set with robust capabilities for assessing disease activity (Yixi Li et al. 2022). Similarly, Zhao et al. used protein array analysis to identify TNF RII and MIP-1b as biomarkers, achieving an AUC of 0.914, thereby effectively distinguishing active lupus from healthy controls (Yafei Zhao et al. 2022).

Emerging biomarkers have further enhanced understanding of SLE pathogenesis. Meng et al. identified MX2 as a biomarker linked to neutrophil infiltration and the NOD-like receptor signaling pathway, highlighting its potential in predicting disease activity (X.-W. Meng et al. 2022). In another study, Zhong et al. utilized ML to identify ABCB1, EIF2AK2, HERC6, and PLSCR1 as diagnostic biomarkers, with significant associations to immune cell infiltration patterns (Zhong et al. 2022).

Chen et al. used a multi-miRNA detection platform in urinary extracellular vesicles, achieving AUC 1.00, demonstrating the potential of non-invasive diagnostics (Xiaofei Chen et al. 2024). Ceccarelli et al. reviewed various ML applications in SLE, emphasizing their capability to handle complex datasets and predict disease outcomes (Ceccarelli et al. 2023).

Further insights into disease mechanisms have been gained through advanced biomarker identification. Wang et al. used protein microarrays to identify citrullinated peptide biomarkers, demonstrating high diagnostic efficiency even in anti-Smith antibody-negative patients (Yao Wang et al. 2019). Similarly, Chen et al. identified DDX60 as a novel biomarker associated with interferon signaling and SLE disease activity, emphasizing its role in improving disease classification (W. Chen et al. 2023).

6 AI TOOLS FOR DISEASE CLASSIFICATION AND PREDICTION

ML-based models made significant strides in SLE diagnostics. Adamichou et al. developed the SLE Risk Probability Index (SLERPI), an ML-based model that utilized 14 clinical features, including thrombocytopenia and proteinuria, achieving an impressive 94.8% diagnostic accuracy (Adamichou et al. 2021). Another study by Chen et al. applied random forest algorithms to gene expression datasets, identifying six key genes with AUC values exceeding 0.95, thus showing the potential of genetic-level identification for SLE (H. Chen et al. 2022).

ML has been effective in predicting and classifying immunological disorders beyond SLE and RA, including MS and type 1 diabetes (T1D). A study by Prietl et al. used ML and automated clustering to analyze immune phenotypes in MS, T1D, SLE, and RA, identifying key differences in immune cell populations, particularly IL7alpha receptor (CD127) positive T cell clusters, which are crucial in disease mechanisms (PRIETL et al. 2023).

Du et al. demonstrated that ML algorithms could accurately classify diseases such as RA, SLE, sicca syndrome, and ankylosing spondylitis based on liquid chromatography-mass spectrometry (LC-MS) metabolomic signatures (Du et al. 2023). For MS, Zhao et al. explored the use of support vector machines (SVM) to predict disease progression by analyzing clinical, demographic, and MRI data. Their findings highlighted the potential of ML in forecasting MS disease course and optimizing treatment strategies (Yijun Zhao et al. 2017).

In RA, a ML model was developed to predict the development of anti-citrullinated peptide antibody (ACPA)-positive RA using genetic data from non-HLA genes such as PTPN22, STAT4, and CD40. This study suggested that ML can improve early detection and preventive approaches for individuals at high risk of developing RA (Dudek et al. 2024).

Additionally, ML techniques have been applied to predict lupus disease activity based on gene expression data. Kegerreis et al. integrated multiple datasets using random forest classifiers to distinguish between active and inactive SLE cases with high accuracy (Kegerreis et al. 2019).

Diagnosing asthma in children under five is challenging due to symptom variability. A study using clinical and demographic data from the Children's Hospital of Philadelphia Care Network achieved 81% accuracy in predicting asthma persistence, aiding early diagnosis and reducing clinician uncertainty (Bose, Kenyon, and Masino 2021). Predicting asthma exacerbations presents another critical application of ML, as it can directly influence therapeutic decisions (Jiao et al. 2022), (Hurst et al. 2022). These studies cover diverse populations, including children and adults, assessed during routine and emergency asthma care. In adults with exacerbations, ML models identify clinical and lab markers, such as peripheral blood eosinophil counts, which strongly predict severe exacerbation risk (Hurst et al. 2022).

AD benefits from AI-driven analysis, improving diagnosis, severity assessment, prediction, and treatment forecasting. SCORAD, once labor-intensive, is now automated using DL and CNN for consistency. ML models leverage patient-reported outcomes and biomarkers to predict severity, identify high-risk patients, and enable targeted management strategies (Silverberg et al. 2021).

Advanced biosensing technologies have also benefited from AI integration. Campuzano et al. explored electrochemical and DNA-based detection methods for allergens, illustrating how AI-enhanced biosensors can streamline allergen detection processes (Campuzano et al. 2020). A study by Ma et al. identified leukotriene A4 hydrolase as a predictive biomarker for the efficacy of allergen immunotherapy using liquid chromatography-tandem mass spectrometry, further emphasizing the role of precision biomarkers in therapy monitoring (Ma et al. 2020).

A comparative study employed machine learning algorithms, including Random Forest and XGBoost, to predict Multiple Sclerosis (MS) progression, with Random Forest achieving an AUC of 0.93 and 87% accuracy. The study highlights MRI and clinical data integration as pivotal in predictive modeling (Haouam and Benmalek 2024). Unsupervised ML classified MS into subtypes based on MRI abnormalities, predicting disease disability progression and relapse rates. This technique demonstrated potential in stratifying patients for tailored treatment approaches (Eshaghi et al. 2021).

6.1 Medical Imaging Analysis

The integration of AI into imaging analysis has significantly improved the speed and accuracy of diagnostic processes, offering automated, precise assessments of immunological conditions. AI-powered imaging analysis enhances disease detection, refines diagnostic precision, and optimizes patient management, ultimately leading to better clinical outcomes (**Figure 2**).

Figure 2. Role of AI-powered medical imaging in immunological disorders

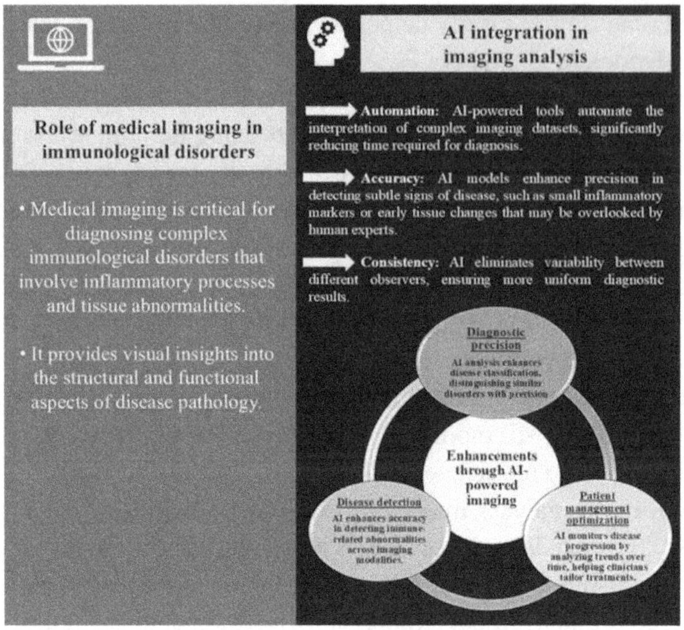

For example, AI-assisted digital pathology and imaging mass cytometry have been used to analyze tumor tissue ecosystems, offering new diagnostic possibilities by identifying spatial immune patterns and cell interactions (Rigamonti et al. 2023).

Zarubin et al. utilized AI-driven multiplex immunofluorescence imaging to characterize the tumor microenvironment, enabling differentiation of immune cell subpopulations and their interactions. This approach is particularly valuable for immunological disorders involving tissue inflammation and immune response modulation (Zarubin et al. 2022). Noaman et al. demonstrated AI-driven histological analysis, where hybrid models achieved 99.7% accuracy in early lung cancer detection. Their findings suggest that similar methodologies could be adapted for diagnosing inflammatory and autoimmune conditions (Noaman et al. 2024).

For autoimmune diseases, AI-based models for analyzing direct immunofluorescence (DIF) images have improved diagnostic accuracy by automating pattern recognition in conditions like autoimmune bullous diseases, reducing variability in interpretation and increasing efficiency (Capurro et al. 2024). AI has also been used in DL-based segmentation of immune infiltrates in histological samples, which aids in the assessment of inflammatory and immune responses in tissue sections (J. Wu and Lin 2021).

Another promising development is AI-assisted flow cytometry, which enables the automated analysis of immune cell populations in primary immunodeficiencies, reducing analysis time and enhancing diagnostic accuracy (Lu et al. 2024).

Another significant study by Jeong et al. introduced an AI-based multi-modal approach that combined H&E staining and CT imaging for predicting immune checkpoint inhibitor responses in non-small cell lung cancer. Their method successfully correlated AI-based image analysis with tumor microenvironment characteristics, demonstrating a high level of accuracy in assessing immune responses (Jeong et al. 2024).

AI-based DL algorithms applied to magnetic resonance imaging (MRI) and synovial tissue analysis have identified inflammation patterns indicative of early RA. These models provide automated quantification of synovitis and joint damage, achieving expert-level diagnostic accuracy (Y. Li et al. 2023). Vascular endothelial growth factor (VEGF)-targeted microbubbles have been utilized in multimodal imaging to detect inflammation in RA (C. Zhao et al. 2020). DL-based pannus localization software classifies synovitis and enhances synovial pannus visualization, supporting its utility in RA disease activity monitoring (Fang et al. 2022).

AI-driven models significantly enhance MS diagnosis and progression prediction using MRI and retinal imaging (Siva Balan R V 2024), (Farabi Maleki et al. 2024). DL models detect MS lesions with 99% precision, surpassing conventional methods (Siva Balan R V 2024). XGBoost improves MS trajectory analysis (Campanioni et al. 2024), while explainable AI models distinguish between relapsing-remitting and progressive MS, aiding clinician interpretation (Nicolaou et al. 2023). AI detects emerging biomarkers like cortical lesions and leptomeningeal contrast enhancement, refining MS progression predictions (Tavazzi et al. 2020). ML-enhanced optical coherence tomography analysis further advances MS diagnosis and patient stratification for personalized care (Farabi Maleki et al. 2024).

Furthermore, AI-driven medical imaging platforms, such as the one described by Eldin & Kaboudan, have revolutionized automated image classification and segmentation, enabling more precise evaluation of inflammation-related disorders, including autoimmune diseases (Salah Eldin and Kaboudan 2023).

AD diagnosis varies across specialties, utilizing distinct methods. Innovative techniques like multiphoton tomography allow noninvasive subcellular 3D imaging, while raster-scanning optoacoustic mesoscopy, successfully used in psoriasis detection, shows promise for AD diagnosis with DL-based CNN models (Aguirre et al. 2017), (Guimarães et al. 2020).

7 CHALLENGES, REGULATORY CONSIDERATIONS AND CLINICAL VALIDATION

While AI offers transformative possibilities for diagnosing immunological disorders, it faces substantial challenges that must be addressed to ensure clinical efficacy and integration. These challenges span data availability and quality, interpretability, and ethical concerns.

7.1 Challenges of AI Implementation in Real-World Applications

Despite significant advancements in AI in medical diagnostics, real-world implementation presents considerable challenges, particularly in ensuring model generalization across diverse patient populations. AI models trained in controlled research environments often fail to maintain accuracy and robustness when applied to real-world clinical settings, which exhibit variability in imaging protocols, laboratory techniques, and demographic diversity (Chinta et al. 2024). These challenges are particularly pronounced in immunological diagnostics, where autoimmune diseases, allergies, and immunodeficiencies vary significantly across ethnic, genetic, and environmental backgrounds, necessitating AI models that can adapt to diverse datasets while maintaining diagnostic accuracy.

One of the major concerns in AI-driven immunology is bias in model training, particularly when AI models are developed using datasets that do not sufficiently represent the global patient population. This lack of diversity can result in misdiagnoses, disparities in diagnostic accuracy, and inconsistent clinical recommendations, especially for underrepresented ethnic groups and rare immunological disorders (R. J. Chen et al. 2022). Addressing these issues requires the implementation of bias mitigation strategies, including adversarial training, where AI models are trained on synthetic and diversified datasets to enhance their ability to generalize across patient populations (Joshi and Burlina 2021). Another effective approach is bias correction algorithms, which utilize domain adaptation techniques to reweight underrepresented patient data, ensuring equitable model performance. Additionally, FL enables AI models to be trained on multi-institutional datasets without compromising patient privacy, facilitating a broader range of immunological data sources and improving diagnostic accuracy (Wen et al. 2023).

To ensure that AI models maintain their diagnostic accuracy and clinical relevance over time, post-market monitoring and real-world evidence generation are essential. Continuous performance tracking, updating models with new clinical data, and identifying potential biases or diagnostic errors through real-world validation are critical steps in refining AI-based immunological diagnostics (Kelly et al. 2019).

Another major barrier to AI adoption in immunology is clinician skepticism and lack of AI literacy, which can hinder trust in AI-powered decision-making tools (Zahraei and Shakeri 2024). Key concerns among healthcare professionals include the lack of explainability in AI models, as clinicians require transparent decision-making frameworks to justify AI-driven diagnoses. Furthermore, over-reliance on AI systems is a concern, as AI should serve as a supportive tool rather than replacing human clinical judgment. Additionally, seamless integration of AI-based diagnostics into hospital systems and EHRs remains a technical challenge, requiring extensive software interoperability and workflow adaptation.

To address these challenges, targeted AI education programs are being developed to improve clinician understanding of AI models and foster a collaborative approach between AI systems and healthcare professionals (Zahraei and Shakeri 2024). Additionally, regulatory agencies such as the FDA and EMA are advocating for the development of explainable AI frameworks, allowing clinicians to audit AI-driven decisions and ensure their reliability in immunological applications.

The successful real-world implementation of AI in immunological diagnostics requires addressing significant challenges, including model generalization, bias mitigation, clinician acceptance, and regulatory compliance. Strategies such as federated learning, adversarial training, and post-market surveillance are essential for enhancing AI robustness, fairness, and clinical reliability. Furthermore, increasing AI literacy among clinicians and integrating AI into existing clinical workflows will be crucial in ensuring successful AI adoption in immunology. By tackling these challenges, AI has the potential to revolutionize immunological diagnostics, leading to more accurate, equitable, and personalized patient care.

7.2 Limitations of AI in Diagnosing Rare Immunological Disorders

Despite the transformative potential of AI in medical diagnostics, its application in rare immunological disorders remains challenging. These disorders, such as primary immunodeficiencies and autoimmune diseases, present a unique set of difficulties due to their low prevalence, complex symptomatology, and limited availability of clinical data. AI models, which rely heavily on large datasets for training, struggle to generalize effectively when dealing with rare diseases, leading to potential misdiagnoses and delays in treatment initiation (Wojtara et al. 2023).

One of the primary challenges in applying AI to rare immunological disorders is the scarcity of high-quality, labeled data. Most AI models are designed to recognize patterns from extensive datasets, yet rare diseases inherently lack sufficient training data. Unlike common conditions where models can be trained on millions of cases, rare diseases often have only a few hundred documented cases, making it difficult for AI to learn robust diagnostic patterns (Hurvitz et al. 2021).

Moreover, AI models tend to overfit to the limited data available, reducing their ability to generalize across diverse patient populations. For instance, deep learning models trained on a specific ethnic or geographic cohort may fail to diagnose the same condition in another population due to genetic and environmental variations (Abdallah et al. 2023). This limitation underscores the need for AI frameworks that can learn from smaller datasets while maintaining diagnostic accuracy.

AI algorithms can inherit biases from the datasets they are trained on, leading to disparities in diagnostic accuracy. Many AI models used in immunology are trained on data from well-resourced medical centers in high-income countries, which may not represent global patient populations. This can result in lower diagnostic accuracy for underrepresented groups and misclassification of rare immunological disorders (Bottini, Emmert-Streib, and Franco 2021).

Additionally, some rare immune disorders share overlapping symptoms with more common diseases, making them difficult for AI models to differentiate. This increases the risk of false negatives, where AI fails to detect a rare disease, leading to diagnostic delays and suboptimal treatment outcomes (Bottini, Emmert-Streib, and Franco 2021).

To overcome these challenges, researchers are exploring several innovative approaches:

- Federated learning (FL): This technique allows AI models to learn from multiple healthcare institutions without directly sharing patient data, thus improving model generalization while preserving data privacy (Hurvitz et al. 2021).
- Synthetic data generation: GANs and other synthetic data techniques are being used to artificially expand training datasets, enabling AI models to recognize rare disease patterns more accurately (Booven et al. 2024).
- XAI: To improve clinician trust and reduce diagnostic errors, explainable AI models are being developed to provide transparent insights into how a diagnosis is reached, rather than operating as a "black box" (Bottini, Emmert-Streib, and Franco 2021).
- Cross-institutional data sharing: Initiatives such as global rare disease registries and multi-center collaborations are crucial for aggregating data and improving AI training models for rare immunological disorders.

While AI holds immense promise for diagnosing rare immunological disorders, current limitations related to data scarcity, model generalization, and algorithmic bias must be addressed. Advances in federated learning, synthetic data generation, and explainable AI are paving the way for more robust and equitable AI-driven diagnostics. However, continued research, regulatory oversight, and interdisciplinary collaboration are essential to fully realize AI's potential in rare disease diagnosis and management.

7.3 Challenges for Integrating AI Into Clinical Workflows for Immunological Diagnostics

The integration of AI into clinical workflows is revolutionizing the diagnosis and management of immunological disorders, including autoimmune diseases, allergies, and immunodeficiencies. AI-based diagnostic models rely on large-scale data processing, Clinical Decision Support Systems (CDSS), and federated learning techniques to enhance diagnostic precision while ensuring patient data privacy

(Dodevski et al. 2024). Despite these advances, the successful deployment of AI-based immunological diagnostics in hospitals and laboratories requires seamless integration with existing clinical workflows, particularly EHR systems. Several challenges hinder the widespread adoption of AI, necessitating technical, ethical, and operational solutions to ensure its efficacy and acceptance.

One of the primary barriers to AI implementation in immunology diagnostics is workflow disruption. AI tools must be clinician-friendly and operate within pre-existing healthcare frameworks to avoid complicating diagnostic procedures (Blezek et al. 2021). Another major challenge is interoperability, as AI-powered immunology models must be compatible with legacy hospital systems and EHR platforms to ensure smooth data integration. Additionally, clinician acceptance is crucial, with healthcare professionals requiring XAI outputs to reduce skepticism and improve trust in AI-generated predictions (Elhaddad et al. 2024). Scalability and data privacy also remain significant concerns, as AI models require access to large and diverse patient datasets while complying with stringent data protection laws such as HIPAA and GDPR (Oakley 2023).

To address these challenges, AI-based Clinical Decision Support Systems (CDSS) are being integrated into EHRs to assist in disease prediction, risk stratification, and treatment recommendations for immunological conditions. These AI-driven CDSS tools provide real-time decision-making support, reducing diagnostic errors and treatment delays, particularly in complex immune-mediated diseases such as systemic SLE, RA, and multiple sclerosis (Elhaddad et al. 2024).

A key technological advancement facilitating AI-driven immunology diagnostics is FL. Unlike traditional ML, which requires centralized patient data, FL enables AI models to be trained collaboratively across multiple healthcare institutions while keeping patient data localized. This approach enhances diagnostic accuracy while ensuring compliance with data privacy regulations (Zhang et al. 2024). FL is particularly beneficial in immunology applications such as early autoimmune disease detection, where AI models trained on multi-institutional datasets can significantly improve disease classification and treatment optimization.

In addition to disease diagnosis, AI is playing a transformative role in personalized immunotherapy. AI-driven models can analyze patient-specific immune responses to biologic drugs, optimizing precision medicine approaches in treating chronic inflammatory diseases (Dodevski et al. 2024). AI-powered risk prediction models for allergic reactions, transplant rejection, and immunodeficiency syndromes are now being embedded into EHRs, allowing clinicians to make data-driven decisions in real time.

Looking ahead, the future of AI integration into clinical workflows for immunological disorders will require continued advancements in transparency, scalability, and data privacy protection. The development of explainable AI models will be crucial in ensuring clinician trust and adoption, while robust federated learning frameworks will enable multi-hospital collaboration without breaching privacy laws (Zhang et al. 2024). Moreover, AI-based CDSS models must be adaptable to work across heterogeneous EHR platforms, enabling real-time, AI-driven immune disease diagnostics. By addressing these critical challenges, AI-driven immunological diagnostics will continue to enhance patient outcomes, streamline clinical workflows, and advance precision medicine in immunology.

7.4 Regulatory Challenges and FDA Approvals

The regulatory landscape for AI in medical diagnostics is evolving as agencies such as the U.S. Food and Drug Administration (FDA), European Medicines Agency (EMA), and Health Canada seek to establish clear guidelines for AI-based medical devices (Reddy 2023). AI-powered diagnostic tools, particularly

ML-based models, pose unique regulatory challenges due to their adaptive learning capabilities, which may lead to continuous changes in model performance over time.

The FDA has categorized AI-driven medical diagnostics under Software as a Medical Device (SaMD), necessitating stringent clinical validation, post-market surveillance, and real-world performance monitoring (Kaladharan, Manayath, and Gopalakrishnan 2024). This is particularly relevant for AI applications in autoimmune disease detection, allergy diagnostics, and immunotherapy response prediction, where evolving datasets necessitate continuous algorithm updates. The challenge lies in ensuring that AI algorithms remain consistent, unbiased, and interpretable when applied across different healthcare settings. The FDA's proposed Predetermined Change Control Plan (PCCP) aims to regulate AI models that evolve over time, allowing developers to predefine how their models can be modified post-approval while maintaining compliance (Oualikene-Gonin et al. 2024). In autoimmune diseases such as RA and lupus, AI models must account for genetic, environmental, and ethnic variations to avoid disparities in diagnostic accuracy. Regulatory agencies now require multicenter clinical trials to validate AI models across different demographic and geographic groups

One significant barrier to AI adoption is data diversity and bias, which can impact regulatory approval. AI models trained on homogeneous datasets may fail to generalize across diverse patient populations, leading to disparities in diagnostic accuracy (Coeckelbergh 2019). Regulators emphasize the need for multicenter clinical trials and external validation studies to assess model performance across various demographic groups.

7.5 Ethical and Biases Concerns

AI-based diagnostic tools must provide interpretable insights for clinicians to ensure trust and effective decision-making. Regulatory approvals and integration with existing healthcare workflows remain significant hurdles. The adoption of AI in immunology faces ethical challenges such as algorithmic bias, data privacy, and interpretability.

One real-world example involves the use of AI for early detection of immunodeficiencies through genetic profiling. Companies offering direct-to-consumer (DTC) genetic testing, such as 23andMe, have faced scrutiny for selling anonymized genomic data to third parties, including pharmaceutical companies, without explicit patient consent (Gilligan 2022). This raises ethical questions about how AI-driven models should balance the need for large-scale immunological datasets with respecting patient confidentiality.

Another significant ethical issue is algorithmic bias in AI-powered immunology diagnostics. AI models trained on non-representative datasets may fail to provide accurate diagnoses for certain racial or ethnic groups, exacerbating existing healthcare disparities (Chinta et al. 2024). In immunological diseases, such as lupus and RA, clinical presentations vary significantly across populations, yet many AI models are trained on datasets dominated by European ancestry populations.

AI models operating in black-box formats limit transparency, raising concerns among clinicians and patients about trust and accountability ("Ethical issues in implementing artificial intelligence in healthcare," n.d.).

A real-world case highlighting this issue involved an AI system used in a hospital setting to predict sepsis risk in immunocompromised patients. Physicians initially followed the AI's recommendations, only to find that the model over-relied on non-clinical factors, such as hospital resource allocation data, leading to inappropriate treatment decisions ("Artificial Intelligence Failure at IBM 'Watson for Oncology' - ProQuest," n.d.). Such cases highlight the need for XAI models that provide justifications for their predictions, allowing physicians and patients to make more informed decisions (Wang and Ma 2025).

AI deployment in clinical settings requires interpretable models that provide actionable insights. Many DL models function as "black boxes," limiting transparency and hindering clinical trust (Ceccarelli et al. 2023). Moreover, regulatory hurdles remain a significant barrier, as AI tools must comply with healthcare standards like the GDPR and HIPAA (Oakley 2023). Integrating AI into existing healthcare workflows also demands significant changes in infrastructure and clinician training. For example, the need for interoperability between AI systems and electronic health records (EHRs) to streamline adoption was recently highlighted (M. and Chacko 2021).

AI-driven immunological diagnostics hold immense promise but also introduce significant ethical concerns, including data privacy risks, algorithmic bias, challenges to patient autonomy, and unclear liability frameworks. Real-world cases illustrate the dangers of biased training data, opaque decision-making, and potential patient harm when AI recommendations are blindly followed. To ensure ethical AI deployment, regulatory agencies, clinicians, and AI developers must collaborate to enhance model transparency, diversify training datasets, and establish clear accountability measures. Ethical considerations must remain at the forefront of AI innovation to ensure fair, safe, and effective immunological diagnostics.

7.6 Barriers to AI Adoption in Clinical Immunology: Resistance and Cost Concerns

Despite the transformative potential of AI in medical diagnostics, its adoption in clinical immunology remains slow due to several practical and economic challenges. Resistance from healthcare professionals, concerns about financial investment, and integration issues with existing workflows are significant barriers that must be addressed to facilitate AI's widespread implementation in immunological diagnostics (Gupta and Srivastava 2024).

One of the primary obstacles to AI adoption in clinical settings is the reluctance of healthcare professionals to trust and rely on AI-driven decision-making. Many clinicians are skeptical about AI's ability to match human expertise, particularly in complex cases of immunological disorders such as autoimmune diseases, primary immunodeficiencies, and allergic conditions (Chaibi and Zaiem 2022). This resistance stems from several factors, including:

- Lack of explainability: Many AI models function as "black boxes," meaning their decision-making processes are not transparent. Clinicians require interpretable AI models that provide a clear rationale for their recommendations.
- Fear of job displacement: Some healthcare professionals view AI as a threat rather than a tool for augmentation. The concern that AI might replace human expertise rather than complement it creates hesitancy in adoption.
- Ethical and legal responsibility: In the event of a misdiagnosis, determining liability remains a challenge. If an AI model makes an incorrect recommendation, it is unclear whether responsibility lies with the clinician, the hospital, or the AI developer (X. Li and Abangbila 2024).

To address these concerns, AI education and training programs for clinicians are being implemented to enhance their trust and familiarity with AI systems. Moreover, regulatory bodies such as the FDA and EMA are pushing for XAI frameworks that make AI-driven decisions more transparent and auditable.

The high cost of AI implementation is another major barrier, particularly for healthcare institutions with limited resources. AI-driven diagnostic tools require significant financial investment for data infrastructure, software and hardware integration, clinical validation and regulatory approval (Hassan, Kushniruk, and Borycki 2024).

A potential solution to financial barriers is the adoption of FL, where AI models are trained across multiple hospitals without requiring centralized data storage. This reduces infrastructure costs while maintaining data privacy.

For AI to be successfully adopted in clinical immunology, it must seamlessly integrate into existing workflows. However, current hospital systems were not designed with AI implementation in mind, leading to challenges such as:

- Interoperability issues: Many AI models struggle to interact with legacy hospital software, resulting in fragmented workflows.
- Alert fatigue: Clinicians are already overwhelmed with alerts from various clinical decision support systems. Adding AI-generated alerts without proper filtering can reduce efficiency rather than enhance it.
- Customization needs: AI models must be tailored to specific clinical environments. A one-size-fits-all approach may not work across different healthcare settings and patient populations (Alshehri, Alahmari, and Alasiry 2024).

To address these issues, AI developers are working on user-friendly interfaces and adaptive learning models that can adjust to different clinical workflows while maintaining high accuracy and reliability.

Despite its potential, AI adoption in immunological diagnostics faces substantial resistance from healthcare professionals, financial constraints, and integration challenges. Addressing these barriers requires targeted AI education, cost-effective deployment strategies, and seamless integration with existing clinical workflows. By overcoming these obstacles, AI can significantly enhance diagnostic accuracy, improve patient outcomes, and reduce healthcare costs in immunology.

8. FUTURE DIRECTIONS AND CONCLUSIONS

Artificial intelligence (AI) has emerged as a transformative tool in immunological diagnostics, offering unprecedented advancements in disease detection, risk assessment, and personalized treatment strategies. The integration of ML, DL, and NLP has significantly enhanced the accuracy and efficiency of diagnosing complex immunological disorders, including autoimmune diseases, primary immunodeficiencies, and inflammatory conditions. AI-driven approaches facilitate rapid and precise analysis of large-scale immunological datasets, enabling early disease identification and improved patient outcomes. The collaboration between advanced analytics and clinical expertise is key to addressing gaps in care and enhancing patient outcomes. Wearable devices and remote patient monitoring (RPM) further advance real-time data collection, aiding in predicting exacerbation risks (Iqbal et al. 2021). Electronic inhaler data, including usage patterns, peak inspiratory flow, inhalation volume, and duration, trained an ML model that predicted asthma exacerbations within five days with an AUC of 0.83, demonstrating strong clinical relevance (Lugogo et al. 2022).

Future applications of ML for exacerbation prediction may integrate data from smart peak flow meters, smartwatches, and indoor air quality monitors (Tsang et al. 2022), (Bae et al. 2022). However, the practical implementation of these technologies will depend on their cost, accessibility, and insurance coverage.

A major challenge in severe AD management is selecting optimal treatments as new therapies emerge. For instance, an ML model analyzing cytokine and chemokine data failed to predict responses to azathioprine or methotrexate accurately (Hurault et al. 2022). Conversely, another ML model trained on demographic and clinical data from patients initiating dupilumab therapy demonstrated greater promise, achieving a 69% accuracy rate in predicting non-responders (Huang et al. 2020).

Despite these advancements, several challenges hinder the full-scale clinical adoption of AI in immunology. Model generalization remains a critical issue, as AI systems often struggle to perform optimally across diverse patient populations due to limited training data, demographic variability, and rare disease complexities. Bias in AI models is another pressing concern, particularly in immunological disorders where genetic, ethnic, and environmental factors play significant roles in disease progression. Efforts such as federated learning, adversarial training, and bias mitigation algorithms are essential to improving AI model fairness and reliability.

Furthermore, regulatory and ethical challenges pose significant barriers to AI deployment in immunology. Ensuring compliance with FDA, EMA, and GDPR guidelines, as well as maintaining patient data privacy and security, is paramount for AI-driven immunological diagnostics. Additionally, clinician resistance and skepticism toward AI technologies highlight the need for XAI frameworks that enhance transparency and interpretability in AI-assisted decision-making. AI education programs and seamless integration into EHRs are critical in fostering acceptance and widespread clinical implementation.

Looking ahead, AI's role in immunology will continue to evolve, with emerging innovations in multi-omics integration, real-world clinical validation, and AI-driven immunotherapies. The use of next-generation AI models, digital pathology, and automated laboratory diagnostics is expected to redefine precision medicine in immunology, leading to more targeted treatments and better patient care. By addressing existing challenges and leveraging AI's potential, the future of AI-enhanced immunological diagnostics promises greater accuracy, efficiency, and accessibility, ultimately revolutionizing how immune-mediated diseases are diagnosed and managed.

ACKNOWLEDGMENTS

The authors acknowledge a grant of the Ministry of Research, Innovation and Digitalization, CNCS—UEFISCDI, project number PN-IV-P2-2.1-TE-2023-0993, within PNCDI IV. The authors also acknowledge the Romanian Ministry of Research, Innovation and Digitalization under the Romanian National Nucleu Program LAPLAS VII—contract No. 30N/2023.

REFERENCES

Abdallah, S., Sharifa, M., Kh, I., Almadhoun, M. K., Khawar, M. M.Sr, Shaikh, U., Balabel, K. M., Saleh, I., Manzoor, A., Mandal, A. K., Ekomwereren, O., Khine, W. M., & Oyelaja, O. T. (2023). The Impact of Artificial Intelligence on Optimizing Diagnosis and Treatment Plans for Rare Genetic Disorders. *Cureus, 15*(10), e46860. DOI: 10.7759/cureus.46860

Adamichou, C., Genitsaridi, I., Nikolopoulos, D., Nikoloudaki, M., Repa, A., Bortoluzzi, A., Fanouriakis, A., Sidiropoulos, P., Boumpas, D. T., & Bertsias, G. K. (2021). Lupus or Not? SLE Risk Probability Index (SLERPI): A Simple, Clinician-Friendly Machine Learning-Based Model to Assist the Diagnosis of Systemic Lupus Erythematosus. *Annals of the Rheumatic Diseases, 80*(6), 758–766. DOI: 10.1136/annrheumdis-2020-219069 PMID: 33568388

Agache, I., Canelo-Aybar, C., Annesi-Maesano, I., Cecchi, L., Rigau, D., Rodríguez-Tanta, L. Y., Nieto-Gutierrez, W., Song, Y., Cantero-Fortiz, Y., Roqué, M., Vasquez, J. C., Sola, I., Biagioni, B., Chung, F., D'Amato, G., Damialis, A., del Giacco, S., Vecillas, L., Dominguez-Ortega, J., & Akdis, C. A. (2024). The Impact of Outdoor Pollution and Extreme Temperatures on Asthma-Related Outcomes: A Systematic Review for the EAACI Guidelines on Environmental Science for Allergic Diseases and Asthma. *Allergy, 79*(7), 1725–1760. DOI: 10.1111/all.16041 PMID: 38311978

Aguirre, J., Schwarz, M., Garzorz, N., Omar, M., Buehler, A., Eyerich, K., & Ntziachristos, V. (2017). Precision Assessment of Label-Free Psoriasis Biomarkers with Ultra-Broadband Optoacoustic Mesoscopy. *Nature Biomedical Engineering, 1*(5), 1–8. DOI: 10.1038/s41551-017-0068

Ahmed, Z., Mohamed, K., Zeeshan, S., & Dong, X. Q. (2020). Artificial Intelligence with Multi-Functional Machine Learning Platform Development for Better Healthcare and Precision Medicine. *Database : The Journal of Biological Databases and Curation, 2020*(January), baaa010. Advance online publication. DOI: 10.1093/database/baaa010 PMID: 32185396

Alag, A. (2019). Machine Learning Approach Yields Epigenetic Biomarkers of Food Allergy: A Novel 13-Gene Signature to Diagnose Clinical Reactivity. *PLoS One, 14*(6), e0218253. DOI: 10.1371/journal.pone.0218253 PMID: 31216310

Almuhanna, H., Alenezi, M., Abualhasan, M., Alajmi, S., Alfadhli, R., & Karar, A. S. (2024). AI Asthma Guard: Predictive Wearable Technology for Asthma Management in Vulnerable Populations. *Applied System Innovation, 7*(5), 78. DOI: 10.3390/asi7050078

Alshehri, S., Alahmari, K. A., & Alasiry, A. (2024). A Comprehensive Evaluation of AI-Assisted Diagnostic Tools in ENT Medicine: Insights and Perspectives from Healthcare Professionals. *Journal of Personalized Medicine*, *14*(4), 354. DOI: 10.3390/jpm14040354 PMID: 38672981

Alter, O., Newman, E., Ponnapalli, S. P., & Tsai, J. W. (2024). AI/ML-Derived Mechanistically Interpretable Whole-Genome Biomarkers of Patient Survival in Pre-Treatment Primary Neuroblastoma Tumors and Whole Blood. *Journal of Clinical Oncology*, *42*(16, suppl), 10043–10043. DOI: 10.1200/JCO.2024.42.16_suppl.10043

Deng, Y. (2024). Application Research of Machine Learning Algorithms in Medical Diagnosis. *Journal of Artificial Intelligence Practice*, *7*(2). Advance online publication. DOI: 10.23977/jaip.2024.070214

Faheem, H., & Dutta, S. (2023). Artificial Intelligence Failure at IBM 'Watson for Oncology' - ProQuest. IUP Journal of Knowledge Management. 21(3). Accessed March 4, 2025. https://www.proquest.com/openview/5d55d56634fb060f97ae707091489ec9/1?pq-origsite=gscholar&cbl=54461

Artsi, Y., & Vera Sorin, B. S. (2024). Advancing Clinical Practice: The Potential of Multimodal Technology in Modern Medicine. *Journal of Clinical Medicine*, *13*(20), 6246. DOI: 10.3390/jcm13206246 PMID: 39458196

Asiniwasis, R., Merati, N., Roesler, J., Simpson, E. L., Aubry, R., McMullen, E., Fraess, L., Choi, U. Y., Hinther, K., Chu, D. K., & Jack, C. (2024). The Social and Home Environment: Impacts of Determinants of Health on Atopic Dermatitis, Pathways Toward Solutions, and Unique Considerations for Rural and Remote North American Indigenous Populations. *The Journal of Allergy and Clinical Immunology. In Practice*, *12*(2), 290–299. DOI: 10.1016/j.jaip.2023.11.034 PMID: 38013155

Aslam, R., Herrles, L., Aoun, R., Pioskowik, A., & Pietrzyk, A. (2024). Link between Gut Microbiota Dysbiosis and Childhood Asthma: Insights from a Systematic Review. *The Journal of Allergy and Clinical Immunology. Global*, *3*(3), 100289. DOI: 10.1016/j.jacig.2024.100289 PMID: 39105129

Bae, W. D., Alkobaisi, S., Horak, M., Park, C.-S., Kim, S., & Davidson, J. (2022). Predicting Health Risks of Adult Asthmatics Susceptible to Indoor Air Quality Using Improved Logistic and Quantile Regression Models. *Life (Chicago, Ill.)*, *12*(10), 1631. DOI: 10.3390/life12101631 PMID: 36295066

Bakare, S. S., Adeniyi, A. O., Akpuokwe, C. U., & Eneh, N. E.Seun Solomon BakareAdekunle Oyeyemi AdeniyiChidiogo Uzoamaka AkpuokweNkechi Emmanuella Eneh. (2024). Data Privacy Laws and Compliance: A Comparative Review Of The Eu GDPR And USA Regulations. *Computer Science & IT Research Journal*, *5*(3), 528–543. DOI: 10.51594/csitrj.v5i3.859

Bakker, D. S., Nierkens, S., Knol, E. F., Giovannone, B., Delemarre, E. M., van der Schaft, J., van Wijk, F., de Bruin-Weller, M. S., Drylewicz, J., & Thijs, J. L. (2021). Confirmation of Multiple Endotypes in Atopic Dermatitis Based on Serum Biomarkers. *The Journal of Allergy and Clinical Immunology*, *147*(1), 189–198. DOI: 10.1016/j.jaci.2020.04.062 PMID: 32526312

Balakrishna, S., & Solanki, V. K. (2024). A Comprehensive Review on AI-Driven Healthcare Transformation. *Ingeniería Solidaria*, *20*(2), 1–30. DOI: 10.16925/2357-6014.2024.02.07

Bellanti, J. A. (2024). IgE and Non-IgE Food Allergy: A Review of Immunological Mechanisms. *Journal of Food Allergy*, *6*(1), 37–46. DOI: 10.2500/jfa.2024.6.240003 PMID: 39257598

Bellinghausen, I., Khatri, R., & Saloga, J. (2022). Current Strategies to Modulate Regulatory T Cell Activity in Allergic Inflammation. *Frontiers in Immunology*, *13*(May), 912529. Advance online publication. DOI: 10.3389/fimmu.2022.912529 PMID: 35720406

Benkirane, H., Pradat, Y., Michiels, S., & Cournède, P.-H. (2023). CustOmics: A Versatile Deep-Learning Based Strategy for Multi-Omics Integration. *PLoS Computational Biology*, *19*(3), e1010921. DOI: 10.1371/journal.pcbi.1010921 PMID: 36877736

Bilsen, J. H. M. (2019). A Network-Based Approach for Identifying Suitable Biomarkers for Oral Immunotherapy of Food Allergy. *BMC Bioinformatics*, *20*(1), 206. DOI: 10.1186/s12859-019-2802-9 PMID: 31014233

Blezek, D. J., Olson-Williams, L., Missert, A., & Korfiatis, P. (2021). AI Integration in the Clinical Workflow. *Journal of Digital Imaging*, *34*(6), 1435–1446. DOI: 10.1007/s10278-021-00525-3 PMID: 34686923

Van Booven, D. J., Chen, C. B., Malpani, S., Mirzabeigi, Y., Mohammadi, M., Wang, Y., & Arora, H. (2024). Synthetic genitourinary image synthesis via generative adversarial networks: enhancing AI diagnostic precision. bioRxiv, 2024-05.

Bose, S., Kenyon, C. C., & Masino, A. J. (2021). Personalized Prediction of Early Childhood Asthma Persistence: A Machine Learning Approach. *PLoS One*, *16*(3), e0247784. DOI: 10.1371/journal.pone.0247784 PMID: 33647071

Bottini, S., Emmert-Streib, F., & Franco, L. (2021). Editorial: AI and Multi-Omics for Rare Diseases: Challenges, Advances and Perspectives. *Frontiers in Molecular Biosciences*, *8*(June), 719978. Advance online publication. DOI: 10.3389/fmolb.2021.719978 PMID: 34277712

Boushehri, S., Sayedali, K. E., Chlis, N.-K., Herter, S., Bacac, M., Theis, F. J., Glasmacher, E., Marr, C., & Schmich, F. (2023). Explainable Machine Learning for Profiling the Immunological Synapse and Functional Characterization of Therapeutic Antibodies. *Nature Communications*, *14*(1), 7888. DOI: 10.1038/s41467-023-43429-2 PMID: 38036503

Campanioni, S., Veiga, C., Prieto-González, J. M., González-Nóvoa, J. A., Busto, L., Martinez, C., Alberte-Woodward, M., García de Soto, J., Pouso-Diz, J., Fernández Ceballos, M. Á., & Agis-Balboa, R. C. (2024). Explainable Machine Learning on Baseline MRI Predicts Multiple Sclerosis Trajectory Descriptors. *PLoS One*, *19*(7), e0306999. DOI: 10.1371/journal.pone.0306999 PMID: 39012871

Campuzano, S., Montiel, V. R.-V., Serafín, V., Yáñez-Sedeño, P., & Pingarrón, J. M. (2020). Cutting-Edge Advances in Electrochemical Affinity Biosensing at Different Molecular Level of Emerging Food Allergens and Adulterants. *Biosensors (Basel)*, *10*(2), 10. DOI: 10.3390/bios10020010 PMID: 32041251

Cañas, J. A., Núñez, R., Cruz-Amaya, A., Gómez, F., Torres, M. J., Palomares, F., & Mayorga, C. (2021). Epigenetics in Food Allergy and Immunomodulation. *Nutrients*, *13*(12), 4345. DOI: 10.3390/nu13124345 PMID: 34959895

Capurro, N., Pastore, V. P., Touijer, L., Odone, F., Cozzani, E., Gasparini, G., & Parodi, A. (2024). A Deep Learning Approach to Direct Immunofluorescence Pattern Recognition in Autoimmune Bullous Diseases. *British Journal of Dermatology*, *191*(2), 261–266. DOI: 10.1093/bjd/ljae142 PMID: 38581445

Ceccarelli, F., Natalucci, F., Picciariello, L., Ciancarella, C., Dolcini, G., Gattamelata, A., Alessandri, C., & Conti, F. (2023). Application of Machine Learning Models in Systemic Lupus Erythematosus. *International Journal of Molecular Sciences*, *24*(5), 4514. DOI: 10.3390/ijms24054514 PMID: 36901945

Chaibi, A., & Zaiem, I. (2022). Doctor Resistance of Artificial Intelligence in Healthcare. [IJHISI]. *International Journal of Healthcare Information Systems and Informatics*, *17*(1), 1–13. DOI: 10.4018/IJHISI.315618

Chakraborty, S., Chopra, H., Akash, S., Chakraborty, C., & Dhama, K. (2023). Advances in Artificial Intelligence (AI)-Based Diagnosis in Clinical Practice—Correspondence. *Annals of Medicine and Surgery (London)*, *85*(7), 3757–3758. DOI: 10.1097/MS9.0000000000000959 PMID: 37427159

Chen, H., Huang, L., Jiang, X., Wang, Y., Bian, Y., Ma, S., & Liu, X. (2022). Establishment and Analysis of a Disease Risk Prediction Model for the Systemic Lupus Erythematosus with Random Forest. *Frontiers in Immunology*, *13*(November), 1025688. Advance online publication. DOI: 10.3389/fimmu.2022.1025688 PMID: 36405750

Chen, R. J., Chen, T. Y., Lipkova, J., Wang, J. J., Williamson, D. F., Lu, M. Y., . . . Mahmood, F. (2021). Algorithm fairness in ai for medicine and healthcare. arXiv preprint arXiv:2110.00603.

Chen, W., Li, Z.-Y., Huang, L., Zhou, D.-H., Luo, W.-Q., Zhang, X.-F., Li, L., Wen, C.-P., & Wang, Q. (2023). Integrative Bioinformatics Analysis Identifies DDX60 as a Potential Biomarker for Systemic Lupus Erythematosus. *Disease Markers*, *8564650*(1), 1–14. DOI: 10.1155/2023/8564650 PMID: 36655136

Chen, X., Xiang, Q., Yan, S., Wang, Y., Su, N., Yang, X., Gao, M., & Zhang, X. (2024). Simultaneous Multi-miRNA Detection in Urinary Small Extracellular Vesicles Using Target-Triggered Locked Hairpin DNA-Functionalized Au Nanoprobes for Systemic Lupus Erythematosus Diagnosis. *Analytical Chemistry*, *96*(41), 16370–16378. DOI: 10.1021/acs.analchem.4c03794 PMID: 39363542

Chen, X., Zhang, D., Liu, Q., Liu, S., Li, H., & Li, Z. (2023). Enzyme-Linked Immunosorbent Assay-Based Microarray on a Chip for Bioaerosol Sensing: Toward Sensitive and Multiplexed Profiling of Foodborne Allergens. *Analytical Chemistry*, *95*(18), 7354–7362. DOI: 10.1021/acs.analchem.3c00591 PMID: 37098245

Chinta, S. V., Wang, Z., Zhang, X., Viet, T. D., Kashif, A., Smith, M. A., & Zhang, W. 2024. "AI-Driven Healthcare: A Survey on Ensuring Fairness and Mitigating Bias." arXiv. https://doi.org//arXiv.2407.19655.DOI: 10.48550

Choi, S., & Kim, S. (2023). Artificial Intelligence in the Pathology of Gastric Cancer. *Journal of Gastric Cancer*, *23*(3), 410–427. DOI: 10.5230/jgc.2023.23.e25 PMID: 37553129

Coeckelbergh, M. (2019, May). Artificial Intelligence: Some Ethical Issues and Regulatory Challenges. *Technology and Regulation*, *31–34*, 31–34. Advance online publication. DOI: 10.71265/a9yxhg88

Cyrielle, N. N. T., Andigema, A. S., Mafo, K. L. D., & Ekwelle, E. (2024). Harnessing The Power Of Artificial Intelligence For Enhanced Point-Of-Care Quality Control In Healthcare. *Asian Journal Of Medical Technology*, *4*(1), 22–33. DOI: 10.32896/ajmedtech.v4n1.22-33

Datta, P., & Rohilla, R. 2019. "An Introduction to Deep Learning Applications In MRI Images." In *2019 2nd International Conference on Power Energy, Environment and Intelligent Control (PEEIC)*, 458–65. DOI: 10.1109/PEEIC47157.2019.8976727

Deepa, R., Arunkumar, S., Jayaraj, V., & Sivasamy, A. (2023). Healthcare's New Frontier: AI-Driven Early Cancer Detection for Improved Well-Being. *AIP Advances*, *13*(11), 115331. DOI: 10.1063/5.0177640

Dodevski, Z., Starič, K. D., Bogdanova, A. M., & Trajkovikj, V. (2024, June). Enhancing Privacy of Clinical Decision Support Systems with Federated Learning. In 2024 9th International Conference on Smart and Sustainable Technologies (SpliTech) (pp. 1-6). IEEE.

Dranove, D., & Garthwaite, C. L. (2022). *Artificial intelligence, the evolution of the healthcare value chain, and the future of the physician (No. c14761)*. National Bureau of Economic Research.

Du, Q., Wang, X., Chen, J., Wang, Y., Liu, W., Wang, L., Liu, H., Jiang, L., & Nie, Z. (2023). Machine Learning Encodes Urine and Serum Metabolic Patterns for Autoimmune Disease Discrimination, Classification and Metabolic Dysregulation Analysis. *Analyst*, *148*(18), 4318–4330. DOI: 10.1039/D3AN01051A PMID: 37547947

Dudek, G., Sakowski, S., Brzezińska, O., Sarnik, J., Budlewski, T., Dragan, G., Poplawska, M., Poplawski, T., Bijak, M., & Makowska, J. (2024). Machine Learning-Based Prediction of Rheumatoid Arthritis with Development of ACPA Autoantibodies in the Presence of Non-HLA Genes Polymorphisms. *PLoS One*, *19*(3), e0300717. DOI: 10.1371/journal.pone.0300717 PMID: 38517871

Kardia. "EKG Anywhere, Anytime". Accessed January 20, 2025. https://www.kardia.com/

Elhaddad, M., Hamam, S., Elhaddad, M., & Hamam, S. (2024). AI-Driven Clinical Decision Support Systems: An Ongoing Pursuit of Potential. *Cureus*, *16*(4). Advance online publication. DOI: 10.7759/cureus.57728 PMID: 38711724

Elsayed, S. A.-R., Kamaly, H. M., & Esmail, M. A. (2022). Co-Positivity of Anti-dsDNA, Anti-Nucleosome, and Anti-Smith Autoantibodies as Serological Biomarkers for Disease Activity in Systemic Lupus Erythematosus. *Egyptian Rheumatology & Rehabilitation*, *49*(1), 8. DOI: 10.1186/s43166-021-00110-0

Erdem, Y., Özkaya, E., Erbilgin, Y., Saritas, M., Sayitoglu, M., Küçük, Ö. S., & Salman, A.. (2025). Filaggrin Gene Variants Among Patients With Atopic Dermatitis in Turkey: A Multicenter Study Investigating Its Relationship With Disease Severity and Clinical/Laboratory Findings. *Dermatitis*, (January), derm.2024.0403. Advance online publication. DOI: 10.1089/derm.2024.0403 PMID: 39772616

Eshaghi, A., Young, A. L., Wijeratne, P. A., Prados, F., Arnold, D. L., Narayanan, S., Guttmann, C. R. G., Barkhof, F., Alexander, D. C., Thompson, A. J., Chard, D., & Ciccarelli, O. (2021). Identifying Multiple Sclerosis Subtypes Using Unsupervised Machine Learning and MRI Data. *Nature Communications*, *12*(1), 2078. DOI: 10.1038/s41467-021-22265-2 PMID: 33824310

Fang, W., An, Y., Sugimori, H., Kiuch, S., & Kamishima, T. (2022). Pos1391 Deep Learning-Based Pannus Localization Software in the Hands of Inflammatory Arthritis Using Time-Intensity Curve (Tic) Shape Classification on Dynamic Mri Dataset. *Annals of the Rheumatic Diseases*, *81*(Suppl 1), 1036–1036. DOI: 10.1136/annrheumdis-2022-eular.2196

Feng, Y., Wang, Y., Zeng, C., & Mao, H. (2021). Artificial Intelligence and Machine Learning in Chronic Airway Diseases: Focus on Asthma and Chronic Obstructive Pulmonary Disease. *International Journal of Medical Sciences*, *18*(13), 2871–2889. DOI: 10.7150/ijms.58191 PMID: 34220314

Fox, T. A., & Booth, C. (2021). Gene Therapy for Primary Immunodeficiencies. *British Journal of Haematology*, *193*(6), 1044–1059. DOI: 10.1111/bjh.17269 PMID: 33336808

Frishberg, M. (2025). Peering Inside AI's Black Box. *Research Technology Management*, *68*(2), 59–60. DOI: 10.1080/08956308.2025.2448388

Gani, R., Isty, M. N., Rimi, R. A., Parsub, W. R., Islam, M. S., Priyanka, M. M., . . . Adnan, M. N. (2024, March). Impact of ai in healthcare services: Analysis using medical synthetic data. In 2024 International Conference on Advances in Computing, Communication, Electrical, and Smart Systems (iCACCESS) (pp. 01-06). IEEE.

Ghodke-Puranik, Y., Olferiev, M., & Crow, M. K. (2024). Systemic Lupus Erythematosus Genetics: Insights into Pathogenesis and Implications for Therapy. *Nature Reviews. Rheumatology*, *20*(10), 635–648. DOI: 10.1038/s41584-024-01152-2 PMID: 39232240

Gilligan, K. C. (2022). Protecting consumers and regulating data: The need for comprehensive federal oversight of the direct-to-consumer genetic testing industry. *Drexel L. Rev.*, *14*, 207.

Guida, G., Bagnasco, D., Carriero, V., Bertolini, F., Fabio, L. M. R., Nicola, S., & Brussino, L.. (2022). Critical Evaluation of Asthma Biomarkers in Clinical Practice. *Frontiers in Medicine*, *9*(October), 969243. Advance online publication. DOI: 10.3389/fmed.2022.969243 PMID: 36300189

Guimarães, P., Batista, A., Zieger, M., Kaatz, M., & Koenig, K. (2020). Artificial Intelligence in Multiphoton Tomography: Atopic Dermatitis Diagnosis. *Scientific Reports*, *10*(1), 7968. DOI: 10.1038/s41598-020-64937-x PMID: 32409755

Gupta, A. K., & Srivastava, M. K. (2024). Framework for AI Adoption in Healthcare Sector: Integrated DELPHI, ISM–MICMAC Approach. *IEEE Transactions on Engineering Management*, *71*, 8116–8131. DOI: 10.1109/TEM.2024.3386580

Haghayegh, F., Norouziazad, A., Haghani, E., Feygin, A. A., Rahimi, R. H., Ghavamabadi, H. A., Sadighbayan, D., Madhoun, F., Papagelis, M., Felfeli, T., & Salahandish, R. (2024). Revolutionary Point-of-Care Wearable Diagnostics for Early Disease Detection and Biomarker Discovery through Intelligent Technologies. *Advancement of Science*, *11*(36), 2400595. DOI: 10.1002/advs.202400595 PMID: 38958517

Han, W., Wang, X., Li, L., Wichuk, S., Hutchings, E., Dadashova, R., Paschke, J., & Maksymowych, W. P. (2020). Thu0105 Isotope-Labeling-Lc-Ms-Based Metabolic Profiling Of Multiple Serum Sample Sets For The Discovery Of High-Confidence Rheumatoid Arthritis Biomarkers. *Annals of the Rheumatic Diseases*, *79*(June), 266–267. DOI: 10.1136/annrheumdis-2020-eular.5189

Hanna, M. G., Pantanowitz, L., Dash, R., Harrison, J. H., Deebajah, M., Pantanowitz, J., & Rashidi, H. H. (2025). Future of Artificial Intelligence (AI) - Machine Learning (ML) Trends in Pathology and Medicine. *Modern Pathology*, *100705*(January), 100705. DOI: 10.1016/j.modpat.2025.100705 PMID: 39761872

Haouam, K.-D., & Benmalek, M. (2024). Machine Learning Algorithms for Early Prediction of Multiple Sclerosis Progression: A Comparative Study. *Advances in Artificial Intelligence and Machine Learning*, *04*(01), 2027–2051. DOI: 10.54364/AAIML.2024.41116

Hardy, L. C., Smeekens, J. M., & Kulis, M. D. (2019). Biomarkers in food allergy immunotherapy. *Current Allergy and Asthma Reports*, *19*, 1–9.

Hasan, S. A., & Farri, O. (2019). Clinical Natural Language Processing with Deep Learning. In Consoli, S., Recupero, D. R., & Petković, M. (Eds.), *Data Science for Healthcare: Methodologies and Applications* (pp. 147–171). Springer International Publishing., DOI: 10.1007/978-3-030-05249-2_5

Hassan, M., Kushniruk, A., & Borycki, E. (2024). Barriers to and Facilitators of Artificial Intelligence Adoption in Health Care: Scoping Review. *JMIR Human Factors*, *11*(1), e48633. DOI: 10.2196/48633 PMID: 39207831

He, Z., Liu, Z., & Gong, L. (2021). Biomarker Identification and Pathway Analysis of Rheumatoid Arthritis Based on Metabolomics in Combination with Ingenuity Pathway Analysis. *Proteomics*, *21*(11–12), 2100037. DOI: 10.1002/pmic.202100037 PMID: 33969925

Ada. "Health Powered by Ada." Accessed January 20, 2025. https://ada.com/

"Healthily: Medically Verified Health Information You Need for Self-Care." n.d. Healthily. Accessed January 20, 2025. https://www.livehealthily.com/

Huang, J., Habib, A.-R., Mendis, D., Chong, J., Smith, M., Duvnjak, M., Chiu, C., Singh, N., & Wong, E. (2020). An Artificial Intelligence Algorithm That Differentiates Anterior Ethmoidal Artery Location on Sinus Computed Tomography Scans. *The Journal of Laryngology and Otology*, *134*(1), 52–55. DOI: 10.1017/S0022215119002536 PMID: 31865928

Hurault, G., Roekevisch, E., Schram, M. E., Szegedi, K., Kezic, S., Middelkamp-Hup, M. A., & Tanaka, R. J. (2022). Can serum biomarkers predict the outcome of systemic immunosuppressive therapy in adult atopic dermatitis patients? *Skin Health and Disease*, *2*(1), ski2–ski77.

Hurst, J. H., Zhao, C., Hostetler, H. P., Gorveh, M. G., Lang, J. E., & Goldstein, B. A. (2022). Environmental and Clinical Data Utility in Pediatric Asthma Exacerbation Risk Prediction Models. *BMC Medical Informatics and Decision Making*, *22*(1), 108. DOI: 10.1186/s12911-022-01847-0 PMID: 35459216

Hurvitz, N., Azmanov, H., Kesler, A., & Ilan, Y. (2021). Establishing a Second-Generation Artificial Intelligence-Based System for Improving Diagnosis, Treatment, and Monitoring of Patients with Rare Diseases. *European Journal of Human Genetics : EJHG*, *29*(10), 1485–1490. DOI: 10.1038/s41431-021-00928-4 PMID: 34276056

Iqbal, F. M., Lam, K., Joshi, M., Khan, S., Ashrafian, H., & Darzi, A. (2021). Clinical Outcomes of Digital Sensor Alerting Systems in Remote Monitoring: A Systematic Review and Meta-Analysis. *NPJ Digital Medicine*, *4*(1), 1–12. DOI: 10.1038/s41746-020-00378-0 PMID: 33420338

Izuhara, K., Nunomura, S., Nakahara, T., & Onozuka, D. (n.d.). The Search for Blood Biomarkers Useful in Treating Atopic Dermatitis Patients. *Expert Review of Clinical Pharmacology*, *0*(0), 1–10. DOI: 10.1080/17512433.2024.2438192 PMID: 39631097

Jang, H., Lee, A. C., Lee, S., & Kwon, S. (2024). Abstract 3533: Spatially Resolved Laser-Activated Cell Sorting (SLACS) and AI Integration for Enhanced Pathological Analysis and Biomarker Discovery. *Cancer Research, 84*(6, Supplement), 3533. DOI: 10.1158/1538-7445.AM2024-3533

Jeong, D. Y., Park, J., Song, H., Moon, J., Lee, T., Ahn, C., Park, S., Lee, S.-H., Ock, C.-Y., & Lee, H. Y. (2024). Abstract 4170: Artificial Intelligence (AI)-Based Multi-Modal Approach Using H&E and CT Image for Predicting Treatment Response of Immune Checkpoint Inhibitor (ICI) in Non-Small Cell Lung Cancer (NSCLC). *Cancer Research, 84*(6, Supplement), 4170. DOI: 10.1158/1538-7445.AM2024-4170

Jiao, T., Schnitzer, M. E., Forget, A., & Blais, L. (2022). Identifying Asthma Patients at High Risk of Exacerbation in a Routine Visit: A Machine Learning Model. *Respiratory Medicine, 198*(July), 106866. DOI: 10.1016/j.rmed.2022.106866 PMID: 35594754

Joshi, N., & Burlina, P. (2021). AI fairness via domain adaptation. arXiv preprint arXiv:2104.01109.

Kaladharan, S., Manayath, D., & Gopalakrishnan, R. (2024). Regulatory Challenges in AI/ML-Enabled Medical Devices: A Scoping Review and Conceptual Framework. *Journal of Medical Devices, 18*(040801), 040801. Advance online publication. DOI: 10.1115/1.4066280

Kamya, P., Ozerov, I. V., Pun, F. W., Tretina, K., Fokina, T., Chen, S., Naumov, V., Long, X., Lin, S., Korzinkin, M., Polykovskiy, D., Aliper, A., Ren, F., & Zhavoronkov, A. (2024). PandaOmics: An AI-Driven Platform for Therapeutic Target and Biomarker Discovery. *Journal of Chemical Information and Modeling, 64*(10), 3961–3969. DOI: 10.1021/acs.jcim.3c01619 PMID: 38404138

Kaplan, A., Cao, H., FitzGerald, J. M., Iannotti, N., Yang, E., Kocks, J. W. H., Kostikas, K., Price, D., Reddel, H. K., Tsiligianni, I., Vogelmeier, C. F., Pfister, P., & Mastoridis, P. (2021). Artificial Intelligence/Machine Learning in Respiratory Medicine and Potential Role in Asthma and COPD Diagnosis. *The Journal of Allergy and Clinical Immunology. In Practice, 9*(6), 2255–2261. DOI: 10.1016/j.jaip.2021.02.014 PMID: 33618053

Karachaliou, C.-E., & Livaniou, E. (2023). Immunosensors for Autoimmune-Disease-Related Biomarkers: A Literature Review. *Sensors (Basel), 23*(15), 6770. DOI: 10.3390/s23156770 PMID: 37571553

Karami, P., Gholamin, D., Fathi, F., Afsar, T., & Johari-Ahar, M. (2024). Anti-CCP Biosensors in Rheumatoid Arthritis. *Clinica Chimica Acta, 561*(July), 119767. DOI: 10.1016/j.cca.2024.119767 PMID: 38857671

Kegerreis, B., Catalina, M. D., Bachali, P., Geraci, N. S., Labonte, A. C., Zeng, C., Stearrett, N., Crandall, K. A., Lipsky, P. E., & Grammer, A. C. (2019). Machine Learning Approaches to Predict Lupus Disease Activity from Gene Expression Data. *Scientific Reports, 9*(1), 9617. DOI: 10.1038/s41598-019-45989-0 PMID: 31270349

Kelly, C. J., Karthikesalingam, A., Suleyman, M., Corrado, G., & King, D. (2019). Key Challenges for Delivering Clinical Impact with Artificial Intelligence. *BMC Medicine, 17*(1), 195. DOI: 10.1186/s12916-019-1426-2 PMID: 31665002

Khan, S., Mohan, K., Muzammil, S., Alam, M. A., & Khayyam, K. U. (2024). Current Prospects in Rheumatoid Arthritis: Pathophysiology, Genetics, and Treatments. *Recent Advances in Anti-infective Drug Discovery, 19*(1), 36–55. DOI: 10.2174/2772434418666230406083149 PMID: 37038682

Khatib, C. M., Klein-Petersen, A. W., Amalie, T. M. R., Egeberg, A., Christensen, M. O., Silverberg, J. I., Thomsen, S. F., Irvine, A. D., & Thyssen, J. P. (2024). Increased Loss-of-Function Filaggrin Gene Mutation Prevalence in Atopic Dermatitis Patients across Northern Latitudes Indicates Genetic Fitness: A Systematic Review and Meta-Analysis. *Experimental Dermatology*, *33*(7), e15130. DOI: 10.1111/exd.15130 PMID: 38989976

Klangkalya, N., Fleisher, T. A., & Rosenzweig, S. D. (2024). Diagnostic Tests for Primary Immunodeficiency Disorders: Classic and Genetic Testing. *Allergy and Asthma Proceedings*, *45*(5), 355–363. DOI: 10.2500/aap.2024.45.240051 PMID: 39294902

Klein, J., Sprague, D., Lane, M., Hart, M., Petrillo, O., do Valle, I. F., Davis, M., Ferguson, A., Allen, A., Jooss, K., & Dhanik, A. (2024). Abstract 904: AI Platform Provides an EDGE and Enables State-of-the-Art Identification of Peptide-HLAs for the Development of T Cell Inducing Vaccines. *Cancer Research*, *84*(6, Supplement), 904. DOI: 10.1158/1538-7445.AM2024-904

Koper-Lenkiewicz, O. M., Sutkowska, K., Wawrusiewicz-Kurylonek, N., Kowalewska, E., & Matowicka-Karna, J. (2022). Proinflammatory Cytokines (IL-1, -6, -8, -15, -17, -18, -23, TNF-α) Single Nucleotide Polymorphisms in Rheumatoid Arthritis—A Literature Review. *International Journal of Molecular Sciences*, *23*(4), 2106. DOI: 10.3390/ijms23042106 PMID: 35216226

Korsunskiy, I., Blyuss, O., Gordukova, M., Davydova, N., Zaikin, A., Zinovieva, N., Zimin, S., Molchanov, R., Salpagarova, A., Eremeeva, A., Filipenko, M., Prodeus, A., Korsunskiy, A., Hsu, P., & Munblit, D. (2020). Expanding TREC and KREC Utility in Primary Immunodeficiency Diseases Diagnosis. *Frontiers in Immunology*, *11*(March), 320. Advance online publication. DOI: 10.3389/fimmu.2020.00320 PMID: 32194560

Kwilinski, A., Szczepanska-Woszczyna, K., Lyulyov, O., & Pimonenko, T. (2024). Digital Public Services: Catalysts for Healthcare Efficiency. *Journal of Open Innovation*, *10*(3), 100319. DOI: 10.1016/j.joitmc.2024.100319

Laigle, L., Chadli, L., & Moingeon, P. (2023). Biomarker-Driven Development of New Therapies for Autoimmune Diseases: Current Status and Future Promises. *Expert Review of Clinical Immunology*, *19*(3), 305–314. DOI: 10.1080/1744666X.2023.2172404 PMID: 36680799

Laska, J., Tota, M., Łacwik, J., Sędek, Ł., & Gomułka, K. (2024). IL-22 in Atopic Dermatitis. *Cells*, *13*(16), 1398. DOI: 10.3390/cells13161398 PMID: 39195286

Lee, H.-S., Hong, S.-H., Kim, G.-H., You, H.-J., Lee, E.-Y., Jeong, J.-H., Ahn, J.-W., & Kim, J.-H. (2024). Generative Models Utilizing Padding Can Efficiently Integrate and Generate Multi-Omics Data. *AI*, *5*(3), 1614–1632. DOI: 10.3390/ai5030078

Lee, K. H., Song, Y., Wu, W., Yu, K., & Zhang, G. (2020). The Gut Microbiota, Environmental Factors, and Links to the Development of Food Allergy. *Clinical and Molecular Allergy : CMA*, *18*(1), 5. DOI: 10.1186/s12948-020-00120-x PMID: 32265597

Li, C., Lu, Y., & Han, X. (2022). Identification of Effective Diagnostic Biomarkers and Immune Cell Infiltration in Atopic Dermatitis by Comprehensive Bioinformatics Analysis. *Frontiers in Molecular Biosciences*, *9*(July), 917077. Advance online publication. DOI: 10.3389/fmolb.2022.917077 PMID: 35911963

Li, X., & Abangbila, L. (2024). Resistance to Medical Artificial Intelligence: Integrating AI Awareness, AI Risks, and Displacement of Responsibility. *Journal of Infrastructure, Policy and Development*, *8*(11), 7923. DOI: 10.24294/jipd.v8i11.7923

Li, Y., Ma, C., Liao, S., Qi, S., Meng, S., Cai, W., Dai, W., Cao, R., Dong, X., Krämer, B. K., Yun, C., Hocher, B., Hong, X., Liu, D., Tang, D., He, J., Yin, L., & Dai, Y. (2022). Combined Proteomics and Single Cell RNA-Sequencing Analysis to Identify Biomarkers of Disease Diagnosis and Disease Exacerbation for Systemic Lupus Erythematosus. *Frontiers in Immunology*, *13*(November), 969509. Advance online publication. DOI: 10.3389/fimmu.2022.969509 PMID: 36524113

Li, Y., Shamonin, D., Hassanzadeh, T., Reijnierse, M., Van der Helm-van Mil, A., & Stoel, B. (2023). Op0002 Exploring the Use of Artificial Intelligence in Predicting Rheumatoid Arthritis, Based on Extremity Mr Scans in Early Arthritis and Clinically Suspect Arthralgia Patients. *Annals of the Rheumatic Diseases*, *82*(Suppl 1), 1–2. DOI: 10.1136/annrheumdis-2023-eular.3531

Libon, F., Caron, J., & Nikkels, A. F. (2024). Biomarkers in Atopic Dermatitis. *Dermatology and Therapy*, *14*(7), 1729–1738. DOI: 10.1007/s13555-024-01193-1 PMID: 38874894

Liu, Y., Zhang, Y., Xie, W., Zhao, J., Dong, Y., Xu, C., Wang, Y., Li, M., Wang, G., Zhu, X., Wang, W., Lin, K., Lu, H., Han, Y., Li, L., Duan, J., Cai, S., Wang, J., & Wang, Z. (2023). IMPACT: A Web Server for Exploring Immunotherapeutic Predictive and Cancer Prognostic Biomarkers. *Clinical and Translational Medicine*, *13*(9), e1354. DOI: 10.1002/ctm2.1354 PMID: 37649319

Liu, Z., Liu, L., Weng, S., Xu, H., Xing, Z., Ren, Y., Ge, X., Wang, L., Guo, C., Li, L., Cheng, Q., Luo, P., Zhang, J., & Han, X. (2023). BEST: A Web Application for Comprehensive Biomarker Exploration on Large-Scale Data in Solid Tumors. *Journal of Big Data*, *10*(1), 165. DOI: 10.1186/s40537-023-00844-y PMID: 37193361

Long, N. P., Park, S., Anh, N. H., Min, J. E., Yoon, S. J., Kim, H. M., Nghi, T. D., Lim, D. K., Park, J. H., Lim, J., & Kwon, S. W. (2019). Efficacy of Integrating a Novel 16-Gene Biomarker Panel and Intelligence Classifiers for Differential Diagnosis of Rheumatoid Arthritis and Osteoarthritis. *Journal of Clinical Medicine*, *8*(1), 50. DOI: 10.3390/jcm8010050 PMID: 30621359

Lu, Z., Morita, M., Yeager, T. S., Lyu, Y., Wang, S. Y., Wang, Z., & Fan, G. (2024). Validation of Artificial Intelligence (AI)-Assisted Flow Cytometry Analysis for Immunological Disorders. *Diagnostics (Basel)*, *14*(4), 420. DOI: 10.3390/diagnostics14040420 PMID: 38396459

Lugogo, N. L., DePietro, M., Reich, M., Merchant, R., Chrystyn, H., Pleasants, R., Granovsky, L., Li, T., Hill, T., Brown, R. W., & Safioti, G. (2022). A Predictive Machine Learning Tool for Asthma Exacerbations: Results from a 12-Week, Open-Label Study Using an Electronic Multi-Dose Dry Powder Inhaler with Integrated Sensors. *Journal of Asthma and Allergy*, *15*(November), 1623–1637. DOI: 10.2147/JAA.S377631 PMID: 36387836

Sreenivasan, M., & Chacko, A. M. (2021). Interoperability issues in EHR systems: Research directions. Data analytics in biomedical engineering and healthcare, 13-28.

Ma, T.-T., Cao, M.-D., Yu, R.-L., Shi, H.-Y., Yan, W.-J., Liu, J.-G., Pan, C., Sun, J., Wei, Q.-Y., Wang, D.-Y., Wei, J.-F., Wang, X.-Y., & Yin, J.-S. (2020). Leukotriene A4 Hydrolase Is a Candidate Predictive Biomarker for Successful Allergen Immunotherapy. *Frontiers in Immunology*, *11*(November), 559746. Advance online publication. DOI: 10.3389/fimmu.2020.559746 PMID: 33329520

Maleki, F., Shadi, M. Y., Afshar, S., Pedrammehr, S., Lim, C. P., Jafarizadeh, A., & Asadi, H. (2024). Artificial Intelligence for Multiple Sclerosis Management Using Retinal Images: Pearl, Peaks, and Pitfalls. *Seminars in Ophthalmology*, *39*(4), 271–288. DOI: 10.1080/08820538.2023.2293030 PMID: 38088176

Mastio, J., Saeed, M. B., Wurzer, H., Krecke, M., Westerberg, L. S., & Thomas, C. (2020). Higher Incidence of B Cell Malignancies in Primary Immunodeficiencies: A Combination of Intrinsic Genomic Instability and Exocytosis Defects at the Immunological Synapse. *Frontiers in Immunology*, *11*(November), 581119. Advance online publication. DOI: 10.3389/fimmu.2020.581119 PMID: 33240268

MyTherapy. "Medication Reminder and Pill Tracker App – MyTherapy." Accessed January 20, 2025. https://www.mytherapyapp.com

Meng, L., Jiang, L., Chen, J., Ren, H., Gao, Z., Wu, F., Wen, Y., & Yang, L. (2021). Transfer RNA-derived Fragment tRF-28-QSZ34KRQ590K in Plasma Exosomes May Be a Potential Biomarker for Atopic Dermatitis in Pediatric Patients. *Experimental and Therapeutic Medicine*, *21*(5), 1–7. DOI: 10.3892/etm.2021.9920 PMID: 33790998

Meng, X.-W., Cheng, Z.-L., Lu, Z.-Y., Tan, Y.-N., Jia, X.-Y., & Zhang, M. (2022). MX2: Identification and Systematic Mechanistic Analysis of a Novel Immune-Related Biomarker for Systemic Lupus Erythematosus. *Frontiers in Immunology*, *13*(August), 978851. Advance online publication. DOI: 10.3389/fimmu.2022.978851 PMID: 36059547

Menzies-Gow, A., Mansur, A. H., & Brightling, C. E. (2020). Clinical Utility of Fractional Exhaled Nitric Oxide in Severe Asthma Management. *The European Respiratory Journal*, *55*(3), 1901633. Advance online publication. DOI: 10.1183/13993003.01633-2019 PMID: 31949116

Mijač, S., Banić, I., Genc, A.-M., Lipej, M., & Turkalj, M. (2024). The Effects of Environmental Exposure on Epigenetic Modifications in Allergic Diseases. *Medicina*, *60*(1), 110. DOI: 10.3390/medicina60010110 PMID: 38256371

Mollaei, N., Cepeda, C., Rodrigues, J., & Gamboa, H. 2025. "Biomedical Text Mining: Applicability of Machine Learning-Based Natural Language Processing in Medical Database." In, 159–66. https://www.scitepress.org/Link.aspx?doi=10.5220/0010819500003123

Muhsen, I. N., Shyr, D., Sung, A. D., & Hashmi, S. K. (2020). Machine Learning Applications in the Diagnosis of Benign and Malignant Hematological Diseases. *Clinical Hematology International*, *3*(1), 13–20. DOI: 10.2991/chi.k.201130.001 PMID: 34595462

Nakagome, K., & Nagata, M. (2024). The Possible Roles of IL-4/IL-13 in the Development of Eosinophil-Predominant Severe Asthma. *Biomolecules*, *14*(5), 546. DOI: 10.3390/biom14050546 PMID: 38785953

Namkung, J.-H., Lee, J.-E., Kim, E., Kim, H.-J., Seo, E.-Y., Jang, H.-Y., Shin, E.-S., Cho, E.-Y., & Yang, J.-M. (2011). Association of Polymorphisms in Genes Encoding IL-4, IL-13 and Their Receptors with Atopic Dermatitis in a Korean Population. *Experimental Dermatology*, *20*(11), 915–919. DOI: 10.1111/j.1600-0625.2011.01357.x PMID: 21913997

Newton, Y., Novak, A. M., Swatloski, T., McColl, D. C., Chopra, S., Graim, K., Weinstein, A. S., Baertsch, R., Salama, S. R., Ellrott, K., Chopra, M., Goldstein, T. C., Haussler, D., Morozova, O., & Stuart, J. M. (2017). TumorMap: Exploring the Molecular Similarities of Cancer Samples in an Interactive Portal. *Cancer Research*, *77*(21), e111–e114. DOI: 10.1158/0008-5472.CAN-17-0580 PMID: 29092953

Nicolaou, A., Pantzaris, M., Loizou, C. P., Kakas, A., & Pattichis, C. S. 2023. "An Explainable AI Model in the Assessment of Multiple Sclerosis Using Clinical Data and Brain MRI Lesion Texture Features *." In *2023 IEEE EMBS International Conference on Biomedical and Health Informatics (BHI)*, 1–4. DOI: 10.1109/BHI58575.2023.10313379

Noaman, N. F., Kanber, B. M., Al Smadi, A., Jiao, L., & Alsmadi, M. K. (2024). Advancing Oncology Diagnostics: AI-Enabled Early Detection of Lung Cancer Through Hybrid Histological Image Analysis. *IEEE Access : Practical Innovations, Open Solutions*, *12*, 64396–64415. DOI: 10.1109/ACCESS.2024.3397040

Oakley, A. (2023). HIPAA, HIPPA, or HIPPO: What Really Is the Heath Insurance Portability and Accountability Act? *Biotechnology Law Report*, *42*(6), 306–318. DOI: 10.1089/blr.2023.29329.aso

Ofek, E., Haj, R., Molchanov, Y., Yacobi, R., Mayer, C., Barliya, T., Gazy, I., Dvir, A., Hayun, I., Zalach, J., Paz Yaacov, N., Peled, N., Bar, J., & Barshack, I. (2023). High-Confidence AI-Based Biomarker Profiling for H&E Slides to Optimize Pathology Workflow in Lung Cancer. *Journal of Clinical Oncology*, *41*(16, suppl), e21207–e21207. DOI: 10.1200/JCO.2023.41.16_suppl.e21207

Miiskin. "Online Dermatologist | Get a Virtual Dermatology Consultation." n.d. Miiskin. Accessed January 20, 2025. https://miiskin.com/

Oualikene-Gonin, W., Jaulent, M.-C., Thierry, J.-P., Oliveira-Martins, S., Belgodère, L., Maison, P., & Ankri, J.The Scientific Advisory Board of ANSM. (2024). Artificial Intelligence Integration in the Drug Lifecycle and in Regulatory Science: Policy Implications, Challenges and Opportunities. *Frontiers in Pharmacology*, *15*(August), 1437167. Advance online publication. DOI: 10.3389/fphar.2024.1437167 PMID: 39156111

Pacillo, L., Giardino, G., Amodio, D., Giancotta, C., Rivalta, B., Rotulo, G. A., Manno, E. C., Cifaldi, C., Palumbo, G., Pignata, C., Palma, P., Rossi, P., Finocchi, A., & Cancrini, C. (2022). Targeted Treatment of Autoimmune Cytopenias in Primary Immunodeficiencies. *Frontiers in Immunology*, *13*(August), 911385. Advance online publication. DOI: 10.3389/fimmu.2022.911385 PMID: 36052091

Palm, V., Norajitra, T., von Stackelberg, O., Heussel, C. P., Skornitzke, S., Weinheimer, O., Kopytova, T., Klein, A., Almeida, S. D., Baumgartner, M., Bounias, D., Scherer, J., Kades, K., Gao, H., Jäger, P., Nolden, M., Tong, E., Eckl, K., Nattenmüller, J., & Wielpütz, M. O. (2022). AI-Supported Comprehensive Detection and Quantification of Biomarkers of Subclinical Widespread Diseases at Chest CT for Preventive Medicine. *Health Care*, *10*(11), 2166. DOI: 10.3390/healthcare10112166 PMID: 36360507

Papanastasiou, G., Scutari, M., Tachdjian, R., Hernandez-Trujillo, V., Raasch, J., Billmeyer, K., Vasilyev, N. V., & Ivanov, V. 2024. "Causal Modeling in Large-Scale Data to Improve Identification of Adults at Risk for Combined and Common Variable Immunodeficiencies." *medRxiv*. DOI: 10.1101/2024.08.08.24311672

Picard, M., Scott-Boyer, M.-P., Bodein, A., Périn, O., & Droit, A. (2021). Integration Strategies of Multi-Omics Data for Machine Learning Analysis. *Computational and Structural Biotechnology Journal*, *19*(January), 3735–3746. DOI: 10.1016/j.csbj.2021.06.030 PMID: 34285775

Poalelungi, D. G., Neagu, A. I., Fulga, A., Neagu, M., Tutunaru, D., Nechita, A., & Fulga, I. (2024). Revolutionizing Pathology with Artificial Intelligence: Innovations in Immunohistochemistry. *Journal of Personalized Medicine*, *14*(7), 693. DOI: 10.3390/jpm14070693 PMID: 39063947

Poirion, O. B., Jing, Z., Chaudhary, K., Huang, S., & Garmire, L. X. (2021). DeepProg: An Ensemble of Deep-Learning and Machine-Learning Models for Prognosis Prediction Using Multi-Omics Data. *Genome Medicine*, *13*(1), 112. DOI: 10.1186/s13073-021-00930-x PMID: 34261540

Prietl, B., Antonio Vera-Ramos, J. O. S. É., Pfeifer, V., Khalil, M., Herbsthofer, L., Sourij, H., & Pieber, T. (2023). 202-OR: Automated Cluster Analysis by Machine Learning Reveals Important Dissimilarities in the Immune Phenotype of T1D, MS, and SLE. Diabetes, 72(Supplement_1).

Qorri, B., Tsay, M. J., Leonchyk, P., Alphs, L., Pani, L., & Geraci, J. (2024). Abstract LB395: NetraAI-Driven Discovery of Novel Biomarkers in MSI-High Colon Cancer for Precision Immunotherapy. *Cancer Research*, *84*(7, Supplement), LB395. Advance online publication. DOI: 10.1158/1538-7445.AM2024-LB395

Raheem, S. S., & Alwandawi, T. (2024). The Relationship Between Human Leukocyte Antigen (HLA) and Autoimmune Diseases : Human Leukocyte Antigen (HLA) and Autoimmune Diseases. [JMOB]. *Journal of Medical and Oral Biosciences*, *1*(4), 36–43. DOI: 10.58564/jmob.66

Raikar, G. V. S., Raikar, A. S., & Somnache, S. N. (2023). Advancements in artificial intelligence and machine learning in revolutionising biomarker discovery. *Brazilian Journal of Pharmaceutical Sciences*, *59*, e23146.

Rajdan, N., Srivastava, B., & Sharma, K. (2024). Rheumatoid Arthritis: Treatments Available at Present. In *Nanotherapeutics for Inflammatory Arthritis*. CRC Press. DOI: 10.1201/9781003348672-13

Rashidi, H. H., Pantanowitz, J., Hanna, M., Tafti, A. P., Sanghani, P., Buchinsky, A., & Fennell, B.. (2025). Introduction to Artificial Intelligence (AI) and Machine Learning (ML) in Pathology & Medicine: Generative & Non-Generative AI Basics. *Modern Pathology*, *100688*(January), •••. DOI: 10.1016/j.modpat.2024.100688 PMID: 39755237

Ray, A., Das, J., & Wenzel, S. E. (2022). Determining Asthma Endotypes and Outcomes: Complementing Existing Clinical Practice with Modern Machine Learning. *Cell Reports Medicine*, *3*(12), 100857. DOI: 10.1016/j.xcrm.2022.100857 PMID: 36543110

Reddy, S. (2023). Navigating the AI Revolution: The Case for Precise Regulation in Health Care. *Journal of Medical Internet Research*, *25*(1), e49989. DOI: 10.2196/49989 PMID: 37695650

Rider, N. L., Cahill, G., Motazedi, T., Wei, L., Kurian, A., Noroski, L. M., Seeborg, F. O., Chinn, I. K., & Roberts, K. (2021). PI Prob: A Risk Prediction and Clinical Guidance System for Evaluating Patients with Recurrent Infections. *PLoS One*, *16*(2), e0237285. DOI: 10.1371/journal.pone.0237285 PMID: 33591972

Rigamonti, A., Viatore, M., Polidori, R., Erreni, M., Fumagalli, M., Rahal, D., Locati, M., Mantovani, A., & Marchesi, F. (2023). Abstract 5783: Integration of AI-Powered Digital Pathology and Imaging Mass Cytometry to Identify Relevant Features of the Tumor Microenvironment. *Cancer Research*, *83*(7, Supplement), 5783. DOI: 10.1158/1538-7445.AM2023-5783

Salah Eldin, W., & Kaboudan, A. (2023). AI-Driven Medical Imaging Platform: Advancements in Image Analysis and Healthcare Diagnosis. *Journal of the ACS Advances in Computer Science*, *14*(1), 0. Advance online publication. DOI: 10.21608/asc.2024.248278.1018

Sayers, I., John, C., Chen, J., & Hall, I. P. (2024). Genetics of Chronic Respiratory Disease. *Nature Reviews. Genetics*, *25*(8), 534–547. DOI: 10.1038/s41576-024-00695-0 PMID: 38448562

Schultes, B., Ernst, B., & Schmid, S. M. (2021). Treating Hypercholesterinemia in a Patient with Maternally Inherited Diabetes and Deafness (MIDD) by the Proprotein Convertase Subtilisin/Kexin Type 9 (PCSK9) Inhibitor Alirocumab. *Acta Diabetologica*, *58*(11), 1575–1577. DOI: 10.1007/s00592-021-01776-w PMID: 34370095

Shamji, M. H., Valenta, R., Jardetzky, T., Verhasselt, V., Durham, S. R., Würtzen, P. A., & Joost van Neerven, R. J. (2021). The Role of Allergen-Specific IgE, IgG and IgA in Allergic Disease. *Allergy*, *76*(12), 3627–3641. DOI: 10.1111/all.14908 PMID: 33999439

Silva, H. E. C. D., Santos, G. N. M., Leite, A. F., Mesquita, C. R. M., Figueiredo, P. T. D. S., Stefani, C. M., & de Melo, N. S. (2023). The use of artificial intelligence tools in cancer detection compared to the traditional diagnostic imaging methods: An overview of the systematic reviews. *PLoS One*, *18*(10), e0292063.

Silverberg, J. I., Lei, D., Yousaf, M., Janmohamed, S. R., Vakharia, P. P., Chopra, R., Chavda, R., Gabriel, S., Patel, K. R., Singam, V., Kantor, R., & Hsu, D. Y. (2021). What Are the Best Endpoints for Eczema Area and Severity Index and Scoring Atopic Dermatitis in Clinical Practice? A Prospective Observational Study*. *British Journal of Dermatology*, *184*(5), 888–895. DOI: 10.1111/bjd.19457 PMID: 32959390

Simon, A. J., Golan, A. C., Lev, A., Stauber, T., Barel, O., Somekh, I., Klein, C., AbuZaitun, O., Eyal, E., Kol, N., Unal, E., Amariglio, N., Rechavi, G., & Somech, R. (2020). Whole Exome Sequencing (WES) Approach for Diagnosing Primary Immunodeficiencies (PIDs) in a Highly Consanguineous Community. *Clinical Immunology (Orlando, Fla.)*, *214*(May), 108376. DOI: 10.1016/j.clim.2020.108376 PMID: 32135276

Singh, A., Jha, S. K., Dwivedi, P. C., Srivastava, U., & Pal, A. (2024). Revolutionizing Healthcare: Integrating Electronics, AI, Traditional, and Conventional Methods. *World Journal of Advanced Research and Reviews*, *23*(3), 2426–2434. DOI: 10.30574/wjarr.2024.23.3.2919

Siva Balan, R. V. (2024). Diagnosis of Multiple Sclerosis Lesion Using Deep Learning Models. *Journal of Electrical Systems*, *20*(3), 2354–2367. DOI: 10.52783/jes.4082

SkinVision. SkinVision | Skin Cancer Melanoma Detection App | SkinVision. Accessed January 20, 2025. https://www.skinvision.com

Sundarraj, P. (2024). Artificial Intelligence in Advance Angiogenesis and Inflammation Research: A Breakthrough in Disease Prediction and Therapy. *Journal of Angiotherapy*, *8*(9), 1–8. DOI: 10.25163/angiotherapy.899861

Suprun, M., Getts, R., Raghunathan, R., Grishina, G., Witmer, M., Gimenez, G., Sampson, H. A., & Suárez-Fariñas, M. (2019). Novel Bead-Based Epitope Assay Is a Sensitive and Reliable Tool for Profiling Epitope-Specific Antibody Repertoire in Food Allergy. *Scientific Reports*, *9*(1), 18425. DOI: 10.1038/s41598-019-54868-7 PMID: 31804555

Suratannon, N., van Wijck, R. T. A., Broer, L., Xue, L., van Meurs, J. B. J., Barendregt, B. H., van der Burg, M., Dik, W. A., Chatchatee, P., Langerak, A. W., Swagemakers, S. M. A., Goos, J. A. C., Mathijssen, I. M. J., Dalm, V. A. S. H., Suphapeetiporn, K., Heezen, K. C., Drabwell, J., Uitterlinden, A. G., van der Spek, P. J., & van Hagen, P. M. (2020). Rapid Low-Cost Microarray-Based Genotyping for Genetic Screening in Primary Immunodeficiency. *Frontiers in Immunology*, *11*(April), 614. Advance online publication. DOI: 10.3389/fimmu.2020.00614 PMID: 32373116

Sutanto, H., & Yuliasih, Y. (2023). Disentangling the Pathogenesis of Systemic Lupus Erythematosus: Close Ties between Immunological, Genetic and Environmental Factors. *Medicina*, *59*(6), 1033. DOI: 10.3390/medicina59061033 PMID: 37374237

Symptomate. "Symptomate – Check Your Symptoms Online." Accessed January 20, 2025. https://symptomate.com/

Tang, C., Fang, M., Tan, G., Zhang, S., Yang, B., Li, Y., Zhang, T., Saxena, R., Mohan, C., & Wu, T. (2022). Discovery of Novel Circulating Immune Complexes in Lupus Nephritis Using Immunoproteomics. *Frontiers in Immunology*, *13*(March), 850015. Advance online publication. DOI: 10.3389/fimmu.2022.850015 PMID: 35419005

Tanvir, R. B., Islam, M. M., Sobhan, M., Luo, D., & Mondal, A. M. (2023). "MOGAT: An Improved Multi-Omics Integration Framework Using Graph Attention Networks." *bioRxiv*. DOI: 10.1101/2023.04.01.535195

Tavazzi, E., Zivadinov, R., Dwyer, M. G., Jakimovski, D., Singhal, T., Weinstock-Guttman, B., & Bergsland, N. (2020). MRI Biomarkers of Disease Progression and Conversion to Secondary-Progressive Multiple Sclerosis. *Expert Review of Neurotherapeutics*, *20*(8), 821–834. DOI: 10.1080/14737175.2020.1757435 PMID: 32306772

Tian, J., Zhang, D., Yang, Y., Huang, Y., Wang, L., Yao, X., & Lu, Q. (2024). Global Epidemiology of Atopic Dermatitis: A Comprehensive Systematic Analysis and Modelling Study. *British Journal of Dermatology*, *190*(1), 55–61. DOI: 10.1093/bjd/ljad339 PMID: 37705227

Tsang, K. C. H., Pinnock, H., Wilson, A. M., Salvi, D., & Shah, S. A. (2022). Predicting Asthma Attacks Using Connected Mobile Devices and Machine Learning: The AAMOS-00 Observational Study Protocol. *BMJ Open*, *12*(10), e064166. DOI: 10.1136/bmjopen-2022-064166 PMID: 36192103

Vasiliev, Y. A., Александрович, В. Ю., Vasiliev, Y. A., Vlazimirsky, A. V., Вячеславович, В. А., Vlazimirsky, A. V., & Omelyanskaya, O. V.. (2023). Methodology for Testing and Monitoring Artificial Intelligence-Based Software for Medical Diagnostics. *Digital Diagnostics*, *4*(3), 252–267. DOI: 10.17816/DD321971

Vetchinkina, E. A., Mikhaylenko, D. S., Kuznetsova, E. B., Deryagina, T. A., Alekseeva, E. A., Bure, I. V., Zamyatnin, A. A.Jr, & Nemtsova, M. V. (2021). Genetic Factors of Predisposition and Clinical Characteristics of Rheumatoid Arthritis in Russian Patients. *Journal of Personalized Medicine*, *11*(6), 469. DOI: 10.3390/jpm11060469 PMID: 34070522

Viswanathan, J., Saranya, N., & Inbamani, A. (2021). Deep learning applications in medical imaging: Introduction to deep learning-based intelligent systems for medical applications. In *Deep Learning Applications in Medical Imaging* (pp. 156–177). IGI Global.

Wang, W., Zhang, X., & Dai, D.-Q. (2021). DeFusion: A Denoised Network Regularization Framework for Multi-Omics Integration. *Briefings in Bioinformatics*, *22*(5), bbab057. Advance online publication. DOI: 10.1093/bib/bbab057 PMID: 33822879

Wang, Y., Liu, H., Fu, Y., Kao, W., Ji, Y., Liu, X., Mu, F., Wu, J., Li, X., & Meng, C. (2019). Novel Biomarkers Containing Citrullinated Peptides for Diagnosis of Systemic Lupus Erythematosus Using Protein Microarrays. *Clinical and Experimental Rheumatology*, *6*, 929–936. PMID: 30789148

Wang, Y., & Ma, Z. (2025). Ethical and Legal Challenges of Medical AI on Informed Consent: China as an Example. *Developing World Bioethics*, *25*(1), 46–54. DOI: 10.1111/dewb.12442 PMID: 38240080

Wen, J., Zhang, Z., Lan, Y., Cui, Z., Cai, J., & Zhang, W. (2023). A Survey on Federated Learning: Challenges and Applications. *International Journal of Machine Learning and Cybernetics*, *14*(2), 513–535. DOI: 10.1007/s13042-022-01647-y PMID: 36407495

Westermann-Clark, E., Meehan, C. A., Meyer, A. K., Dasso, J. F., Amre, D., Ellison, M., Patel, B., Betensky, M., Hauk, C. I., Mayer, J., Metts, J., Leiding, J. W., Sriaroon, P., Kumar, A., Ayala, I., & Walter, J. E. (2021). Primary Immunodeficiency in Children With Autoimmune Cytopenias: Retrospective 154-Patient Cohort. *Frontiers in Immunology*, *12*(April), 649182. Advance online publication. DOI: 10.3389/fimmu.2021.649182 PMID: 33968040

Wojtara, M., Rana, E., Rahman, T., Khanna, P., & Singh, H. (2023). Artificial Intelligence in Rare Disease Diagnosis and Treatment. *Clinical and Translational Science*, *16*(11), 2106–2111. DOI: 10.1111/cts.13619 PMID: 37646577

Wu, J., & Lin, D. (2021). A Review of Artificial Intelligence in Precise Assessment of Programmed Cell Death-Ligand 1 and Tumor-Infiltrating Lymphocytes in Non−Small Cell Lung Cancer. *Advances in Anatomic Pathology*, *28*(6), 439–445. DOI: 10.1097/PAP.0000000000000322 PMID: 34623343

Wu, Y., Gu, C., Wang, S., Yin, H., Qiu, Z., Luo, Y., Li, Z., Wang, C., Yao, X., & Li, W. (2023). Serum Biomarker-Based Endotypes of Atopic Dermatitis in China and Prediction for Efficacy of Dupilumab. *British Journal of Dermatology*, *188*(5), 649–660. DOI: 10.1093/bjd/ljad032 PMID: 36756674

Wu, Y., & Xie, L. (2024). "AI-Driven Multi-Omics Integration for Multi-Scale Predictive Modeling of Causal Genotype-Environment-Phenotype Relationships." arXiv. https://doi.org//arXiv.2407.06405 .DOI: 10.48550

Xu, Z., Wang, X., Zeng, S., Ren, X., Yan, Y., & Gong, Z. (2021). Applying Artificial Intelligence for Cancer Immunotherapy. *Acta Pharmaceutica Sinica. B*, *11*(11), 3393–3405. DOI: 10.1016/j.apsb.2021.02.007 PMID: 34900525

Yu, L., & Li, L. (2022). Potential Biomarkers of Atopic Dermatitis. *Frontiers in Medicine*, *9*(November), 1028694. Advance online publication. DOI: 10.3389/fmed.2022.1028694 PMID: 36465933

Zahraei, P. S., & Shakeri, Z. (2024). "Detecting Bias and Enhancing Diagnostic Accuracy in Large Language Models for Healthcare." arXiv. https://doi.org//arXiv.2410.06566.DOI: 10.48550

Zarubin, D., Belotskiy, V., Xiang, Z., Varlamova, A., Ovcharov, P., Galkin, I., Polyakova, M., Svekolkin, V., Perelman, G., Bruttan, M., Brown, J. H., Postovalova, E., Bagaev, A., & Fowler, N. (2022). A Clinical AI-Driven Multiplex Immunofluorescence Imaging Pipeline to Characterize Tumor Microenvironment Heterogeneity. *Journal of Clinical Oncology*, *40*(16, suppl), 3020–3020. DOI: 10.1200/JCO.2022.40.16_suppl.3020

Zeb, S., Fnu, N., Abbasi, N., & Fahad, M. (2024). AI in Healthcare: Revolutionizing Diagnosis and Therapy. *International Journal of Multidisciplinary Sciences and Arts*, *3*(3), 118–128. DOI: 10.47709/ijmdsa.v3i3.4546

Zhang, Y., Joly, R., Beecy, A. N., Principe, S., Satpathy, S., Gore, A., & Reilly, T.. (2024). Implementation of a Machine Learning Risk Prediction Model for Postpartum Depression in the Electronic Health Records. *AMIA Joint Summits on Translational Science Proceedings AMIA Summit on Translational Science*, *2024*(October), 1057–1066. PMID: 39444417

Zhao, C., Zhang, R., Luo, Y., Liu, S., Tang, T., Yang, F., Zhu, L., He, X., Yang, M., & Jiang, Y. (2020). Multimodal VEGF-Targeted Contrast-Enhanced Ultrasound and Photoacoustic Imaging of Rats with Inflammatory Arthritis: Using Dye-VEGF-Antibody-Loaded Microbubbles. *Ultrasound in Medicine & Biology*, *46*(9), 2400–2411. DOI: 10.1016/j.ultrasmedbio.2020.05.007 PMID: 32522458

Zhao, Y., Healy, B. C., Rotstein, D., Guttmann, C. R. G., Bakshi, R., Weiner, H. L., Brodley, C. E., & Chitnis, T. 2017. "Exploration of Machine Learning Techniques in Predicting Multiple Sclerosis Disease Course." Edited by Sreeram V. Ramagopalan. *PLOS ONE* 12 (4): e0174866. DOI: 10.1371/journal.pone.0174866

Zhao, Y., Qi, Y., Liu, X., Cui, Y., & Zhao, Z. (2022). Efficiency of Disease and Disease Activity Diagnosis Models of Systemic Lupus Erythematosus Based on Protein Array Analysis. *Journal of Immunology Research*, *1830431*(1), 1–14. DOI: 10.1155/2022/1830431 PMID: 35966818

Zhong, Y., Zhang, W., Hong, X., Zeng, Z., Chen, Y., Liao, S., Cai, W., Xu, Y., Wang, G., Liu, D., Tang, D., & Dai, Y. (2022). Screening Biomarkers for Systemic Lupus Erythematosus Based on Machine Learning and Exploring Their Expression Correlations With the Ratios of Various Immune Cells. *Frontiers in Immunology*, *13*(June), 873787. Advance online publication. DOI: 10.3389/fimmu.2022.873787 PMID: 35757721

Chapter 4
AI Technologies for Predicting Susceptibility and Outcomes of Immunological Disorders

R. Keerthana
https://orcid.org/0009-0001-4898-4075
K.S.R. College of Engineering, India

S. Savitha
https://orcid.org/0000-0002-4914-8386
K.S.R. College of Engineering, India

K. Logeswaran
https://orcid.org/0000-0001-8161-7376
Kongu Engineering College, India

A. Rajivkannan
K.S.R. College of Engineering, India

M. Namasivayam
https://orcid.org/0000-0002-7215-272X
K.S.R. College of Engineering, India

ABSTRACT

AI improves immune disease prediction by examining clinical and genomic information to determine biomarkers, enhance diagnoses, individualize treatment, and predict outcomes. Challenges include scarce high-quality data, integrating genomic and environmental variables, privacy legislation, bias, and deep learning transparency lowering clinician confidence. Federated learning maintains privacy but grapples with data quality, and explainable AI (XAI) assists interpretability but remains clinically irrelevant. SVMs, RF, CNNs, and RNNs are AI models that help in disease tracking and diagnosis. Clustering and Bayesian networks evaluate risks. Maximizing the potential of AI requires enhancing data quality, model interpretability, and clinician-data scientist collaboration to improve immunological disorder prediction.

DOI: 10.4018/979-8-3693-9725-1.ch004

1. INTRODUCTION TO AI IN IMMUNOLOGY

Artificial Intelligence (AI) is revolutionizing the prediction of susceptibility and outcomes in immunological diseases by processing large volumes of clinical, genomic, and biomarker data. Machine learning algorithms detect patterns in immune system function, allowing for early disease detection and risk prediction (Smith & Lee, 2021). These AI-based insights assist in diagnosing autoimmune diseases, allergies, and immunodeficiency disorders with increased accuracy and efficiency. AI technologies also augment treatment approaches by individualizing immunotherapy and streamlining drug discovery.

1.1 Literature Survey

Savitha et.al, 2025 highlights that Artificial intelligence has transformed immunology through the improvement of disease forecasting, biomarker identification, and personalized treatment approaches. Deep learning algorithms examine immune reactions, machine learning forecasts the risk of autoimmune diseases, and AI-based multi-omics integration enhances diagnosis. Artificial intelligence encounters challenges of biased data sets, non-interpretable results, regulatory issues, and difficulty in clinical uptake.

Deep learning models process medical imaging, and predictive analytics evaluate patient reactions to immunomodulatory therapies. Through the combination of AI with electronic health records (EHRs) and multi-omics data, healthcare professionals can make data-driven decisions, enhancing disease control and patient care (Kim & Cho, 2021). Though it has progressed, AI in immunology also has its shortcomings, including data bias, privacy issues, and the requirement of more interpretable models. Mitigating these drawbacks through responsible AI development and interaction between clinicians and data scientists is important. As AI evolves further, it has great potential to transform immunological studies and clinical care into more accurate and anticipatory healthcare interventions (Shrikaant Kulkarni.,et.al, 2023).

Abu-Shanab et.al, 2020 discuss the application of AI in the diagnosis of infectious diseases and outbreak prediction. The research focuses on machine learning and deep learning models applied to early detection, epidemiological forecasting, and response to outbreaks. It highlights the ability of AI to handle large amounts of data, such as clinical history and environmental variables, to enhance disease surveillance. The authors touch on issues like data quality, AI model bias, and clinical validation requirements. The authors conclude that although AI improves infectious disease management, its integration into public health frameworks needs more research.

Stephen et.al, 2020 offer a detailed review of basic immunology concepts and their translation into clinical practice. The work delves into critical immune system elements, which involve innate and adaptive immunity, cytokine signaling, and immune tolerance. It touches on recent progress in immunotherapy, for instance, monoclonal antibodies and checkpoint inhibitors, for the management of autoimmune disorders and cancers. The authors offer insights into upcoming issues in immunological research, which include individualized treatment approaches and identification of biomarkers. The article emphasizes the need to merge immunological understanding with AI-based strategies for enhanced diagnostics and therapeutic interventions.

1.2 Role of AI in Drug Discovery and Immunotherapy Development

AI speeds up drug discovery through the analysis of biological data, the prediction of drug-target interactions, and the optimization of immunotherapy candidates. AI-based methods allow for accurate molecular docking, biomarker discovery, and drug repurposing, which shortens the time and cost of drug development.

Key Contributions of AI in Drug Discovery

- **Target Identification and Validation**: AI identifies promising drug targets by analyzing genomic and proteomic data.
- **Molecular Docking and Simulation**: AI predicts drug molecule interactions to optimize binding efficiency.
- **Drug Repurposing**: AI models evaluate existing drugs for potential immunotherapy applications.
- **Biomarker Discovery**: AI enhances the identification of biomarkers for predicting treatment responses.

Examples:

- DeepMind's AlphaFold predicts protein structures, aiding in immunotherapy design.
- Benevolent AI mines biomedical literature to discover new drug candidates.
- IBM Watson for Drug Discovery identifies cancer immunotherapy targets.
- BioNTech and Moderna leverage AI for mRNA vaccine development, enabling AI-powered cancer vaccines.

1.3. Overview of Immunological Disorders

Immunological disorders involve a wide range of conditions affecting the immune system and causing a distorted immune response. Immunological disorders can be classified into three main categories:

1.**Autoimmune Diseases** – These occur when the immune system mistakenly attacks the body's own cells and tissues. Examples include:

- **Rheumatoid Arthritis (RA):** A chronic inflammatory disorder affecting joints.
- **Systemic Lupus Erythematosus (SLE):** A multisystem autoimmune disease with widespread inflammation.
- **Type 1 Diabetes (T1D):** An autoimmune attack on insulin-producing beta cells in the pancreas.

1. **Allergic Diseases** – These result from hypersensitive immune reactions to normally harmless substances (allergens). Examples include:
    - **Asthma:** Chronic airway inflammation triggered by allergens or irritants.
    - **Anaphylaxis:** A severe, life-threatening allergic reaction.
    - **Atopic Dermatitis and Food Allergies:** Immune overreactions to environmental or dietary substances.

2. **Immune Deficiency Disorders** – These conditions arise from a weakened or malfunctioning immune system, making individuals more susceptible to infections. Examples include:
   - **Primary Immunodeficiency Disorders (PIDs):** Genetic disorders affecting immune function (e.g., Severe Combined Immunodeficiency - SCID).
   - **Acquired Immunodeficiency's:** Conditions like HIV/AIDS that weaken the immune system over time.

1.4 Importance of Early Prediction and Outcome Assessment

Early detection and outcome assessment are crucial in immunological disorders for several reasons:

- **Improved Patient Prognosis:** Early diagnosis allows for timely interventions, reducing complications and slowing disease progression.
- **Personalized Treatment Plans:** Predicting susceptibility helps tailor treatments to individual patients, optimizing therapeutic outcomes.
- **Prevention of Severe Manifestations:** Identifying at-risk individuals enables preventive measures, such as lifestyle modifications or early administration of immunomodulatory drugs.
- **Reduced Healthcare Burden:** Early prediction minimizes hospitalizations, long-term disability, and healthcare costs by initiating appropriate interventions at an early stage.
- **Better Disease Management:** AI-driven risk assessment can help stratify patients into different risk groups, ensuring targeted and efficient healthcare delivery.

Artificial Intelligence is transforming the field of immunology by enhancing disease prediction, diagnosis, and therapy. AI tools improve immunological research and clinical applications in the following ways:

- **Machine Learning (ML) Algorithms:** AI models analyze genetic, proteomic, and biomarker data to predict susceptibility to diseases like lupus or multiple sclerosis.
- **Deep Learning for Imaging:** AI-powered image recognition detects early signs of autoimmune disorders in medical imaging (e.g., joint inflammation in RA using MRI scans).
- **Natural Language Processing (NLP):** AI processes electronic health records (EHRs) to identify early symptoms and risk factors.
- **Predictive Analytics for Immunotherapy Response:** AI models predict how patients will respond to biologics or immunosuppressive drugs, leading to precision medicine.
- **Drug Discovery:** AI accelerates the development of immunomodulatory drugs by analyzing vast datasets to identify potential therapeutic targets.
- **Adaptive Clinical Trials:** AI-driven models optimize clinical trial designs, ensuring faster and more efficient testing of new therapies.

1.5. AI in Personalized Medicine and Treatment Optimization

AI is transforming personalized medicine by utilizing patient-specific genetic, molecular, and clinical information to tailor treatment for enhanced efficacy. Machine learning and deep learning algorithms process enormous datasets to find disease biomarkers, forecast disease progression, and suggest targeted therapies based on an individual's distinctive biological profile (Gao & Li, 2020). This strategy is most effective in oncology, autoimmune conditions, and infectious diseases, where precision medicine maximizes treatment outcomes. AI-based models also aid in predicting drug response, allowing adaptive treatment plans that respond dynamically to real-time patient data. This reduces side effects while optimizing therapeutic effect. AI-based clinical decision support systems (CDSS) also aid clinicians in selecting the most appropriate interventions by combining medical history, imaging, and lab data. By streamlining treatment protocols, AI not only improves patient care but also speeds up drug development and decreases healthcare expenses, making precision medicine more affordable and efficient (Rajan & Mehta, 2020).

AI adoption in immunology faces regulatory hurdles, integration issues with existing clinical workflows, and the need for clinician trust in AI-driven insights. Real-world deployment requires standardized protocols, ethical AI governance, and extensive validation in diverse patient populations. Rigorous validation of AI models in immunology is necessary to ensure reliability, generalizability, and reproducibility across different datasets and patient demographics.

External benchmarking, real-world clinical trials, and explainability techniques are essential for regulatory approval and physician acceptance. AI enhances precision immunotherapy by predicting patient-specific immune responses, optimizing treatment strategies, and identifying novel therapeutic targets. Machine learning models can analyze biomarkers, genetic profiles, and immune system interactions to personalize cancer immunotherapy and autoimmune disease treatments (Thangarasan.,et.al., 2022).

1.6. AI in Immunological Research

AI is transforming immunological research by combining multi-omics data genomics, transcriptomics, and proteomics to reveal disease mechanisms and biomarkers for precision medicine. Machine learning algorithms examine immune responses, forecast treatment outcomes, and enable personalized immunotherapy (DeepMind, 2021). In epidemiology, predictive modeling using AI assists in monitoring disease outbreaks, evaluating environmental impacts on allergies, and improving public health surveillance. With the help of massive datasets and sophisticated algorithms, AI expedites drug discovery, enhances vaccine development, and deepens our knowledge of immune system dynamics, setting the stage for more effective treatments and diagnostics (Moderna, 2021).

1.6.1. Multi-Omics Integration

AI is essential in the integration of multi-omics data, such as genomics, transcriptomics, proteomics, metabolomics, and epigenomics. This holistic strategy aids in the discovery of new disease mechanisms, biomarker identification, and treatment response prediction (Watson & Anderson, 2022).

- **Genomics:** Machine learning-based algorithms examine big-data genomic sequencing data to identify genetic mutations, single nucleotide polymorphisms (SNPs), and structural variations associated with immune diseases like autoimmune disorders and cancer.
- **Transcriptomics:** From an analysis of the RNA patterns of expression, AI determines various differently expressed genes (DEGs) that have involvement in activation of the immune system, inflammation, and the pathogenesis of a disease. Techniques in Natural Language Processing are even employed in analysis of the literature and gathering outcomes of independent investigations.

- **Proteomics:** Machine learning algorithms analyze mass spectrometry and protein interaction data to chart immune cell signaling networks, identify immune system dysregulation, and discover therapeutic targets for diseases such as rheumatoid arthritis, multiple sclerosis, and immunodeficiencies.
- **Metabolomics & Epigenomics:** Computational models based on AI assist in the comprehension of metabolic alterations and epigenetic changes that affect immune responses. This supports precision medicine by individualizing treatments according to personal molecular profiles (White & Green, 2021).

1.6.2. AI-Powered Epidemiology

Artificial intelligence is transforming the field of epidemiology as it allows for predictive modeling of disease outbreaks, estimation of risk factors, and elucidation of environmental and genetic interactions on immune disorders.

- **Predictive Disease Modeling:** AI models use past health data, climate information, and socioeconomic variables to forecast disease outbreaks, including influenza, COVID-19, and allergic diseases.
- **Influence of Environment on Allergies:** AI assesses pollution levels, temperature fluctuation, humidity, and exposure to allergens to identify correlations between environmental trends and the incidence of allergies. This assists in predicting allergy seasons and recommending health interventions.
- **Public Health Surveillance:** AI-based systems scan social media trends, real-time health reports, and wearable sensor data to identify early warning signs of disease outbreaks, allowing proactive interventions to curb their spread.
- **Immunotherapy:** AI combines epidemiological information with patient-specific immune reactions to create tailored treatment plans for immunotherapy in diseases such as cancer, asthma, and autoimmune disorders.

2. AI TECHNIQUES IN IMMUNOLOGICAL DISORDER PREDICTION

The AI Utilization to forecast immunological diseases is reshaping early disease detection, disease risk assessment, and tailored therapies. AI algorithms, especially ML and deep neural models, decipher sophisticated immunologic information, identify hidden patterns, and enhance healthcare decisions. Major AI methods and feature engineering methodology adopted in disease forecasting are detailed below.

Figure 1. AI techniques in immunological disorder prediction

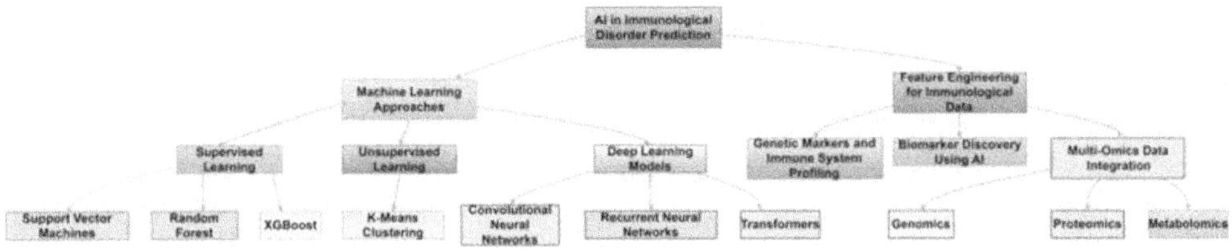

2.1 Machine Learning (ML) Approaches

Machine learning employs algorithms through which computers learn from data and predict outcomes. In immunology, ML enables us to detect patterns in immune system data in order to forecast disorders (Patel & Sharma, 2022).. Below are the key types of ML strategies:

2.1.1. Supervised Learning

Supervised learning, the computer is taught from labelled data (data for which we already have the outcomes). The algorithm becomes aware of the connection between inputs (e.g., genetic information or biomarkers) and outputs (e.g., whether someone has an immune disorder) (Banerjee & Patel, 2022).

Examples:

- **Support Vector Machines (SVM)**: A powerful tool for classification tasks, like distinguishing between healthy and diseased immune systems.
- **Random Forest**: Uses multiple decision trees to make predictions. It's like asking a group of experts for advice and using the most common answer.
- **XGBoost**: A popular technique for making predictions based on structured data. It helps boost the accuracy of predictions.

2.1.2. Unsupervised Learning

Unsupervised learning, the computer is provided with data with unlabeled outcomes. The aim is to discover hidden structures or patterns within the data(Thomas & Evans, 2023)..

Example: **Clustering Techniques** (like K-means): These methods group similar data together. For example, it might help identify patterns in immune system responses that lead to disorders, even if we don't know what those patterns are in advance.

2.2. Deep Learning Models

Deep learning is a more advanced form of machine learning that uses neural networks with many layers. It's great for analysing complex data, such as images, genetic sequences, or protein structures (Smith & Lee, 2021).

Examples:

- **Convolutional Neural Networks (CNNs)**: These are particularly good at analysing images or data with a grid-like structure (e.g., scans of tissue samples or gene sequences).
- **Recurrent Neural Networks (RNNs)**: These are used for analysing sequential data, like gene expression over time or patient health data in a time series.
- **Transformers**: A newer and highly efficient model, especially useful for processing long sequences of data, like DNA sequences, and understanding the context in which different genes or proteins interact.

2.3. Feature Engineering for Immunological Data

Feature engineering involves choosing, changing, or constructing new features (data attributes) that will aid AI models to make better predictions. For immunological disorders, this is most important because data tends to be complex and high-dimensional. Consider some significant features for immunological prediction(Gao & Li, 2020)

1.**Genetic Markers and Immune System Profiling**

- Genetic markers are particular genes or mutations associated with immune disorders. By characterizing an individual's immune system (e.g., by blood tests or genetic tests), we can determine which markers or gene expressions are correlated with a higher risk of developing an immune-related disorder.

2.Biomarker Discovery Using AI

- Biomarkers are biological markers (such as proteins or enzymes) that can indicate the existence of a disease. AI can be applied to search through enormous volumes of biological information (such as blood samples) to identify new biomarkers for autoimmune diseases or allergies, allowing physicians to diagnose patients sooner.

3.Multi-Omics Data Integration

- The term "multi-omics" refers to integrating different layers of biological data, such as:
  - **Genomics**: Information from a person's genes and DNA.
  - **Proteomics**: Data about the proteins produced in the body, which are crucial in immune responses.
  - **Metabolomics**: Data on metabolites, which are chemicals involved in metabolism that can indicate disease states.

2.4. AI-Based Treatment Optimization Algorithm

AI-based treatment optimization algorithms apply machine learning and reinforcement learning methods to tailor treatments to specific patients(Johnson & Peters, 2020).. The following is a general algorithm that integrates patient information, predictive modeling, and optimization methods.

Algorithm: AI-Based Treatment Optimization

Input:

- Patient medical history P
- Genetic, molecular, and clinical data D

- Available treatments T={T1,T2,...,Tn}
- Treatment efficacy model E(T)
- Cost function C(T) (including side effects, financial cost, etc.)
- Regularization parameter λ

Output:

Optimized treatment plan T*

Steps:

1. Data Preprocessing:
   - Collect patient-specific data D, including genomic, proteomic, and clinical parameters.
   - Normalize and encode features for AI models.
2. Predictive Modeling:
   - Use machine learning models (e.g., Random Forest, Neural Networks) to predict treatment efficacy E(T) for each available option.
   - Compute potential side effects and patient-specific risks using statistical models.
3. Optimization Function:
   - Define the objective function:$T^{*} = \textit{arg max\_}T[E(T) - \lambda \cdot C(T)]$
   - Apply reinforcement learning (e.g., Q-learning, Deep Q Networks) or Bayesian optimization to iteratively improve treatment recommendations.
4. Adaptive Learning:
   - Monitor real-time patient response to the selected treatment T^{*}
   - Update the AI model with feedback (e.g., biomarker changes, side effect occurrence).
5. Decision Support & Recommendation:
   - Rank treatments based on predicted efficacy and patient compatibility.
   - Provide recommendations to healthcare professionals for final decision-making.
6. Continuous Improvement:
   - Integrate new patient data to refine future treatment predictions.
   - Use federated learning techniques to update AI models across multiple hospitals while maintaining patient privacy(Shrikaant Kulkarni.,et.al, 2023)..

3. AI-BASED RISK ASSESSMENT AND SUSCEPTIBILITY PREDICTION

The application of Artificial Intelligence in medicine has transformed disease prediction, risk evaluation, and tailored treatment. AI-based models provide substantial improvements in the identification of susceptibility to immune disorders, genetic predisposition analysis, and disease epidemiology modeling. This chapter discusses how AI-based technologies assist in risk evaluation and susceptibility prediction, laying the groundwork for early detection and prevention.

3.1 AI Models for Predicting Individual Susceptibility to Immune Disorders

Immune disorders such as autoimmune disorders, allergies, and immunodeficiency afflict millions across the globe. They occur as a result of intricate interactions among genetic, environmental, and lifestyle factors. Foretelling one's risk of immune disorders is important in initiating early intervention, targeted therapy, and preventive care. Artificial intelligence models, more specifically machine learning and deep learning techniques, have transformed disease prediction through the processing of enormous quantities of genomic, clinical, and environmental information (Sun & Zhou, 2022). AI models improve risk assessment by detecting patterns that may not be detectable by conventional statistical means (Qian & Wu, 2023).

3.1.1 Role of AI in Disease Prediction

AI employs machine learning and deep learning techniques to analyze vast datasets, identifying patterns and correlations that may not be evident through traditional methods. By leveraging AI algorithms, healthcare professionals can predict an individual's likelihood of developing immune-related diseases based on genetic, environmental, and lifestyle factors.

3.1.2 Machine Learning Techniques in Immune Disorder Prediction

- Supervised Learning: Utilized for classification tasks, such as differentiating between high-risk and low-risk individuals.
- Unsupervised Learning: Helps in discovering unknown disease subtypes and clustering similar patient profiles.
- Reinforcement Learning: Optimizes decision-making processes for risk assessment.

3.1.3. Biomarkers and Clinical Data Utilization

AI models integrate multiple sources of patient data, including:

- Genetic Markers

Genetic markers are specific DNA sequences that help identify variations associated with disease susceptibility, drug response, and immune system function. These markers, including single nucleotide polymorphisms (SNPs) and copy number variations (CNVs), play a crucial role in precision medicine by enabling early diagnosis and targeted treatments. AI-driven genomic analysis allows researchers to identify genetic predispositions to autoimmune diseases, cancers, and infectious diseases, helping personalize therapies based on an individual's genetic makeup. By integrating genetic markers with multi-omics data, researchers can improve risk assessment, drug efficacy predictions, and treatment personalization (Zhang & Wang, 2021)

Figure 2. Genetic markers

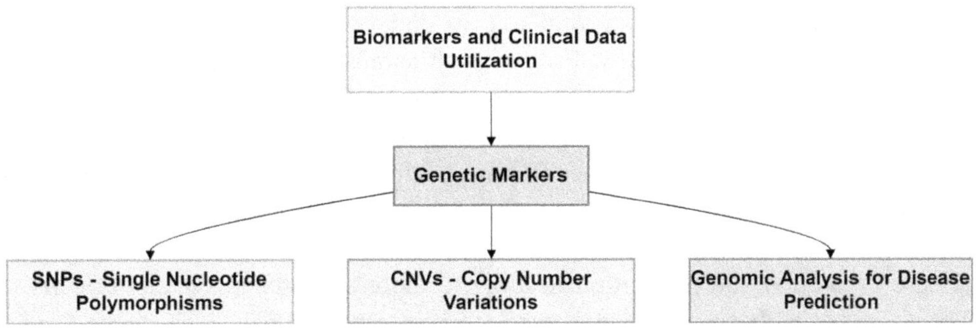

- **Immunological Biomarkers**

Immunological biomarkers are quantifiable markers of immune system function, employed to identify, diagnose, and track diseases. They encompass cytokines, chemokines, antibodies, and immune cell subsets, which are useful in the understanding of conditions like autoimmune diseases, infections, and cancer. AI-based biomarker analysis improves early disease detection and treatment optimization through the identification of aberrant immune responses. For instance, in cancer immunotherapy, biomarkers such as PD-L1 expression and T-cell activation levels predict patient response to checkpoint inhibitors (Watson & Anderson, 2022). Machine learning combined with biomarker data facilitates precision medicine strategies, allowing for more efficient and personalized treatment plans.

- **Electronic Health Records (EHR)**

Electronic Health Records (EHR) hold rich patient data on medical history, diagnostic results, prescriptions, and treatment outcomes. AI-driven analysis of EHR data reveals disease progression patterns, streamlines treatment plans, and improves predictive models (Qian & Wu, 2023). Machine learning algorithms analyze massive EHR databases to suggest patient-specific interventions, identify early indications of chronic disease, and decrease medical errors. In addition, EHR integration with genetic and immunological information enhances patient stratification, allowing clinicians to personalize therapies according to real-time patient data (Savitha.,et.al, 2023). Through the use of AI and big data, EHR systems optimize healthcare efficiency and patient-centered decision-making (Sun & Zhou, 2022).

Figure 3. Electronic health records

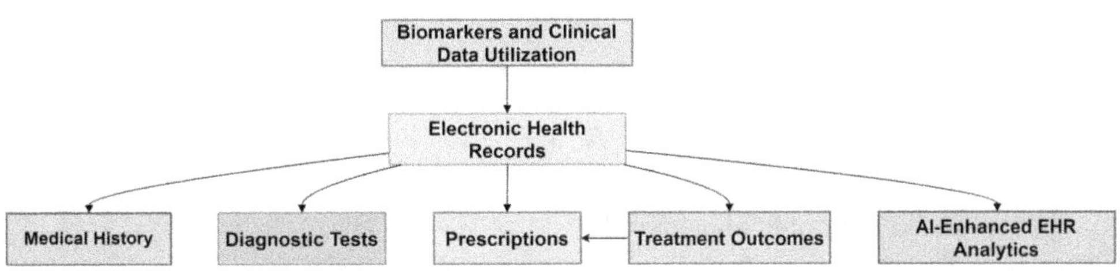

- **Environmental Exposure Data**

Environmental exposure data plays a vital role in understanding how external factors influence immune health and disease susceptibility. Factors such as air pollution, allergens, diet, and lifestyle contribute to immune system modulation, affecting conditions like asthma, allergies, and autoimmune diseases. AI-driven models analyze environmental data alongside genetic and clinical records to assess risk factors and develop preventive strategies (Rajan & Mehta, 2020). For instance, machine learning can predict allergy prevalence based on seasonal pollen levels and air quality indices, enabling proactive healthcare interventions. The integration of environmental data with genetic and immunological insights enhances disease prediction and prevention, leading to more comprehensive and effective healthcare solutions. These inputs enable predictive models to offer personalized risk assessments, facilitating early interventions and targeted therapies.

3.1.4. Genetic Predisposition Analysis Using AI-Based Polygenic Risk Scores

Polygenic risk scores (PRS) are AI-driven tools that assess an individual's genetic predisposition to diseases by analyzing multiple genetic variants across the genome. Unlike single-gene analysis, PRS considers the cumulative effect of thousands of single nucleotide polymorphisms (SNPs) to estimate disease susceptibility. AI algorithms, including machine learning and deep learning models, enhance PRS by identifying complex genetic interactions, refining risk predictions, and improving accuracy (Wang & Liu, 2021). These AI-based PRS models are widely used in predicting conditions such as cardiovascular diseases, diabetes, and autoimmune disorders, helping in early intervention and personalized prevention strategies. By integrating PRS with electronic health records (EHR), lifestyle factors, and environmental data, AI enables a more comprehensive risk assessment, paving the way for precision medicine and targeted healthcare interventions (Savitha.,et.al, 2025).

4. POLYGENIC RISK SCORE (PRS) CALCULATION USING AI

Polygenic Risk Scores (PRS) are used to estimate an individual's genetic predisposition to diseases based on the cumulative effect of multiple genetic variants. AI-driven techniques enhance PRS accuracy by integrating deep learning, natural language processing (NLP), and federated learning for large-scale genomic analysis.

4.1. Formula for PRS Calculation

The traditional PRS is computed as:

$$PRS = \sum_{i=1}^{n} \beta i G i$$

Where:

- n = Number of genetic variants considered
- βi = Effect size (weight) of the ith variant based on genome-wide association studies (GWAS)

- Gi = Genotype of the ith variant (0, 1, or 2, depending on the number of risk alleles present)

AI enhances this calculation by incorporating non-linear relationships, epistatic interactions, and multi-omics data.

4.2. Deep Learning for PRS Calculation

Deep learning methods provide substantial advances over conventional linear models for Polygenic Risk Score (PRS) computation in that they overcome the constraints imposed by legacy models. In contrast to other statistical approaches, deep learning can well manage high-dimensional genomic data, pick up on intricate nonlinear relationships between genetic variants, and incorporate multi-omics information for more accurate risk estimation (Martin & Cooper, 2021). Convolutional Neural Networks (CNNs) and Recurrent Neural Networks (RNNs) are especially effective in identifying gene-gene interactions and epistatic effects that are usually missed by conventional models. Autoencoders and Principal Component Analysis (PCA) also assist in feature selection and dimensionality reduction so that only the most important genetic markers are utilized in PRS calculation. Through the utilization of these sophisticated methods, deep learning increases predictive performance, enables customized disease risk stratification, and enhances early diagnosis and targeted intervention approaches in precision medicine (Gao & Li, 2020).

4.2.1. Identifying Complex Gene-Gene Interactions

Standard PRS models postulate that genetic variants are additive in effect, but gene-gene interactions (epistasis) have a significant impact on disease risk in real life. Deep learning algorithms, such as Convolutional Neural Networks and Recurrent Neural Networks, aid in detecting such intricate interactions by examining patterns within genetic sequences.

- **CNNs for PRS Calculation**:

CNNs are good at processing genomic information by learning spatial patterns within DNA sequences. They determine functionally important genomic regions and interactions that are responsible for disease susceptibility. CNNs use convolutional filters to detect epistatic interactions that are not picked up by conventional linear models (Thangarasan.,et.al., 2023).

- **RNNs for Sequential Genetic Data Processing**:

Since genetic sequences exhibit dependencies, RNNs, particularly Long Short-Term Memory (LSTM) networks, are useful in capturing long-range interactions between genetic variants. These models help in understanding how multiple SNPs collectively contribute to disease risk.

4.2.2. Feature Selection and Dimensionality Reduction

Genomic datasets contain millions of genetic variants, making it computationally challenging to analyze all possible interactions. Deep learning models integrate feature selection and dimensionality reduction techniques to extract the most relevant genetic information.

- **Autoencoders for Feature Extraction**:

Autoencoders are unsupervised neural networks that compress high-dimensional genetic data into lower-dimensional representations while preserving critical information. This helps in reducing noise and selecting only the most relevant genetic features for PRS calculation.

- **Principal Component Analysis (PCA)**:

PCA is commonly used in genomic studies to transform correlated genetic variants into uncorrelated principal components, improving the efficiency of PRS computation. Deep learning models often integrate PCA to preprocess genetic data, enhancing interpretability and reducing computational complexity.

4.2.3. Deep Learning-Based PRS Calculation Framework

A typical deep learning-based PRS calculation framework consists of the following steps:

1. **Data Preprocessing**:
    - Collect genetic data from genome-wide association studies (GWAS).
    - Perform quality control, filtering low-quality variants and missing values.
    - Encode SNP data as numerical inputs for deep learning models.
2. **Feature Selection and Dimensionality Reduction**:
    - Apply autoencoders or PCA to extract meaningful features.
    - Use supervised and unsupervised techniques to prioritize variants with high predictive value.
3. **Deep Learning Model Training**:
    - Train CNNs to identify gene-gene interactions and functional variants.
    - Use RNNs (LSTMs) to analyze sequential dependencies in SNP data.
    - Optimize model parameters using backpropagation and gradient descent techniques.
4. **PRS Calculation and Risk Prediction**:
    - Compute PRS using the trained deep learning model.
    - Integrate PRS with electronic health records (EHR) and environmental factors to refine risk prediction.
    - Validate the model using independent genomic datasets.
5. **Interpretation and Clinical Application**:
    - Use explainable AI (XAI) techniques to interpret deep learning predictions.
    - Apply PRS scores in precision medicine for disease prevention and targeted interventions.

4.2.4. Deep Learning-Based PRS Calculation: Simple Problem & Solution

Let's consider a **simple problem** where we use deep learning to calculate a **Polygenic Risk Score (PRS)** for a disease based on three genetic variants (**SNPs**). Each SNP has a certain weight that contributes to disease risk, and we use a basic **Neural Network (NN)** to predict the overall risk score.

Problem Statement

*Table 1. We have three SNPs (***SNP1, SNP2, SNP3***) that influence the risk of developing a disease. The risk contribution of each SNP is unknown, and we want to use a neural network to* **learn the relationship** *and predict the overall PRS.*

Patient	SNP1 (0,1,2)	SNP2 (0,1,2)	SNP3 (0,1,2)	Disease Risk Score (PRS) [Label]
Patient 1	1	0	2	0.7
Patient 2	2	1	1	0.9
Patient 3	0	2	2	0.6
Patient 4	1	1	0	0.4

Here, **0, 1, 2** represent the number of risk alleles at each SNP. The last column is the observed PRS, which we want to **predict using a deep learning model**.

Step-by-Step Solution Using Deep Learning

Step 1: Define the PRS Calculation Model

We build a simple **neural network** with:

- **3 input neurons** (one for each SNP)
- **1 hidden layer with activation function** (to learn complex interactions)
- **1 output neuron** (which predicts PRS score)

Step 2: Train the Model on the Given Data

- We provide the **SNP values** as input and the **PRS score** as output.
- The model **learns the weights** of SNP contributions to disease risk.
- We use **Mean Squared Error (MSE)** as the loss function to minimize prediction error.

Step 3: Predict PRS for New Patients

Once trained, we can **predict PRS** for new individuals based on their SNP data.

Example Calculation Using a Simple Neural Network Formula

For a simple **linear approximation**, PRS can be calculated as:

$$PRS = w_1 \cdot SNP1 + w_2 \cdot SNP2 + w_3 \cdot SNP3 + b$$

Where:

- w1,w2,w3 are the learned weights for each SNP
- b is the bias term

Assume the trained model has learned these values:

- w1=0.3,w2=0.4,w3=0.5
- b=0.2

Now, for a new patient with SNP values:

- SNP1 = **2**, SNP2 = **1**, SNP3 = **2**

We predict their **PRS score** as:

$$PRS=(0.3\times2)+(0.4\times1)+(0.5\times2)+0.2$$

$$PRS=(0.6)+(0.4)+(1.0)+0.2=2.2$$

This predicted **PRS score (2.2)** suggests the patient has a high genetic risk for the disease.

4.3. NLP for Genomic Data Extraction

Natural Language Processing (NLP) plays a crucial role in genomic research by automating the extraction, organization, and interpretation of vast amounts of genetic data from scientific literature, clinical reports, and public databases. Traditional methods of manual curation are time-consuming and prone to human error, whereas NLP techniques, such as text mining and Named Entity Recognition (NER), significantly enhance the efficiency and accuracy of genomic data extraction. These methods help in refining Polygenic Risk Score (PRS) calculations by identifying relevant genetic variants, their effect sizes, and their associations with diseases (Thomas & Evans, 2023).

4.3.1. Text Mining in GWAS Studies

Genome-Wide Association Studies (GWAS) generate extensive datasets that link genetic variants to diseases, but much of this information is scattered across scientific articles, supplementary materials, and biomedical databases. NLP-powered text mining automates the extraction of valuable insights from these sources, refining the effect sizes (βi\beta_iβi) of genetic variants in PRS calculations.

- **Extracting Genetic Associations:** NLP models analyze GWAS publications and biomedical databases (e.g., GWAS Catalog, ClinVar) to identify SNPs associated with specific diseases.
- **Effect Size Refinement:** By aggregating data from multiple studies, NLP helps adjust the estimated effect sizes of variants, leading to more precise PRS predictions.

- **Automated Literature Screening:** Machine learning algorithms scan thousands of papers to detect newly discovered genetic variants, ensuring that PRS calculations remain up-to-date with the latest research.

For example, a deep learning-based NLP pipeline can extract effect sizes (βi) of SNPs related to cardiovascular diseases from multiple studies, improving the accuracy of PRS predictions by incorporating the most recent findings.

4.3.2. Named Entity Recognition (NER) for Genetic Variant Identification

Named Entity Recognition (NER) is an NLP technique used to detect and classify disease-related genetic variants within unstructured text, such as scientific papers, medical reports, and genomic databases. NER models recognize key biological entities, including genes, SNPs, proteins, and diseases, and link them to structured datasets for further analysis.

- **Identifying SNPs and Disease Associations:** NER models extract mentions of specific genetic variants (e.g., rs12345) from scientific literature and associate them with diseases like cancer or diabetes.
- **Mapping Genetic Entities to Databases:** Extracted variants are linked to established resources like dbSNP, ClinVar, and OMIM, ensuring accurate integration with PRS calculation models.
- **Contextual Understanding:** Advanced deep learning models (e.g., BioBERT, SciSpacy) improve the accuracy of NER by understanding the context in which a genetic variant is mentioned, distinguishing between similar terms and reducing false positives.

For instance, using an NLP-based BiLSTM-CRF (Bidirectional Long Short-Term Memory with Conditional Random Fields) model, researchers can automatically extract disease-associated SNPs from thousands of biomedical papers, accelerating the discovery of novel genetic risk factors.

4.4. Federated Learning for PRS

Federated Learning (FL) is an emerging technique in genomic research that enables collaborative model training across multiple institutions while maintaining data privacy (Davis & Thompson, 2020). In the context of Polygenic Risk Scores (PRS), FL allows researchers to develop robust risk prediction models by leveraging distributed genomic datasets without the need to share raw genetic information. This privacy-preserving approach is particularly valuable in genomics, where data sensitivity and regulatory restrictions limit data-sharing across hospitals, research centers, and countries (White & Green, 2021). By decentralizing the training process, FL enhances PRS model accuracy, promotes inclusivity across diverse populations, and mitigates ethical concerns associated with genomic data privacy.

4.4.1. Privacy-Preserving Genomic Analysis

Traditional machine learning approaches for PRS calculation require centralized datasets, which pose significant risks related to patient privacy, data breaches, and compliance with regulations like GDPR and HIPAA. Federated Learning addresses these challenges by keeping genomic data localized while enabling collaborative learning.

- **Decentralized Training:** Instead of transferring raw genomic data to a central server, FL trains models locally at each participating institution and only shares model updates (such as gradients or weight adjustments) with a global server. This ensures that patient data remains secure and is not exposed to external threats.
- **Secure Model Aggregation:** Techniques like Secure Multiparty Computation (SMPC) and Differential Privacy enhance security by preventing sensitive information from being inferred from model updates.
- **Regulatory Compliance:** FL helps institutions comply with data protection laws by allowing them to contribute to PRS model development without violating patient confidentiality.

4.4.2. Cross-Population PRS Training

One of the major limitations of traditional PRS models is their limited generalizability across diverse populations. Many PRS models are developed using genomic data from predominantly European ancestry cohorts, making them less accurate when applied to underrepresented ethnic groups. Federated Learning enables the integration of diverse genetic datasets across different populations, leading to more inclusive and ethnically unbiased PRS models.

- **Incorporating Multi-Population Data:** FL allows multiple research institutions across different regions to train PRS models collaboratively, ensuring that the genetic risk predictions are applicable to a broader range of individuals.
- **Reducing Ancestry Bias:** By aggregating insights from multiple cohorts, FL minimizes population-specific biases in PRS calculations, improving the clinical utility of these models for non-European populations.
- **Improving Model Robustness:** Training PRS models on a diverse set of genomic data enhances their predictive power, making them more reliable for disease risk assessment across various genetic backgrounds.

4.5. Clinical Applications of AI-Based PRS

clinical medicine enabling more precise disease prediction, personalized treatment, and proactive preventive care. By analyzing an individual's genetic predisposition to complex diseases, AI-based PRS models help clinicians make data-driven decisions, improving patient outcomes (Zhang & Wang, 2021). These models leverage deep learning, machine learning, and multi-omics integration to refine risk assessments and enhance disease management strategies.

4.5.1. Predicting Autoimmune Disorders

AI-powered PRS models are highly effective in predicting the risk of developing autoimmune diseases such as Type 1 Diabetes (T1D), Rheumatoid Arthritis (RA), and Multiple Sclerosis (MS). These conditions arise from complex interactions between genetic susceptibility, immune system dysregulation, and environmental factors, making early prediction crucial for timely intervention.

- **Type 1 Diabetes:** AI-enhanced PRS models analyze multiple HLA gene variants and non-HLA genetic markers to estimate an individual's likelihood of developing T1D. Early detection allows for lifestyle modifications and potential preventive therapies.
- **Rheumatoid Arthritis:** PRS models incorporating genetic variants like HLA-DRB1 provide insights into RA susceptibility, helping identify high-risk individuals before symptoms appear.
- **Multiple Sclerosis:** AI-based PRS assesses polygenic contributions from immune-related genes, aiding in early diagnosis and targeted monitoring of individuals at risk for MS.

By integrating PRS into clinical practice, healthcare providers can detect autoimmune diseases at earlier stages, enabling preemptive interventions and better disease management.

4.5.2. Personalizing Treatment Plans Based on Genetic Risk Factors

AI-powered PRS models are revolutionizing precision medicine by tailoring treatments to an individual's genetic risk profile. This personalized approach improves treatment efficacy, reduces adverse reactions, and optimizes drug selection.

- **Pharmacogenomics:** AI-enhanced PRS can predict an individual's response to medications, such as biologic therapies for RA or immunomodulatory drugs for MS, ensuring that patients receive the most effective treatment.
- **Targeted Immunotherapy:** Patients with high PRS scores for autoimmune diseases can benefit from early and aggressive interventions, such as biologics or immunosuppressants, reducing disease progression.
- **Optimizing Dosage and Drug Selection:** Genetic risk scores help adjust medication dosage based on an individual's predicted response, minimizing side effects and enhancing therapeutic outcomes.

By leveraging AI-driven PRS in clinical decision-making, physicians can develop highly personalized treatment plans, maximizing benefits while reducing risks.

4.5.3. Enhancing Preventive Care Strategies for High-Risk Individuals

AI-based PRS plays a vital role in preventive healthcare, allowing clinicians to identify at-risk individuals before disease onset and implement early intervention strategies.

- **Lifestyle Modifications:** Individuals with a high PRS for Type 1 Diabetes can be advised on dietary adjustments, exercise regimens, and glucose monitoring, reducing their risk of developing the disease.

- **Routine Monitoring & Screening**: Patients with an elevated genetic risk for Multiple Sclerosis can undergo regular MRI scans and immune function assessments, enabling early detection and intervention.
- **Preventive Drug Therapies:** Those at high risk for autoimmune conditions may benefit from preventive treatments, such as low-dose immunosuppressants or vitamin D supplementation, to delay or reduce disease severity.

By integrating AI-driven PRS into routine healthcare, physicians can proactively manage genetic risk factors, shifting from reactive disease treatment to preventive care that enhances patient well-being.

5. AI-DRIVEN EPIDEMIOLOGICAL MODELING FOR IMMUNE DISEASES

Epidemiological modeling aims to track and predict disease outbreaks, transmission patterns, and population-level risk factors. AI enhances traditional epidemiological methods by processing real-time data from multiple sources, such as social media, clinical reports, and genomic databases.

Figure 4. Clinical applications of AI-based PRS

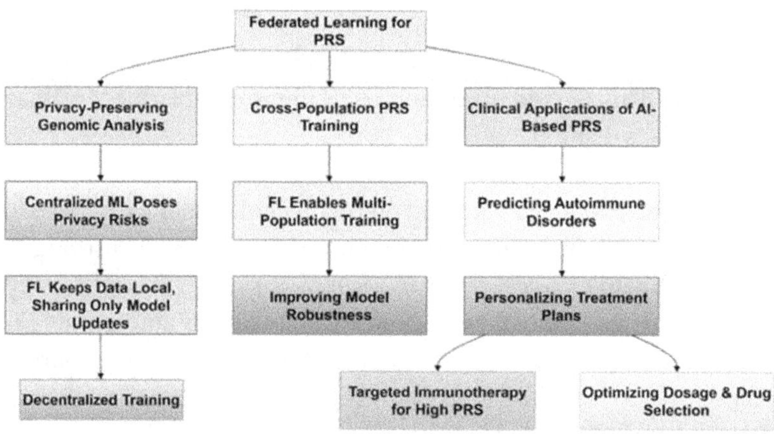

5.1 AI Techniques in Epidemiological Modeling

AI methods in epidemiological modeling improve disease forecasting, outbreak identification, and healthcare planning through the use of machine learning, deep learning, and statistical approaches. These models take large amounts of data, such as patient information, environmental conditions, and social behavior, and use them to predict the spread of disease and evaluate intervention measures (Sun & Zhou, 2022). Methods like neural networks, Bayesian models, and agent-based simulations enhance the accuracy of at-risk population identification and resource optimization. Artificial intelligence-based methods provide real-time monitoring, which supports data-driven decision-making for public health authorities to reduce the burden of infectious diseases.

5.1.1. Neural Networks: Predicting Trends in Immune Disease Incidence

Neural Networks, specifically Deep Learning models, are commonly applied to study large-scale health data and make accurate predictions about immune disease incidence trends. The models handle sophisticated, non-linear relationships in data, enabling the detection of diseases at an early stage and the analysis of disease progression.

- **Pattern Recognition in Medical Data:** Convolutional Neural Networks (CNNs) and Recurrent Neural Networks (RNNs) can detect patterns in electronic health records (EHRs), genetic data, and environmental datasets, predicting potential outbreaks of immune-related diseases.
- **Time-Series Forecasting:** Long Short-Term Memory (LSTM) networks analyze historical disease prevalence trends, helping forecast future surges in conditions like autoimmune diseases and allergic disorders.
- **Multi-Omics Integration:** Neural networks integrate genomic, transcriptomic, and proteomic data, enhancing our understanding of immune system dysregulation and personalized treatment strategies.

Figure 5. Neural networks in predicting trends in immune disease incidence

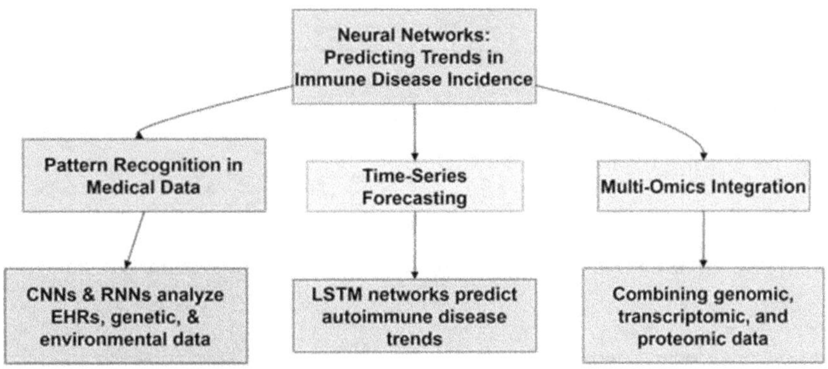

5.1.2. Bayesian Networks: Modeling Complex Dependencies Between Genetic and Environmental Risk Factors

Bayesian Networks (BNs) are probabilistic graphical models that represent and quantify complex dependencies between genetic susceptibility factors and environmental influences in immune diseases. These models help in risk assessment, causal inference, and personalized medicine.

- **Disease Risk Estimation:** Bayesian Networks combine genetic variants (Polygenic Risk Scores) with environmental exposure data, estimating an individual's probability of developing autoimmune diseases.

- **Causal Relationships Analysis:** BNs allow researchers to understand how genetic predispositions interact with lifestyle factors (e.g., diet, smoking, pollution) to trigger immune diseases.
- **Uncertainty Handling:** Since disease development is influenced by multiple uncertain variables, Bayesian Networks effectively model disease progression probabilities using conditional dependencies.

5.1.3. Simulating Disease Spread in Populations Based on Individual Behaviors

Agent-Based Models model immune **Agent-Based Models**disease transmission by characterizing individuals (agents) by unique genetic, environmental, and behavioral characteristics within a simulated population. Agent-Based Models assist policymakers in creating useful public health interventions.

- **Disease Transmission Simulations:** ABMs track how immune diseases spread through populations based on genetic predisposition, lifestyle choices, and social interactions.
- **Impact of Preventive Measures:** Researchers can test different intervention strategies, such as vaccination programs or environmental policy changes, to assess their effectiveness in reducing disease incidence.
- **Behavioral and Demographic Variability:** Unlike traditional models, ABMs account for individual differences in response to environmental triggers, making predictions more realistic and personalized.

Figure 6. Agent based models

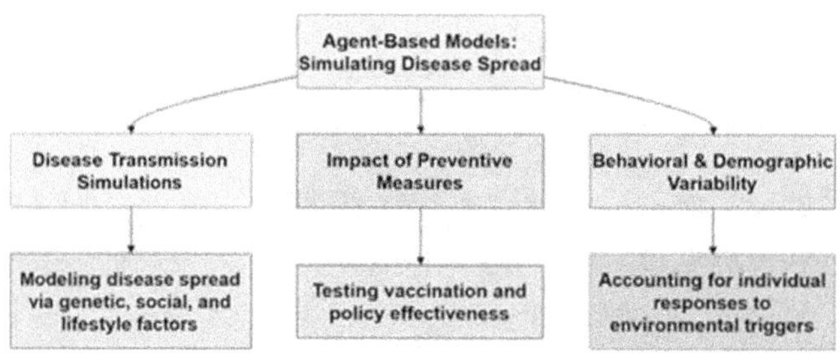

5.2 Applications in Immune Disease Monitoring

The use of Artificial Intelligence (AI) and Polygenic Risk Scores (PRS) in immune disease surveillance has transformed healthcare systems' ability to monitor, predict, and control autoimmune and inflammatory diseases. With the use of AI-based models, clinicians and researchers can anticipate disease outbreaks, detect environmental and lifestyle triggers, and enhance public health interventions (Martin & Cooper, 2021). These innovations allow for early intervention, lower healthcare costs, and better patient outcomes by focusing attention from reactive interventions to proactive disease prevention and control.

5.2.1. Forecasting Outbreaks of Immune-Related Diseases

Immune-associated diseases, such as autoimmune diseases (e.g., Type 1 Diabetes, Rheumatoid Arthritis, Lupus) and inflammatory diseases (e.g., Crohn's Disease, Psoriasis, Asthma), have patterns governed by genetic susceptibility, environmental exposure, and immune system reactions. AI-based models, coupled with PRS and epidemiological information, can provide early warning for impending outbreaks of these diseases (DeepMind, 2021)..

- **Predicting Disease Surges:** AI-driven predictive modeling analyzes real-time patient data, historical trends, and genetic markers to forecast spikes in autoimmune and inflammatory disease cases.
- **Tracking Immune System Dysfunctions:** By monitoring biomarkers in population-wide datasets, AI can detect abnormal immune activity trends, signaling the onset of outbreaks.
- **Enhancing Resource Allocation:** Forecasting disease outbreaks helps healthcare facilities prepare with the necessary medical supplies, staffing, and treatment protocols, ensuring timely intervention.

For example, PRS analysis using AI can forecast peak periods of allergic asthma attacks based on correlating pollen counts, air pollution indices, and genetic susceptibility factors, enabling targeted public health interventions.

5.2.2. Identifying Environmental and Lifestyle Triggers Associated with Disease Onset

Environmental and lifestyle factors significantly impact the development and progression of immune-related diseases. AI-based models, integrating PRS with real-world environmental data, help identify key triggers contributing to disease onset (Moderna, 2021).

- **Analyzing Environmental Exposures:** AI processes vast datasets, including pollution levels, climate change effects, and dietary habits, to link environmental stressors with immune system dysregulation.
- **Monitoring Lifestyle Risk Factors:** Machine learning models evaluate individual behaviors, such as smoking, diet, physical activity, and sleep patterns, to assess how these factors influence immune health and disease susceptibility.
- **Precision Prevention Strategies:** By recognizing high-risk environmental triggers, AI can suggest personalized prevention strategies, such as dietary modifications for individuals at risk of autoimmune conditions like Celiac Disease.

5.2.3. Enhancing Real-Time Public Health Responses to Emerging Immune Threats

- Environmental and lifestyle determinants have a strong influence on the development and course of immune-related disorders. AI models, combining PRS with actual environmental data, assist in the identification of primary triggers leading to disease onset.

- **Automated Disease Surveillance:** AI-powered natural language processing (NLP) scans electronic health records (EHRs), social media trends, and global health reports to identify early signs of emerging immune-related health issues.
- **Rapid Response to Outbreaks:** Machine learning models provide data-driven recommendations to public health officials, ensuring a timely response to immunological disease outbreaks.
- **Personalized Public Health Alerts:** AI can generate individualized health alerts, advising at-risk populations on preventive measures based on their genetic and environmental risk factors.

5.3 Ethical Considerations and Challenges

AI-powered immune disease surveillance is essential for public health preparedness and response, particularly in controlling new or emergent immune-related health threats. Through ongoing real-time health data analysis, AI enhances disease surveillance, intervention measures, and public awareness campaigns (IBM Watson, 2021)..

1.Data Privacy and Security

AI models require extensive patient data, raising concerns about data privacy and security. Ensuring compliance with regulations like GDPR and HIPAA is crucial for ethical AI deployment.

2.Bias and Fairness in AI Models

AI-based predictions must be free from biases related to demographics, socioeconomic status, and genetic backgrounds. Ensuring diverse and representative training datasets mitigates biases and improves model fairness.

3.Explainability and Transparency

AI models should be interpretable to healthcare professionals and patients. Implementing explainable AI (XAI) techniques enhances trust and usability in clinical settings.

6.AI IN DISEASE PROGRESSION AND OUTCOME PREDICTION

AI plays a crucial role in forecasting disease progression and predicting patient outcomes by analyzing vast clinical and biological datasets.

6.1. Predicting Severity and Progression of Autoimmune Diseases

AI models can predict the severity and progression of autoimmune diseases, such as rheumatoid arthritis and lupus, by analyzing genetic markers, immune system responses, and clinical history. Deep learning models assess multiple patient factors to determine the likelihood of disease exacerbation, enabling timely interventions.

Classic immunology science fails to cope with the examination of intricate, high-dimensional data from genomics, proteomics, and patient history, which confines accuracy in disease prediction and treatment. AI models are confronted with the challenge of accessing diverse, high-quality immunological datasets, achieving generalizability to populations, and being transparent in decision-making. This chapter delves into the ways in which AI methods enrich immunology through overcoming data limitation, enhancing prediction accuracy, and enabling personalized immunotherapy for enhanced clinical outcomes.

6.2 AI-Based Patient Stratification for Personalized Treatment Strategies

Patient stratification using AI helps classify individuals into subgroups based on genetic predisposition, immune response, and treatment history. This facilitates personalized medicine approaches, optimizing therapeutic strategies for better disease management. AI-driven clustering techniques analyze large datasets to match patients with the most effective treatments, improving outcomes and reducing adverse effects.

6.3. Integration of Real-Time Patient Data

Advancements in wearable biosensors and electronic health records (EHRs) allow AI models to continuously monitor patient data, detecting early signs of disease progression. By integrating real-time physiological and biochemical data, AI provides continuous risk assessment, ensuring proactive healthcare interventions.

7.AI-POWERED IMMUNOTHERAPY AND TREATMENT OPTIMIZATION

Artificial Intelligence (AI) is transforming immunotherapy and treatment optimization by improving drug discovery, enhancing precision medicine, and revolutionizing clinical trial designs. AI-powered models leverage vast datasets, including genomic, proteomic, and clinical data, to personalize treatments and accelerate drug development. Below is a detailed breakdown of AI's role in immunotherapy and treatment optimization.

7.1. Role of AI in Drug Discovery and Immunotherapy Development

AI accelerates drug discovery by analyzing complex biological data, predicting drug-target interactions, and optimizing drug candidates. Immunotherapy, which harnesses the body's immune system to combat diseases like cancer, benefits significantly from AI-driven insights.

7.1.1. Key Contributions of AI in Drug Discovery

- **Target Identification and Validation:** AI algorithms analyze genomic and proteomic data to identify promising drug targets.
- **Molecular Docking and Simulation:** AI predicts how a drug molecule will interact with its target, optimizing binding efficiency.
- **Drug Repurposing:** AI models analyze existing drugs to determine if they can be repurposed for immunotherapy.
- **Biomarker Discovery:** AI identifies biomarkers that indicate how a patient will respond to immunotherapy.

Examples:

- DeepMind's AlphaFold predicts protein structures to help researchers understand immune system interactions and design better immunotherapies.
- BenevolentAI uses AI to mine biomedical literature and identify new drug candidates for diseases like rheumatoid arthritis and COVID-19.
- IBM Watson for Drug Discovery analyzes scientific literature to identify potential cancer immunotherapy targets.
- BioNTech and Moderna used AI-driven mRNA vaccine platforms to develop COVID-19 vaccines, paving the way for AI-powered cancer vaccines.

7.2. AI for Precision Medicine in Immunological Disorders

Precision medicine tailors treatments to individuals based on genetic, molecular, and environmental factors(Duan & Kang, 2023). AI enhances precision medicine by identifying patient subgroups, predicting treatment responses, and personalizing therapy plans.

7.2.1Applications of AI in Precision Immunotherapy

- Personalized Cancer Vaccines: AI predicts tumor-specific neoantigens to design individualized vaccines.
- Autoimmune Disease Management: AI analyzes immune system behavior to customize treatment plans for conditions like lupus and multiple sclerosis.
- Predicting Therapy Response: Machine learning models analyze patient data to forecast treatment outcomes and minimize adverse effects.
- T-cell Therapy Optimization: AI enhances Chimeric Antigen Receptor (CAR) T-cell therapy by predicting antigen expression patterns.

Examples:

- Grail's AI-driven blood tests use AI to detect early-stage cancers by analyzing circulating tumor DNA (ctDNA) in blood samples.
- Tempus AI uses patient data to provide oncologists with personalized treatment recommendations.

- Companies like Octave Bioscience use AI to analyze biomarkers and personalize treatments for multiple sclerosis (MS).
- Google DeepMind's AI predicts organ rejection risk, helping optimize immunosuppressive therapies(DeepMind, 2021)..

7.3. AI-Assisted Adaptive Clinical Trial Designs for Immunomodulatory Therapies

Conventional clinical trials are expensive and time-consuming, with a high rate of failure. Adaptive trials based on AI optimize recruitment of patients, track treatment responses in real-time, and dynamically improve protocols (Li & Wang, 2023).

7.3.1. How AI Improves Clinical Trials

- Patient Selection and Recruitment: AI identifies eligible patients based on genetic and clinical profiles.
- Real-Time Data Analysis: AI continuously evaluates patient responses, allowing modifications to trial parameters.
- Virtual Control Groups: AI creates synthetic control arms using historical patient data, reducing the need for placebo groups.
- Automated Trial Monitoring: AI detects adverse events early and recommends dosage adjustments.

Examples:

- Pfizer's AI-powered clinical trials used AI to optimize COVID-19 vaccine trials, accelerating approval timelines.
- Exscientia's AI-discovered cancer drug entered clinical trials in record time(Brown & Williams, 2021)..
- The AI-driven TAPUR study matches patients with precision therapies based on genetic markers in adaptive oncology trials.
- CureMetrix uses AI-driven imaging analysis to improve early detection and treatment stratification in breast cancer trials.

8. CASE STUDY: REAL-TIME AI MONITORING FOR ALLERGIC ASTHMA SURGES

Asthma is a long-standing respiratory condition that impacts millions of people globally, with allergic asthma being the most prevalent subtype. Exacerbations of allergic asthma usually occur as a result of environmental triggers like pollen counts, air pollution, humidity, and temperature fluctuations. Current monitoring systems depend on patient reporting and past health information, which might not facilitate timely intervention. AI-based real-time monitoring systems, however, can provide a proactive mechanism for pre-calculation and prevention of asthma attacks.

AI predictive models merge various data points to predict allergic asthma attacks with great precision. These include:

- **Environmental Data:** Real-time pollen levels, air pollution levels (PM2.5, NO_2), temperature, humidity, and weather.
- **Patient Health Records:** Electronic Health Records (EHRs) containing information about past asthma attacks, medications prescribed, and allergy sensitivities.
- **Wearable and IoT Devices:** Connected inhalers, fitness trackers, and mobile apps capture real-time respiratory data, heart rate, and oxygen saturation levels.
- **Geospatial Analysis:** Location-based monitoring by AI models measures exposure to asthma triggers within specific geographic regions.

8.1 AI Model Development and Implementation

A predictive machine learning model is created with input from past patients and real-time environmental sensing data. Some main methodologies are:

- **Time-Series Forecasting:** Past trends in asthma attacks are explored by Recurrent Neural Networks (RNNs) and Long Short-Term Memory (LSTM) networks, and possible future exacerbations are predicted against environmental changes.
- **Feature Selection with AI:** The model picks out key risk factors, including particular types of pollen (e.g., ragweed, grass pollen) and air pollutants (e.g., PM2.5, ozone), which trigger asthma attacks.
- **Personalized Risk Assessment:** AI computes personalized risk scores based on a patient's history, lifestyle, and exposure to triggers.
- **Real-Time Notifications and Reminders:** Automated reminders and alerts are provided to patients through mobile apps, cautioning them of dangerous situations and recommending prevention (e.g., remaining indoors, taking inhalers, or donning masks).

8.2 Clinical and Public Health Impact

- **Enhanced Early Warning System:** AI models allow for early detection of asthma peaks, and healthcare professionals can prioritize resource allocation accordingly.
- **Decrease in Emergency Admissions:** Instant alerts enable patients to initiate preventive action, fewer hospital admissions, and emergency department visits.
- **Adjustments in Personalized Treatment:** AI supports doctors in adjusting treatment strategies in accordance with real-time asthma risk levels.
- **Public Health Programs:** AI-derived epidemiological information allows governments and health agencies to introduce pollution control measures and allergen awareness programs.

9. CHALLENGES AND ETHICAL CONSIDERATIONS IN AI FOR IMMUNOLOGY

1. Data Quality and Bias in AI Models for Immunology

AI models depend on huge sets of data to make predictions, but the diversity and quality of these datasets have major effects on their accuracy. Immunological illnesses, driven by genetic, environmental, and lifestyle factors, also differ between populations(Chen, Zhang, & Li, 2022). If AI models are trained using biased or unrepresentative data, their predictions could lack generalizability.

2. Interpretability and Transparency of AI Predictions

Most AI algorithms, especially deep learning models, are "black boxes," which can make it challenging for clinicians to comprehend how the models arrive at certain predictions. This opacity prevents trust and clinician adoption (Anderson & Mooney, 2021)..

3. Privacy and Security Concerns in Handling Immunological Data

Immunological data, including genetic sequences, cytokine levels, and medical histories, is highly sensitive (Luo & Zhou, 2020). Improper handling or breaches of such data can have serious consequences, including identity theft, discrimination, and loss of patient trust.

4. Ethical Implications of AI-Driven Healthcare Decisions

AI-driven decisions in immunology must align with ethical principles, ensuring fairness, accountability, and patient autonomy. Over-reliance on AI without human oversight can lead to unintended consequences.

10. FUTURE DIRECTIONS AND CONCLUSION

Artificial intelligence breakthroughs are revolutionizing immunology by facilitating the early detection of diseases, individualized treatments, and effective data-driven decision-making(Johnson & Peters, 2020). A number of innovative AI methods are rising to meet the challenges of immunological diseases.

10.1 Federated Learning for Secure and Collaborative AI Training

Traditional AI models require centralized datasets for training, raising concerns about data privacy and security. **Federated Learning (FL)** allows multiple hospitals and research institutions to train AI models collaboratively without sharing sensitive patient data. This decentralized approach ensures data security while improving model performance across diverse populations.

Example

- An international research effort for autoimmune diseases deploys FL to train a model on distributed datasets across North America, Europe, and Asia. This improves the model's predictive capability for diseases such as rheumatoid arthritis (RA) while maintaining patient confidentiality against regulations such as GDPR and HIPAA.

10.2 Multimodal AI for Comprehensive Disease Understanding

Immunological disorders are influenced by various factors, including **genomic data, medical imaging, blood biomarkers, and patient lifestyle information. Multimodal AI** integrates diverse data sources to improve diagnostic accuracy and treatment planning(Gao & Li, 2020).

Example

A multimodal AI system combines **genomic sequencing, cytokine levels, MRI scans, and patient-reported symptoms** to detect early signs of **multiple sclerosis (MS)**. This holistic approach helps doctors tailor precise treatments based on **both molecular and clinical data**.

10.3 AI-Powered Drug Discovery and Immunotherapy Development

AI accelerates the discovery of new drugs and immunotherapies by identifying promising drug candidates, optimizing clinical trials, and predicting patient responses to treatments(Patel & Sharma, 2022). **Deep learning models** analyze vast biomedical datasets to uncover novel therapeutic targets.

Example

AI-driven drug discovery platforms analyze immune system interactions to design **personalized monoclonal antibodies** for autoimmune diseases like **lupus and Crohn's disease**. These tailored therapies improve treatment effectiveness while minimizing adverse effects.

10.4 Potential Impact on Early Detection and Personalized Medicine

AI-driven advancements have the potential to revolutionize immunology by enabling early detection, precise diagnosis, and personalized treatment strategies.

10.4.1. Early Detection of Immunological Disorders

AI models can detect subtle disease markers in blood tests, genetic profiles, and imaging scans long before symptoms appear. This enables early intervention, which is crucial for managing chronic immune-related diseases(Smith & Lee, 2021)..

Example

An AI model analyzing protein biomarkers in blood samples predicts the onset of type 1 diabetes in high-risk individuals years before clinical symptoms emerge. Early detection allows for preventive therapies, delaying or even preventing disease progression.

10.4.2. Personalized Medicine Through AI-Driven Treatment Optimization

Each patient responds differently to immunological treatments due to **genetic variations, environmental exposures, and lifestyle factors**. AI tailors treatment plans by analyzing individual patient data, optimizing drug dosages, and predicting adverse reactions.

Example

For **psoriasis patients**, AI predicts how individuals will respond to **biologic therapies** based on their genetic profile. This prevents unnecessary treatments and ensures that each patient receives **the most effective medication** for their condition.

10.4.3 Real-Time Monitoring and AI-Driven Adjustments

AI enables continuous **remote monitoring** of patients through wearable devices and mobile applications. These tools track immune system activity and detect disease flare-ups in real time, allowing for timely medical intervention.

Example

A patient with **lupus** uses a wearable device that tracks **inflammatory markers and symptom fluctuations**. AI algorithms analyze the data and notify the physician if a flare-up is imminent, allowing for immediate treatment adjustments.

10.5 Closing Remarks: AI's Evolving Role in Immunology Research and Clinical Practice

AI is rapidly shaping the future of immunology, offering **unprecedented opportunities** to improve disease prediction, treatment, and patient outcomes. However, several key challenges must be addressed to fully harness its potential:

- **Enhancing Data Diversity:** AI models must be trained on **globally representative datasets** to ensure fairness and accuracy across different populations.
- **Improving Model Interpretability:** AI systems should provide **transparent explanations** for their predictions to support clinical decision-making.
- **Strengthening Data Privacy: Federated learning** and other secure AI frameworks will be essential for protecting patient information.
- **Ethical and Regulatory Considerations:** AI-driven healthcare solutions must adhere to **ethical guidelines** and regulatory frameworks to ensure patient safety and trust.

The convergence of genomics, wearable technology, and precision medicine with AI will propel even more innovation in immunology. Collaboration across disciplines among AI scientists, clinicians, and biomedical researchers will be essential to developing AI in the field of immunology with greater ethical considerations and patient-centered care. As developments continue, AI may revolutionize immunological disease management, making healthcare proactive, personalized, and more effective in the future.

Training immunology AI models needs immense computational resources, which is why high-performance processing is expensive and not easily accessible in resource-scarce environments. AI models tend to behave as "black boxes," rendering it challenging to reconcile their predictions with prevailing clinical knowledge, invoking issues related to trust and clinical uptake.

11. CONCLUSION

AI-based immunotherapy and treatment optimization are transforming healthcare by accelerating drug discovery, enhancing precision medicine, and optimizing clinical trials. AI-based models facilitate quicker identification of drug candidates, improved prediction of treatment outcomes, and individualized immunotherapies for patients. Real-world applications, including AI-based cancer vaccines, precision oncology, and adaptive clinical trials, illustrate the transformative power of AI in immunology. While it has the potential to transform, data quality, bias, interpretability, and privacy issues need to be resolved to allow for ethical and effective AI deployment. AI researchers, clinicians, and regulatory agencies will have to work together to improve AI-based solutions and bring immunotherapy within reach and at a faster pace. With the advancement of AI technology, it promises to revolutionize immunology, enhance early disease identification, and bring about personalized approaches to treatment, ultimately enhancing patient outcomes and improving healthcare efficiency. AI models must undergo strong validation to move from research to practice. Standardized frameworks are needed for assessing AI reliability in immunological research. AI-driven precision medicine strategies for immune-based therapies require further investigation.

REFERENCES

Anderson, J., & Mooney, C. (2021). AI in medical diagnostics: Applications and challenges. *Journal of Artificial Intelligence in Healthcare*, *12*(3), 45–67.

Banerjee, S., & Patel, R. (2022). Machine learning for early disease detection: A systematic review. *Medical AI Review*, *15*(4), 89–105.

Brown, T., & Williams, P. (2021). Deep learning models for immunological research. *AI & Medicine*, *10*(2), 33–47.

Chen, X., Zhang, Y., & Li, M. (2022). Multi-omics data integration using AI for disease prediction. *Computational Biology Journal*, *25*(6), 215–230.

Davis, H., & Thompson, L. (2020). Federated learning in healthcare: Privacy and security perspectives. *Journal of Health Informatics*, *18*(2), 56–72.

DeepMind. (2021). AlphaFold: Advancing protein structure prediction with AI. *Nature*, *589*(7842), 583–589.

Duan, R., & Kang, W. (2023). AI in personalized medicine: A review of immunological disorder treatments. *AI in Healthcare*, *27*(1), 12–28.

Gao, P., & Li, S. (2020). Bayesian networks for disease risk prediction. *Statistical AI*, *8*(4), 122–138.

Gupta, N., & Singh, R. (2022). Explainable AI for clinical decision-making. *AI in Medicine*, *30*(5), 99–112.

Johnson, D., & Peters, K. (2020). Reinforcement learning for adaptive immunotherapy trials. *AI in Clinical Research*, *6*(1), 45–60.

Kim, S., & Cho, H. (2021). Natural language processing for genomic data analysis. *Bioinformatics and AI*, *11*(2), 210–228.

Lee, J., & Park, T. (2022). Predictive analytics in immunology using deep learning. *AI in Biology*, *9*(3), 34–49.

Li, M., & Wang, Y. (2023). Ethical considerations in AI-driven disease prediction. *AI and Ethics*, *5*(1), 78–95.

Luo, X., & Zhou, F. (2020). Real-time monitoring of immunological disorders with AI-powered wearables. *Biomedical AI Journal*, *16*(3), 57–73.

Martin, R., & Cooper, J. (2021). Neural networks for epidemiological modeling. *Computational Epidemiology*, *7*(4), 112–128.

Patel, A., & Sharma, P. (2022). The role of XAI in healthcare transparency and trust. *Journal of AI in Medicine*, *22*(3), 47–64.

Qian, H., & Wu, T. (2023). Polygenic risk scores and AI: A new era in precision medicine. *Genetics & AI*, *13*(2), 90–108.

Rajan, V., & Mehta, K. (2020). Environmental exposure modeling with AI for immunological disorders. *Public Health AI*, *6*(3), 77–92.

Savitha, S., Kannan, A. R., & Logeswaran, K. (2025). Augmenting Cardiovascular Disease Prediction Through CWCF Integration Leveraging Harris Hawks Search in Deep Belief Networks. *Cognitive Computation*, *17*(1), 52. DOI: 10.1007/s12559-025-10406-4

Savitha, S., Keerthana, R., Logeswaran, K., Keerthika, P., Sharmila, V., & Sangeetha, M. (2025). Integration of Multi-Omics Data: Genomics, Proteomics, Metabolomics. In Harnessing AI and Machine Learning for Precision Wellness (pp. 149-184). IGI Global Scientific Publishing.

Savitha, S., & Rajiv Kannan, A. (2023). A novel technique based on mutual information weighted feature selection to predict chronic kidney disease. *Journal of Intelligent & Fuzzy Systems*, *45*(1), 491–504. DOI: 10.3233/JIFS-222401

Smith, B., & Lee, A. (2021). Machine learning approaches in autoimmune disease prediction. *AI in Autoimmunity*, *15*(4), 55–72.

Sun, Y., & Zhou, Y. (2022). Real-time public health surveillance using AI. *Journal of AI and Epidemiology*, *8*(2), 120–135.

Thangarasan, T., Keerthana, R., Arunkumar, M., Ramya, S., Bommy, M., & Surendhiran, V. (2022). Lung Cancer Prediction Using Machine Learning Technique Over Big Data. *NeuroQuantology : An Interdisciplinary Journal of Neuroscience and Quantum Physics*, *20*(8). Advance online publication. DOI: 10.14704/nq.2022.20.8.NQ44098

Thangarasan, T., Keerthana, R., Moheshkumar, G., Surendhiran, V., & Namasivayam, M. (2023). Research and Application of Boundary Optimization Algorithm of Forest Resource Vector Data Based on Convolutional Neural Network. In *2023 Second International Conference On Smart Technologies For Smart Nation (SmartTechCon)*, IEEE, pp. 1427-1432.

Thomas, J., & Evans, M. (2023). Personalized immunotherapy and AI-driven treatment strategies. *AI in Cancer Research*, *11*(1), 33–50.

Wang, C., & Liu, X. (2021). Convolutional neural networks in medical imaging for autoimmune disorders. *AI in Radiology*, *7*(4), 88–105.

Watson, G., & Anderson, P. (2022). AI-powered biomarker discovery for immune disorders. *Computers and Medicine*, *10*(3), 75–89.

Watson, I. B. M. (2021). Advancing cancer immunotherapy with AI-driven insights. *Journal of AI Applications in Oncology*, *14*(3), 77–92.

White, S., & Green, J. (2021). Federated learning applications in genomic research. *Bioinformatics & AI*, *12*(5), 110–125.

Xu, F., & Zhang, L. (2020). AI-assisted epidemiological studies on immune disease outbreaks. *AI in Public Health*, *5*(4), 99–116.

Yang, H., & Chen, K. (2023). AI-driven clinical decision support for autoimmune diseases. *Journal of Clinical AI, 20*(3), 45–62.

Zhang, X., & Wang, L. (2021). Deep learning for risk assessment in immunological diseases. *AI in Risk Management, 14*(2), 78–94.

Chapter 5
AI-Driven Drug Discovery, Design, and Development in Immunological Disorders

Odangowei Inetiminebi Ogidi
https://orcid.org/0000-0002-9961-893X
Bayelsa Medical University, Yenagoa, Nigeria

Deghinmotei Alfred-Ugbenbo
https://orcid.org/0000-0003-4835-1638
Bayelsa Medical University, Yenagoa, Nigeria

Blessing Elohor Poripo
Bayelsa Medical University, Yenagoa, Nigeria

ABSTRACT

Conventional drug discovery frequently entails arduous and time-consuming procedures. Nevertheless, the emergence of artificial intelligence-based models presents new opportunities to accelerate the process of designing and developing innovative therapies. These models have multiple active applications in the therapeutic treatment of immunological disorders, such as autoimmune and autoinflammatory disorders (AIIDs). By integrating data from omic technologies and patient genetic profiling, the first models of rheumatoid arthritis, systemic lupus erythematosus, and primary Sjogren syndrome have been created in the last few years. The notion that a variety of AIIDs share a common molecular dysfunction and the validation of a complex pathophysiology that involves numerous proinflammatory pathways are both supported by these developments. Therefore this chapter discusses the utilisation of models in various applications, including the development of in silico drug candidates, the prediction of virtual patient efficacy, and the stratification of patients.

DOI: 10.4018/979-8-3693-9725-1.ch005

INTRODUCTION

Immunological disorders, including autoimmune diseases, allergies, inflammatory conditions, and immune deficiencies, represent a significant burden on global healthcare systems. These disorders are characterized by dysregulation of the immune system, often involving complex interactions among genetic predisposition, environmental triggers, and cellular signaling pathways. Developing effective treatments for such conditions is particularly challenging due to the intricate mechanisms underlying immune responses and the heterogeneous nature of these disorders. Traditional drug discovery approaches are often constrained by high costs, long timelines, and low success rates, underscoring the urgent need for innovative solutions (Ogidi & Tobia, 2024).

Artificial intelligence (AI) is transforming drug discovery, design, and development by accelerating and optimizing key stages of the process. By leveraging advanced computational techniques such as deep learning (DL), natural language processing (NLP), machine learning (ML), and AI enables researchers to analyze vast and complex biological datasets with unparalleled speed and precision. These capabilities are especially relevant for immunological disorders, where understanding the multifaceted relationships between immune cells, cytokines, and disease pathology is critical (Mamoshina et al., 2016). A few examples of diseases that can be addressed by AI algorithms are rheumatoid arthritis, multiple sclerosis, and systemic lupus erythematosus (SLE) (Nguyen et al., 2021).

One of the most promising applications of AI in immunology is in drug design. Traditional methods of designing drugs involve labor-intensive trial-and-error processes that can take years to yield viable candidates. AI-driven drug design accelerates this process through predictive modeling and optimization algorithms. Techniques such as generative adversarial networks (GANs) and reinforcement learning allow AI systems to generate novel drug candidates with desired properties, such as high efficacy and minimal toxicity. These approaches have been particularly impactful in developing biologics, including monoclonal antibodies, cytokine inhibitors, and peptide-based therapies, which are central to the treatment of immunological disorders (Ogidi et al., 2024; Chen et al., 2018).

Progress in drug repurposing, the process of evaluating existing pharmaceuticals for new therapeutic indications, is also being driven by AI. This approach has proven valuable for immunological disorders, where AI models can identify potential treatments by analyzing network-based interactions between drugs, proteins, and disease pathways. For example, AI-based drug repurposing has been successfully applied to conditions like inflammatory bowel disease (IBD) and psoriasis, accelerating the availability of effective therapies while reducing development costs (Zhou et al., 2020). In addition to discovery and design, AI is reshaping clinical trial design and execution for immunological therapies. Predictive analytics powered by AI enables more accurate patient stratification, ensuring that trials are targeted to specific subgroups with the greatest likelihood of benefit. AI can also model trial outcomes based on patient characteristics and biomarker data, reducing trial duration and increasing the likelihood of success. These advancements are particularly important for immune-modulating therapies, which often require highly personalized approaches due to the variability in immune responses among individuals (Topol, 2019).

The integration of AI into drug discovery for immunological disorders offers immense potential, but it also presents challenges. High-quality datasets are essential for training AI models, and inconsistencies in data standardization and accessibility can hinder progress. Furthermore, the interpretability of AI-generated insights is critical for gaining regulatory approval and ensuring clinical applicability. Despite these hurdles, advancements in explainable AI (XAI) and interdisciplinary collaboration between computational scientists and immunologists are addressing these limitations, paving the way for more reliable and impactful applications. As the global prevalence of immunological disorders continues to rise, driven by factors such as environmental pollution, stress, and aging populations, the need for innovative therapeutic solutions becomes increasingly urgent. This chapter explores the transformative role of AI in the drug discovery, design, and development pipeline for immunological disorders, highlighting its potential to revolutionize treatment paradigms and improve patient outcomes.

Objectives of the Chapter

The aims of this chapter are as follows:

(1) To evaluate the overview of Artificial Intelligence.
(2) To discuss the application of AI in drug discovery.
(3) To review the AI-based tools in drug discovery.
(4) To evaluate the AI-based models to support better targeted therapies for immune diseases.
(5) To X-ray the AI-based predictive models to design and evaluate therapeutic drug candidates for AIIDs.
(6) To discuss the case studies of AI-driven drug discovery, design, and development in immunological disorders
(7) To review the challenges and future perspectives.

Organization of the Chapter

The rest of this chapter is organized as follows: Section 2 explores the overview of Artificial Intelligence. Section 3 discusses the application of AI in drug discovery. Section 4 traverse the AI-based tools in drug discovery. Section 5 discusses the AI-based models to support better targeted therapies for immune diseases. Section 6 X-ray the AI-based predictive models to design and evaluate therapeutic drug candidates for AIIDs. Section 7 discusses the case studies of AI-driven drug discovery, design, and development in immunological disorders. Finally, a review on the challenges and future perspectives and a concluding section summarizes the AI-driven drug discovery, design, and development in immunological disorders.

ARTIFICIAL INTELLIGENCE OVERVIEW

The utilisation of digital data within the pharmaceutical industry has significantly increased in recent years. The acquisition, analysis, and application of knowledge to address complex healthcare issues present challenges associated with digitalisation (Ramesh et al., 2004). This facilitates the use of AI, capable of handling large volumes of data with enhanced automation (Miles & Walker, 2006). Machines utilising artificial intelligence (AI) can learn and address problems similarly to humans. Nonetheless, it does not present a significant risk of entirely replacing the necessity for human interaction (Yang & Siau, 2018; Wirtz et al., 2019). AI utilises software and systems capable of learning from data inputs and making independent judgements to accomplish its objectives. This chapter outlines the ongoing expansion of its applications within the pharmaceutical industry. The rapid advancement of AI-driven automation is anticipated to significantly transform societal perspectives on work, according to the McKinsey Global Institute (Smith & Farquhar, 2000).

Along with reasoning, knowledge representation, and solution search, Machine Learning is one of the many fields that make up Artificial Intelligence. In order to find patterns in a dataset that has already been classified, machine learning (ML) uses algorithms. Machine learning includes deep learning, which makes use of ANNs. They consist of a complex network of "perceptons" (Beneke & Mackenrodt, 2019) and function similarly to the way electrical impulses go through the human brain. In order to solve issues, Artificial Neural Networks (ANNs) use a network of linked nodes to take in data as inputs and turn it into outputs, either alone or in conjunction with other nodes (Steels & Brooks, 2019). It is possible to train ANNs using either supervised or unsupervised approaches; such examples are multilayer perceptrons (MLPs), convolutional neural networks (CNNs), and recurrent neural networks (RNNs) (Bielecki & Bielecki, 2019). An MLP network can be trained using unidirectional supervised procedures and then used as a universal pattern classifier. Pattern recognition, optimisation tools, process identification, and controls are all examples of possible applications (Kalyane et al., 2020).

The capacity to remember and store data is a property of closed-loop networks, which include RNNs, Boltzmann machines, and Hopfield networks (Kalyane et al., 2020). Convolutional neural networks (CNNs) are topologically described as a collection of dynamic systems with local connections (Hanggi & Moschytz, 2000). They have diverse applications, such as image and video processing, pattern recognition, biological system modelling, and complicated signal processing. Networks such as ADALINE, counter-propagation, LVQ, RBF, and Kohonen are examples of advanced kinds (Bielecki & Bielecki, 2019). The building blocks of AI systems, especially networks, have been the focus of multiple resources. One example of a tool driven by artificial intelligence is the IBM Watson supercomputer, which was developed in the USA by International Business Machines in New York. Cancer therapy alternatives can be found by analysing and correlating a patient's medical records with a huge database. Quick identification of illnesses is made possible by this method. The fact that breast cancer can be detected in as little as 60 seconds is proof of this (Ogidi & Tawariowei, 2023; Rouse, 2017; Ogidi et al., 2024).

Artificial intelligence (AI) has the potential to play a crucial role in the whole pharmaceutical product life cycle, from research to patient care, thanks to its abilities to handle clinical data for future drug development, aid in decision-making, and enable rational medication design. Through the use of machine learning algorithms and an intuitive user interface, E-VAI, an artificial intelligence platform created by Eularis, aids marketing executives in allocating resources optimally to increase market share, reverse falling sales, and anticipate investment possibilities. In order to provide analytical roadmaps, the platform takes into account the present market share, important stakeholders, and rivals (Baronzio et al., 2015).

APPLICATION OF AI IN DRUG DISCOVERY

Artificial intelligence significantly influences the pharmaceutical industry by enhancing efficiency, reducing costs, and improving effectiveness. The process of developing new medications can be enhanced through the application of AI at various stages. The integration of AI technology has enabled substantial progress in pharmaceutical research through its exceptional capabilities in data processing, pattern recognition, and decision-making (Khan et al., 2021; Chen et al., 2021). This analysis examines the impact of artificial intelligence (AI) on drug discovery processes. This discussion will examine advancements in drug design, polypharmacology, chemical synthesis, drug repurposing, and screening, as well as other critical components of drug development. Table 1 shows AI-driven drug discovery, design, and development in immunological disorders, it provides in-depth insights into how AI technologies revolutionize each phase of drug discovery and development for immunological disorders, with real-world applications and examples. Figure 1 illustrates some applications of AI in drug discovery.

Figure 1. Application of AI in drug discovery

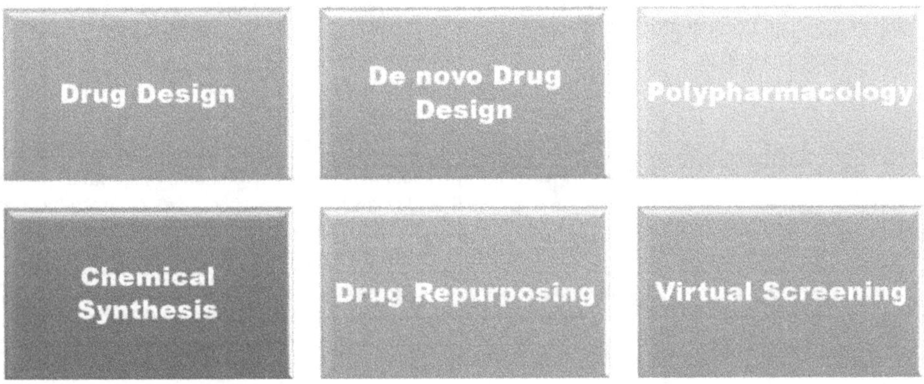

Table 1. AI-driven drug discovery, design, and development in immunological disorders

Phase	AI Application	Immunological Disorder	Key Benefits	AI Techniques/Tools Used	Examples and Case Studies
Drug Target Identification	Identifying molecular targets for drug development	Rheumatoid Arthritis (RA)	Speeds up discovery of novel targets, enhances accuracy in identifying relevant pathways	Deep learning, graph-based algorithms	AI tools like AtomNet identifying JAK-STAT and NF-κB pathways for RA
		Psoriasis	Unveils hidden molecular interactions, reducing manual work	Protein-protein interaction networks	AI mapping IL-23 and TNF-α as critical targets in psoriasis
Hit Compound Discovery	Screening large chemical libraries for potential drug candidates	Systemic Lupus Erythematosus (SLE)	Reduces time and cost, identifies promising leads efficiently	Virtual screening, molecular docking	GANs predicting small molecules targeting B-cell receptor signaling in SLE
		Asthma	Accelerates discovery of anti-inflammatory compounds	High-throughput screening (HTS) simulations	DeepChem identifying novel corticosteroid analogs with fewer side effects

continued on following page

Table 1. Continued

Phase	AI Application	Immunological Disorder	Key Benefits	AI Techniques/Tools Used	Examples and Case Studies
Lead Optimization	Refining chemical structures for improved efficacy and safety	Inflammatory Bowel Disease (IBD)	Improves binding affinity predictions, reduces off-target effects	Quantitative structure-activity relationship (QSAR) models	AI refining IL-12/ IL-23 inhibitors like ustekinumab for better efficacy
Drug Design	Generating novel molecules with desired properties	Type 1 Diabetes (T1D)	Enables design of highly specific drugs, reduces dependency on trial-and-error	Reinforcement learning, GANs	Insilico Medicine using GANs to design molecules targeting autoimmunity pathways
		Psoriatic Arthritis	Tailors molecular designs for specific disease subtypes	Evolutionary algorithms	Novel compounds targeting TNF-α and IL-17 pathways
Preclinical Testing	Predicting drug toxicity and pharmacokinetics	Multiple Sclerosis (MS)	Identifies potential safety risks early, reduces animal testing	Machine learning (ML) for ADMET (absorption, distribution, metabolism, excretion, toxicity) predictions	AstraZeneca using AI for hepatotoxicity screening during MS drug development
Clinical Trial Design	Patient stratification and optimal trial design	Inflammatory Bowel Disease (IBD)	Enhances trial efficiency, improves success rates by identifying suitable candidates	Clustering algorithms, survival analysis	IBM Watson Health identifying biomarkers for Crohn's disease trial optimization
		Lupus	Reduces trial costs by optimizing dosage and patient selection	Predictive analytics, Bayesian optimization	AI-driven stratification in belimumab clinical trials for lupus
Repurposing Existing Drugs	Identifying new therapeutic uses for existing drugs	Type 1 Diabetes (T1D)	Speeds up development process, reduces cost	NLP, deep learning	AI identifying methotrexate for potential use in T1D to modulate immune response
		Psoriasis	Saves years of research by finding alternative applications for approved drugs	Knowledge graphs, data mining	Baricitinib repurposed for severe psoriasis using AI-driven repurposing tools
Biologics Design	Designing antibodies, peptides, and other biologics	HIV/AIDS	Customizes biologics for better specificity and efficacy	Neural networks for antibody structure prediction	DeepMind's AlphaFold accurately predicting antibody structures targeting HIV

continued on following page

Table 1. Continued

Phase	AI Application	Immunological Disorder	Key Benefits	AI Techniques/Tools Used	Examples and Case Studies
		Cancer Immunotherapy	Optimizes T-cell receptor (TCR) designs for improved immune targeting	ML-based affinity prediction models	AI improving chimeric antigen receptor (CAR) T-cell therapies
Immune System Modeling	Simulating immune responses to predict drug effects	Multiple Sclerosis (MS)	Provides insights into immune-drug interactions, reduces need for extensive in vivo studies	Agent-based modeling, systems biology approaches	AI predicting immune response to interferon beta treatment in MS
Post-Market Surveillance	Monitoring real-world drug efficacy and adverse effects	Allergies, Autoimmune Diseases	Enhances drug safety, supports regulatory compliance	NLP, real-time data processing	NLP analyzing electronic health records (EHRs) for side effects of biologics like adalimumab

Drug Design

Artificial intelligence (AI) significantly enhances the identification of potential lead compounds in the pharmaceutical sector, thereby substantially reducing the duration required for drug development (Hasselgren, 2024). AI has expedited the transition from concept to clinical application by automating the analysis of diverse chemical configurations and predicting their potential binding affinities (Deng et al., 2022). The identification of small molecules that fulfil specific critical criteria is central to the process of drug design. The innovative spirit necessary for securing intellectual property rights for economic viability, along with pharmacological efficacy, a favourable safety profile, and acceptable chemical and biological characteristics, are critical factors (Santos-Filho et al., 2024). Conventional methods encounter several challenges, such as prolonged input durations, substantial computational expenses, and variable reliability (Lavecchia & Cerchia, 2016; Hasselgren, 2024), whereas computational tools have revolutionised drug design and discovery processes.

AI presents a promising solution to address these challenges and enhance the effectiveness and applicability of computational methods in drug development. Protein dysfunction is linked to numerous diseases, making the study of protein architectures a crucial aspect of therapeutic development. Structural drug design aims to identify small compounds capable of binding to specific proteins. Historically, predicting the three-dimensional (3D) structure of proteins has been a challenging and costly endeavour, with de novo predictions demonstrating low accuracy (Dara et al., 2022). The field of medication design has been significantly altered by the emergence of artificial intelligence, particularly through feature extraction tools and deep learning methodologies. The advancements in these technologies have improved our understanding of the relationship between structure and sequence, facilitating precise predictions of secondary protein structures and the mapping of protein interactions (Dara et al., 2022; Spencer et al., 2015). The primary purpose of employing deep learning in this context are to investigate protein-protein interactions (PPI) and enhance structural drug design by yielding more precise predictions of 3D protein structures (Dara et al., 2022). The integration of AI into medication design represents a significant advancement, with the potential to enhance the efficiency, speed, and cost-effectiveness of drug development efforts (Hasselgren, 2024). Artificial intelligence drug design categorization is shown in Figure 2.

Figure 2. Artificial intelligence drug design categorization

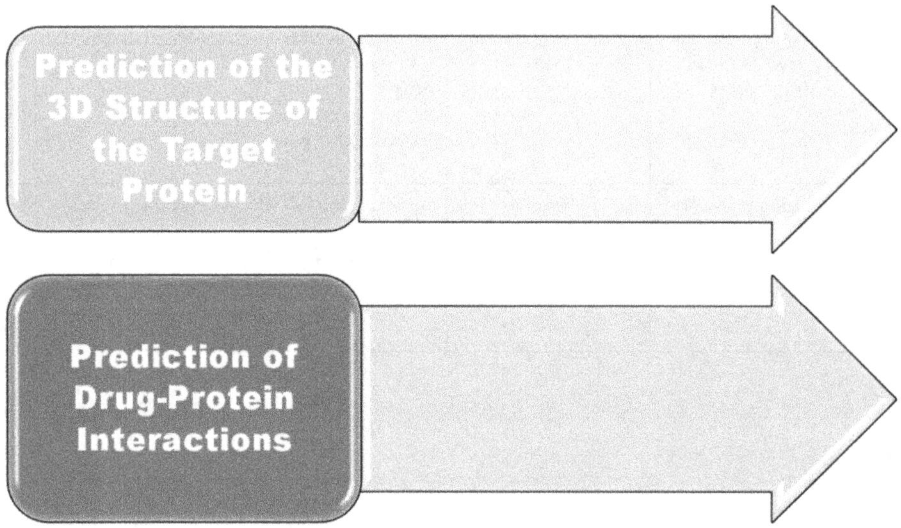

Prediction of the 3D Structure of the Target Protein

An essential component of structure-based drug design and discovery is the precise prediction of the three-dimensional (3D) structure of target proteins. To address this challenge, AI techniques, including machine learning and deep learning algorithms, have become essential (Sarkar et al., 2023; Dara et al., 2022). The accumulation of extensive structural and sequence data from various sources is fundamental to AI-driven protein structure prediction. The complex relationships between amino acid sequences and their three-dimensional structures can be incorporated into AI models utilising this dataset (Liu et al., 2019). Artificial intelligence models, particularly those utilising deep learning, have shown significant proficiency in identifying complex patterns in protein data through advanced computational techniques (Khan et al., 2021). Models can predict protein 3D structures from sequences by meticulously extracting features related to amino acid characteristics, structural motifs, and evolutionary background (Jumper et al., 2021; Qureshi et al., 2023;Moult et al., 2014). Google DeepMind's AlphaFold marks a significant advancement in the field of AI-based protein structure prediction (Narayanan et al., 2022).

AlphaFold predicts the three-dimensional structure of target proteins by analysing peptide bond angles and the distances between adjacent amino acids (Jumper et al., 2021). In a recent evaluation, AlphaFold accurately predicted 25 out of 43 protein structures, underscoring its potential in structure-based drug discovery (Khan et al., 2021). Traditional methods of protein structure determination, while precise, tend to be resource-intensive (Sarkar et al., 2023). AI facilitates the rapid and cost-effective generation of reliable 3D structures from sequence data. This advancement enables early prediction of medication effectiveness and safety through design aligned with the target protein's structure (Gaudelet et al., 2021).

Molecular dynamics (MD) simulations and various AI methods can utilise predicted three-dimensional structures of drugs and proteins from databases like DrugBank and the Protein Data Bank (PDB) to investigate the dynamics, geometry, binding efficacy, and stability of protein-drug complexes. This may elucidate the complexities of their interactions over time (Qureshi et al., 2023). Graph machine learning algorithms have shown potential in modelling complex interactions within biomedical data (Gaudelet et al., 2021). These techniques represent molecular systems as graphs, where atoms serve as fundamental units. This enables the identification of intricate patterns and relationships among medications, diseases, PPI, and drug side effects. This may facilitate drug repurposing and enhance response prediction (Gaudelet et al., 2021).

Prediction of Drug-Protein Interactions

Artificial intelligence (AI) can significantly enhance drug development by improving the prediction of drug-protein interactions (DPIs) (Jimenes-Vargas et al., 2024). Artificial intelligence (AI) facilitates the analysis of large chemical and biological datasets through the application of advanced computational techniques, including deep learning and machine learning (Jimenes-Vargas et al., 2024). These datasets are meticulously organised into comprehensive databases that detail well-documented drug-protein interactions (DPIs), encompassing molecular structures, chemical properties, and experimental binding affinities. These repositories provide a valuable resource for artificial intelligence algorithms to analyse and identify the intricate patterns that dictate the interactions between drug compounds and protein targets (Dhakal et al., 2022). Through the analysis of molecular data, AI models effectively identify critical factors influencing DPIs and can predict potential interactions for new drug candidates based on their chemical compositions (Dhakal et al., 2022). Artificial intelligence enhances the drug development process by enabling scientists to prioritise potential drug candidates based on anticipated safety and efficacy. This results in more effective and efficient treatments, significantly reducing the time and financial resources required for testing (Qiu et al., 2024; Borkakoti & Thornton, 2023).

The ongoing development of new treatments and the repurposing of existing medications for various clinical applications contribute to a dynamic pharmaceutical landscape, underscoring the significance of studying DPIs. Investing significant time and resources in the development of a new medicine through traditional biological research presents considerable challenges and demands extensive effort. Consequently, computational methods, including AI techniques, have emerged as crucial tools for accurately predicting DPIs, resulting in significant advancements in high-precision prediction methodologies. In recent years, DPI prediction has undergone a transformation, with a shift from traditional machine learning methods to the more complex domain of deep learning. Research into DPI predictions is increasingly motivated by the enhanced accuracy of deep learning architectures such as RNNs, CNNs, and deep neural networks (DNNs) in comparison to previous methodologies (Zhang et al., 2022; Yingkai-Gao et al., 2018; Tian et al., 2016;Mayr et al., 2018). Accurate prediction of ligand-protein interactions is essential for understanding therapeutic efficacy, facilitating drug repurposing, and reducing the risks associated with polypharmacology (Cichonska et al., 2024; Avorn, 2015). The utilisation of AI approaches has enabled accurate predictions of these interactions, resulting in enhanced therapy outcomes. An example is the model developed by researchers, which was trained on 15,000 protein-ligand interactions (Mayr et al., 2018; Reddy & Zhang, 2013).

This model identified nine novel compounds and their interactions with four significant targets by utilising primary protein sequences and the structural characteristics of small molecules. Furthermore, considering potential off-target effects, AI methodologies can aid in the development of new compounds that align with polypharmacology principles, resulting in the formulation of safer medication candidates (Reddy & Zhang, 2013). The integration of extensive databases with AI platforms, such as self-organising maps (SOMs), enables the association of multiple substances with diverse objectives and off-targets. Bayesian classifiers and SEA algorithms enhance the understanding and prediction of DPIs by establishing connections between drug pharmacological characteristics and their potential targets (Yingkai-Gao et al., 2018).

AI In De Novo Drug Design

De novo drug design involves the creation of novel molecular structures that resemble drugs, without utilising existing compounds or templates (Blaschke et al., 2020). This method may successfully explore the vast chemical space, estimated to encompass between 10^60 and 10^100 drug-like compounds (Jiménez-Luna et al., 2021). AI, particularly machine learning and deep learning methods, has played a significant role in addressing the challenges associated with de novo design. This has the potential to transform the discovery process of new therapeutic agents (Jiménez-Luna et al., 2021). Traditional de novo design methods often face two significant challenges: complex synthetic routes and the difficulty of predicting the bioactivity of new compounds. Artificial intelligence seeks to address these limitations through advanced computational models and algorithms that analyse extensive biological and chemical datasets to identify patterns connecting pharmaceutical effects to molecular structures (Hessler & Baringhaus, 2018). Generative adversarial networks (GANs) and variational autoencoders (VAEs) are particularly effective models within this sector of generative AI. Through the analysis of molecular representation distributions, these models are capable of generating novel chemical entities that align with user-defined characteristics (Chen et al., 2018; Agu & Obulose, 2024).

Gómez-Bombarelli et al. (2018), proposed a VAE-based method to translate chemical structures into a continuous latent space, thereby enhancing the production of novel molecules through the optimisation of latent representations. Additionally, de novo drug design has utilised deep reinforcement learning (DRL). The Reinforcement Learning for Structural Evolution (RLSE) program employs both models: one that proposes new structures and another that assesses their attributes, utilising both types of deep neural networks (DNNs) to generate new molecules. Compounds targeting specific receptors, including retinoid X and PPAR agonists, have been developed through DRL techniques, demonstrating the anticipated therapeutic benefits (Merk et al., 2018; Segler et al., 2018). Artificial intelligence (AI) enhances the efficiency of lead discovery and optimisation via computer-aided synthesis planning, which identifies numerous synthesizable structures and delineates potential synthesis pathways. Techniques including strategic synthesis planning, continuous data refinement, and online learning platforms facilitate this process (Dara et al., 2022). In addition to the synthesis of small molecules, artificial intelligence has extensive applications in the de novo design of pharmaceuticals. Symbolic AI has been employed alongside techniques such as deep neural networks (DNNs) and Monte Carlo tree searches (MTCS) for the purposes of reaction prediction and mechanism elucidation. This has facilitated more rapid exploration of chemical space compared to traditional methods (Klucznik et al., 2018; Segler et al., 2018).

PPI prediction, a relatively underexplored therapeutic area, has shown potential for AI applications. AI-driven tools facilitate the study of protein-protein interaction (PPI) interfaces, enhancing our understanding of the structural factors governing these interactions. This knowledge can be utilised to develop novel medicinal therapies that specifically target PPIs. Significant efforts have been made to advance AI in de novo drug design; however, considerable progress remains necessary. The efficient exploration of the vast chemical space, the synthesis of accessible compounds, and the accurate prediction of bioactivity for novel molecules present significant challenges (Popova et al., 2018; Schneider-Clark, 2019). The application of artificial intelligence (AI) techniques in the development of new medications represents a transformative approach that has the potential to accelerate the creation of safe and effective pharmaceuticals.

AI In Polypharmacology

Polypharmacology, which examines the interactions between multiple medications and various targets, is supplanting the traditional "one drug, one target" model in the pharmaceutical development sector (Reddy & Zhang, 2013). The rationale for this change is to enhance the management of complex diseases and to increase treatment efficacy (Chaudhari et al., 2020). Polypharmacology has advanced significantly due to artificial intelligence (AI), which facilitates the analysis of extensive biological datasets and identifies new candidates with polypharmacological potential (Lavecchia & Cerchia, 2016). Polypharmacology has become increasingly relevant as our understanding of disease aetiology and molecular complexities has advanced (Lavecchia & Cerchia, 2016). Extensive databases such as ZINC, PubChem, and DrugBank have played a crucial role in facilitating this transformation (Chaudhari et al., 2020). These resources integrate extensive data on chemical characteristics, binding affinities, and molecular pathways, offering a substantial foundation for artificial intelligence algorithms to explore and comprehend the intricate connections within (Mak & Pichika, 2019; Ryu et ak., 2018). Platforms such as DeepDDI demonstrate the impact of AI by elucidating drug-drug interactions and predicting alternative therapeutic applications with reduced side effects. Furthermore, AI has the capability to predict off-target interactions, thereby enhancing our understanding of a drug's comprehensive effects and facilitating the development of safer, more effective therapies (Chaudhari et al., 2020; Mak & Pichika, 2019; Ryu et ak., 2018).

Drug repurposing, off-target toxicity prediction, and the rational design of multi-target medicines (MTDs) are domains that can benefit from the shift towards polypharmacology. Computational approaches powered by artificial intelligence (AI) have demonstrated significant efficacy in two domains: predicting polypharmacological profiles and facilitating medication repurposing (Lavecchia & Cerchia, 2016). The realisation that targeting multiple nodes within complex biological networks may yield greater success than focussing on a single node has driven the shift towards polypharmacology, especially for multifactorial disorders. This method offers a comprehensive perspective on drug development by integrating characteristics of biological networks, including connectedness, redundancy, and pleiotropy (Lavecchia & Cerchia, 2016). Furthermore, polypharmacology may facilitate medication repurposing or drug reprofiling, potentially reducing drug development costs and time by identifying new applications for existing approved pharmaceuticals. Reports indicate successful pharmacological repositioning, with artificial intelligence approaches aiding in the identification of new repurposing potentials (Lavecchia & Cerchia, 2016).

AI In Chemical Synthesis

In the search for new pharmaceuticals, the efficiency and sustainability of chemical synthesis are critical. The introduction of AI has significantly transformed this field, enhancing reaction conditions and enabling remarkably accurate predictions of results. The integration of chemical knowledge with artificial intelligence facilitates the rapid synthesis of complex medicinal compounds, thereby enhancing the potential for new medication discoveries (Struble et al., 2020). The integration of AI into chemical synthesis enhances the accuracy and efficiency of synthetic processes, marking a substantial advancement in drug discovery (Struble et al., 2020). Numerous studies indicate that AI significantly impacts the rapid identification of optimal reaction conditions and the achievement of error-free autonomous synthesis (Struble et al., 2020; Ryu et al., 2018). The integration of AI, real-time reaction monitoring, and automation enhances the speed and reliability of experimental workflows (Ryu et al., 2018). The reliance on automated systems and AI algorithms poses the risk of oversimplifying the complex nature of chemical reactions. The thorough integration of AI technologies with a comprehensive understanding of chemical concepts is crucial, as oversimplification may lead to inaccurate interpretations of reaction dynamics (Ryu et al., 2018).

AI In Drug Repurposing

Drug repurposing, drug repositioning, or retasking refers to the process of identifying new therapeutic applications for medications initially developed for different medical conditions (Lotfi-Shahreza et al., 2018). This method has garnered significant attention due to its potential to reduce the time required for the development of new treatments, decrease associated costs, and expedite patient access compared to traditional drug discovery pipelines (Parvathaneni et al., 2019). AI has emerged as a crucial instrument in drug repurposing due to its robust analytical capabilities. It has the capability to analyse extensive datasets encompassing genomic information, clinical records, and pharmacological databases. This approach facilitates the identification of new disease targets and the establishment of novel associations between existing drugs (Yadav et al., 2024). Different AI strategies, including feature-based, network-based, and matrix-based approaches, enable drug repurposing (Yadav et al., 2024). Due to established safety profiles from previous studies, AI-driven drug repurposing can bypass early-phase clinical trials and toxicological assessments. The effectiveness reduces development times and costs substantially, allowing repurposed medications to bypass Phase I trials and proceed directly to Phase II trials for new indications (Corsello et al., 2017; Hernandez et al., 2017).

Deep neural networks (ANNs) and generative adversarial networks (GANs) represent significant artificial intelligence techniques with substantial potential in pharmacological property prediction, novel molecule synthesis, and the classification of complex drug action mechanisms (Aliper et al., 2016; Mak & Pichika, 2019). GANs are capable of generating novel molecular structures derived from actual data, whereas DNNs can categorise pharmaceuticals into therapeutic classes based on their functional characteristics, efficacy, therapeutic applications, and toxicity, potentially transforming drug design. A notable advantage of reinforcement learning, a distinct AI approach, is its reduced dependence on learning from datasets. Conversely, these algorithms can identify trends in the strategic design of pharmacological molecules, potentially leading to the development of medications with minimised adverse effects. AI algorithms can enhance the safety profiles of repurposed medications by accurately differentiating between cardiotoxic and non-cardiotoxic compounds (Mak & Pichika, 2019).

Furthermore, by facilitating the creation of therapeutic compounds tailored to specific genetic profiles and disease subtypes, AI demonstrates its potential in precision medicine. This individualised strategy is anticipated to enhance treatment outcomes and reduce side effects (Kadurin et al., 2017). Contemporary artificial intelligence (AI) techniques offer advanced applications in information science for the definition of diseases, medications, and therapies, as well as for target identification, minimising the potential for error in the context of big data and network medicine. Researchers have utilised extensive knowledge graphs to identify potential drugs for disorders like COVID-19, mapping the relationships among publications, biological processes, and targets (Ogidi, 2024; Tripathi et al., 2021; Ogidi, 2022).

Obstacles remain in the application of AI for medication repurposing, including the requirement for advanced computational resources to manage and analyse extensive networks. Additionally, identifying specific areas for further research may lead to innovative strategies, such as the development of machine-learning models focused on medication side effects, which could illuminate new pathways for drug repurposing (Struble et al., 2020). The application of artificial intelligence in drug repurposing signifies the onset of a transformative era in drug discovery. This era will accelerate the development of innovative therapeutic agents, decrease costs, and enhance the delivery of effective medications. This is especially relevant for complex and rare diseases that presently have limited treatment options.

AI In Virtual Screening

Virtual screening is a critical computational strategy in contemporary drug discovery pipelines. To identify compounds effective against a specific biological target, rapid evaluation of extensive chemical libraries is facilitated (Tripathi et al., 2021; Chen et al., 2017; Kusumoto et al., 2022). This technique typically employs a series of computational procedures to identify small molecules with specific biological activities from extensive compound libraries (Wu et al., 2019). Virtual screening methods are generally categorised into two main types: structure-based virtual screening (SBVS) and ligand-based virtual screening (LBVS). SBVS methodologies commonly employ molecular docking simulations to examine the three-dimensional structure of target proteins, aiming to identify compounds that may bind effectively to their active sites (Tripathi et al., 2021).

Conversely, LBVS methodologies utilise a repository of known active ligands to identify structurally similar compounds through various molecular representations, such as two-dimensional fingerprints, pharmacophore models, and three-dimensional shape similarities (Tripathi et al., 2021). Artificial intelligence, particularly deep learning and machine learning techniques, can significantly enhance the efficiency and accuracy of virtual screening campaigns. The substantial data generated by virtual screening, including molecular structures, binding affinities, and target-ligand interactions, can be analysed, allowing for the extraction of valuable insights through AI algorithms (Tripathi et al., 2021). SBVS has employed AI methodologies, including boosting algorithms, support vector machines (SVMs), and random forests (RFs), to enhance current scoring systems by establishing non-linear correlations between molecular characteristics and target-ligand interactions (Tripathi et al., 2021). Deep learning architectures, such as CNNs, have shown exceptional efficacy in virtual screening applications by automatically identifying relevant features from molecular data. DeepVS employs CNNs for screening compounds against targets, while PTPD utilises them for constructing peptide-based molecules (Wu et al., 2019; Tripathi et al., 2021). Artificial intelligence methods have demonstrated efficacy in LBVS by categorising and predicting the bioactivities of chemicals based on their physicochemical properties and geographical similarities to known active ligands. The expanding chemical space and the growing volume of publicly available data necessitate the use of deep learning techniques for the efficient and precise processing of large datasets (Tripathi et al., 2021).

Artificial intelligence in virtual screening offers several advantages, including enhanced hit rates relative to traditional screening methods, the ability to predict ADME/Tox properties and "drug-likeness" during the screening process, and the potential to explore interactions between all existing molecules and prospective targets. To validate virtual screening results, it is essential to complement them with relevant laboratory tests and clinical investigations (Wu et al., 2019). Virtual screening utilising artificial intelligence has emerged as a crucial method in the discovery of novel pharmaceuticals, particularly those exhibiting anticancer characteristics. The identification of potential anticancer lead compounds from natural sources has been facilitated by the ability to efficiently screen libraries of natural products, encompassing terpenes, alkaloids, coumarins, flavonoids, lignans, quinones, and tannins (Wu et al., 2019).

Prediction Of Physicochemical Properties

Accurate forecasting of the physicochemical properties of potential therapeutic candidates is essential in the dynamic field of drug research. AI has significantly enhanced features such as solubility, permeability, and stability, demonstrating a substantial impact in this domain. To ensure that a medication effectively reaches its target and exerts therapeutic effects, these qualities are essential (Zang et al., 2017). Solubility significantly influences medication pharmacokinetics and formulation, prompting AI-driven prediction efforts (Agu & Obulose, 2024; Zang et al., 2017). Research into AI-based solutions for addressing the resource-intensive and time-consuming challenges associated with traditional experimental methods for measuring solubility has commenced (Agu & Obulose, 2024). Various deep learning methods, including SchNet, fully connected neural networks, recurrent neural networks (RNNs), and graph neural networks, have demonstrated effectiveness in accurately predicting solubility. The investigations have highlighted the efficacy of 2D molecular descriptors, as evidenced by the superior performance of fully connected neural networks employing these descriptors (Agu & Obulose, 2024). A broader range of physicochemical parameters, including intrinsic permeability, degree of ionisation, and partition coefficient (logP), can also be predicted by AI, alongside solubility (Zang et al., 2017).

The overall pharmacokinetic profile and interaction with target receptor families are influenced by these features (Zang et al., 2017; Yang et al., 2019). Workflows for Quantitative Structure-Property Relationship (QSPR) and neural networks have been established to predict essential properties, including lipophilicity and the acid dissociation constant, thereby demonstrating the utility of AI in drug design (Yang et al., 2019). AI tools utilise extensive datasets from prior compound optimisations to train models capable of generating and predicting viable molecules and their properties. This process employs molecular descriptors such as SMILES strings, potential energy measurements, and electron density. Various prediction models have been employed to estimate the intestinal absorptivity of drugs, considering factors such as molecular volume, logP, and solubility index (Kumar et al., 2017).

An example includes the use of convolutional neural networks (CNN) and undirected graph recursive neural networks for simulating solubility. AI has significantly advanced the prediction of pharmacological properties through rapid candidate screening, detection of potential drug-drug interactions, and assessments of drug metabolism and toxicity. Artificial intelligence (AI) has the potential to enhance and accelerate drug development processes, as evidenced by sophisticated AI frameworks and predictive models such as ImageMol for analysing drug-drug interactions. Before the initiation of clinical trials, these advancements illuminate drug behaviour and interactions, facilitating a more efficient drug development process (Kumar et al., 2017).

Drug Toxicity Prediction

The emergence of AI has significantly advanced drug toxicity prediction, improving the identification of potential side effects in new medication candidates. AI models are meticulously trained and validated to outline toxicity profiles, emphasising potential damage to specific organs or biological processes. This capability allows for the prioritisation of molecules with reduced side effects, resulting in the selection of safer medication candidates (Hessler & Baringhaus, 2018). Assessing toxicity is a critical factor in the development of new pharmaceuticals (Agu & Obulose, 2024). In vivo animal testing is frequently employed for conventional toxicity evaluations; however, it incurs high costs and raises ethical concerns (Agu & Obulose, 2024; Basile et al., 2019). Computational methods utilising AI represent an efficient and cost-effective strategy for assessing chemical toxicity (Agu & Obulose, 2024). The Tox21 challenge and similar initiatives illustrate the efficacy of diverse computational techniques, with artificial intelligence notably excelling in accurately predicting substance toxicity (Raises & Bajic, 2016; Agu & Obulose, 2024).

In comparative experiments, the DeepTox algorithm, utilising a DNN architecture, surpassed traditional models in predicting substance toxicity, highlighting the potential of AI in this domain (Agu & Obulose, 2024). Artificial intelligence is employed to predict toxicity, thereby mitigating the risks associated with drug development. Early anticipation of negative effects during the development process is achievable through tools such as DeepTox, which effectively assesses drug toxicity and aids in the detection and management of toxicological issues (Santos-Filho et al., 2024). AI's predictive capabilities significantly improve pre-market medication safety by enabling the anticipation of side effects, therapeutic targets, and safety profiles before the initiation of clinical trials. This preventative measure enhances medication safety and decreases post-marketing adverse effects by reducing the likelihood of trial failures due to unforeseen toxicity (Santos-Filho et al., 2024; Basile et al., 2019; Lysenko et al., 2018). The use of AI for toxicity prediction offers enhanced efficiency in assessing cytotoxicity, mitochondrial toxicity, off-target toxicity, genotoxicity, organ toxicity, and other related areas (Santos-Filho et al., 2024). Artificial intelligence algorithms can effectively predict in vivo toxicity outcomes by analysing extensive datasets that encompass gene expression and cell imaging information. Quantitative structure-activity relationship (QSAR) models utilising ensemble techniques such as support vector machines (SVMs) and random forests (RF) demonstrate superior toxicity prediction accuracy and robustness compared to traditional methods (Pattewicz & Fitzpatrick, 2016; Santos-Filho et al., 2024).

Drug Bioactivity Prediction

Artificial intelligence (AI) possesses the capacity to transform drug discovery through enhancements in drug screening methodologies and, specifically, in the prediction of bioactivity. AI is transforming the evaluation of therapeutic potential and the understanding of mechanisms of action for drug candidates by predicting a compound's affinity for specific proteins or receptors and identifying potential interactions (Hasselgren, 2024). Many drugs derived from natural sources may lack efficacy due to insufficient bioactivity, making the evaluation of bioactivity a significant challenge in drug development (Khan et al., 2021). Traditional methods for assessing a drug's bioactivity depend on costly and lengthy in vitro and in vivo experiments. AI methodologies have emerged as effective tools for predicting pharmacological activities, including antibacterial, antiviral, and anticancer properties, due to their efficiency and cost-effectiveness (Agu & Obulose, 2024; Strokes et al., 2020).

Stokes et al. (2020) introduced a directed message-passing neural network model as a novel application of AI for predicting antibiotic activity. This model evaluates a molecule's antibacterial potential by constructing chemical graphs from SMILES notations and extracting detailed feature vectors. A simplified method for the discovery of new antimicrobial drugs is presented (Agu & Obulose, 2024). Forecasting a drug's target binding affinity (DTBA) is essential for assessing its effectiveness. AI-powered approaches utilise two interaction types: feature-based interactions, which consider the pharmacological characteristics of both the medication and the target, and similarity-based interactions, which posit that pharmaceuticals with analogous characteristics will interact with corresponding targets (Ozturk et al., 2018). Reliable forecasting of DTBA has employed tools such as ChemMapper and SEA, alongside machine learning and deep learning methods including KronRLS, SimBoost, DeepDTA, and PADME. Artificial intelligence (AI) tools have enhanced the capacity for predicting drug-protein interactions through advanced computational models that do not rely on the availability of three-dimensional (3D) protein structures (Ozturk et al., 2018).

Deep learning models such as DeepAffinity and PADME can predict drug-target interactions by incorporating comprehensive drug and target characteristics (Karimi et al., 2019). For instance, Deep Affinity combines RNN and CNN with both labelled and unlabelled data to create a comprehensive representation of DPIs (Karimi et al., 2019). PADME employs feed-forward neural networks to estimate the strength of drug-target protein interactions, facilitating more accurate predictions of treatment efficacy and mechanisms of action (Ozturk et al., 2018). Furthermore, AI can predict ADME (Absorption, Distribution, Metabolism, and Excretion) properties, which are crucial for understanding the pharmacokinetics of drug molecules. Tools such as XenoSite and SMARTCyp enhance the prediction of drug clearance pathways and contribute to the understanding of drug metabolism by identifying metabolic sites and specific CYP450 isoforms involved in this process (Karimi et al., 2019).

AI-BASED TOOLS IN DRUG DISCOVERY

Artificial intelligence is set to transform the drug development industry by enhancing the exploration of large databases, facilitating the creation of new chemical structures, and improving the prediction of the efficacy of potential drug candidates (Qureshi et al., 2023). Figure 3 and Table 2 highlights how various AI-based tools accelerate and optimize the drug discovery process, from target identification to lead optimization, showcasing their real-world applications is shown below.

Figure 3. Some AI-based tools in drug discovery and development

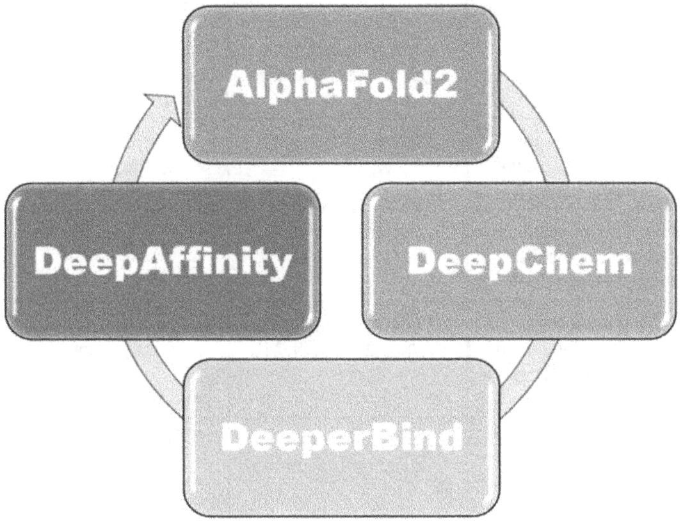

Table 2. AI-based tools in drug discovery

AI Tool	Function	Key Features	Applications in Drug Discovery	Examples of Use Cases
AtomNet	Predicts binding of small molecules to proteins	Deep learning, convolutional neural networks	Target identification, lead discovery	Identified novel drug candidates for Ebola and multiple sclerosis
DeepChem	Provides machine learning models for molecular property prediction	Open-source, supports cheminformatics	Virtual screening, ADMET predictions	Used for predicting solubility, toxicity, and bioactivity of compounds
AlphaFold	Predicts protein 3D structures with high accuracy	Deep neural networks, attention mechanisms	Protein structure prediction	Solved previously uncharacterized protein structures for novel drug targets
Generative Adversarial Networks (GANs)	Generates novel drug-like molecules	Generative modeling, reinforcement learning	De novo drug design, lead optimization	Designed novel compounds for kinase inhibitors and antibiotics
Schrödinger	Molecular modeling and simulation software	Quantum mechanics, machine learning	Lead optimization, binding affinity prediction	Optimized HIV-1 protease inhibitors and other antiviral compounds
BenevolentAI	Identifies potential drug targets and repurposing opportunities	Knowledge graphs, deep learning	Target discovery, drug repurposing	Repurposed baricitinib for COVID-19 treatment
Exscientia	AI-driven automated drug design	Reinforcement learning, multi-parameter optimization	Lead optimization, compound prioritization	Developed the first AI-designed drug, DSP-1181, for obsessive-compulsive disorder (OCD)

continued on following page

Table 2. Continued

AI Tool	Function	Key Features	Applications in Drug Discovery	Examples of Use Cases
Insilico Medicine	AI-powered platform for generative biology and chemistry	Deep learning, generative modeling	Drug target discovery, de novo drug design	Identified potential anti-aging and anti-fibrotic drug candidates
Cresset	Uses computational chemistry for molecular design	Electrostatics, shape analysis	Hit-to-lead optimization	Used for designing improved inhibitors for cancer and neurodegenerative diseases
GENTRL	Generates novel chemical structures for specific biological targets	Variational autoencoders (VAEs), RL	De novo drug design	Designed DDR1 kinase inhibitors within 46 days
IBM Watson for Drug Discovery	Analyzes scientific literature and biomedical data to identify patterns	Natural language processing (NLP), ML	Target identification, repurposing	Used to identify novel drug-disease associations in oncology and autoimmune disorders
OpenEye	Provides tools for molecular modeling and visualization	Molecular docking, ligand optimization	Virtual screening, lead discovery	Accelerated structure-based drug design for various oncology targets
BioSymetrics	Combines AI with biomedical data to find actionable insights	Multi-modal data integration, ML	Biomarker discovery, target validation	Identified biomarkers and drug targets for inflammatory diseases
Cyclica	Predicts polypharmacology of small molecules	AI-driven ligand prediction	Drug repurposing, target deconvolution	Successfully repurposed drugs for rare genetic diseases

Fold2 Developed By AlphaFold2

The prediction of protein three-dimensional structures based on amino acid sequences presents a highly complex challenge. DeepMind's AlphaFold2, accessible through Google Colab, has achieved a significant breakthrough in accuracy (Jumper et al., 2021).

DeepChem

DeepChem, a TensorFlow wrapper, facilitates and enhances the analysis of chemical datasets (Subramanian et al., 2016). Research on one-shot deep-learning algorithms for medication development and application projects, such as BACE-1 inhibitor modelling, has utilised it (Subramanian et al., 2016). DeepChem enables the counting of cells in microscopic images, the prediction of solubility for small molecule medications and their binding affinity to targets, as well as the analysis of protein structures. MoleculeNet, as part of its DeepChem package, now encompasses the properties of 700,000 chemicals (Subramanian et al., 2016).

DeeperBind

A long-short-term recurrent convolutional network, termed DeeperBind, models the interaction between transcription factors (TF) and their respective DNA/RNA binding sites by predicting protein binding specificity concerning DNA probes (Alipanahi et al., 2015). DeeperBind provides insights into the behaviour of probe sequences. Datasets comprising sequences of differing lengths are applicable for both training and testing purposes (Alipanahi et al., 2015).

DeepAffinity

DeepAffinity employs a semi-supervised model that combines convolutional and recurrent neural networks to predict the binding affinity of a drug to target sequences (Karimi et al., 2019). The model combines labelled and unlabelled data to produce distinct, structurally annotated representations of protein sequences that encapsulate molecular representations. DeepAffinity outperformed RNN-CNN models, ensemble methods, and random forests (Karimi et al., 2019).

AI-BASED MODELS TO SUPPORT BETTER TARGETED THERAPIES FOR IMMUNE DISEASES

Representation of the Complexity of Immune Disorders

The initial phase of implementing precision medicine involves creating models to understand and represent patient heterogeneity. Recent advancements in high-throughput multi-omics technology have enabled complete molecular profiling of patient cohorts comprising thousands of individuals (Barturen et al., 2021; Lee & Cleynen, 2019; Moingeon, 2023). This facilitates the documentation of dysregulated biological processes in blood and target organs. The integration and analysis of high-dimensional data, previously challenging for traditional bioinformatics methods, is now feasible due to advancements in AI and ML. This enables researchers to categorise patients into comparable clusters and subsequently identify the distinct molecular markers associated with each cluster. These signals may serve as biomarkers in precision medicine, facilitating patient selection, predicting disease progression, assessing treatment responses, and identifying potential treatment-related risks. Table 3 illustrate AI-based predictive models and their applications in the study of immunological diseases.

Selection of Relevant Therapeutic Targets

After patients are grouped according to their risk factors, a detailed map of dysregulated genes or proteins in blood or target organs is created for each cluster. This map is then compared to a healthy control group. Pathway enrichment approaches facilitate the assembly of disease-associated components into canonical molecular pathways (Moingeon et al., 2022). The subsequent step involves performing network computational analysis to identify dysregulated pathways that may contribute to the causation of the disease. An interactome can be constructed to document the relative significance of each gene and protein in relation to other components of the disrupted biological system. This offers compelling evidence for a causative role in the disease by facilitating the identification of hubs, master regulators, and driver mutations essential for regulating the entire disease system (Moingeon et al., 2023).

Identification and Optimization of Drug Candidates

Once therapeutic targets have been identified, the next step in using AI to create and optimise new drugs can begin. To forecast target-binding and pharmacological effects from virtual libraries of tiny chemical compounds, AI-enhanced computational chemistry uses quantitative structure-activity relationships (QSAR). In order to associate and predict the pharmacological properties of a large number of possible medicinal compounds, artificial neural networks are trained using a large number of chemical structures (Moingeon et al., 2022). With the help of AI, chemists can foretell how a molecule will dissolve in water, how it will break down in the body, whether it will be harmful or not, and whether it will have an agonistic or antagonistic effect. The use of artificial neural networks to forecast the characteristics of synthetic antisense oligonucleotides and tiny chemical compounds is on the rise, while monoclonal antibodies are a major tool in the fight against infectious diseases (Mason et al., 2021). Some immunological illnesses, such as Sjogren's disease, allergies, inflammatory bowel disease, and systemic lupus erythematosus, are characterised by dysregulation of many proinflammatory molecular pathways, according to recent modelling research. This highlights the importance of researching and developing new drug combinations for the treatment of patients with complicated IDs (Desvaux et al., 2022). The use of computational approaches in the design and selection of combination medicines can increase the likelihood of success in confirmatory clinical studies.

In Silico Trial Simulation in Virtual Patients

AI can be useful in determining whether potential drugs for infectious diseases are safe and effective. Improvements in patient selection, data integration, analysis, and clinical trial design are made possible by the application of AI. One area where AI has recently found use is in the realm of clinical trial simulation using in silico drug performance predictions (Moingeon et al., 2023). To achieve this goal, virtual patients are created using data acquired from real patients or electronic health records. On the flip side, investigational drugs for autoimmune illnesses can be tested on virtual patients created using AI-enhanced quantitative system pharmacology (QSP) models (Moingeon et al., 2023).

One alternative makes use of digital twins, an idea originally developed for the automotive and aerospace sectors, to build a VR that mimics the operation of a real-life system with linked parts. Digital twins serve as organ models for medical applications, constructed from multi-level physiological data and medical imaging. These models may be specific to cells, tissues, or organs. Medical devices exhibiting mechanical effects, such as human heart models, are more effectively assessed through digital twins compared to medications that influence biological processes, as the latter do not currently utilise extensive molecular data (Moingeon et al., 2023). Despite the ongoing challenges in simulating the complexity of the immune system, preliminary efforts have been undertaken to create an immunological digital twin capable of replicating immune responses in both healthy individuals and those with immunodeficiency disorders (Moingeon, 2023). Finally, employing AI-based causal models of ID pathophysiology enables the simulation of medication effects through the analysis of their interactions with key drivers of the disrupted biological system.

Table 3. AI-based predictive models and their applications in the study of immunological diseases

Model Type	Application	Immunological Disease	Key Features
Random Forest	Predicting disease susceptibility and biomarker discovery	Rheumatoid Arthritis (RA)	Feature selection, handles high-dimensional data, interpretable outputs
Support Vector Machine	Classifying disease stages and patient stratification	Multiple Sclerosis (MS)	Effective in small sample sizes, kernel-based learning
Neural Networks	Modeling immune response and drug efficacy prediction	Type 1 Diabetes (T1D)	High predictive accuracy, captures complex non-linear relationships
Convolutional Neural Networks (CNN)	Image-based analysis of immune cells	Psoriasis, Lupus	Processes medical images (e.g., histology), automates feature extraction
Recurrent Neural Networks (RNN)	Predicting disease progression using sequential data	Inflammatory Bowel Disease (IBD)	Captures temporal patterns, useful for longitudinal patient data
Gradient Boosting Machines	Identifying genetic variants linked to immune diseases	Ankylosing Spondylitis	High performance in classification and regression tasks, robust to overfitting
Bayesian Networks	Modeling causal relationships in immune pathways	Asthma, Allergies	Incorporates uncertainty, useful for probabilistic inferences
k-Nearest Neighbors (k-NN)	Classifying patient groups based on immune profiles	Systemic Lupus Erythematosus	Simple, interpretable, works well with small datasets
Autoencoders	Dimensionality reduction and anomaly detection in immune data	HIV/AIDS	Identifies rare patterns, compresses complex data efficiently
Transformers	Predicting immune responses from sequence data	Cancer Immunotherapy	Processes large-scale sequence data, captures long-range dependencies

AI-BASED PREDICTIVE MODELS TO DESIGN AND EVALUATE THERAPEUTIC DRUG CANDIDATES FOR AIIDS

Model-Based Design and Optimization of Drug Candidates

Using AI-based models to better understand the pathophysiology of patient subgroups, current drugs can be assessed for their potential as AIID therapeutics. In order to find new molecular targets for current drugs, this method employs network-based deep learning to examine databases of cellular, genetic, phenotypic, and chemical data. Treatments for severe COVID-19 strains have been identified through the use of drug repurposing, and research into artificial influenza immunodeficiency virus (AIID) medications is ongoing (Desvaux et al., 2021; Ogidi et al., 2021). In order to create and optimise new drugs to treat AIIDs, it is crucial to identify important targets involved in their aetiology. Through the use of properties like quantitative structure-activity relationships (QSARs) to forecast target binding and activity, artificial intelligence (AI) in computational chemistry may search virtual libraries of small molecules for possible pharmaceuticals that interact with therapeutic targets (Moingeon et al., 2022).

Predicting three-dimensional protein structures from readily available primary amino acid sequences has become much easier with the latest release of the DeepMind AlphaFold algorithm (Jumper et al., 2021).

In a chemical environment containing millions of chemicals, deep learning is used to train convolutional neural networks on ligand-based virtual screens to find and improve drugs that interact with possible therapeutic targets (Vamathevan et al., 2019; Rube et al., 2022). To train neural networks to predict the functional properties of tiny chemical compounds, the SMILES (Simple Molecular Input Line Entry System) technique converts the structure of each molecule. Current deep learning capabilities allow for the simultaneous prediction of numerous properties, including as pharmacological activity, high-affinity target binding, and ADMET (absorption, distribution, metabolism, excretion, and toxicity) factors (Vamathevan et al., 2019). Predictions about the functional properties and improvements to the ornamentation of these molecules allow for further optimisation in silico after leads have been identified. With the help of adversarial neural network-based generative AI, scientists can learn how to synthesise new chemicals and create new substances altogether, a process known as retrosynthesis (Moingeon et al., 2022).

Employing AI-based approaches for drug candidate design offers numerous benefits. A significant aspect is its extensive coverage of chemical space. For confirmatory testing in wet-lab experiments, it is sufficient to synthesise a limited number of molecules with predicted suitable properties, which are likely to succeed. A limitation of contemporary deep learning neural network methodologies is their optimal application in predicting the properties of synthetic antisense oligonucleotides and small chemical entities (Moingeon et al., 2022).

In Silico Evaluation of the Efficacy and Safety of Drug Candidates

AI has multiple applications in the assessment of safety and efficacy for potential AIID drugs. AI can enhance the planning of clinical trials by improving data collection and analysis during monitoring, as well as assisting in the identification of eligible patients for participation (Subbiah, 2023). Digital devices utilised by patients during their daily activities can facilitate the collection of patient-reported outcomes in decentralised clinical trials (Burnester, 2018; Capobianco & Meroni, 2021). In trials with a limited number of placebo recipients, artificial intelligence can facilitate the creation of virtual placebo groups or parallel control arms (Thorlund et al., 2020; Subbiah, 2023).

Using real-world data sources, such as electronic health records, this program creates virtual patients based on real-life subjects that meet the trial's inclusion and exclusion criteria and have documented responses to standard treatment. A lot of people are looking into in silico trial simulations right now, using different kinds of virtual models of patients' illnesses. Several models are being investigated as substitutes for real patients in order to ascertain the efficacy and security of tailored medications. The aerospace and automotive sectors were the first to use the idea of a digital twin, which is a way to simulate physical reality by using a system of linked components (Corral-Acero et al., 2020; Kamel-Boulos & Peng, 2021). At the cellular, tissue, and organ-wide levels, digital twins are representations of organ-specific models built from physiological and medical imaging data (Corral-Acero et al., 2020; Kamel-Boulos & Peng, 2021). By faithfully reproducing anatomical details and blood flow dynamics during simulated cardiac activity, a living human heart model was successfully created using MRI images, demonstrating the efficiency of pacemakers and stents. For the time being, digital twins are better suited for testing mechanically active medical devices than drugs that alter biological processes due to a lack of complete molecular data. One major reason why organ-specific AIIDs using digital twins have not been developed yet is the difficulty of correctly simulating the immune system. A recently suggested paradigm for constructing an immune digital twin makes it possible to mimic immune responses in both healthy individuals and those with diverse immunological diseases (Laubenbacher et al., 2022).

This model captures the inherent diversity in immune responses observed in humans, which is impacted by variables like age, ethnicity, genes, environment, and microbiome composition (Nedelec et al., 2016; Clemente et al., 2018; Ogidi & Felagha, 2024). Information gathered from healthy groups that were exposed to natural triggers or vaccinations could provide support for this approach (Thomas et al., 2015; Brodin & Davis, 2017). Virtual patients are an alternative sort of model that are built using data that is unique to each patient, such as their medical history, lifestyle decisions, and the results of multiomic profiling. This approach takes into account the individual characteristics of each patient in order to improve and personalise treatment results (Voigt et al., 2021). In the field of AI-enhanced quantitative systems pharmacology (QSP), the goal of developing virtual patients is to forecast how well investigational medications will work against AIIDs. The core components of a QSP model include a drug candidate's pharmacokinetic and pharmacodynamic characteristics, clinical symptom data, and information about different biological processes in blood and tissues (Aghamiri et al., 2022). By simulating the system with the help of ordinary differential equations, we can predict how the medicine will affect the biological system and, hopefully, how it would reduce symptoms (Zhang et al., 2022). Finding biomarkers for patient categorisation and monitoring, determining dosage regimens and administration procedures, and selecting clinical objectives for future studies are all made easier with QSP models. By realistically altering biological and clinical features, virtual patient cohorts can be generated by AI thanks to its ability to incorporate large and multimodal data. This allows for the recreation of the variability observed in real patients, for example, in multiomic profiling (Aghamiri et al., 2022).

CASE STUDIES OF AI-DRIVEN DRUG DISCOVERY, DESIGN, AND DEVELOPMENT IN IMMUNOLOGICAL DISORDERS

The revolutionary impact of AI in streamlining and improving the drug development process is demonstrated in case studies of AI-driven drug discovery, design, and development in immunological disorders. Drug targeting, chemical structure optimisation, toxicity prediction, and drug repurposing are all areas where artificial intelligence (AI) technologies like deep learning, generative models, and reinforcement learning come into play. As an example, BenevolentAI repurposed the rheumatoid arthritis drug baricitinib and used it to treat COVID-19 (Ogidi, 2020). Artificial intelligence (AI) has the ability to generate new treatments; for example, Exscientia developed DSP-1181, the first AI-designed medication, to treat obsessive-compulsive disorder (OCD) (Hasselgren, 2024).

Artificial intelligence models have enhanced the creation of biologics like IL-6 inhibitors and personalised T-cell treatments for autoimmune illnesses like multiple sclerosis (MS) and systemic lupus erythematosus (SLE). Insilico Medicine's platform for inflammatory bowel disease is only one example of how AI has improved preclinical testing by predicting the safety and efficacy of medication candidates. In addition, convolutional neural networks (CNNs) can now categorise psoriasis subtypes, which helps in developing individualised treatment plans, all thanks to AI. These examples demonstrate how AI can simplify and expedite the treatment of immunological illnesses while simultaneously enhancing their outcomes (Santos-Filho et al., 2024). In order to demonstrate concrete results and progress, Table

4 details real-world case studies that show how AI has greatly aided in the discovery, design, and development of drugs for immunological illnesses.

Table 4. Case studies of AI-driven drug discovery, design, and development in immunological disorders

Case Study	AI Tool/Model Used	Disease	Application	Outcome/Impact	Example
Baricitinib for COVID-19 (Repurposed)	BenevolentAI	Rheumatoid Arthritis (RA), COVID-19	Drug repurposing	Identified JAK inhibitor (baricitinib) as an effective treatment for COVID-19 inflammation	BenevolentAI's repurposing of baricitinib for cytokine storm-related conditions
DSP-1181 for OCD	Exscientia	Obsessive-Compulsive Disorder (OCD)	AI-driven drug design	First AI-designed drug to enter human trials, targeting serotonin receptors	Collaboration between Exscientia and Sumitomo Dainippon Pharma
Anti-TNF Biologics Optimization	DeepChem	Rheumatoid Arthritis (RA)	Lead optimization	Improved binding affinity and reduced immunogenicity of TNF inhibitors	AI optimizing etanercept and adalimumab formulations
IL-6 Inhibitor Development	Schrödinger	Systemic Lupus Erythematosus (SLE)	Virtual screening, molecular docking	Identified new IL-6 receptor inhibitors to reduce cytokine storm	Schrödinger's molecular modeling tools
Neoantigen Vaccine Design	DeepImmune	Cancer Immunotherapy	Personalized immunotherapy	Predicted T-cell epitopes for personalized neoantigen vaccines	Used in designing patient-specific vaccines for melanoma
T-cell Therapy for MS	AlphaFold	Multiple Sclerosis (MS)	Protein structure prediction	Modeled myelin protein structures to enhance T-cell receptor specificity	AI tools helping improve chimeric antigen receptor (CAR) T-cell therapies
Drug Toxicity Prediction	Insilico Medicine	Inflammatory Bowel Disease (IBD)	Preclinical testing	Predicted hepatotoxicity and off-target effects of new anti-inflammatory compounds	Insilico's AI platform for toxicity and ADMET predictions
Small Molecule Inhibitors for SLE	Generative Adversarial Networks (GANs)	Systemic Lupus Erythematosus (SLE)	De novo drug design	Designed novel small molecules targeting B-cell pathways	GAN-generated inhibitors tested in preclinical studies
Cancer Immunotherapy Antibody Design	AlphaFold	Cancer Immunotherapy	Antibody optimization	Improved structure and binding affinity of immune checkpoint inhibitors	AI designing PD-1 and CTLA-4 checkpoint inhibitors
Autoimmune Thyroiditis Biomarker Discovery	Cyclica	Hashimoto's Thyroiditis	Target discovery	Identified novel biomarkers and therapeutic targets for thyroid inflammation	Cyclica's Ligand Express platform identifying thyroid-specific protein interactions
Asthma Biologics Development	Reinforcement Learning Models	Asthma	Lead optimization	Optimized IL-5 inhibitors for eosinophilic asthma	AI refining mepolizumab and benralizumab formulations

continued on following page

Table 4. Continued

Case Study	AI Tool/Model Used	Disease	Application	Outcome/Impact	Example
Psoriasis Subtype Classification	Convolutional Neural Networks (CNN)	Psoriasis	Image-based patient stratification	Automated classification of psoriasis severity and subtypes using skin biopsy images	AI-enhanced diagnostic tools assisting in personalized treatment plans
Biologic for Ankylosing Spondylitis (AS)	Bayesian Optimization	Ankylosing Spondylitis (AS)	Protein engineering	Engineered biologics targeting HLA-B27 protein with reduced immunogenicity	AI streamlining the development of TNF-α and IL-17 inhibitors

CHALLENGES AND FUTURE PERSPECTIVES

Artificial intelligence-based AIID models are being used more and more in drug development to aid in important decisions like finding the best therapeutic target based on in-depth pathophysiology insights, choosing the best drug out of millions of virtual candidates, and predicting which patient subsets will have the best recovery. Predictive algorithms connect patient data to virtual medication qualities based on anticipated characteristics; computational precision medicine is the outcome of AIID-specific medicines being implemented more quickly. In response to the revolutionary effect of AI-driven models on medication development, pharmaceutical firms are constructing high-throughput computational platforms to uncover potential targets and choose treatment methods. Advanced computational analytics and big data are facilitating a paradigm shift that enhances patient care by accelerating the discovery of improved, personalised treatments across various therapeutic areas (Jayatunga et al., 2022).

Multiple factors must be considered when implementing a model-informed drug development strategy. Regulatory bodies require more reliable and acceptable anticipated results, necessitating improvements and validation of computer models. The importance of standardised validation best practices, cross-validation, and independent testing for AI and ML models applied to AIIDs is underscored by the observation that merely 8.3% of published studies have performed thorough evaluations of these models (Stafford et al., 2020). To ensure that virtual models of specific patients' diseases yield reliable predictions, clinical trials with actual patients are now necessary. Reduced necessity for clinical investigations and increased likelihood of success will occur if regulatory bodies consistently recognise these models as evidence of medication efficacy, given their reliability in meeting standardised criteria is increasingly validated. Future prediction models are expected to combine other data sources, such as multiomic data, high-resolution imaging data, environmental and lifestyle data, and others, even if first-generation models show excellent performance (Stafford et al., 2020). More lifelike digital twins of the human body and better virtual patients are now within reach, thanks to these innovations. More sophisticated models are required to reproduce 'healthy' immune responses after vaccination or spontaneous infection in order to precisely characterise pathogenic dysregulation in autoimmune immune deficiency diseases (AIIDs). Drug candidates that interact with components of pathways resulting in bad outcomes can have their safety issues investigated using causative illness models based on systems biology, in addition to therapeutic efficacy assessment (Ankley et al., 2018).

Given the impracticality of assessing every potential combination therapy in clinical trials, there is a need for more effective computational tools to evaluate the efficacy of medications. The development of these complex models necessitates increased computational power, and regulators will seek validation of these models. In the realm of data management, curation, and preprocessing, along with effective simulation methods, several established recommendations exist (Boehme et al., 2019; Wilkinson et al., 2016). Supportive predictive computer modelling will play a significant supplementary role in the development of new medications and the demonstration of their safety and effectiveness. The integration of outcomes from predictive computer models with data from actual drug development processes represents the most effective strategy for discovering new treatments for AIIDs within a mixed reality framework (USFDA. 2021).

CONCLUSION

AI-driven technologies are revolutionising the medication research and discovery pipeline, particularly in the context of addressing the complexities of immune disorders. By employing advanced machine learning models, neural networks, and generative algorithms, artificial intelligence enables the precise optimisation of biologics, the rapid identification of therapeutic targets, and the efficient design of novel drug candidates. These technologies can be employed to streamline and enhance the efficiency of the traditional drug development process, while also enhancing the accuracy of predictions regarding the medicine's efficacy, safety, and individual responses in patients. AI has also facilitated the process of drug repurposing, as evidenced by the repurposing of baricitinib for COVID-19. This enables the modification of previously approved pharmaceuticals for novel immunological applications. Artificial intelligence models, such as AlphaFold, are decoding complex protein structures for autoimmune disorders like rheumatoid arthritis and systemic lupus erythematosus, which is bringing about intriguing new opportunities in the production of biologics and antibodies. The field of immunology is poised to capitalise on the growing sophistication of AI tools, which will facilitate the development of personalised treatment, improve patient outcomes, and increase healthcare equity on a global scale. Researchers in the field must maintain open lines of communication with pharmaceutical companies and physicians in order to ensure that patients have access to treatments that are more efficient, effective, and tailored to their specific needs. This will allow them to make the most of AI.

REFERENCES

Aghamiri, S. S., Amin, R., & Helikar, T. (2022). Recent applications of quantitative systems pharmacology and machine learning models across diseases. *Journal of Pharmacokinetics and Pharmacodynamics, 49*(1), 19–37. DOI: 10.1007/s10928-021-09790-9 PMID: 34671863

Agu, P. C., & Obulose, C. N. (2024). Piquing artificial intelligence towards drug discovery: Tools, techniques, and applications. *Drug Development Research, 85*(2), e22159. DOI: 10.1002/ddr.22159 PMID: 38375772

Alipanahi, B., Delong, A., Weirauch, M. T., & Frey, B. J. (2015). Predicting the sequence specificities of DNA- and RNA-binding proteins by deep learning. *Nature Biotechnology, 33*(8), 831–838. DOI: 10.1038/nbt.3300 PMID: 26213851

Aliper, A., Plis, S., Artemov, A., Ulloa, A., Mamoshina, P., & Zhavoronkov, A. (2016). Deep Learning Applications for Predicting Pharmacological Properties of Drugs and Drug Repurposing Using Transcriptomic Data. *Molecular Pharmaceutics, 13*(7), 2524–2530. DOI: 10.1021/acs.molpharmaceut.6b00248 PMID: 27200455

Ankley, G. T., & Edwards, S. W. (2018). The Adverse Outcome Pathway: A Multifaceted Framework Supporting 21st Century Toxicology. *Current Opinion in Toxicology, 9*, 1–7. DOI: 10.1016/j.cotox.2018.03.004 PMID: 29682628

Avorn, J. (2015). The $2.6 billion pill—Methodologic and policy considerations. *The New England Journal of Medicine, 372*(20), 1877–1879. DOI: 10.1056/NEJMp1500848 PMID: 25970049

Baronzio, G., Parmar, G., & Baronzio, M. (2015). Overview of Methods for Overcoming Hindrance to Drug Delivery to Tumors, with Special Attention to Tumor Interstitial Fluid. *Frontiers in Oncology, 5*, 165. DOI: 10.3389/fonc.2015.00165 PMID: 26258072

Barturen, G., Babaei, S., Català-Moll, F., Martínez-Bueno, M., Makowska, Z., Martorell-Marugán, J., Carmona-Sáez, P., Toro-Domínguez, D., Carnero-Montoro, E., Teruel, M., Kerick, M., Acosta-Herrera, M., Le Lann, L., Jamin, C., Rodríguez-Ubreva, J., García-Gómez, A., Kageyama, J., Buttgereit, A., Hayat, S., & Alarcón-Riquelme, M. E. (2021). Integrative Analysis Reveals a Molecular Stratification of Systemic Autoimmune Diseases. *Arthritis & Rheumatology (Hoboken, N.J.), 73*(6), 1073–1085. DOI: 10.1002/art.41610 PMID: 33497037

Basile, A. O., Yahi, A., & Tatonetti, N. P. (2019). Artificial Intelligence for Drug Toxicity and Safety. *Trends in Pharmacological Sciences, 40*(9), 624–635. DOI: 10.1016/j.tips.2019.07.005 PMID: 31383376

Beneke, F., & Mackenrodt, M. O. (2019). Artificial intelligence and collusion. *IIC Int. Rev. IIC; International Review of Industrial Property and Copyright Law, 50*(1), 109–134. DOI: 10.1007/s40319-018-00773-x

Bielecki, A., & Bielecki, A. (2019). Foundations of artificial neural networks. In Kacprzyk, J. (Ed.), *Models of Neurons and Perceptrons: Selected Problems and Challenges* (pp. 15–28). Springer International Publishing. DOI: 10.1007/978-3-319-90140-4_3

Blaschke, T., Arús-Pous, J., Chen, H., Margreitter, C., Tyrchan, C., Engkvist, O., Papadopoulos, K., & Patronov, A. (2020). REINVENT 2.0: An AI Tool for De Novo Drug Design. *Journal of Chemical Information and Modeling*, *60*(12), 5918–5922. DOI: 10.1021/acs.jcim.0c00915 PMID: 33118816

Boehme, P., Hansen, A., Roubenoff, R., Scheeren, J., Herrmann, M., Mondritzki, T., Ehlers, J., & Truebel, H. (2019). How soon will digital endpoints become a cornerstone for future drug development? *Drug Discovery Today*, *24*(1), 16–19. DOI: 10.1016/j.drudis.2018.07.001 PMID: 30009955

Borkakoti, N., & Thornton, J. M. (2023). AlphaFold2 protein structure prediction: Implications for drug discovery. *Current Opinion in Structural Biology*, *78*, 102526. DOI: 10.1016/j.sbi.2022.102526 PMID: 36621153

Brodin, P., & Davis, M. M. (2017). Human immune system variation. *Nature Reviews. Immunology*, *17*(1), 21–29. DOI: 10.1038/nri.2016.125 PMID: 27916977

Burmester, G. R. (2018). Rheumatology 4.0: Big data, wearables and diagnosis by computer. *Annals of the Rheumatic Diseases*, *77*(7), 963–965. DOI: 10.1136/annrheumdis-2017-212888 PMID: 29802224

Capobianco, E., & Meroni, P. L. (2021). Value of digital biomarkers in precision medicine: Implications in cancer, autoimmune diseases, and COVID-19. *Expert Review of Precision Medicine and Drug Development*, *6*(4), 235–238. DOI: 10.1080/23808993.2021.1924055

Chaudhari, R., Fong, L. W., Tan, Z., Huang, B., & Zhang, S. (2020). An up-to-date overview of computational polypharmacology in modern drug discovery. *Expert Opinion on Drug Discovery*, *15*(9), 1025–1044. DOI: 10.1080/17460441.2020.1767063 PMID: 32452701

Chen, H., Engkvist, O., Wang, Y., Olivecrona, M., & Blaschke, T. (2018). The rise of deep learning in drug discovery. *Drug Discovery Today*, *23*(6), 1241–1250. DOI: 10.1016/j.drudis.2018.01.039 PMID: 29366762

Chen, H., Engkvist, O., Wang, Y., Olivecrona, M., & Blaschke, T. (2018). The rise of deep learning in drug discovery. *Drug Discovery Today*, *23*(6), 1241–1250. DOI: 10.1016/j.drudis.2018.01.039 PMID: 29366762

Chen, H., Zhou, X., Gao, Y., Chen, H., & Zhou, J. (2017). Fragment-based drug design: Strategic advances and lessons learned. *Comprehensive Medicinal Chemistry III*, 2–8, 212–232. .DOI: 10.1016/B978-0-12-409547-2.12319-4

Chen, Z., Liu, X., Hogan, W., Shenkman, E., & Bian, J. (2021). Applications of artificial intelligence in drug development using real-world data. *Drug Discovery Today*, *26*(5), 1256–1264. DOI: 10.1016/j.drudis.2020.12.013 PMID: 33358699

Cichońska, A., Ravikumar, B., & Rahman, R. (2024). AI for targeted polypharmacology: The next frontier in drug discovery. *Current Opinion in Structural Biology*, *84*, 102771. DOI: 10.1016/j.sbi.2023.102771 PMID: 38215530

Clemente, J. C., Manasson, J., & Scher, J. U. (2018). The role of the gut microbiome in systemic inflammatory disease. *BMJ (Clinical Research Ed.)*, *360*, j5145. DOI: 10.1136/bmj.j5145 PMID: 29311119

Corral-Acero, J., Margara, F., Marciniak, M., Rodero, C., Loncaric, F., Feng, Y., Gilbert, A., Fernandes, J. F., Bukhari, H. A., Wajdan, A., Martinez, M. V., Santos, M. S., Shamohammdi, M., Luo, H., Westphal, P., Leeson, P., DiAchille, P., Gurev, V., Mayr, M., & Lamata, P. (2020). The 'Digital Twin' to enable the vision of precision cardiology. *European Heart Journal, 41*(48), 4556–4564. DOI: 10.1093/eurheartj/ehaa159 PMID: 32128588

Corsello, S. M., Bittker, J. A., Liu, Z., Gould, J., McCarren, P., Hirschman, J. E., Johnston, S. E., Vrcic, A., Wong, B., Khan, M., Asiedu, J., Narayan, R., Mader, C. C., Subramanian, A., & Golub, T. R. (2017). The Drug Repurposing Hub: A next-generation drug library and information resource. *Nature Medicine, 23*(4), 405–408. DOI: 10.1038/nm.4306 PMID: 28388612

Dara, S., Dhamercherla, S., Jadav, S. S., Babu, C. M., & Ahsan, M. J. (2022). Machine Learning in Drug Discovery: A Review. *Artificial Intelligence Review, 55*(3), 1947–1999. DOI: 10.1007/s10462-021-10058-4 PMID: 34393317

Deng, J., Yang, Z., Ojima, I., Samaras, D., & Wang, F. (2022). Artificial intelligence in drug discovery: Applications and techniques. *Briefings in Bioinformatics, 23*(1), bbab430. Advance online publication. DOI: 10.1093/bib/bbab430 PMID: 34734228

Desvaux, E., Aussy, A., Hubert, S., Keime-Guibert, F., Blesius, A., Soret, P., Guedj, M., Pers, J. O., Laigle, L., & Moingeon, P. (2022). Model-based computational precision medicine to develop combination therapies for autoimmune diseases. *Expert Review of Clinical Immunology, 18*(1), 47–56. DOI: 10.1080/1744666X.2022.2012452 PMID: 34842494

Desvaux, E., Hamon, A., Hubert, S., Boudjeniba, C., Chassagnol, B., Swindle, J., Aussy, A., Laigle, L., Laplume, J., Soret, P., Jean-François, P., Dupin-Roger, I., Guedj, M., & Moingeon, P. (2021). Network-based repurposing identifies anti-alarmins as drug candidates to control severe lung inflammation in COVID-19. *PLoS One, 16*(7), e0254374. DOI: 10.1371/journal.pone.0254374 PMID: 34293006

Dhakal, A., McKay, C., Tanner, J. J., & Cheng, J. (2022). Artificial intelligence in the prediction of protein-ligand interactions: Recent advances and future directions. *Briefings in Bioinformatics, 23*(1), bbab476. Advance online publication. DOI: 10.1093/bib/bbab476 PMID: 34849575

Gao, Y., K., Fokoue, A., Luo, H., Iyengar, A., Dey, S., & Zhang, P. (2018). Interpretable drug target prediction using deep neural representation. *IJCAI International Joint Conference on Artificial Intelligence*, 7, 3371– 3377. https://doi.org/DOI: 10.24963/ijcai.2018/468

Gaudelet, T., Day, B., Jamasb, A. R., Soman, J., Regep, C., Liu, G., Hayter, J. B. R., Vickers, R., Roberts, C., Tang, J., Roblin, D., Blundell, T. L., Bronstein, M. M., & Taylor-King, J. P. (2021). Utilizing graph machine learning within drug discovery and development. *Briefings in Bioinformatics, 22*(6), bbab159. Advance online publication. DOI: 10.1093/bib/bbab159 PMID: 34013350

Gómez-Bombarelli, R., Wei, J. N., Duvenaud, D., Hernández-Lobato, J. M., Sánchez-Lengeling, B., Sheberla, D., Aguilera-Iparraguirre, J., Hirzel, T. D., Adams, R. P., & Aspuru-Guzik, A. (2018). Automatic Chemical Design Using a Data-Driven Continuous Representation of Molecules. *ACS Central Science, 4*(2), 268–276. DOI: 10.1021/acscentsci.7b00572 PMID: 29532027

Hanggi, M., & Moschytz, G. S. (2000). *Cellular Neural Networks: Analysis, Design and Optimization*. Springer Science & Business Media. DOI: 10.1007/978-1-4757-3220-7

Hasselgren, C., & Oprea, T. I. (2024). Artificial Intelligence for Drug Discovery: Are We There Yet? *Annual Review of Pharmacology and Toxicology*, *2024*(64), 527–550. DOI: 10.1146/annurev-pharmtox-040323-040828 PMID: 37738505

Hernandez, J. J., Pryszlak, M., Smith, L., Yanchus, C., Kurji, N., Shahani, V. M., & Molinski, S. V. (2017). Giving Drugs a Second Chance: Overcoming Regulatory and Financial Hurdles in Repurposing Approved Drugs as Cancer Therapeutics. *Frontiers in Oncology*, *7*, 291479. DOI: 10.3389/fonc.2017.00273 PMID: 29184849

Hessler, G., & Baringhaus, K. H. (2018). Artificial Intelligence in Drug Design. *Molecules (Basel, Switzerland)*, *23*(10), 2520. DOI: 10.3390/molecules23102520 PMID: 30279331

Jayatunga, M. K. P., Xie, W., Ruder, L., Schulze, U., & Meier, C. (2022). AI in small-molecule drug discovery: A coming wave? *Nature Reviews. Drug Discovery*, *21*(3), 175–176. DOI: 10.1038/d41573-022-00025-1 PMID: 35132242

Jimenes-Vargas, K., Pazos, A., Munteanu, C. R., Perez-Castillo, Y., & Tejera, E. (2024). Prediction of compound-target interaction using several artificial intelligence algorithms and comparison with a consensus-based strategy. *Journal of Cheminformatics*, *16*(1), 1–13. DOI: 10.1186/s13321-024-00816-1 PMID: 38449058

Jiménez-Luna, J., Grisoni, F., Weskamp, N., & Schneider, G. (2021). Artificial intelligence in drug discovery: Recent advances and future perspectives. *Expert Opinion on Drug Discovery*, *16*(9), 949–959. DOI: 10.1080/17460441.2021.1909567 PMID: 33779453

Jumper, J., Evans, R., Pritzel, A., Green, T., Figurnov, M., Ronneberger, O., Tunyasuvunakool, K., Bates, R., Žídek, A., Potapenko, A., Bridgland, A., Meyer, C., Kohl, S. A. A., Ballard, A. J., Cowie, A., Romera-Paredes, B., Nikolov, S., Jain, R., Adler, J., & Hassabis, D. (2021). Highly accurate protein structure prediction with AlphaFold. *Nature*, *596*(7873), 583–589. DOI: 10.1038/s41586-021-03819-2 PMID: 34265844

Kadurin, A., Nikolenko, S., Khrabrov, K., Aliper, A., & Zhavoronkov, A. (2017). druGAN: An Advanced Generative Adversarial Autoencoder Model for de Novo Generation of New Molecules with Desired Molecular Properties in Silico. *Molecular Pharmaceutics*, *14*(9), 3098–3104. DOI: 10.1021/acs.molpharmaceut.7b00346 PMID: 28703000

Kalyane, D., Sanap, G., Paul, D., Shenoy, S., Anup, N., Polaka, S., Tambe, V., & Tekade, R. K. (2020). Artificial intelligence in the pharmaceutical sector: current scene and future prospect. In Tekade, R. K. (Ed.), *The Future of Pharmaceutical Product Development and Research* (pp. 73–107). Elsevier. DOI: 10.1016/B978-0-12-814455-8.00003-7

Kamel Boulos, M. N., & Zhang, P. (2021). Digital Twins: From Personalised Medicine to Precision Public Health. *Journal of Personalized Medicine*, *11*(8), 745. DOI: 10.3390/jpm11080745 PMID: 34442389

Karimi, M., Wu, D., Wang, Z., & Shen, Y. (2019). DeepAffinity: Interpretable deep learning of compound-protein affinity through unified recurrent and convolutional neural networks. *Bioinformatics (Oxford, England), 35*(18), 3329–3338. DOI: 10.1093/bioinformatics/btz111 PMID: 30768156

Karimi, M., Wu, D., Wang, Z., & Shen, Y. (2019). DeepAffinity: Interpretable deep learning of compound-protein affinity through unified recurrent and convolutional neural networks. *Bioinformatics (Oxford, England), 35*(18), 3329–3338. DOI: 10.1093/bioinformatics/btz111 PMID: 30768156

Khan, S. R., Al Rijjal, D., Piro, A., & Wheeler, M. B. (2021). Integration of AI and traditional medicine in drug discovery. *Drug Discovery Today, 26*(4), 982–992. DOI: 10.1016/j.drudis.2021.01.008 PMID: 33476566

Kumar, R., Sharma, A., Siddiqui, M. H., & Tiwari, R. K. (2017). Prediction of Human Intestinal Absorption of Compounds Using Artificial Intelligence Techniques. *Current Drug Discovery Technologies, 14*(4), 244–254. DOI: 10.2174/1570163814666170404160911 PMID: 28382857

Kusumoto, D., Yuasa, S., & Fukuda, K. (2022). Induced Pluripotent Stem Cell-Based Drug Screening by Use of Artificial Intelligence. *Pharmaceuticals (Basel, Switzerland), 15*(5), 562. DOI: 10.3390/ph15050562 PMID: 35631387

Laubenbacher, R., Niarakis, A., Helikar, T., An, G., Shapiro, B., Malik-Sheriff, R. S., Sego, T. J., Knapp, A., Macklin, P., & Glazier, J. A. (2022). Building digital twins of the human immune system: Toward a roadmap. *NPJ Digital Medicine, 5*(1), 64. DOI: 10.1038/s41746-022-00610-z PMID: 35595830

Lavecchia, A., & Cerchia, C. (2016). In silico methods to address polypharmacology: Current status, applications and future perspectives. *Drug Discovery Today, 21*(2), 288–298. DOI: 10.1016/j.drudis.2015.12.007 PMID: 26743596

Lee, H. S., & Cleynen, I. (2019). Molecular Profiling of Inflammatory Bowel Disease: Is It Ready for Use in Clinical Decision-Making? *Cells, 8*(6), 535. DOI: 10.3390/cells8060535 PMID: 31167397

Liu, B., He, H., Luo, H., Zhang, T., & Jiang, J. (2019). Artificial intelligence and big data facilitated targeted drug discovery. *Stroke and Vascular Neurology, 4*(4), 206–213. DOI: 10.1136/svn-2019-000290 PMID: 32030204

Lotfi Shahreza, M., Ghadiri, N., Mousavi, S. R., Varshosaz, J., & Green, J. R. (2018). A review of network-based approaches to drug repositioning. *Briefings in Bioinformatics, 19*(5), 878–892. DOI: 10.1093/bib/bbx017 PMID: 28334136

Lysenko, A., Sharma, A., Boroevich, K. A., & Tsunoda, T. (2018). An integrative machine learning approach for prediction of toxicity-related drug safety. *Life Science Alliance, 1*(6), e201800098. DOI: 10.26508/lsa.201800098 PMID: 30515477

Mak, K. K., & Pichika, M. R. (2019). Artificial intelligence in drug development: Present status and future prospects. *Drug Discovery Today, 24*(3), 773–780. DOI: 10.1016/j.drudis.2018.11.014 PMID: 30472429

Mamoshina, P., Vieira, A., Putin, E., & Zhavoronkov, A. (2016). Applications of deep learning in biomedicine. *Molecular Pharmaceutics, 13*(5), 1445–1454. DOI: 10.1021/acs.molpharmaceut.5b00982 PMID: 27007977

Mason, D. M., Friedensohn, S., Weber, C. R., Jordi, C., Wagner, B., Meng, S. M., Ehling, R. A., Bonati, L., Dahinden, J., Gainza, P., Correia, B. E., & Reddy, S. T. (2021). Optimization of therapeutic antibodies by predicting antigen specificity from antibody sequence via deep learning. *Nature Biomedical Engineering*, *5*(6), 600–612. DOI: 10.1038/s41551-021-00699-9 PMID: 33859386

Mayr, A., Klambauer, G., Unterthiner, T., Steijaert, M., Wegner, J. K., Ceulemans, H., Clevert, D. A., & Hochreiter, S. (2018). Large-scale comparison of machine learning methods for drug target prediction on ChEMBL. *Chemical Science (Cambridge)*, *9*(24), 5441–5451. DOI: 10.1039/C8SC00148K PMID: 30155234

Merk, D., Friedrich, L., Grisoni, F., & Schneider, G. (2018). De Novo Design of Bioactive Small Molecules by Artificial Intelligence. *Molecular Informatics*, *37*(1-2), 1700153. DOI: 10.1002/minf.201700153 PMID: 29319225

Mikulak-Klucznik, B., Gołębiowska, P., Bayly, A. A., Popik, O., Klucznik, T., Szymkuć, S., Gajewska, E. P., Dittwald, P., Staszewska-Krajewska, O., Beker, W., Badowski, T., Scheidt, K. A., Molga, K., Mlynarski, J., Mrksich, M., & Grzybowski, B. A. (2020). Computational planning of the synthesis of complex natural products. *Nature*, *588*(7836), 83–88. DOI: 10.1038/s41586-020-2855-y PMID: 33049755

Miles, J., & Walker, A. (2006). The potential application of artificial intelligence in transport. IEE Proc. *Intell. Transport Syst.* 153, 183–198 DOI: 10.1049/ip-its:20060014

Moingeon, P. (2023). Artificial intelligence-driven drug development against autoimmune diseases. *Trends in Pharmacological Sciences*, *44*(7), 411–424. DOI: 10.1016/j.tips.2023.04.005 PMID: 37268540

Moingeon, P., Chenel, M., Rousseau, C., Voisin, E., & Guedj, M. (2023). Virtual patients, digital twins and causal disease models: Paving the ground for in silico clinical trials. *Drug Discovery Today*, *28*(7), 103605. DOI: 10.1016/j.drudis.2023.103605 PMID: 37146963

Moingeon, P., Kuenemann, M., & Guedj, M. (2022). Artificial intelligence-enhanced drug design and development: Toward a computational precision medicine. *Drug Discovery Today*, *27*(1), 215–222. DOI: 10.1016/j.drudis.2021.09.006 PMID: 34555509

Moingeon, P., Kuenemann, M., & Guedj, M. (2022). Artificial intelligence-enhanced drug design and development: Toward a computational precision medicine. *Drug Discovery Today*, *27*(1), 215–222. DOI: 10.1016/j.drudis.2021.09.006 PMID: 34555509

Moult, J., Fidelis, K., Kryshtafovych, A., Schwede, T., & Tramontano, A. (2014). Critical assessment of methods of protein structure prediction (CASP)--round x. *Proteins, 82 Suppl 2*(0 2), 1–6. https://doi.org/DOI: 10.1002/prot.24452

Narayanan, R. R., Durga, N., & Nagalakshmi, S. (2022). Impact of Artificial Intelligence (AI) on Drug Discovery and Product Development. *Indian Journal of Pharmaceutical Education and Research*, *56*(3s), s387–s397. DOI: 10.5530/ijper.56.3s.146

Nédélec, Y., Sanz, J., Baharian, G., Szpiech, Z. A., Pacis, A., Dumaine, A., Grenier, J. C., Freiman, A., Sams, A. J., Hebert, S., Pagé Sabourin, A., Luca, F., Blekhman, R., Hernandez, R. D., Pique-Regi, R., Tung, J., Yotova, V., & Barreiro, L. B. (2016). Genetic Ancestry and Natural Selection Drive Population Differences in Immune Responses to Pathogens. *Cell, 167*(3), 657–669.e21. DOI: 10.1016/j.cell.2016.09.025 PMID: 27768889

Nguyen, L., Moni, M. A., & Lio, P. (2021). Machine learning approaches in drug discovery: Methods and applications. *Molecular Diversity*, *25*(4), 1307–1322. DOI: 10.1007/s11030-021-10181-z

Ogidi, O. I. (2020). A review on the use of Herbal Remedies and Clinical Therapeutics for the Management of Covid-19 Pandemic. *ASIO Journal of Pharmaceuical & Herbal Medicines Research*, 6(2): 68-77. http://doi.org/doilink/10.2020.85722646/

Ogidi, O. I. (2022). Omicron (B.1.1.529): Variant of Concern- A Mini Review. *Biomedical Journal of Scientific & Technical Research,* 41(5), 33106- 33112. https://www.doiDOI: 10.26717/BJSTR.2022.41.006672

Ogidi, O. I. (2024). Therapeutic Role of Biomaterials in the Study of Severe Acute Respiratory Syndrome Corona Virus 2 (Sars-Cov-2). In: Advances in Sustainable Biomaterials: Bioprocessing 4.0, Characterizations and Application. *CRC Press, Taylor and Francis Group, Florida, USA.*

Ogidi, O. I., Barwant, M. M., & Okara, E. (2024). Biomarker Discovery: Protein Phosphorylation State. In *Spatially Variable Genes in Cancer: Development, Progression, and Treatment Response*. IGI Global., DOI: 10.4018/979-8-3693-7728-4.ch005

Ogidi, O.I., Berefagha, W.L., & Okara, E. (2021). Covid-19 vaccination: The pros and cons. *World Journal of Biology Pharmacy and Health Sciences,* 07(01), 015–022. https://doi.org/DOI: 10.30574/wjbphs.2021.7.1.0072

Ogidi, O. I., Deghinmotei, A. U., & Omolora, S. O. (2024). Anti-Diabetic and Lipid Profile Effect of Ethanol Extract of Ocimum tenuiflorum (Holy Basil) in Albino Rats. *Pharma Sci Analytical Res J*, *6*(3), 180070.

Ogidi, O. I., & Felagha, I. (2024). Gut Microbiome and Diet Interaction. In *Nutrition Controversies and Advances in Autoimmune Disease*. IGI Global. DOI: 10.4018/979-8-3693-5528-2.ch012

Ogidi, O. I., & Tawariowei, A. M. (2023). Endocrine Disrupting Chemicals and their Role in Cancer-A review. *Molecular Sciences and Applications.*, *3*, 5–14. DOI: 10.37394/232023.2023.3.2

Ogidi, O. I., & Tobia, P. S. (2024). Harnessing Artificial Intelligence (AI) Techniques for the prevention of Microbial Disease in Humans. In *Artificial Intelligence in Microbiology: scopes and Challenges*. Elsevier.

Öztürk, H., Özgür, A., & Ozkirimli, E. (2018). DeepDTA: Deep drug-target binding affinity prediction. *Bioinformatics (Oxford, England)*, *34*(17), i821–i829. DOI: 10.1093/bioinformatics/bty593 PMID: 30423097

Parvathaneni, V., Kulkarni, N. S., Muth, A., & Gupta, V. (2019). Drug repurposing: A promising tool to accelerate the drug discovery process. *Drug Discovery Today*, *24*(10), 2076–2085. DOI: 10.1016/j.drudis.2019.06.014 PMID: 31238113

Patlewicz, G., & Fitzpatrick, J. M. (2016). Current and Future Perspectives on the Development, Evaluation, and Application of in Silico Approaches for Predicting Toxicity. *Chemical Research in Toxicology*, *29*(4), 438–451. DOI: 10.1021/acs.chemrestox.5b00388 PMID: 26686752

Popova, M., Isayev, O., & Tropsha, A. (2018). Deep reinforcement learning for de novo drug design. *Science Advances*, *4*(7), eaap7885. Advance online publication. DOI: 10.1126/sciadv.aap7885 PMID: 30050984

Qiu, X., Li, H., Ver Steeg, G., & Godzik, A. (2024). Advances in AI for Protein Structure Prediction: Implications for Cancer Drug Discovery and Development. *Biomolecules*, *14*(3), 339. DOI: 10.3390/biom14030339 PMID: 38540759

Qureshi, R., Irfan, M., Gondal, T. M., Khan, S., Wu, J., Hadi, M. U., Heymach, J., Le, X., Yan, H., & Alam, T. (2023). AI in drug discovery and its clinical relevance. *Heliyon*, *9*(7), e17575. DOI: 10.1016/j.heliyon.2023.e17575 PMID: 37396052

Raies, A. B., & Bajic, V. B. (2016). In silico toxicology: Computational methods for the prediction of chemical toxicity. *Wiley Interdisciplinary Reviews. Computational Molecular Science*, *6*(2), 147–172. DOI: 10.1002/wcms.1240 PMID: 27066112

Ramesh, A. N., Kambhampati, C., Monson, J. R., & Drew, P. J. (2004). Artificial intelligence in medicine. *Annals of the Royal College of Surgeons of England*, *86*(5), 334–338. DOI: 10.1308/147870804290 PMID: 15333167

Reddy, A. S., & Zhang, S. (2013). Polypharmacology: Drug discovery for the future. *Expert Review of Clinical Pharmacology*, *6*(1), 41–47. DOI: 10.1586/ecp.12.74 PMID: 23272792

Rouse, M. (2017) IBM Watson Supercomputer. 2017. Accessed 13 October 2024 https://searchenterpriseai.techtarget.com/definition/ IBM-Watson-supercomputer

Rube, H. T., Rastogi, C., Feng, S., Kribelbauer, J. F., Li, A., Becerra, B., Melo, L. A. N., Do, B. V., Li, X., Adam, H. H., Shah, N. H., Mann, R. S., & Bussemaker, H. J. (2022). Prediction of protein-ligand binding affinity from sequencing data with interpretable machine learning. *Nature Biotechnology*, *40*(10), 1520–1527. DOI: 10.1038/s41587-022-01307-0 PMID: 35606422

Ryu, J. Y., Kim, H. U., & Lee, S. Y. (2018). Deep learning improves prediction of drug-drug and drug-food interactions. *Proceedings of the National Academy of Sciences of the United States of America*, *115*(18), E4304–E4311. DOI: 10.1073/pnas.1803294115 PMID: 29666228

Santos-Filho, A., Dhudum, R., Ganeshpurkar, A., & Pawar, A. (2024). Revolutionizing Drug Discovery: A Comprehensive Review of AI Applications. *Drugs and Drug Candidates*, *3*(1), 148–171. DOI: 10.3390/ddc3010009

Sarkar, C., Das, B., Rawat, V. S., Wahlang, J. B., Nongpiur, A., Tiewsoh, I., Lyngdoh, N. M., Das, D., Bidarolli, M., & Sony, H. T. (2023). Artificial Intelligence and Machine Learning Technology Driven Modern Drug Discovery and Development. *International Journal of Molecular Sciences*, *24*(3), 2026. DOI: 10.3390/ijms24032026 PMID: 36768346

Schneider, G., & Clark, D. E. (2019). Automated De Novo Drug Design: Are We Nearly There Yet? *Angewandte Chemie International Edition*, *58*(32), 10792–10803. DOI: 10.1002/anie.201814681 PMID: 30730601

Segler, M. H. S., Kogej, T., Tyrchan, C., & Waller, M. P. (2018). Generating Focused Molecule Libraries for Drug Discovery with Recurrent Neural Networks. *ACS Central Science*, *4*(1), 120–131. DOI: 10.1021/acscentsci.7b00512 PMID: 29392184

Segler, M. H. S., Preuss, M., & Waller, M. P. (2018). Planning chemical syntheses with deep neural networks and symbolic AI. *Nature*, *555*(7698), 604–610. DOI: 10.1038/nature25978 PMID: 29595767

Smith, R. G., & Farquhar, A. (2000). The road ahead for knowledge management: An AI perspective. *AI Magazine*, *21*, 17–17.

Spencer, M., Eickholt, J., & Cheng, J. (2015). A Deep Learning Network Approach to ab initio Protein Secondary Structure Prediction. *IEEE/ACM Transactions on Computational Biology and Bioinformatics*, *12*(1), 103–112. DOI: 10.1109/TCBB.2014.2343960 PMID: 25750595

Stafford, I. S., Kellermann, M., Mossotto, E., Beattie, R. M., MacArthur, B. D., & Ennis, S. (2020). A systematic review of the applications of artificial intelligence and machine learning in autoimmune diseases. *NPJ Digital Medicine*, *3*(1), 30. DOI: 10.1038/s41746-020-0229-3 PMID: 32195365

Steels, L., & Brooks, R. (2018). *The Artificial Life Route to Artificial Intelligence: Building Embodied, Situated Agents*. Routledge. DOI: 10.4324/9781351001885

Stokes, J. M., Yang, K., Swanson, K., Jin, W., Cubillos-Ruiz, A., Donghia, N. M., MacNair, C. R., French, S., Carfrae, L. A., Bloom-Ackermann, Z., Tran, V. M., Chiappino-Pepe, A., Badran, A. H., Andrews, I. W., Chory, E. J., Church, G. M., Brown, E. D., Jaakkola, T. S., Barzilay, R., & Collins, J. J. (2020). A Deep Learning Approach to Antibiotic Discovery. *Cell*, *180*(4), 688–702.e13. DOI: 10.1016/j.cell.2020.01.021 PMID: 32084340

Struble, T. J., Alvarez, J. C., Brown, S. P., Chytil, M., Cisar, J., DesJarlais, R. L., Engkvist, O., Frank, S. A., Greve, D. R., Griffin, D. J., Hou, X., Johannes, J. W., Kreatsoulas, C., Lahue, B., Mathea, M., Mogk, G., Nicolaou, C. A., Palmer, A. D., Price, D. J., & Jensen, K. F. (2020). Current and Future Roles of Artificial Intelligence in Medicinal Chemistry Synthesis. *Journal of Medicinal Chemistry*, *63*(16), 8667–8682. DOI: 10.1021/acs.jmedchem.9b02120 PMID: 32243158

Subbiah, V. (2023). The next generation of evidence-based medicine. *Nature Medicine*, *29*(1), 49–58. DOI: 10.1038/s41591-022-02160-z PMID: 36646803

Subramanian, G., Ramsundar, B., Pande, V., & Denny, R. A. (2016). Computational Modeling of β-Secretase 1 (BACE-1) Inhibitors Using Ligand Based Approaches. *Journal of Chemical Information and Modeling*, *56*(10), 1936–1949. DOI: 10.1021/acs.jcim.6b00290 PMID: 27689393

Thomas, S., Rouilly, V., Patin, E., Alanio, C., Dubois, A., Delval, C., Marquier, L. G., Fauchoux, N., Sayegrih, S., Vray, M., Duffy, D., Quintana-Murci, L., Albert, M. L., Abel, L., Alcover, A., Bousso, P., Bruhns, P., Cumano, A., Daëron, M., & Albert, M. L.Milieu Intérieur Consortium. (2015). The Milieu Intérieur study - an integrative approach for study of human immunological variance. *Clinical Immunology (Orlando, Fla.)*, *157*(2), 277–293. DOI: 10.1016/j.clim.2014.12.004 PMID: 25562703

Thorlund, K., Dron, L., Park, J. J. H., & Mills, E. J. (2020). Synthetic and External Controls in Clinical Trials - A Primer for Researchers. *Clinical Epidemiology*, *12*, 457–467. DOI: 10.2147/CLEP.S242097 PMID: 32440224

Tian, K., Shao, M., Wang, Y., Guan, J., & Zhou, S. (2016). Boosting compound-protein interaction prediction by deep learning. *Methods (San Diego, Calif.)*, *110*, 64–72. DOI: 10.1016/j.ymeth.2016.06.024 PMID: 27378654

Topol, E. J. (2019). High-performance medicine: The convergence of human and artificial intelligence. *Nature Medicine*, *25*(1), 44–56. DOI: 10.1038/s41591-018-0300-7 PMID: 30617339

Tripathi, M. K., Nath, A., Singh, T. P., Ethayathulla, A. S., & Kaur, P. (2021). Evolving scenario of big data and Artificial Intelligence (AI) in drug discovery. *Molecular Diversity*, *25*(3), 1439–1460. DOI: 10.1007/s11030-021-10256-w PMID: 34159484

US Food and Drug Administration. (2021). *Assessing the Credibility of Computational Modeling and Simulation in Medical Device Submissions*. FDA.

Vamathevan, J., Clark, D., Czodrowski, P., Dunham, I., Ferran, E., Lee, G., Li, B., Madabhushi, A., Shah, P., Spitzer, M., & Zhao, S. (2019). Applications of machine learning in drug discovery and development. *Nature Reviews. Drug Discovery*, *18*(6), 463–477. DOI: 10.1038/s41573-019-0024-5 PMID: 30976107

Voigt, I., Inojosa, H., Dillenseger, A., Haase, R., Akgün, K., & Ziemssen, T. (2021). Digital Twins for Multiple Sclerosis. *Frontiers in Immunology*, *12*, 669811. DOI: 10.3389/fimmu.2021.669811 PMID: 34012452

Wilkinson, M. D., Dumontier, M., Aalbersberg, I. J., Appleton, G., Axton, M., Baak, A., Blomberg, N., Boiten, J. W., da Silva Santos, L. B., Bourne, P. E., Bouwman, J., Brookes, A. J., Clark, T., Crosas, M., Dillo, I., Dumon, O., Edmunds, S., Evelo, C. T., Finkers, R., & Mons, B. (2016). The FAIR Guiding Principles for scientific data management and stewardship. *Scientific Data*, *3*(1), 160018. DOI: 10.1038/sdata.2016.18 PMID: 26978244

Wirtz, B. W., Weyere, J. C., & Geyer, C. (2019). Artificial intelligence and the public sector—Applications and challenges. *International Journal of Public Administration*, *42*(7), 596–615. DOI: 10.1080/01900692.2018.1498103

Wu, C., Gao, R., Zhang, Y., & De Marinis, Y. (2019). PTPD: Predicting therapeutic peptides by deep learning and word2vec. *BMC Bioinformatics*, *20*(1), 1–8. DOI: 10.1186/s12859-019-3006-z PMID: 31492094

Yadav, S., Singh, A., Singhal, R., & Yadav, J. P. (2024). Revolutionizing drug discovery: The impact of artificial intelligence on advancements in pharmacology and the pharmaceutical industry. *Intelligent Pharmacy*, *2*(3), 367–380. DOI: 10.1016/j.ipha.2024.02.009

Yang, X., Wang, Y., Byrne, R., Schneider, G., & Yang, S. (2019). Concepts of Artificial Intelligence for Computer-Assisted Drug Discovery. *Chemical Reviews*, *119*(18), 10520–10594. DOI: 10.1021/acs.chemrev.8b00728 PMID: 31294972

Yang, Y., & Siau, K. (2018). *A Qualitative Research on Marketing and Sales in the Artificial Intelligence Age*. MWAIS.

Zang, Q., Mansouri, K., Williams, A. J., Judson, R. S., Allen, D. G., Casey, W. M., & Kleinstreuer, N. C. (2017). In Silico Prediction of Physicochemical Properties of Environmental Chemicals Using Molecular Fingerprints and Machine Learning. *Journal of Chemical Information and Modeling*, *57*(1), 36–49. DOI: 10.1021/acs.jcim.6b00625 PMID: 28006899

Zhang, T., Androulakis, I. P., Bonate, P., Cheng, L., Helikar, T., Parikh, J., Rackauckas, C., Subramanian, K., Cho, C. R., Androulakis, I. P., Bonate, P., Borisov, I., Broderick, G., Cheng, L., Damian, V., Dariolli, R., Demin, O., Ellinwood, N., Fey, D., & Cho, C. R.Working Group. (2022). Two heads are better than one: current landscape of integrating QSP and machine learning: An ISoP QSP SIG white paper by the working group on the integration of quantitative systems pharmacology and machine learning. *Journal of Pharmacokinetics and Pharmacodynamics*, *49*(1), 5–18. DOI: 10.1007/s10928-022-09805-z PMID: 35103884

Zhang, Y., Hu, Y., Li, H., & Liu, X. (2022). Drug-protein interaction prediction *via* variational autoencoders and attention mechanisms. *Frontiers in Genetics*, *13*, 1032779. DOI: 10.3389/fgene.2022.1032779 PMID: 36313473

Zhou, Y., Wang, F., Tang, J., & Nussinov, R. (2020). Artificial intelligence in COVID-19 drug repurposing. *Nature Machine Intelligence*, *2*(7), 347–365. DOI: 10.1038/s42256-020-0182-0 PMID: 32984792

Chapter 6
AI-Assisted Vaccine Design and Development in Immunological Disorders

Neha Tavare
https://orcid.org/0009-0002-2364-1065
Amity University, Maharashtra, India

Rajshri Singh
https://orcid.org/0000-0001-5748-5799
Amity University, Maharashtra, India

Sagar H. Barage
https://orcid.org/0000-0003-0752-6948
Amity University, Maharashtra, India

ABSTRACT

Artificial Intelligence (AI)-driven methodologies in vaccine design and development offer transformational abilities for the identification of immunogen, antigen selection, epitope prediction, and tailored vaccine production. AI-driven multi-omics integration facilitates the combination of genomic, transcriptomic, and proteomic datasets for the creation of comprehensive models of immune responses assessing immunogenicity and prioritizing antigens for experimental evolution. Immunological disorders characterized by abnormalities in immune system dysfunction pose considerable challenges in vaccine development. We explored and examined AI approaches and technologies to enhance our comprehension and management of vaccine design. AI algorithms support epitope mapping for precise targeting in vaccine design based on genotypic and phenotypic profiles. The data analysis and pattern recognition in AI enables the identification of distinct, unique immune response profiles across various immunological conditions, including autoimmune diseases, immunodeficiencies, and hypersensitivity reactions.

DOI: 10.4018/979-8-3693-9725-1.ch006

INTRODUCTION

Vaccine stands as one of the most remarkable developments in medical history, crucial in saving numerous lives and alleviating the global impact on various diseases. Currently, vaccines are extensively regarded as one of the most powerful and economical community tools, playing a pivotal role in controlling and even eliminating wide infectious diseases. The traditional method is time-consuming and detailed process, which includes numerous stages such as isolating the pathogen, identifying the antigen, formulating the immunogen, and conducting clinical trials. After characterising the pathogen, researchers should search appropriate immunogens keep up accelerate an immune response without any detrimental effect. This step often requires extensive trial-and-error experimentation, which can be challenging, resource-demanding and unpredictable. (Olawade, et al.,2024) Once the antigen is identified, the consequent hurdle is creating an immunogen that can accurately replicate the pathogen and stimulate a strong immune response. This requires an in-depth understanding of immunology and how antigens are presented to the immune system to ensure the vaccine produces the intended effect. (Gorki V & Medhi B, 2024) Furthermore, the formulation must be secure, stable, and capable of being produced on a large scale (Gulati et al.,2023). Recently, the field of vaccine development has been revolutionized with the rise of artificial intelligence (AI) and computational methods. These advanced technologies efficiency, provides opportunities to speed up vaccine design, enhance immunogen formulations, and predict immune responses with improved accuracy and reliable effectiveness (Aileni et al.,2022) Leveraging AI technologies for tasks such as selecting antigens, predicting epitopes, identifying adjuvants, and refining optimization methods has the potential to significantly streamline the vaccine development process. (Olawade et al.,2024). By using AI to better understand how the immune system works, we can more effectively identify the right targets for vaccines, forecast how the body will respond, and optimize the ingredients in the vaccine. This technology can help create vaccines that are not only more effective but also safer for individuals with immune system issues. As AI continues to evolve, it offers great potential for developing treatments for autoimmune diseases, immunodeficiencies, and other immunological conditions, ultimately improving the lives of affected person. Artificial Intelligence (AI) involves the mimicking of human-like intelligence in machines that are assigned to think, learn, and establish decisions on their own. (Subramanian et al.,2020) Autoimmune diseases have a significant impact on individuals and caregivers, leading to high healthcare costs. These conditions are expected to become more prevalent in the future, highlighting the need for increased research and resources. To better understand their causes and risk factors, and to improve diagnosis, treatment, and prevention, urgent action is required. Failing to address this now will result in greater future health burdens and costs. By investing in these efforts today, we can reduce the long-term impact of autoimmune diseases. (Miller et al., 2023) Understanding the complexities of immune responses, including genetic variability and pathogen diversity, is crucial not only for vaccine development but also for addressing immunological disorders, as it helps identify underlying mechanisms and potential therapeutic strategies for better disease management. The immune system's complexity, involving multiple cells, tissues, and signaling pathways, complicates our understanding of how these components work together. Systems biology and vaccinomics aim to bridge this gap by studying immune responses at a systemic level, enabling more accurate predictions and improving vaccine development. Genetic differences among individuals significantly affect vaccine responses. Genome-wide association studies (GWAS) (Uffelmann et al.,2021) can be used to identify genetic variants linked to immune variations, helping to develop more personalized vaccines and improve efficacy by targeting specific immune pathways. Genetic diversity in pathogens, including antigenic shifts and mutations, complicates vaccine development. Genome sequencing helps identify conserved pathogen regions, facilitating the design of vaccines targeting stable epitopes, thus improving vaccine effectiveness and safety. New vaccine development must address both public health needs and safety concerns. By leveraging genomics, systems vaccinology, and AI, researchers can predict vaccine responses, understand genetic and environmental factors, and improve safety profiles, leading to more effective and personalized vaccines. (Kennedy, et al.,2020)

ARTIFICIAL INTELLIGENCE AND COMPUTATIONAL BIOLOGY

Artificial Intelligence (AI) and Computational Biology refer to the integration of advanced algorithms and computational techniques to study biological data, particularly in the context of understanding complex biological systems and processes. Computational biology is an interdisciplinary field that applies mathematical models, computational algorithms, and statistical methods to understand biological systems. It aims to simulate, model, and analyse biological processes like gene expression, protein folding, and immune system responses. The use of computational models helps researchers predict outcomes, identify biomarkers, and discover potential drug targets. Artificial intelligence (AI), Machine learning (ML) and deep learning (DL) are coordinated fields. AI is a broad discipline dedicated to building system that can perform task obtain human like intelligence, including as reasoning, decision making and problem solving. ML is a subset that canters on allow machines to learn and improve from data without explicit programming, using algorithms to identify patterns and make predictions. DL is a specialized subclass of ML, utilize multilayered Neural networks to evaluate large and compound datasets. (Patil et al.,2024, Xu et al., 2021) In the context of disease diagnosis and vaccine design, these technologies are revolutionizing approaches at the genetic level by identifying genetic mutations, mapping pathogen genomes, predicting immunological epitopes, and personalized vaccine formulations to target specific populations and high-risk groups effectively.

The immune system comprises a complex network of proteins, cells, and signalling pathways that safeguard the body against viruses, infections, autoimmune disorders, cancer, and inflammation. When the immune system is disrupted, it can lead to challenging-to-diagnose conditions, such as primary immunodeficiencies (PIDs) (Giardino et al., 2026) These disorders are marked by impaired immune responses, making individuals more vulnerable to infections, autoimmune diseases, and inflammatory processes. Understanding the immune system is vital for uncovering the mechanisms of cellular defence, devising innovative treatments, and enhancing overall health outcomes.

The discipline of Computational Immunology has grown significantly with advancements in computational biology and multi-omics technologies. (Pappalardo et al.,2026) These approaches leverage high-throughput genomic tools and bioinformatics to convert complex immunological data into interpretable and actionable insights. (Ghosh,2020). Key areas in computational immunology include next-generation sequencing, structural bioinformatics, integrative data analysis, and the use of bioinformatics in drug discovery. Artificial intelligence also plays a pivotal role in diagnosing primary immunodeficiencies, offering innovative solutions to complex diagnostic challenges. These advancements, coupled with emerging trends, highlight the transformative potential of computational approaches in understanding immune system dynamics and addressing immunological disorders. Artificial intelligence techniques can support both large-scale population risk evaluations and personalized assessments to facilitate the diagnosis of diseases.

AI-driven prediction of B-cell and T-cell epitopes, along with the identification of new vaccine candidates, is significantly advancing immunoinformatic methodologies, leading to the creation of more sophisticated AI- and ML-powered prediction platforms. In immunology, the prediction of epitopes for B- and T-cell receptors is a crucial application of structural bioinformatics. Structural bioinformatics is a discipline that employs databases and computational tools to investigate the molecular folding, evolution, binding interactions, and structure–function connections of macromolecules such as proteins, RNA, and DNA

An antigen is a molecule capable of binding to an antibody, initiating an immune response. This interaction occurs at the antigen-binding site (paratope) of the antibody, which recognizes a specific amino acid sequence on the antigen, known as an epitope. Epitopes can be classified into two types: conformational epitopes, which depend on the three-dimensional structure of the antigen for binding, and linear epitopes, which consist of a specific sequence of amino acids that a T-cell receptor or antibody recognizes. (Bukhari et al., 2022).

Various widely recognized Artificial intelligence and machine learning methods includes Logistic regression (LR), Support Vector machines (SVM), Random Forests (RF), and a range of neural network architectures (Table 1). These networks encompass convolutional neural networks (CNN), recurrent neural networks (RNN), multilayer perceptron's (MLP) and deep neural networks (DNN), among others. (Kaushik et al., 2023)

Table 1. Application of AI models in biological complex system components identification.

AI system	Use	Reference
Deep learning	Structural analysis of proteins, predicting epitope binding	(Zhang et al.,2023)
Machine learning.	Prediction, classification, pattern recognition	(Bravi et al.,2024)
Hidden Markov Models (HMMs)	Modelling vaccine interactions with immune cells	(Tong et al.,2013)
Neural Networks (NNs)	Identifying complex patterns in immunological data	(Karthika et al.,2023)
Generative Models	Designing novel antigens and optimizing vaccine formulations	(Elshafei et al.,2024) (Khan et al.,2021) (Kaushik et al.,2023)
SAR Models	Adjuvant designing	
Molecular Dynamics (MD)	Simulating antigen interactions with immune system components	

Immunity is a body's ability to recognize the foreign particle and defend against the harmful substances such as toxins, biological pathogens, abnormal cells etc. immunity majorly classified as of two types of Innate immunity and Adaptive immunity. Innate serves as a first line of defence it is nonspecific, involves physical barrier to block the entry of harmful agents whereas adaptive immunity generate over the time involves T & B lymphocytes that remember and respond to specific antigens. Immunological disorders arise due to dysregulation of immune system it can be due to over reactivity, under reactivity or loss of function. Various components of immune systems such as lymphocytes, macrophages, dendritic cells (Antigen presenting cells), complement molecules, cytokines, chemokines, whereas body organs such as bone marrow, thymus, spleen, lymph nodes also play an important role in body's homeostasis functional regulation. In immunological disorders hyperactivity caused by overproduction of cytokines or antibodies causes autoimmune diseases, under reactivity leads to immunodeficiencies, ineffective immune regulation can lead to chronic disorders. Genetic variations influence immune cell function of recognition and respond mechanism to pathogens, autoantigens, and environmental factors. This variation plays a vital role in determination of susceptibility to disease and effectiveness of immune response. Human Leukocyte antigen genes (HLA Genes), part of MHC is essential and critical for antigen presentation, autoimmune diseases such as Type 1 diabetes, rheumatoid arthritis, multiple sclerosis occurs due to defect in these regions. Cytokines which are proteinaceous molecules mediating immune communication the polymorphism of Cytokine gene leads to Crohn's disease, psoriasis. Toll like receptors which recognizes the pathogen associated molecular patterns, mutation in TLR genes causes increased susceptibility to pathogens. Environmental factors such as infections, pollutions, genetic predispositions can also contribute to immune Malfunctioning. for example -primary immunodeficiencies occur due to Mutation in genes like Bruton's tyrosine kinase (BTK) causes X linked to a gammaglobulinemia characterized by impaired antibody production (Pinder et al.,2020). Allergies and asthma can arise due to polymorphism in IL-4 and IL-13 genes showing increased allergic responses (Shirkani et al.,2019). Auto antiglated disease systemic lupus erythematous characterized(Gao et al.,2024)by the production of autoantibodies against nuclear components leads to organ damage double stranded DNA and histones are recognized as a autoantigens, citrullinated proteins as a foreign molecules due to post translational modification in rheumatoid arthritis(Gao et al.,2024) type 1 diabetes where autoantibody and autoreactive T cells target pancreatic beta cells, leading to insulin deficiency, multiple sclerosis where the immune system encounter the neuronal myelin sheath, causing neurological dysfunction, enzyme linked autoantigen- thyroid autoantigen is a immune condition resulting in chronic inflammation and dysfunction of thyroid gland. (Rapoport et al.,2001)AI algorithms having ability to analyse large datasets such as gene expression profiles immune system dynamics to predict the immune response to pathogens, vaccines and drugs.

IMMUNOINFORMATIC

The immune system has been evolved significantly and modulation of immune system led to generate many pathways to combat with diseases. There are several online resources available for immune pathways, allergens, epitopes, and antigens (Table 2). Tunning between these intrinsic pathways and immune response at an individual personal level shows the prominent way to cure the diseases at personalized level with precise designing of therapies.

Table 2. Immunological databases and source link.

Immunological database	characteristics	Source	Reference
IMGT	Includes antibody, T cell Receptor, data	http://www.imgt.org/IMGTindex/databases.php	(Lane et al.,2010)
Innate DB	Innate immune response analysis. Integrating pathways, interactions and gene annotation.	https://www.innatedb.com/	(Breuer et al., 2013)
ImmuneSpace	Curated data on human immune response, vaccines, infections, diseases.	https://immunespace.org/	(Sauteraud et al., 2016)

continued on following page

Table 2. Continued

Immunological database	characteristics	Source	Reference
Innate Data Discovery Index	Search engine for immunology datasets across repositories includes ImmPort, ImmuneSpace,ITN TrialShare, IEDB, and ImmGen. supported by NIAID.	https://immunedata.org/	(Deng, et al., 2022)
VDJdb	Database of immune receptor sequences from T cell receptors	https://vdjdb.cdr3.net/	(Shugayet al., 2018)
ImmPort (Immunology Database and Analysis Portal)	System immunology analysis	https://www.immport.org/shared/home	(Bhattacharya et al., 2018)
IEDB	Experimentally verified immune epitope information- T cell, B cell, MHC ligands.	https://www.iedb.org/	(Fleri et al., 2017)
Allergen online	Data on allergenic proteins and associated sequences.	http://www.allergenonline.org/	(Goodman et al., 2016)
Human Immunome Project (HIP)	mapping of immune receptor sequences and immune system diversity.	https://www.humanimmunomeproject.org/	(Human Immunome Project, 2020)
NEPdb (Neoantigen Peptide Database)	Curated database of validated neoantigens and ineffective neoepitopes for HLA.	http://nep.whu.edu.cn/	(Xia et al., 2021)

VACCINE AND IMMUNOLOGICAL DISORDERS

Immunological disorders, which occur when the immune system malfunctions or is unable to adequately protect the body from infections and diseases, are a significant challenge in modern medicine. These disorders, including autoimmune diseases, immunodeficiencies, and hypersensitivity reactions, often complicate the effectiveness of vaccines. In individuals with weakened or overactive immune systems, the body may fail to respond properly to vaccination or may even react adversely. For example, autoimmune conditions can trigger inappropriate immune responses to vaccines, leading to inflammation or tissue damage. On the other hand, people with immunodeficiencies may not mount a sufficient immune response to produce protective immunity after vaccination. Understanding the complexities of immunological disorders is crucial for developing more effective and personalized vaccines. Advanced technologies, such as systems vaccinology and AI-driven computational models, allow researchers to identify genetic, environmental, and immune system factors that influence vaccine response, leading to more tailored immunization strategies that can better address the needs of individuals with immunological disorders(Smith, & Germolec 1999, Marshall et al, 2024)Vaccinomics is a field that combines immunogenetics and immunogenomics to study how genetic variations affect immune responses to vaccines. It focuses on understanding how gene polymorphisms influence different types of immune responses, such as humoral, cell-mediated, and innate immunity, both at the individual and population levels (Poland et al.,2008, Kennedy et al.,2020, Ovsyannikova & Poland, 2011).

Fundamentals of Immunological Disorders

Immunology is the foundational field of study for designing vaccines against immunological disorders, focusing on understanding the immune system's structure and function. It involves knowledge of both the innate and adaptive immune responses, where immune cells such as T cells, B cells, dendritic cells, and macrophages play pivotal roles. Understanding how these cells interact and how they respond to pathogens or altered self-molecules (autoantigens in autoimmune diseases) is crucial. Additionally, the concept of immune tolerance is fundamental, as it explains the mechanisms by which the body prevents its immune system from attacking itself. This includes central and peripheral tolerance, which, when disrupted, can lead to autoimmune disorders. Further, knowledge of cytokine networks, which regulate immune responses, inflammation, and immune cell activation, is essential for designing vaccines that either boost immune responses or suppress them when dealing with autoimmune disorders. The ability to manipulate immunological memory is another key aspect, as vaccines often aim to create long-lasting immunity through memory B cells and T cells, ensuring a rapid response upon subsequent exposures to the antigen.

Molecular biology plays a key role in vaccine design, particularly in understanding antigen presentation, where antigens are processed by antigen-presenting cells (APCs) and presented to T cells via MHC molecules. The genetic regulation of immune responses involves comprehending how immune cells express genes and respond to infections or autoimmune conditions. Additionally, recombinant DNA technology enables the cloning and expression of antigens in host cells for vaccine development. Autoimmunity and immunopathology focus on diseases where the immune system mistakenly attacks the body's tissues, such as rheumatoid arthritis or lupus. It's essential to understand immune dysregulation, where failure in immune tolerance triggers autoimmune reactions, and how vaccines can modulate these processes. Chronic inflammation in conditions like asthma and inflammatory bowel disease also requires attention, as it complicates immune responses.

Vaccine science methodologies encompass various types of vaccines, including mRNA, DNA, and live-attenuated vaccines, each tailored to modulate immune responses. The use of adjuvants enhances these responses, especially when immune reactions need to be either amplified or controlled. In vaccine development, immune system modulation is critical to either strengthen or suppress immune reactions, particularly in autoimmune diseases. Lastly, biochemistry and protein engineering are pivotal for designing antigens that can trigger immune responses, understanding protein folding, and using molecular modelling tools to predict how antigens will interact with immune receptors. (Caradonna & Schmidt, 2021).

APPROACHES TO DESIGN NOVEL VACCINE

The unparalleled adaptability of artificial intelligence serves as the basis of driving the development of unique outcomes across the domains. Dynamic learning, continuous optimization and real time adaptation to complex biological data with self-learning principles enables rapid evolution of predictive models and enhancing the field of healthcare. This adaptability mainly allows AI driven models to integrate diverse immunological patterns, parameters, novel biomarker identification and tailor interventions to analyse unique immune profile of individuals in case of immunological disorders. To understand the pathophysiology of immune related diseases computational techniques such as deep learning and multi omics approach enables researchers to gain deeper insights, thus AI possessing property as a crucial tool to revolutionize diagnosis, management and treatment.

- **Reverse vaccinology:**

Reverse vaccinology is a transforming approach, with the integration AI complement modern vaccine design. Reverse vaccinology utilizes the identification of antigen by genome sequencing without cultivating microorganism, although reverse vaccinology not limited to pathogen, it can help to determine allergenic proteins and design modified epitope to desensitize the immune system response. This therapeutic approach can reduce the allergic response while maintain the immune system integrity. Reverse vaccinology focuses on computational analysis of genome of individual to predict potential vaccine target such as surface exposed or secretory proteins. In context of immunology, reverse vaccinology leverages the integration of genomic and immunological insights to pinpoint significant protein antigens for developing diagnostics or vaccines. Within the framework, epitopes targeted by CD4+ T cells or CD8+ T cells mapping, can serve as a reverse approach to uncover novel antigens (Sette & Rappuoli 2010). Integration of AI/ML with this approach will help to identify and analyse large datasets brought about enhancing production of antigens with higher accuracy.

- **Personalized vaccines in Immunological Disorders Using AI:**

Personalized vaccines for immunological disorders aim to modulate the immune system uniquely for each patient, addressing conditions like autoimmune diseases, allergies, and certain immune deficiencies. Personalized medicine aims to enhance patient outcomes by leveraging genomic analysis, identifying biomarkers, assessing risks, implementing individualized treatment plans, and enabling ongoing monitoring. This approach strives to optimize therapeutic effectiveness, minimize side effects, and lower healthcare expenses (Lin et al.,2023) Artificial intelligence plays a transformative role in developing such vaccines by enabling data-driven customization.

- **Machine learning and Deep learning-based models:**

Machine learning (ML) is emerging as a powerful tool to enhance vaccine design, especially given that the molecular and cellular mechanisms underlying the efficacy and long-term protection of many vaccines are still not fully understood. ML is being increasingly used in systems immunology and proteomics to generate predictions that provide valuable insights into immune responses, enabling more precise vaccine development. It is particularly useful in the discovery of B and T cell epitopes, which are crucial for activating immune responses. By characterizing how the adaptive immune system responds to these epitopes at the molecular level, ML helps uncover new biological insights. Additionally, ML models are applied in vaccine construction and preclinical validation of selected vaccine targets, further contributing to rational vaccine design. These models offer predictive capabilities that improve the understanding of immune reactions and help identify optimal vaccine candidates. While many comprehensive reviews cover ML methods in detail, this area continues to evolve with ongoing challenges and future research directions focused on refining predictions for more effective vaccines.

Machine learning (ML) is used to analyse large immunological datasets, detecting patterns that reveal protein structure and function. It allows the development of models to predict the relationship between protein sequences and their outcomes, such as binding specificity. ML can be applied through supervised (classification, regression) or unsupervised (clustering) learning, uncovering meaningful features. In epitope discovery, ML generates prediction scores that assess the likelihood of residues being part of an epitope, aiding in the prioritization of vaccine targets. Machine learning (ML) techniques for B and T cell epitope prediction utilize both sequence-based and structure-based approaches. Sequence-based methods focus on linear epitopes, while structure-based methods, like RoseTTAFold, AlphaFold and trRosetta, are better suited for conformational epitopes by analysing protein folding and 3D interactions. These tools enhance vaccine design and TCR/antibody engineering. ML models, including deep learning and graph-based models, capture complex patterns and key features such as physico-chemical properties, surface accessibility, and evolutionary data. Advances in representation learning, like using language models, improve predictions by identifying inter-residue dependencies. While structure-based methods offer better performance, sequence-based methods are faster. ML also aids in optimizing antigen-antibody interactions and enhancing protein stability, though further research is needed to refine these methods (Baek, et al,2023, Bravi 2024).

- **Structural vaccinology:**

Structural vaccinology involves understanding the three-dimensional structure of antigens and using this information to design vaccines that can effectively stimulate an immune response. By gaining insights into how antigens interact with immune receptors, researchers can develop vaccines with greater precision. AI plays a key role in this field, particularly through structural prediction tools like AlphaFold, which can predict protein structures directly from amino acid sequences. This AI-driven approach enables researchers to better understand the molecular dynamics of antigens, facilitating the design of more targeted and effective vaccines (Lim, 2024)

Sequence alignment, model interaction prediction, and molecular docking are fundamental tasks in structural vaccinology and protein engineering, and AI can significantly enhance these processes.

Sequence alignment involves comparing protein sequences to identify similarities and evolutionary relationships. AI can automate and optimize this process, identifying conserved motifs or patterns that are essential for vaccine design. AI-driven algorithms, like deep learning models, can speed up sequence alignment and improve the detection of functional regions that might otherwise be missed.

Model interaction prediction refers to predicting how proteins, such as antigens and antibodies, interact with each other. AI techniques, particularly those based on machine learning, can predict interactions with higher accuracy by learning from large datasets of known protein-protein interactions. This allows for more precise modelling of immune responses and better targeting in vaccine development (Ye et al.,2021)

Molecular docking is used to predict how two molecules, such as a potential drug or vaccine candidate and a receptor, will bind together. AI enhances molecular docking by improving the accuracy of predictions and speeding up the process. Deep learning algorithms can predict binding affinity, optimize docking simulations, and help researchers identify the most promising candidates for further testing.

By combining AI with these methods, researchers can accelerate vaccine design and development, making the process more efficient and accurate. AI enables better understanding and prediction of the complex molecular interactions involved in immune responses, paving the way for more effective and tailored vaccines.

AI IN ANTIGEN SELECTION AND IMMUNOGEN DESIGN

AI has ability to identify and analyse the attributes from information provided for making decision on new data, referring to previous data with high accuracy. Use of AI in identifying novel antigen shown pivotal importance of AI algorithms (Abdelmageed et al.,2020). Ai powered methodologies utilize sophisticated computational approaches tools to process extensive datasets. It also helps in discovering protein structures their architectures and help to learn dynamics of immune system, enabling the discovery of promising vaccine candidate. Prediction of antigenic determinants, epitopes can be easily overseen by Using ML algorithms. (Bravi et al.,2024) Algorithms helps to examine features such as elemental physiochemical resources, structural characteristics specifically region where the binding or change are responsible for elicit the immune response.(Rahman et al.,2020) Increased stability, immunogenicity has been increased with molecular dynamics models and AI-generative model for the designing immunogens(Rakitina et al.,2023) Generative Adversarial networks (GANs) have used for improved antigenicity and cross reactivity. It can generate unique immunogenic sequence along with appropriate properties referring to existing allowing for super antigenicity and epitope presentation ability (Kim et al., 2024). Neoantigen that identifies immunogenic epitope binding to MHC molecule which led to elicit T cells for active immune response (Hutchison et al.,2018). Recently, AI and ML neoantigen prediction pipelines have been developed based on different inputs data (Table 3). Among them, the peptide MHC binding characteristics by using ML is also possible referring to previous training data such as Immune Epitope Database (IEDB Database)(Cai et al.,2022). One of the major cause immunological disorders are repositioning between genetic sequences. Somatic mutations such as single nucleotide variants, gene fusions, exon-exon junctions, splice variants, non-coding regions, endogenous variation, Unannotated open reading frames. (Ouspenskaia et al.,2022)

Peptide MHC binding is essential feature for immunotherapies. Tools such as NetMHC with help of ANN used to predict and identify peptide MHC I bind affinity by referring allele specific epitope. MHCflurry 2.0 tool give advantage of two processing predictors such as Antigen processing (MHC-Allele independent approach) predictor and presentation (binding affinity predictions) predictor(Ouspenskaia, et al.,2022) For Peptide and MHC II binding prediction methods such as NetMHCII, TEPITOPEpan, NetMHCIIpan, RANKPEP, ANN based methods highly enhanced performance of in sillico prediction strategies by utilizing algorithms. As MHCII is greatly shows variable regions, the training data availability is low(Hutchison et al.,2018) trans allelic prediction model can be used for quantitative binding which gives the peptide-MHCII actual explanation by using existing dataset(Degoot et al.,2018) DeepSeq PanII was used to predict peptide HLAII binding by using HLA alpha and beta chains it is a LSTM-CNN model(Liu et al.,2022) Another ERGO model is used for studying complete set of peptide using a deep learning with the help of algorithm based on long short-term memory. CD3and peptides used as input source data for training neural network. TCR – peptide binding model NetTCR CNN model is sequence-based method for TCR α and TCR ß (Montemurro et al.,2021). pAVseq is developed using ANN for identification and focus on neoantigen originating from DNA or RNA seq data (Hundal et al.,2016).

Table 3. Neoantigen prediction pipeline and key features.

Source	Input Data (Neoantigen source)	Filtering & ML tool	References.
FRED2	RNA seq, SNV	-Gene expression -Allelic variation -Peptide-MHC I/II binding affinity. -Fold change -gene fusion. -mutant allele frequency.	(Schubert et al., 2016)
Tlminer			(Tappeiner et al.,2016)
Vaxrank			(Rubinsteyn et al.,2017)
Scan Neo	RNA seq		(Wang et al.,2019)
NeoPredPipe	Somatic variant cells		(Schenck et al.,2019)
Neosplice	RNA seq		(Chai et al.,2022)
NeoantigenR	DNA/RNA seq		(Tang et al.,2017)

Another pipelines such as Neopepsee uses Random forest, Gaussian naive bayes scoring system (Kim et al.,2018) pTuneos uses random forest ML system(Zhou et al.,2019), DeepAntigen uses sparse learning(Shi et al.,2020), TruNeo(Tang et al .,2020), DeepImmuno -CNN(Li et al.,2021), ML algorithms with key features of immunogenicity score, rank, combined score, peptide entropy, expression, amino acid physiochemical features, mutation in RNA seq, IEDB immunogenicity score, T cell interaction with residue hydrophobicity, exome analysis.

AI in Epitope Prediction

Epitope is an antigenic determinant site of an antigen that composed of protein or polysaccharide it is recognized by T cells, B cells and antibodies. It plays pivotal role in immune response initiation. They allow the immunological cascade to recognize a respond to foreign bodies like mutant cell, pathogens, viruses, etc. T cell receptors are presented and processed by classes of MHC molecules during immune response. Epitope represents central role in vaccine design and development as it stimulates the responsive mechanisms. Al based algorithmic methodologies uses structural characteristic information, sequence information for epitope prediction(Sela-Culang et al., 2013) patient specific genomics and proteomics data processing with AI-ML identifies Neoantigens, autoantigenic specificity leading to personalized medicine and vaccines.(Ott et al.,2017), tissues or cell specific antibodies, monoclonal antibodies, antibody drug combination conjugates, visionary (chimeric)antigen receptors are the most significant forms of biological drugs that can be used for infectious diseases, immune related- autoimmune diseases(Ott et al.,2017, Chen et al.,2012) Epitopes found in two forms such as conformational and linear, they are formed due to 3d folding of proteins and linear chains of amino acids. 90% of B cel epitopes are in conformational structure such as folded protein this information for paratope and epitope designing & mapping can be greatly leveraged to design the therapeutic molecules for specific disease (Caoili et al.,2014). Peptide microarray data, phage display data libraries techniques showed advantage to characterize the epitopes on proteins. The nonfunctional epitopes consist of polysaccharides, proteins and DNA termed as a naïve epitope can be replaced by mimicking the peptides and this can be used as a therapeutic molecule in immunological disorders (Zeng et al.,2023). Linear epitope prediction Zengcan be done using early prediction methods such as BcePred, (Saha et al.,2004), ABCPred (Saha et al.,2006), iBCE-EL 1 (Manavalan et al,2018). iBCE-EL ensemble method is used to generate randomized tree and algorithm to state probable class and value of a query peptide. ML algorithms such as SVM, RF, ERT, GB, AB and k-NN approached to select appropriate features of B Cell epitopes and B non-cell epitopes depicted in Table 4 (Manavalan et al.,2018). Deep neural network designed to recognize patterns and relationship between datasets. Short protein fragments to identify specific regions recognized as a linear B cell epitope. Sequence only approach uses the amino acid sequence of input data which is faster and focuses only on amino acid sequence, thus using deep learning at an individual patient level is useful in immunological disorders management and more approachable towards the vaccine designing (Collatz et al.,2021) EpiDope model is based on DNA and trained on IEDB Linear Epitope Dataset, which contains information about experimentally validated B cell epitopes it gives information about the Part of protein that can elicit the response aiding vaccine design.(Ras-Carmona et al.,2022). Conformational epitope prediction includes regions of antigen identification that are ranged spatially and get recognized by immune system, they are generated from X-ray crystallography or cryo-electron microscopy. Tools such as Discotope, Elipro, BePro used to predict conformational epitope(Yao et al,2013) Mechanisms such as supervised learning that algorithm predict epitope by analysing structural and sequence features, Convolutional Neural network (CNNs) works with surface accessibility, Graph Neural Networks(GNNs) (Collatz et al.,2021) predicting conformational epitope by learning about relationship within 3D antigenic surfaces, Recurrent Neural networks(RNNs) used in integration of sequence and structural data (Cia et al.,2023). Structural Epitope Mapping and Analysis (SEMA) is widely used computational tool for predicting epitope particularly for conformational B cell epitope forming antigen- antibody structures. It employs algorithm to identify region of antigen interact with antibody to map the antigenic determinants. It identifies the residues at the binding interface between antigen antibody complexes aiding to distinguish between the epitope and non-epitope regions. (Shashkova et al.,2022, Yao et al.,2013)

Table 4. ML techniques used for modelling antigen antibody interaction.

ML techniques	Characteristics	References
Support Vector Machines (SVMs)	Classify residues as interacting or non-interacting Hydrophobicity, residue proximity analysis.	(Ye et al.,2021) (Huang et al.,2022) (da Silva et al.,2022)
Graph neural network.	Study Amino acid properties to predict Ag-Ab interaction.	
Recurrent Neural Network		
Random Forest (RF)		
Gradient Boosting Ensemble model	Combines weak model for increasing prediction accuracy.	
Transfer Learning	Pre trained models. Alpha fold models for Ag-Ab interaction. Protein interaction.	

A deep learning-based model Paratope epitope convolutional antibody network (PECAN) helps to predict epitope through paratope prediction. PECAN incorporates the interaction between the binding site that is antibody's paratope and epitope, leveraging this component to improve prediction accuracy (Pittala et al.,2020) uses transfer learning. dysregulated paratope-epitope interaction results in antibodies targeting self-antigens leading to autoimmune conditions, it also exploited in therapies such as immune checkpoint inhibitors, antibody drug conjugates to target tumors antigens while sparing healthy cells or tissue. In allergic conditions epitope binding to specific IgE paratopes triggers histamine release and hypersensitivity reactions. Therapeutics generated to neutralize allergenic epitopes, can be helpful in allergic responses reduction. Chronic infections such as HIV hepatitis manipulate this epitope paratope interaction to evade immune detection. Vaccines can be designed to expose conserved epitopes inducing neutralizing antibodies.

Docking assisted methods including ML techniques are crucial for refining and analysing docking molecules generated by ClusPro and Rosetta algorithms, predicting strength and stability of antibody antigen interactions. ML methods can predict binding affinity and stability for vaccine production. (Rohl et al.,2004) Computational techniques gave revolutionized antibody development making it faster, cheaper, and more customizable(Guarra et al.,2023) Combining Rosetta structural modelling with AI ability to analyse immune system data can better predict how the body will respond to various canine, ai can process complex immunological data to predict the likelihood of a vaccine generating robust immune response.(Jones et al.,2022, Porter et al.,2017) Sphinx combines ab Initio and knowledge-based loop structural predictions outperforming the Rosetta in some cases. Ab generated antibody structures without relying on sequence homology. Making it more suitable for modelling rare CDR conformations. (Guarra et al.,2023)

AI IN ADJUVANT MODELLING FOR VACCINE PRODUCTION

Adjuvant helps in enhancing the immune response to a vaccine. They are the substances that added to improve the immune response to the antigen. They are widely used in vaccine development, because of their ability to generate the immune response qualitatively and quantitatively ensuring greater efficacy and durability of vaccines. For the patients with immunological disorders like autoimmune diseases, adjuvants help overcome immunodeficiencies or enhance the effectiveness of vaccines that may not otherwise induce a strong immune response(Zhao et al.,2023) For chronic immunological conditions where the immune response may diminish over the time thus the bioavailability is increased, adjuvants are essential in maintaining long term immunity(Hemmati et al.,2024) Machine learning tool like neural network and random forest help to identify adjuvant with desirable qualities like controlled toxicity, high stability. AI techniques like virtual screening, docking simulations, structure activity relationship models test many compounds to see which may bound to immune receptor and affect immune pathway, docking help to better design adjuvants (Alawam et al.,2024). AI also allows scientists to design adjuvants specifically for certain vaccines or patients group, making vaccines more effective and personalized. Many kinds of receptors and proteins as a target adjuvant have been developed using traditional as well as with the help of AI. Toll like receptors (Meneveau et al,2021), interferon gene stimulators (STING) (Wilson et al., 2018), Programmed cell death protein 1, apoptotic ligand 1(Gibney et al.,2015, Meneveau et al,2021). AI assisted tool such as Deep Chem, PotentialNet, DeepNeuralNetQSAR, DeepTox, PotentialNet, Gene Ways, are used for the adjuvant development (zhang et al.,2024). GM-CSF act as an adjuvant for enhancing antigen presentation by dendritic cells, IL-12 persuade Activation of cytotoxic T cells & NK cells combining with Immune checkpoint inhibitor used to treat solid neoplasm and provide long resilient immune response (Charychet al.,216). Various factors such as genetics, environment, age, sex can also contribute to immunogenicity. using MLP DeepChem model is developed using python to investigate appropriate adjuvant. DeepTox capable of predicting toxicity of drug (Ciallella et al.,2019, Schubert et al.,2016.)

"De novo Design" (Hartenfeller et al.,2011) using AI in drug discovery is widely used in adjuvant discovery. Reinforcement deep learning algorithms named as ReLeaSE uses deep learning networks for predicting molecular properties (Popova et al.,2018). Virtual screening methods such as ligand based, or structural based screening (LB/SBVS) is based on computing device drug discovery methods that do prediction of binding ability and affinity between protein of interest (Banegas-Luna et al.,2018) In present time AI systems focuses on deep learning method or deep neural networks. It includes drug design and molecular dynamics progress. (Lipinski et al.,2019) alongside evolution of personalized medicine AI can be effectively leveraged for selecting most suitable adjuvant and attain personalized immunotherapies schemes improving effectual and efficacious of adjuvant design.

Figure 1. AI software and tools used in vaccine development.

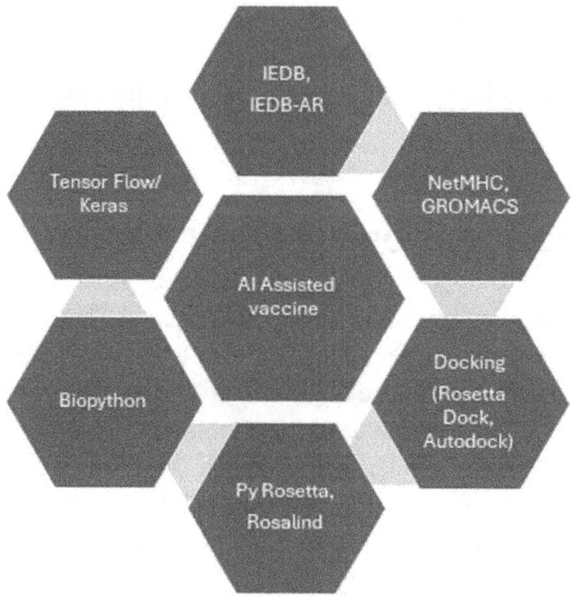

There are several AI based tool has been developed in last decade for vaccine development (Figure 1). AI algorithms assisted precision vaccines for specific pathogen, host population, and immune profile can be generated by analysing genomics, proteomics and interaction between the immune systems. (Li et al.,2024, Li et al., 2021) It enables to forecast immunogenic targets such as proteins, carbohydrate or any other moieties to which the Antibody fragment interact. It also enables to search for specific biomarkers, immune signatures targeted by variability in vaccine response (Abelin et al.,2017).

CONCLUSION

AI has revolutionized vaccine design by accelerating antigen selection, optimizing formulations, and predicting immune responses with unparalleled precision. Machine learning models analyze vast datasets, enabling rapid adaptation to emerging pathogens. AI-driven simulations enhance preclinical testing, reducing reliance on costly experiments. Personalized immunization strategies improve efficacy across diverse populations. Real-time surveillance predicts outbreaks, ensuring timely interventions. Open-source AI tools democratize research, fostering global collaboration. As computational advancements continue,

AI will further refine vaccine development, making it faster, more efficient, and universally accessible. This synergy between AI and vaccinology paves the way for a future of rapid, effective disease prevention.

REFERENCES

Abdelmageed, M. I., Abdelmoneim, A. H., Mustafa, M. I., Elfadol, N. M., Murshed, N. S., Shantier, S. W., & Makhawi, A. M. (2020). Design of a multiepitope-based peptide vaccine against the E protein of human COVID-19: An immunoinformatics approach. *BioMed Research International, 2683286*(1), 2683286. Advance online publication. DOI: 10.1155/2020/2683286 PMID: 32461973

Abelin, J. G., Keskin, D. B., Sarkizova, S., Hartigan, C. R., Zhang, W., Sidney, J., Stevens, J., Lane, W., Zhang, G. L., Eisenhaure, T. M., Clauser, K. R., Hacohen, N., Rooney, M. S., Carr, S. A., & Wu, C. J. (2017). Mass spectrometry profiling of HLA-associated peptidomes in mono-allelic cells enables more accurate Epitope prediction. *Immunity, 46*(2), 315–326. DOI: 10.1016/j.immuni.2017.02.007 PMID: 28228285

Aileni, M., Rohela, G. K., Jogam, P., Soujanya, S., & Zhang, B. (2022). Biotechnological perspectives to combat the COVID-19 pandemic: Precise diagnostics and inevitable vaccine paradigms. *Cells, 11*(7), 1182. DOI: 10.3390/cells11071182 PMID: 35406746

Alawam, A. S., & Alwethaynani, M. S. (2024). Construction of an aerolysin-based multi-epitope vaccine against Aeromonas hydrophila: An in-silico machine learning and artificial intelligence-supported approach. *Frontiers in Immunology, 15*, 1369890. DOI: 10.3389/fimmu.2024.1369890 PMID: 38495891

Baek, M., DiMaio, F., Anishchenko, I., Dauparas, J., Ovchinnikov, S., Lee, G. R., … Baker, D. (2021). Accurate prediction of protein structures and interactions using a three-track neural network. *Science (New York, N.Y.), 373*(6557), 871–876. doi:. abj8754DOI: 10.1126/science

Banegas-Luna, A. J., Cerón-Carrasco, J. P., & Pérez-Sánchez, H. (2018). A review of ligand-based virtual screening web tools and screening algorithms in large molecular databases in the age of big data. *Future Medicinal Chemistry, 10*(22), 2641–2658. DOI: 10.4155/fmc-2018-0076 PMID: 30499744

Bhattacharya, S., Dunn, P., Thomas, C. G., Smith, B., Schaefer, H., Chen, J., & Butte, A. J. (2018). ImmPort, toward repurposing of open access immunological assay data for translational and clinical research. *Scientific Data, 5*(1), 180015. DOI: 10.1038/sdata.2018.15 PMID: 29485622

Bravi, B. (2024). Development and use of machine learning algorithms in vaccine target selection. *NPJ Vaccines, 9*(1), 15. DOI: 10.1038/s41541-023-00795-8 PMID: 38242890

Breuer, K., Foroushani, A. K., Laird, M. R., Chen, C., Sribnaia, A., Lo, R., & Lynn, D. J. (2013). InnateDB: Systems biology of innate immunity and beyond—recent updates and continuing curation. *Nucleic Acids Research, 41*(Database issue), D1228–D1233. DOI: 10.1093/nar/gks1147 PMID: 23180781

Bukhari, S. N. H., Jain, A., Haq, E., Mehbodniya, A., & Webber, J. (2022). Machine Learning Techniques for the Prediction of B-Cell and T-Cell Epitopes as Potential Vaccine Targets with a Specific Focus on SARS-CoV-2 Pathogen: A Review. *Pathogens (Basel, Switzerland), 11*(2), 146. DOI: 10.3390/pathogens11020146 PMID: 35215090

Cai, Y., Chen, R., Gao, S., Li, W., Liu, Y., Su, G., & Zhang, X. (2022). Artificial intelligence applied in neoantigen identification facilitates personalized cancer immunotherapy. *Frontiers in Oncology, 12*, 1054231. DOI: 10.3389/fonc.2022.1054231 PMID: 36698417

Caoili, S. E. C. (2014). Hybrid methods for B-cell epitope prediction. *Methods in Molecular Biology (Clifton, N.J.)*, *1184*, 245–283. DOI: 10.1007/978-1-4939-1115-8_14 PMID: 25048129

Caradonna, T. M., & Schmidt, A. G. (2021). Protein engineering strategies for rational immunogen design. *NPJ Vaccines*, *6*(1), 154. DOI: 10.1038/s41541-021-00417-1 PMID: 34921149

Chai, S., Smith, C. C., Kochar, T. K., Hunsucker, S. A., Beck, W., Olsen, K. S., & Vincent, B. G. (2022). NeoSplice: A bioinformatics method for prediction of splice variant neoantigens. *Bioinformatics Advances*, *2*(1), vbac032. Advance online publication. DOI: 10.1093/bioadv/vbac032 PMID: 35669345

Charych, D. H., Hoch, U., Langowski, J. L., Lee, S. R., Addepalli, M. K., Kirk, P. B., & Doberstein, S. K. (2016). NKTR-214, an engineered cytokine with biased IL2 receptor binding, increased tumor exposure, and marked efficacy in mouse tumor models. *Clinical Cancer Research*, *22*(3), 680–690. DOI: 10.1158/1078-0432.CCR-15-1631 PMID: 26832745

Chen, W., Feng, Y., Zhao, Q., Zhu, Z., & Dimitrov, D. S. (2012). Human monoclonal antibodies targeting nonoverlapping epitopes on insulin-like growth factor II as a novel type of candidate cancer therapeutics. *Molecular Cancer Therapeutics*, *11*(7), 1400–1410. DOI: 10.1158/1535-7163.MCT-12-0172 PMID: 22553356

Cia, G., Pucci, F., & Rooman, M. (2023). Critical review of conformational B-cell epitope prediction methods. *Briefings in Bioinformatics*, *24*(1), bbac567. Advance online publication. DOI: 10.1093/bib/bbac567 PMID: 36611255

Ciallella, H. L., & Zhu, H. (2019). Advancing computational toxicology in the big data era by artificial intelligence: Data-driven and mechanism-driven modeling for chemical toxicity. *Chemical Research in Toxicology*, *32*(4), 536–547. DOI: 10.1021/acs.chemrestox.8b00393 PMID: 30907586

Collatz, M., Mock, F., Barth, E., Hölzer, M., Sachse, K., & Marz, M. (2021). EpiDope: A deep neural network for linear B-cell epitope prediction. *Bioinformatics (Oxford, England)*, *37*(4), 448–455. DOI: 10.1093/bioinformatics/btaa773 PMID: 32915967

da Silva, B. M., Myung, Y., Ascher, D. B., & Pires, D. E. V. (2022). epitope3D: A machine learning method for conformational B-cell epitope prediction. *Briefings in Bioinformatics*, *23*(1), bbab423. Advance online publication. DOI: 10.1093/bib/bbab423 PMID: 34676398

Degoot, A. M., Chirove, F., & Ndifon, W. (2018). Trans-Allelic model for prediction of peptide:MHC-IIinteractions. *Frontiers in Immunology*, *9*, 1410. Advance online publication. DOI: 10.3389/fimmu.2018.01410 PMID: 29988560

Deng, N., Wu, C., Yaseen, A., & Wu, H. (2022). ImmuneData: An integrated data discovery system for immunology data repositories. *Database : The Journal of Biological Databases and Curation*, *2022*, baac003. Advance online publication. DOI: 10.1093/database/baac003 PMID: 35262674

Elshafei, S. O., Mahmoud, N. A., & Almofti, Y. A. (2024). Immunoinformatics, molecular docking and dynamics simulation approaches unveil a multi epitope-based potent peptide vaccine candidate against avian leukosis virus. *Scientific Reports*, *14*(1), 2870. DOI: 10.1038/s41598-024-53048-6 PMID: 38311642

Fleri, W., Paul, S., Dhanda, S. K., Mahajan, S., Xu, X., Peters, B., & Sette, A. (2017). The Immune Epitope Database and Analysis Resource in Epitope discovery and synthetic vaccine design. *Frontiers in Immunology*, *8*, 278. DOI: 10.3389/fimmu.2017.00278 PMID: 28352270

Gao, Y., Zhang, Y., & Liu, X. (2024). Rheumatoid arthritis: Pathogenesis and therapeutic advances. *MedComm*, *5*(3), e509. DOI: 10.1002/mco2.509 PMID: 38469546

Ghosh, S. (2020). *Computational Immunology: Applications* (1st ed.). CRC Press., DOI: 10.1201/9781351023504

Giardino, G., Gallo, V., Prencipe, R., Gaudino, G., Romano, R., De Cataldis, M., & Pignata, C. (2016). Unbalanced immune system: Immunodeficiencies and autoimmunity. *Frontiers in Pediatrics*, *4*, 107. DOI: 10.3389/fped.2016.00107 PMID: 27766253

Gibney, G. T., Kudchadkar, R. R., DeConti, R. C., Thebeau, M. S., Czupryn, M. P., Tetteh, L., & Weber, J. S. (2015). Safety, correlative markers, and clinical results of adjuvant nivolumab in combination with vaccine in resected high-risk metastatic melanoma. *Clinical Cancer Research*, *21*(4), 712–720. DOI: 10.1158/1078-0432.CCR-14-2468 PMID: 25524312

Goodman, R. E., Ebisawa, M., Ferreira, F., Sampson, H. A., van Ree, R., Vieths, S., Baumert, J. L., Bohle, B., Lalithambika, S., Wise, J., & Taylor, S. L. (2016). AllergenOnline: A peer-reviewed, curated allergen database to assess novel food proteins for potential cross-reactivity. *Molecular Nutrition & Food Research*, *60*(5), 1183–1198. DOI: 10.1002/mnfr.201500769 PMID: 26887584

Gorki, V., & Medhi, B. (2024). Use of artificial intelligence in vaccine development against pathogens: Challenges and future directions. *Indian Journal of Pharmacology*, *56*(2), 77–79. DOI: 10.4103/ijp.ijp_259_24 PMID: 38687309

Guarra, F., & Colombo, G. (2023). Computational methods in immunology and vaccinology: Design and development of antibodies and immunogens. *Journal of Chemical Theory and Computation*, *19*(16), 5315–5333. DOI: 10.1021/acs.jctc.3c00513 PMID: 37527403

Gulati, S., Mattsson, A. H., Schussek, S., Zheng, B., DeOliveira, R. B., Shaughnessy, J., & Ram, S. (2023). Preclinical efficacy of a cell division protein candidate gonococcal vaccine identified by artificial intelligence. *mBio*, *14*(6), e0250023. DOI: 10.1128/mbio.02500-23 PMID: 37905891

Hartenfeller, M., & Schneider, G. (2011). Enabling future drug discovery by *de novo* design. *Wiley Interdisciplinary Reviews. Computational Molecular Science*, *1*(5), 742–759. DOI: 10.1002/wcms.49

Hemmati, S., Saeidikia, Z., Seradj, H., & Mohagheghzadeh, A. (2024). Immunomodulatory peptides as vaccine adjuvants and antimicrobial agents. *Pharmaceuticals (Basel, Switzerland)*, *17*(2), 201. DOI: 10.3390/ph17020201 PMID: 38399416

Huang, Y., Zhang, Z., & Zhou, Y. (2022). AbAgIntPre: A deep learning method for predicting antibody-antigen interactions based on sequence information. *Frontiers in Immunology*, *13*, 1053617. DOI: 10.3389/fimmu.2022.1053617 PMID: 36618397

Human Immunome Project. (2020, December 16). Retrieved February 8, 2025, from Human Immunome Project website: https://www.humanimmunomeproject.org/

Hundal, J., Carreno, B. M., Petti, A. A., Linette, G. P., Griffith, O. L., Mardis, E. R., & Griffith, M. (2016). pVAC-Seq: A genome-guided in silico approach to identifying tumor neoantigens. *Genome Medicine*, *8*(1), 11. DOI: 10.1186/s13073-016-0264-5 PMID: 26825632

Hutchison, S., & Pritchard, A. L. (2018). Identifying neoantigens for use in immunotherapy. *Mammalian Genome*, *29*(11–12), 714–730. DOI: 10.1007/s00335-018-9771-6 PMID: 30167844

Jones, G., Jindal, A., Ghani, U., Kotelnikov, S., Egbert, M., Hashemi, N., & Kozakov, D. (2022). Elucidation of protein function using computational docking and hotspot analysis by ClusPro and FTMap. *Acta Crystallographica. Section D, Structural Biology*, *78*(Pt 6), 690–697. DOI: 10.1107/S2059798322002741 PMID: 35647916

Karthika, R., Muthusamy, S., & Prabhu, P. R. (2023). InflANNet: A neural network predictor for Influenza A CTL and HTL epitopes to aid robust vaccine design. *Bulletin of the National Research Center*, *47*(1), 129. Advance online publication. DOI: 10.1186/s42269-023-01101-1

Kaushik, R., Kant, R., & Christodoulides, M. (2023). Artificial intelligence in accelerating vaccine development - current and future perspectives. *Frontiers in Bacteriology*, *2*, 1258159. Advance online publication. DOI: 10.3389/fbrio.2023.1258159

Kennedy, R. B., Ovsyannikova, I. G., Palese, P., & Poland, G. A. (2020). Current challenges in vaccinology. *Frontiers in Immunology*, *11*, 1181. DOI: 10.3389/fimmu.2020.01181 PMID: 32670279

Khan, M. T., Islam, M. J., Parihar, A., Islam, R., Jerin, T. J., Dhote, R., & Halim, M. A. (2021). Immunoinformatic and molecular modeling approach to design a universal multi-epitope vaccine for SARS-CoV-2. *Informatics in Medicine Unlocked*, *24*(100578), 100578. DOI: 10.1016/j.imu.2021.100578 PMID: 33898733

Kim, D. N., McNaughton, A. D., & Kumar, N. (2024). Leveraging artificial intelligence to expedite antibody design and enhance antibody-antigen interactions. *Bioengineering (Basel, Switzerland)*, *11*(2), 185. DOI: 10.3390/bioengineering11020185 PMID: 38391671

Kim, S., Kim, H. S., Kim, E., Lee, M. G., Shin, E.-C., Paik, S., & Kim, S. (2018). Neopepsee: Accurate genome-level prediction of neoantigens by harnessing sequence and amino acid immunogenicity information. *Annals of Oncology : Official Journal of the European Society for Medical Oncology*, *29*(4), 1030–1036. DOI: 10.1093/annonc/mdy022 PMID: 29360924

Lane, J., Duroux, P., & Lefranc, M.-P. (2010). From IMGT-ONTOLOGY to IMGT/LIGMotif: The IMGT standardized approach for immunoglobulin and T cell receptor gene identification and description in large genomic sequences. *BMC Bioinformatics*, *11*(1), 223. DOI: 10.1186/1471-2105-11-223 PMID: 20433708

Li, G., Iyer, B., Prasath, V. B. S., Ni, Y., & Salomonis, N. (2021). DeepImmuno: Deep learning-empowered prediction and generation of immunogenic peptides for T-cell immunity. *Briefings in Bioinformatics*, *22*(6), bbab160. Advance online publication. DOI: 10.1093/bib/bbab160 PMID: 34009266

Li, Y., Wu, X., Fang, D., & Luo, Y. (2024). Informing immunotherapy with multi-omics driven machine learning. *NPJ Digital Medicine*, *7*(1), 67. DOI: 10.1038/s41746-024-01043-6 PMID: 38486092

Lim, C. P., Leow, C. H., Lim, H. T., Kok, B. H., Chuah, C., Oliveira, J. I. N., & Leow, C. Y. (2024). Insights into structural vaccinology harnessed for universal coronavirus vaccine development. *Clinical and Experimental Vaccine Research*, *13*(3), 202–217. DOI: 10.7774/cevr.2024.13.3.202 PMID: 39144127

Lin, F., Lin, E. Z., Anekoji, M., Ichim, T. E., Hu, J., Marincola, F. M., Jones, L. D., Kesari, S., & Ashili, S. (2023). Advancing personalized medicine in brain cancer: Exploring the role of mRNA vaccines. *Journal of Translational Medicine*, *21*(1), 830. DOI: 10.1186/s12967-023-04724-0 PMID: 37978542

Lipinski, C. F., Maltarollo, V. G., Oliveira, P. R., da Silva, A. B. F., & Honorio, K. M. (2019). Advances and perspectives in applying deep learning for drug design and discovery. *Frontiers in Robotics and AI*, *6*, 108. DOI: 10.3389/frobt.2019.00108 PMID: 33501123

Liu, J., Yang, S., Cao, B., Zhou, G., Zhang, F., Wang, Y., Wang, R., Zhu, L., Meng, Y., Hu, C., Liang, H., Lin, X., Zhu, K., Chen, G., Luo, K. Q., Di, L., & Zhao, Q. (2021). Targeting B7-H3 via chimeric antigen receptor T cells and bispecific killer cell engagers augments antitumor response of cytotoxic lymphocytes. *Journal of Hematology & Oncology*, *14*(1), 21. DOI: 10.1186/s13045-020-01024-8 PMID: 33514401

Liu, Z., Jin, J., Cui, Y., Xiong, Z., Nasiri, A., Zhao, Y., & Hu, J. (2022). DeepSeqPanII: An interpretable recurrent neural network model with attention mechanism for peptide-HLA class II binding prediction. *IEEE/ACM Transactions on Computational Biology and Bioinformatics*, *19*(4), 2188–2196. DOI: 10.1109/TCBB.2021.3074927 PMID: 33886473

Manavalan, B., Govindaraj, R. G., Shin, T. H., Kim, M. O., & Lee, G. (2018). IBCE-EL: A new ensemble learning framework for improved linear B-cell Epitope prediction. *Frontiers in Immunology*, *9*, 1695. Advance online publication. DOI: 10.3389/fimmu.2018.01695 PMID: 30100904

Marshall, J. S., Upton, J. E. M., Vliagoftis, H., Hildebrand, K. J., Byrne, A., & Watson, W. (2024). Introduction to immunology and immune disorders. *Allergy, Asthma, and Clinical Immunology : Official Journal of the Canadian Society of Allergy and Clinical Immunology*, *20*(S3, Suppl 3), 69. DOI: 10.1186/s13223-024-00932-5 PMID: 39702433

Meneveau, M. O., Petroni, G. R., Salerno, E. P., Lynch, K. T., Smolkin, M., Woodson, E., & Slingluff, C. L. (2021). Immunogenicity in humans of a transdermal multipeptide melanoma vaccine administered with or without a TLR7 agonist. *Journal for Immunotherapy of Cancer*, *9*(5), e002214. DOI: 10.1136/jitc-2020-002214 PMID: 34035112

Miller, F. W. (2023). The increasing prevalence of autoimmunity and autoimmune diseases: An urgent call to action for improved understanding, diagnosis, treatment, and prevention. *Current Opinion in Immunology*, *80*(102266), 102266. DOI: 10.1016/j.coi.2022.102266 PMID: 36446151

Montemurro, A., Schuster, V., Povlsen, H. R., Bentzen, A. K., Jurtz, V., Chronister, W. D., & Nielsen, M. (2021). NetTCR-2.0 enables accurate prediction of TCR-peptide binding by using paired TCRα and β sequence data. *Communications Biology*, *4*(1), 1060. DOI: 10.1038/s42003-021-02610-3 PMID: 34508155

Olawade, D. B., Teke, J., Fapohunda, O., Weerasinghe, K., Usman, S. O., Ige, A. O., & Clement David-Olawade, A. (2024). Leveraging artificial intelligence in vaccine development: A narrative review. *Journal of Microbiological Methods*, *224*(106998), 106998. DOI: 10.1016/j.mimet.2024.106998 PMID: 39019262

Ott, P. A., Hu, Z., Keskin, D. B., Shukla, S. A., Sun, J., Bozym, D. J., Zhang, W., Luoma, A., Giobbie-Hurder, A., Peter, L., Chen, C., Olive, O., Carter, T. A., Li, S., Lieb, D. J., Eisenhaure, T., Gjini, E., Stevens, J., Lane, W. J., & Wu, C. J. (2017). An immunogenic personal neoantigen vaccine for patients with melanoma. *Nature*, *547*(7662), 217–221. DOI: 10.1038/nature22991 PMID: 28678778

Ouspenskaia, T., Law, T., Clauser, K. R., Klaeger, S., Sarkizova, S., Aguet, F., & Regev, A. (2022). Unannotated proteins expand the MHC-I-restricted immunopeptidome in cancer. *Nature Biotechnology*, *40*(2), 209–217. DOI: 10.1038/s41587-021-01021-3 PMID: 34663921

Ovsyannikova, I. G., & Poland, G. A. (2011). Vaccinomics: Current findings, challenges and novel approaches for vaccine development. *The AAPS Journal*, *13*(3), 438–444. DOI: 10.1208/s12248-011-9281-x PMID: 21671143

Pappalardo, F., Brusic, V., Pennisi, M., & Zhang, G. (2015). Advances in computational immunology. *Journal of Immunology Research*, *170920*, 1–3. Advance online publication. DOI: 10.1155/2015/170920 PMID: 26844232

Patil, D., Rane, N. L., Desai, P., & Rane, J. (2024). Machine learning and deep learning: Methods, techniques, applications, challenges, and future research opportunities. In *Trustworthy Artificial Intelligence in Industry and Society*. DOI: 10.70593/978-81-981367-4-9_2

Pinder, M., Fry, R. C., & Alexis, N. E. (2020). Environmental contaminants and the immune system: A systems perspective. In *Environmental Epigenetics in Toxicology and Public Health* (pp. 217–237). DOI: 10.1016/B978-0-12-819968-8.00009-3

Pittala, S., & Bailey-Kellogg, C. (2020). Learning context-aware structural representations to predict antigen and antibody binding interfaces. *Bioinformatics (Oxford, England)*, *36*(13), 3996–4003. DOI: 10.1093/bioinformatics/btaa263 PMID: 32321157

Poland, G. A., Ovsyannikova, I. G., & Jacobson, R. M. (2008). Personalized vaccines: The emerging field of vaccinomics. *Expert Opinion on Biological Therapy*, *8*(11), 1659–1667. DOI: 10.1517/14712598.8.11.1659 PMID: 18847302

Popova, M., Isayev, O., & Tropsha, A. (2018). Deep reinforcement learning for de novo drug design. *Science Advances, 4*(7), eaap7885. doi:. aap7885DOI: 10.1126/sciadv

Porter, K. A., Xia, B., Beglov, D., Bohnuud, T., Alam, N., Schueler-Furman, O., & Kozakov, D. (2017). ClusPro PeptiDock: Efficient global docking of peptide recognition motifs using FFT. *Bioinformatics (Oxford, England)*, *33*(20), 3299–3301. DOI: 10.1093/bioinformatics/btx216 PMID: 28430871

Rahman, M. S., Hoque, M. N., Islam, M. R., Akter, S., Rubayet Ul Alam, A. S. M., Siddique, M. A., Saha, O., Rahaman, M. M., Sultana, M., Crandall, K. A., & Hossain, M. A. (2020). Epitope-based chimeric peptide vaccine design against S, M and E proteins of SARS-CoV-2, the etiologic agent of COVID-19 pandemic: An in-silico approach. *PeerJ*, *8*(e9572), e9572. DOI: 10.7717/peerj.9572 PMID: 33194329

Rakitina, T., Smirnova, E., Podshivalov, D., Timofeev, V., Komolov, A., Vlaskina, A., & Kovalchuk, M. (2023). An algorithm for the development of a recombinant antiherpetic subunit vaccine combining the crystal structure analysis, AlphaFold2-based modeling, and immunoinformatics. *Crystals*, *13*(10), 1416. DOI: 10.3390/cryst13101416

Rapoport, B., & McLachlan, S. M. (2001). Thyroid autoimmunity. *The Journal of Clinical Investigation*, *108*(9), 1253–1259. DOI: 10.1172/JCI14321 PMID: 11696565

Ras-Carmona, A., Lehmann, A. A., Lehmann, P. V., & Reche, P. A. (2022). Prediction of B cell epitopes in proteins using a novel sequence similarity-based method. *Scientific Reports*, *12*(1), 13739. DOI: 10.1038/s41598-022-18021-1 PMID: 35962028

Rohl, C. A., Strauss, C. E. M., Misura, K. M. S., & Baker, D. (2004). Protein structure prediction using Rosetta. In *Methods in Enzymology. Methods in Enzymology* (pp. 66–93). DOI: 10.1016/S0076-6879(04)83004-0

Rubinsteyn, A., Hodes, I., Kodysh, J., & Hammerbacher, J. (2017). Vaxrank: A computational tool for designing personalized cancer vaccines. DOI: 10.1101/142919

Saha, S., & Raghava, G. P. S. (2004). BcePred: Prediction of continuous B-cell epitopes in antigenic sequences using physico-chemical properties. In *Lecture Notes in Computer Science. Lecture Notes in Computer Science* (pp. 197–204). DOI: 10.1007/978-3-540-30220-9_16

Saha, S., & Raghava, G. P. S. (2006). Prediction of continuous B-cell epitopes in an antigen using recurrent neural network. *Proteins*, *65*(1), 40–48. DOI: 10.1002/prot.21078 PMID: 16894596

Sauteraud, R., Dashevskiy, L., Finak, G., & Gottardo, R. (2016). ImmuneSpace: Enabling integrative modelling of human immunological data. *The Journal of Immunology, 196*(1_Supplement), 124.65-124.65. DOI: 10.4049/jimmunol.196.Supp.124.65

Schenck, R., Lakatos, E., Gatenbee, C., Graham, T. A., & Anderson, A. R. A. (2019). NeoPredPipe: High throughput neoantigen prediction and recognition potential pipeline. *BMC Bioinformatics*, *20*(1), 264. DOI: 10.1186/s12859-019-2876-4 PMID: 31117948

Schubert, B., Walzer, M., Brachvogel, H.-P., Szolek, A., Mohr, C., & Kohlbacher, O. (2016). FRED 2: An immunoinformatic framework for Python. *Bioinformatics (Oxford, England)*, *32*(13), 2044–2046. DOI: 10.1093/bioinformatics/btw113 PMID: 27153717

Sela-Culang, I., Kunik, V., & Ofran, Y. (2013). The structural basis of antibody-antigen recognition. *Frontiers in Immunology*, *4*, 302. DOI: 10.3389/fimmu.2013.00302 PMID: 24115948

Sette, A., & Rappuoli, R. (2010). Reverse vaccinology: Developing vaccines in the era of genomics. *Immunity*, *33*(4), 530–541. DOI: 10.1016/j.immuni.2010.09.017 PMID: 21029963

Shashkova, T. I., Umerenkov, D., Salnikov, M., Strashnov, P. V., Konstantinova, A. V., Lebed, I., & Ivanisenko, N. V. (2022). SEMA: Antigen B-cell conformational epitope prediction using deep transfer learning. *Frontiers in Immunology*, *13*, 960985. DOI: 10.3389/fimmu.2022.960985 PMID: 36189325

Shi, Y., Guo, Z., Su, X., Meng, L., Zhang, M., Sun, J., & Han, Z.-G. (2020). DeepAntigen: A novel method for neoantigen prioritization via 3D genome and deep sparse learning. *Bioinformatics (Oxford, England)*, *36*(19), 4894–4901. DOI: 10.1093/bioinformatics/btaa596 PMID: 32592462

Shirkani, A., Mansouri, A., Farid Hosseini, R., Jabbari Azad, F., Alsadat Mahmoudian, R., Montazer, M., & Gholamin, M. (2019). The role of interleukin-4 and 13 gene polymorphisms in allergic rhinitis: A case control study. *Reports of Biochemistry & Molecular Biology*, *8*(2), 111–118. https://www.ncbi.nlm.nih.gov/pubmed/31832433 PMID: 31832433

Shugay, M., Bagaev, D. V., Zvyagin, I. V., Vroomans, R. M., Crawford, J. C., Dolton, G., Komech, E. A., Sycheva, A. L., Koneva, A. E., Egorov, E. S., Eliseev, A. V., Van Dyk, E., Dash, P., Attaf, M., Rius, C., Ladell, K., McLaren, J. E., Matthews, K. K., Clemens, E. B., & Chudakov, D. M. (2018). VDJdb: A curated database of T-cell receptor sequences with known antigen specificity. *Nucleic Acids Research*, *46*(D1), D419–D427. DOI: 10.1093/nar/gkx760 PMID: 28977646

Smith, D. A., & Germolec, D. R. (1999). Introduction to immunology and autoimmunity. *Environmental Health Perspectives*, *107*(suppl 5), 661–665. DOI: 10.1289/ehp.99107s5661 PMID: 10502528

Subramanian, M., Wojtusciszyn, A., Favre, L., Boughorbel, S., Shan, J., Letaief, K. B., & Chouchane, L. (2020). Precision medicine in the era of artificial intelligence: Implications in chronic disease management. *Journal of Translational Medicine*, *18*(1), 472. DOI: 10.1186/s12967-020-02658-5 PMID: 33298113

Tang, S., & Madhavan, S. (2017). neoantigenR: An annotation-based pipeline for tumor neoantigen identification from sequencing data. DOI: 10.1101/171843

Tang, Y., Wang, Y., Wang, J., Li, M., Peng, L., Wei, G., & Gao, Z. (2020). TruNeo: An integrated pipeline improves personalized true tumor neoantigen identification. *BMC Bioinformatics*, *21*(1), 532. DOI: 10.1186/s12859-020-03869-9 PMID: 33208106

Tappeiner, E., Finotello, F., Charoentong, P., Mayer, C., Rieder, D., & Trajanoski, Z. (2017). TIminer: NGS data mining pipeline for cancer immunology and immunotherapy. *Bioinformatics (Oxford, England)*, *33*(19), 3140–3141. DOI: 10.1093/bioinformatics/btx377 PMID: 28633385

Tong, J. C., & Ranganathan, S. (2013). Computational T cell vaccine design. In *Computer-Aided Vaccine Design* (pp. 59–86). DOI: 10.1533/9781908818416.59

Uffelmann, E., Huang, Q. Q., Munung, N. S., de Vries, J., Okada, Y., Martin, A. R., Martin, H. C., Lappalainen, T., & Posthuma, D. (2021). Genome-wide association studies. *Nature Reviews. Methods Primers*, *1*(1), 59. DOI: 10.1038/s43586-021-00056-9

Uffelmann, E., Huang, Q. Q., Munung, N. S., de Vries, J., Okada, Y., Martin, A. R., Martin, H. C., Lappalainen, T., & Posthuma, D. (2021). Genome-wide association studies. *Nature Reviews. Methods Primers*, *1*(1), 59. DOI: 10.1038/s43586-021-00056-9

Wang, T.-Y., Wang, L., Alam, S. K., Hoeppner, L. H., & Yang, R. (2019). ScanNeo: Identifying indel-derived neoantigens using RNA-Seq data. *Bioinformatics (Oxford, England)*, *35*(20), 4159–4161. DOI: 10.1093/bioinformatics/btz193 PMID: 30887025

Wilson, D. R., Sen, R., Sunshine, J. C., Pardoll, D. M., Green, J. J., & Kim, Y. J. (2018). Biodegradable STING agonist nanoparticles for enhanced cancer immunotherapy. *Nanomedicine; Nanotechnology, Biology, and Medicine*, *14*(2), 237–246. DOI: 10.1016/j.nano.2017.10.013 PMID: 29127039

Xia, J., Bai, P., Fan, W., Li, Q., Li, Y., Wang, D., Yin, L., & Zhou, Y. (2021). NEPdb: A Database of T-Cell Experimentally-Validated Neoantigens and Pan-Cancer Predicted Neoepitopes for Cancer Immunotherapy. *Frontiers in Immunology*, *12*, 644637. DOI: 10.3389/fimmu.2021.644637 PMID: 33927717

Xu, Y., Liu, X., Cao, X., Huang, C., Liu, E., Qian, S., & Zhang, J. (2021). Artificial intelligence: A powerful paradigm for scientific research. *Innovation (Cambridge (Mass.))*, *2*(4), 100179. DOI: 10.1016/j.xinn.2021.100179 PMID: 34877560

Yao, B., Zheng, D., Liang, S., & Zhang, C. (2013). Conformational B-cell epitope prediction on antigen protein structures: A review of current algorithms and comparison with common binding site prediction methods. *PLoS One*, *8*(4), e62249. DOI: 10.1371/journal.pone.0062249 PMID: 23620816

Ye, C., Hu, W., & Gaeta, B. (2021). Machine learning prediction of Antibody-Antigen binding: dataset, method and testing (p. 2021.03.19.435772). DOI: 10.1101/2021.03.19.435772

Zeng, X., Bai, G., Sun, C., & Ma, B. (2023). Recent progress in antibody Epitope prediction. *Antibodies (Basel)*, *12*(3), 52. Advance online publication. DOI: 10.3390/antib12030052 PMID: 37606436

Zhang, W.-Y., Zheng, X.-L., Coghi, P. S., Chen, J.-H., Dong, B.-J., & Fan, X.-X. (2024). Revolutionizing adjuvant development: Harnessing AI for next-generation cancer vaccines. *Frontiers in Immunology*, *15*, 1438030. DOI: 10.3389/fimmu.2024.1438030 PMID: 39206192

Zhang, Y., Huffman, A., Johnson, J., & He, Y. (2023). Vaxign-DL: A deep learning-based method for vaccine design and its evaluation. DOI: 10.1101/2023.11.29.569096

Zhao, T., Cai, Y., Jiang, Y., He, X., Wei, Y., Yu, Y., & Tian, X. (2023). Vaccine adjuvants: Mechanisms and platforms. *Signal Transduction and Targeted Therapy*, *8*(1), 283. DOI: 10.1038/s41392-023-01557-7 PMID: 37468460

Zhou, C., Wei, Z., Zhang, Z., Zhang, B., Zhu, C., Chen, K., & Liu, Q. (2019). pTuneos: Prioritizing tumor neoantigens from next-generation sequencing data. *Genome Medicine*, *11*(1), 67. DOI: 10.1186/s13073-019-0679-x PMID: 31666118

Zhou, X.-J., MacLeod, A. S., & Tsoi, L. C. (2022). Editorial: Advances in using big data and artificial intelligence to understand heterogeneity in inflammatory responses.

Chapter 7
AI-Driven Precision Medicine and Personalized Healthcare for Immunological Disorders

Sharon Anthony Poovathanathil
Amity University, Maharashtra, India

Sagar Barage
https://orcid.org/0000-0003-0752-6948
Amity University, Maharashtra, India

Rajshri Singh
https://orcid.org/0000-0001-5748-5799
Amity University, Maharashtra, India

ABSTRACT

Immunological disorders arise from dysfunctions in the immune system, leading to either an overactive or weakened response, and can manifest as autoimmune diseases, allergies, or immunodeficiencies, each presenting unique challenges in diagnosis and treatment. The considerable heterogeneity of immunological disorders suggests that individual patients may present with unique pathogenetic pathways. This diversity underscores the need to explore these varying mechanisms, potentially leading to the development of personalized therapeutic approaches, precision-based strategies along with adoption of Artificial Intelligence (AI) technologies. Precision medicine with AI seeks to target the medical treatment based upon the specific characteristics of each patient. This chapter includes various AI technologies and elaborates on how several AI technologies can be integrated with precision medicine in personalized healthcare to treat immunological disorders.

1. INTRODUCTION

Healthcare has seen a drastic shift from traditional treatment methods to a technology and AI based method. AI in healthcare is transforming precision medicine by making it possible to personalize treatment regimens for immunological diseases. Due to the complex and dynamic dysregulation of the immune

DOI: 10.4018/979-8-3693-9725-1.ch007

system underlying many illnesses, universally applicable therapies must give way to highly personalized ones. Advanced AI methods for data analysis, pattern recognition, and predictive modelling may clarify complex biological networks that underlie these conditions. A better patient outcome, personalized treatments, and accurate diagnoses will emerge from using these methods (Peng et al., 2021).

2. OVERVIEW OF IMMUNOLOGICAL DISORDERS

Immunological diseases are the disorders that fall under a category where the immune system is imbalanced and either targets the person's own tissues, referred to as autoimmune diseases, or is unable to defend against infections, known as immune deficiencies. Examples include rheumatoid arthritis, systemic lupus erythematosus (SLE), and primary immunodeficiency disorders. These conditions disrupt the delicate balance of the immune system. Hyperactive responses, as found in autoimmune diseases, entail chronic inflammation and tissue damage. Immunodeficiency conditions with suppressed immune responses make the individuals vulnerable to infections, cancers, and delayed recovery (O'Driscroll & Jeggo, 2002). Immunological diseases are a major burden globally in millions of patients, and autoimmune diseases affect 3–5% of the population and tend to occur more frequently in women. Billions are spent each year on diagnostics, treatments, and management of complications (Marshall et al., 2018).

The complex human immune system plays a vital role in maintaining balance and protecting the body from harmful infections. It consists of two primary components: innate and adaptive immunity. Innate immunity serves as the body's first line of defence, providing a rapid but nonspecific response to various infections. Its key elements include physical barriers like the skin and mucous membranes, along with cellular defences involving macrophages, neutrophils, and natural killer cells. While these mechanisms act quickly, they lack the ability to remember past pathogens (Turvey & Broide, 2010). In contrast, adaptive immunity responds more slowly at first but is highly specific and capable of developing immunological memory. It customizes its defence by activating lymphocytes—T cells, which coordinate immune responses, and B cells, which produce antibodies to neutralize pathogens. Following exposure of the body to a pathogen, the adaptive immune system "remembers" it. The faster and stronger response on subsequent exposures is due to memory by the adaptive immune system. Combining innate and adaptive immunity forms a whole, coordinated defence system that protects the body from infection and disease (Bonilla &Oettgen, 2010).

However, dysfunction in this very complex system often leads to diseases. While underactivity in this network results in immunodeficiency, which leaves the body susceptible to infections, overactivity causes autoimmune disorders by the immune system attacking otherwise seemingly healthy tissues. The intricacy of this network frequently relies on massive cell populations, signalling molecules, and pathways that need to coordinate with one another (van der Pouw Kraan & Verweij, 2008). This relationship and the immune system's dynamic response make it difficult to research and control such reactions, necessitating the use of strong tools like artificial intelligence (AI) to interpret and forecast its behaviour.

3. TYPES OF IMMUNOLOGICAL DISORDERS

3.1 Hypersensitivity Reactions

Hypersensitivity reactions are exaggerated or inappropriate immune system reactions to various antigens that interact with the body, that can lead to tissue damage and malfunction. The etiology of most immune illnesses depends on these overreactions or misdirected reactions that damage the host's own tissues. The pathophysiology of the disease is influenced by the immune system's cells, antibodies, and inflammatory mediators (Greenberger & Grammer, 2012).

3.1.1 Type I Hypersensitivity

Type I reactions, or immediate hypersensitivity, are of central importance in allergic diseases such as asthma, allergic rhinitis, and anaphylaxis (Greenberger & Grammer, 2012). Such reactions are caused by exposure to allergens which stimulates the release of IgE produced by plasma cells. The IgE associates with receptors on mast and basophils cells sensitizing them. Subsequent allergen exposure leads to cross-linking of bound IgE, degranulation, and release of inflammatory mediators like histamine, prostaglandins, and leukotrienes. These mediators cause vasodilation, contraction of smooth muscles, and increased vascular permeability, thus inducing symptoms like wheezing, itching, and swelling. Severe manifestation: anaphylaxis in the form of systemic release of these mediators, leading to life-threatening airway obstruction and cardiovascular collapse (Abbas, 2000).

3.1.2 Type II Hypersensitivity

IgG and IgM antibodies are involved in the type II hypersensitivity reaction; they attach to cell surface antigens and identify the cells for phagocytosis or the complement system to destroy. Immunological conditions including autoimmune haemolytic anaemia, in which red blood cells are attacked and killed, and Goodpasture syndrome, in which antibodies target the kidney and lung basement membranes, are characterized by similar reactions. Complement activation causes cell lysis, inflammation, and eventually organ dysfunction through tissue damage (Uzzaman& Cho, 2012).

3.1.3 Type III Hypersensitivity

In Type III reactions, IgG and IgM antibodies form immune complexes with soluble antigens. These complexes deposit in tissues, especially where there is high blood filtration, including the kidneys, joints, and small blood vessels. Such immune complex deposition leads to disorders such as systemic lupus erythematosus (SLE) and serum sickness by activating complement, recruiting neutrophils, and causing tissue inflammation. Chronic stimulation of this pathway results in progressive damage, as seen in lupus nephritis and rheumatoid arthritis (Chinen et al., 2008).

3.1.4 Type IV Hypersensitivity

In contrast to the antibody-mediated ones, type IV hypersensitivity is cell-mediated by hyperactivation of T cells and macrophages. Delayed-type hypersensitivity reactions are often seen in conditions such as contact dermatitis (e.g., exposure to poison ivy) and autoimmune diseases such as diabetes mellitus type 1, in which T cells destroy pancreatic beta cells. Prolonged stimulation of the T cells leads to release of cytokines and development of inflammation and tissue destruction (Ditto, 2009).

3.2 Immunodeficiency and Other Immune Disorders

Immunodeficiency is conditions where there is a weakness in the immune system; patients are extremely prone to infections. Immunodeficiency can be classified as primary, which are mainly caused by genetic mutations (e.g., SCID and DiGeorge syndrome), or secondary, resulting from external factors like HIV/AIDS or chemotherapy. Primary immunodeficiencies include isolated defects in cellular and humoral immune responses that are inherited, while secondary immunodeficiencies are caused by acquired damage to the immune components (Casanova & Abel, 2007)

Other immune disorders include immune system cancers, such as leukaemia, lymphomas, and myelomas, which disrupt normal immune cell production and function. These cancers weaken the immune defences and may bring on serious health complications (Mortaz et al., 2016). Additionally, hyperinflammatory syndromes are a spectrum of immune dysfunction characterized by exaggerated responses. For example, cytokine storms or an uncontrollable release of inflammatory molecules can lead to tissue damage and organ failure due to severe infections such as COVID-19 (Tuano et al., 2021).

3.3 Autoimmune Disorders

Autoimmune disorders are disorder in which the immune system instead of defending the body against harmful invaders, targets its own healthy cells and tissues (Wang et al., 2015).

3.3.1 Rheumatoid Arthritis

The synovium, the lining of the membranes surrounding the joints, is incorrectly targeted by the immune system in rheumatoid arthritis (RA), a chronic inflammatory disease. This causes chronic inflammation, which over time can cause bone and cartilage degradation as well as joint discomfort, stiffness, and oedema. The condition can spread to major joints like the wrists, knees, hips, and shoulders after beginning with smaller ones like the fingers and toes. In addition to affecting joints, RA can also cause systemic issues by affecting other bodily systems like the skin, eyes, lungs, heart, and blood vessels. Although the precise origin of RA is unknown, a mix of immune system dysregulation, environmental triggers, and genetic predispositions may be involved. Without proper management, RA can lead to significant joint deformity, reduced mobility, and a decreased quality of life, underscoring the importance of early diagnosis and tailored treatment strategies. (Radu &Bungau, 2021).

3.3.2 Systemic Lupus Erythematosus (SLE)

In systemic lupus erythematosus (SLE), a chronic autoimmune illness, the body's own tissues and organs are attacked by the immune system, causing extensive inflammation and damage. SLE can impact several organ systems, such as the skin, joints, kidneys, heart, lungs, brain, and blood vessels, in contrast to other autoimmune diseases that may only affect one or a few. The ailment is frequently called a "great imitator" because its symptoms, which include fever, joint pain, exhaustion, and skin rashes, can be difficult to diagnose because they resemble those of other conditions. One characteristic is the "butterfly-shaped" rash that some individuals get on their nose and cheeks. The etiology of SLE is complicated and includes genetic susceptibility, environmental variables such exposure to sunlight, infections, hormone changes, and some drugs. The severity of the ailment varies greatly; some people have moderate symptoms, while others suffer from potentially fatal organ damage, especially to the cardiovascular system or kidneys (lupus nephritis). Immunosuppressive medications and corticosteroids are commonly used to manage SLE, reducing inflammation and enhancing quality of life through individualized treatment plans (Borchers et al., 2010).

3.3.3 Type 1 Diabetes

The immune system of the body mistakenly attacks and kills the beta cells in the pancreas that produce insulin in type 1 diabetes, a chronic autoimmune illness. An essential hormone that helps cells absorb glucose for energy synthesis, insulin controls blood sugar levels. When these beta cells are destroyed, little or no insulin is produced, which leads to hyperglycemia, or an accumulation of glucose in the blood. To keep glucose levels within a safe range, management entails lifetime insulin therapy, blood sugar monitoring, and careful meal planning. Early diagnosis and tailored care are crucial to preventing complications and enhancing quality of life (Belle et al., 2010).

3.3.4 Multiple Sclerosis (MS)

The immune system unintentionally targets the myelin sheath, the protective layer that envelops nerve fibres in the central nervous system (CNS), in multiple sclerosis (MS), a chronic autoimmune disease. Effective electrical signal transmission between the brain, spinal cord, and the rest of the body depends on myelin. Numerous neurological symptoms can result from a disruption in the brain-body communication caused by myelin breakdown. Fatigue, muscle weakness, issues with balance and coordination, tingling or numbness, blurred vision, and cognitive impairments are some of the symptoms, which can differ significantly from person to person. As scar tissue (sclerosis) develops in the afflicted areas over time, the damage may become irreparable, resulting in gradual impairment and irreversible nerve loss. Although the precise origin of multiple sclerosis is still unknown, environmental variables like viral infections or vitamin D insufficiency are thought to have a role in addition to genetic predisposition. Depending on how it develops, multiple sclerosis is usually divided into progressive and relapsing-remitting forms. Although there isn't a cure, medicines include corticosteroids, immunomodulatory therapy, and lifestyle changes try to control symptoms, prevent relapses, and delay the disease's course. For people with MS, better results and a higher quality of life depend on early diagnosis and individualized treatment (Goldenberg, 2012).

4. PRECISION MEDICINE

Precision medicine is reshaping the future of healthcare by shifting the focus from generalized treatment plans to highly personalized solutions tailored to individual patients. Precision medicine is personalized according to an individual's genetics, lifestyle and environmental exposures to provide more accurate diagnosis and much better health outcomes (Kopp et al., 2017). By integrating Artificial Intelligence (AI), evolving medical science is delivered with speed and efficiency in converting precision medicines into a very potent biomedical tool to manage the multifarious applications related to complicated diseases (Mesko, 2017)

Precision medicine, which is driven by AI, holds transformative potential to address this challenge. It promises better outcomes and lower healthcare costs because therapies would be given according to an individual's immune profile rather than the general population, thus paving the way for more effective and equitable healthcare systems across the world. Our current understanding of the immune system is continuously expanded by newer breakthroughs, which form how it operates to defend the body against infection (Marshall et al.,2018).

Precision medicine tailors treatments based on individual genetics, lifestyle, and environment for improved health outcomes. With AI integration, it enhances the speed and accuracy of diagnosing and managing complex diseases. This approach promises more effective, cost-efficient, and equitable healthcare by focusing on personalized immune profiles.

5. THE ROLE OF PRECISION MEDICINE IN IMMUNOLOGICAL DISORDERS

By determining the molecular, genetic, and immunological causes of illnesses, precision medicine aims to provide individualized and focused treatments. To categorize patients and forecast how they will react to treatments, it uses technologies including proteomics, genetics, and sophisticated imaging (Ashley, 2016).

5.1 Key Components of Precision Medicine

Precision medicine uses a range of cutting-edge technologies to customize care according to each patient's unique needs. Understanding the underlying disease mechanisms and tailoring interventions are critical in immunological disorders, where the immune system is malfunctioning and either attacking the body's own tissues (autoimmune diseases) or failing to mount adequate defences (immunodeficiencies). An extensive examination of these essential elements and how they relate to immunological illnesses is provided below (Ashley, 2016).

5.1.1 Biomarkers

Biomarkers are biological characteristics or molecules that can be tested to determine whether a disease is present, how it is progressing, or how well a treatment is working. Biomarkers are crucial for prognosis, early diagnosis, and tracking the effectiveness of treatment in immunological illnesses. Clinicians can customize therapy regimens for each patient by identifying particular biomarkers.

For example, in rheumatoid arthritis biomarkers such as rheumatoid factor (RF) and anti-citrullinated protein antibodies (ACPA) are used to track treatment response and forecast the severity of the disease. When choosing disease-modifying antirheumatic medications (DMARDs) or biologic therapy, elevated ACPA levels are frequently linked to more severe types of RA. Inflammatory indicators such as erythrocyte sedimentation rate (ESR) and C-reactive protein (CRP) are useful for evaluating disease activity and flare-ups (Atzeni et al., 2017). Another example is of Multiple Sclerosis. One important biomarker for multiple sclerosis (MS) is the presence of oligoclonal bands (OCBs) in cerebrospinal fluid (CSF), which show immunological activity in the central nervous system. Furthermore, a promising biomarker for tracking neurodegeneration and forecasting the course of disease is neurofilament light chain (NFL). In MS, biomarkers are especially crucial for identifying the best disease-modifying treatments (DMTs), such as natalizumab, fingolimod, or interferons (Housley et al., 2015)

5.1.2 Omics Technologies

“Omics” technologies involve the comprehensive study of molecules in the body—such as genes (genomics), proteins (proteomics), and RNA (transcriptomics)—to better understand the complexities of diseases, including immunological disorders (Schneider& Orchard, 2011).

5.1.2.1 Genomics

The study of a person's genome with an emphasis on locating genetic mutations, variances, and susceptibilities that lead to the development of disease is known as genomics. Genomic analysis in autoimmune disorders enables the identification of genetic polymorphisms and susceptibility genes that raise the risk of developing particular ailments. For example, variations in the HLA-DRB1 gene, which regulates the immune system, impact genetic risk in rheumatoid arthritis. Determining who may be at risk of getting RA through the identification of these genetic variants may result in earlier intervention or preventive measures (Song & Lin, 2017). Numerous loci linked to immune response modulation in SLE have also been identified by Genome-Wide Association Study (GWAS), including genes implicated in complement system regulation and type I interferon signalling. The creation of targeted treatments, such IFN or BAFF inhibitors, which are intended for patients with certain genetic profiles, is guided by these insights (Fernández et al., 2012).

5.1.2.2 Proteomics

The large-scale study of proteins, especially those implicated in signalling cascades and immunological responses, is known as proteomics. Protein microarrays and mass spectrometry are two proteomic technologies that are used to detect alterations in protein expression and function that take place in immunological disorders. Changes in immune response proteins, such as cytokines that contribute to inflammation, such as IL-17 and IL-23, can be detected by proteomics in multiple sclerosis. Clinicians can identify which patients are most likely to benefit from treatments that target these pathways by assessing these protein levels (Farias et al., 2014). In type I diabetes, proteomic research can detect alterations in beta-cell function or insulin secretion, which aids in tracking the course of the disease and assessing the efficacy of novel immunotherapies meant to maintain beta-cell function in T1D (Crèvecoeur et al., 2017).

5.1.2.3 Transcriptomics

In order to comprehend how genes are activated or silenced in response to disease, transcriptomics focuses on examining RNA expression. Researchers can learn more about how immune responses are activated and regulated in autoimmune illnesses by looking at the expression profiles of immune cells. Certain gene profiles linked to tissue damage, inflammation, and immune cell activation have been found through transcriptome analysis of synovial tissue in RA patients. Targeted treatments like JAK inhibitors and B-cell depletion treatments (like rituximab) are used in accordance with these gene expression profiles (Song & Lin, 2017). The identification of genes implicated in demyelination and neuroinflammation in multiple sclerosis is aided by transcriptome analysis of the brain and spinal cord. The development of treatments that alter the immune system's activity in the central nervous system is made possible by an understanding of the interactions between T cells, B cells, and microglia in multiple sclerosis (Goldenberg, 2012).

5.1.3 Artificial Intelligence

Large volumes of data produced by transcriptomics, proteomics, genomes, and clinical records are being analysed more and more using AI technology. Specifically, machine learning algorithms assist in identifying patterns in intricate datasets that human analysts would miss. AI has the potential to enhance immunological problem diagnosis, forecast disease progression, and customize therapy regimens. Clinical and biomarker data can be analyzed by AI algorithms to forecast which patients will react most well to particular treatments. AI, for instance, can assist in identifying patients who would benefit from biologics that target TNF, IL-6, or other immune pathways by examining gene expression data and inflammatory markers. Large volumes of data, including genetic, transcriptomic, and clinical data, can be processed by AI technologies to customize treatment plans and forecast illness flares. By finding hidden patterns in big datasets, AI can also help find new biomarkers for SLE (Rubinger et al., 2023).

Precision medicine in immunological disorders focuses on identifying molecular, genetic, and immune-related causes to offer personalized treatments. It leverages advanced tools like biomarkers, genomics, proteomics, and transcriptomics to understand disease mechanisms and tailor therapies. Biomarkers help track disease activity and treatment responses in conditions like rheumatoid arthritis and multiple sclerosis. Genomics uncovers genetic susceptibilities, guiding early interventions and targeted therapies. Proteomics and transcriptomics reveal protein and gene expression changes, aiding in diagnosis and treatment planning. Artificial Intelligence enhances precision medicine by analyzing complex datasets to predict disease progression, treatment responses, and discover new biomarkers.

6. IMPORTANCE OF AI

AI has completely changed the concept of diseases diagnosis and hospitals treatment in the modern world. This means that this technology is like how the human brains act; that is using computational techniques based on functions. These additions to many different possibilities in its applications-across even fields such as immunology, precision medicine, and health-care-all lead to some major changes. AI has-taken shape-for becoming one's reliable assistant in the healthcare sector; time is up to the point of blurring the line between a sea of data and some enlightening knowledge (Shaheen, 2021).

The creation of data in the medical sciences has increased exponentially over the past ten years because of developments in imaging, proteomics, genomics, and electronic health records. In terms of sheer amount and complexity, such data vastly surpasses human analytical capabilities, yet offering a richer understanding of disease causes and patient care. AI is, in this sense, a very important facilitator (Mann et al, 2021). Machine learning, natural language processing, and neural networks are the techniques whereby AI can speedily and accurately process vast amounts of data in original applications. The technology can also relate incomprehensibly disparate patterns and data that would have otherwise gone unnoticed (Rubinger et al., 2023). That is why AI represents a major transformation and enhances all parts of health care delivery, not just a tool.

Creating vaccines is yet another use of AI in immunology. Traditional vaccine development sometimes takes years and involves several costly procedures, including finding the correct antigens, testing them, and, of course, scaling up manufacture. AI was crucial in accelerating this process during the COVID-19 pandemic (Goh et al, 2020). The time required to generate and evaluate vaccine candidates was significantly decreased when machine learning models searched viral genomes for possible targets. In addition to infectious diseases, AI can create individualized cancer vaccines by tailoring them to the patient's tumor profile using neoantigen-based or immune checkpoint inhibitors (Olawade et al., 2024).

AI also plays a crucial role in achieving accurate diagnoses in modern healthcare. This is of much concern in immunology and many other areas. The outcomes are often worse than ideal due to most allergic diseases misdiagnosed as overlapping or vague symptoms. AI- however, drives the changes with its diagnostic technologies that yield biomarkers and interpret images. Most biomarkers, analysed by AI systems on patients, can detect early signs of illnesses like multiple sclerosis or inflammatory bowel disease, whereas provided deep learning models trained on medical images can detect tiny abnormalities in tissues or organs that may indicate malfunctioning immune systems (Zhao et al., 2021).

Patient data tends to be very dismembered, such as genomic data kept in research labs, clinical data in hospitals, and lifestyle data in wearable technologies in the instance of the healthcare sector. AI systems can bridge the gap from that using multiple sources of information to yield useful insights. For example, an AI interface could connect immune cell profiles, genomic sequencing information, and details of the patient's lifestyle in immunological research to identify novel disease mechanisms or treatment targets. This type of integrative effort supplements fundamental knowledge of the immune system with the possibility for therapies that are much more precise and effective (Mohammed et al., 2024).

Another instance in which immunology, AI, and precision medicine converge is drug discovery. AI will manage all of this in a new way by predicting effects of drugs and identifying promising drug candidates with unprecedented levels of accuracy (Nayarisseri et al., 2021). Platforms powered by AI are now being harnessed in immunology to screen putative compounds that alter immune responses, including immune stimulants targeting cancer immunotherapy or small-molecule inhibitors for autoimmune diseases. AI hastens the process of drug discovery, reduces failure rates, and is involved in the efficient commercialization of such novel therapies. (Boniolo et al., 2021)

The application of AI in healthcare, however, is not without challenges. Primarily, the ethical implications of AI should be considered in sensitive areas such as immunology and precision medicine. The security and privacy of data will take more emphasis as use of patient data information wrongly may result in grave repercussions. Another urgent issue is the impartiality of AI driven medical innovations, with the risk of widening already existing gaps due to unequal access to advanced technologies. The interpretability of AI models is a major challenge that remains-they should be understandable and trusted by clinicians so that the recommendations given by AI-related systems could be adequately actualized in patient care (Zhao et al., 2021).

Advancement in algorithms of machine learning along with improved processing capacities and ways of obtaining data push forward the boundaries of feasibility. It seems that AI will continue to advance and integrate itself more into the understanding, prevention, and treatment of disease (Mohammed et al., 2024).

AI is revolutionizing healthcare by enabling faster, more accurate disease diagnosis, personalized treatment, and accelerated drug and vaccine development. It processes massive, complex medical data from genomics, imaging, and health records, uncovering patterns beyond human ability. In immunology, AI aids in detecting early biomarkers, designing individualized cancer vaccines, and discovering new treatments. It integrates fragmented patient data to deliver precise insights, advancing precision medicine. However, challenges like data privacy, bias, and model interpretability must be addressed. With ongoing advancements, AI will continue to transform disease understanding, prevention, and care.

7. APPLICATIONS OF AI IN IMMUNOLOGICAL DISORDERS

An innovative method for identifying, treating, and managing illnesses is the use of artificial intelligence (AI) in immunological disorders. From autoimmune diseases to immunodeficiencies, immunological disorders are complicated ailments impacted by lifestyle, environmental, and hereditary variables. The complexities of these disorders are frequently not adequately addressed by traditional approaches, which results in gaps in long-term care, individualized treatment, and early detection. AI provides a suitable answers to these problems because of its capacity to handle and evaluate enormous quantities (Chaplin, 2010)

With AI technologies like machine learning, natural language processing, and predictive analytics, precision medicine can be applied to immune illnesses more successfully. This section goes into additional detail about particular uses of AI in illness management, individualized treatment, and personalized diagnostics for various complicated disorders (Lu et al., 2024).

7.1 Personalised Diagnostics

Since each patient is unique, many diseases necessitate personalized therapies tailored to individual needs. This can range from simple recommendations, such as selecting the most suitable multivitamins for those with weakened immunity, to more complex decisions involving the specific types and dosages of medications required for acute conditions (Kyrarini et al., 2021). Personalized diagnosis has the most potential applications of AI in immunological disorders. The care of immune-related disorders greatly depends on early and correct diagnosis; however, conventional diagnostic techniques may not be able to identify subtle patterns or combine various data sources. These constraints are addressed by AI-driven systems that provide extensive genomic and proteomic analysis and biomarker development (Pandya et al., 2021)

7.2 AI-Powered Biomarker Discovery

For the diagnosis and tracking of immunological diseases, biomarkers are essential. A trait that can be tested and assessed objectively as a sign of pathogenic processes, normal biological processes, or pharmacologic reactions to a therapeutic intervention is called a biomarker (Willis & Lord, 2015). Large-scale datasets can be analysed by AI technology, particularly machine learning algorithms, to find new biomarkers. AI-driven biomarker discovery enhances overall patient outcomes by facilitating the development of targeted medicines and increasing diagnostic accuracy (Willis & Lord, 2015).

7.2.1 Data Pattern Recognition

AI systems can analyse omics data (transcriptomics, proteomics, and genomes) and find patterns that are associated with particular illnesses. AI finds genes that are upregulated or downregulated in response to immunological diseases by analysing RNA expression patterns. For instance, AI techniques have found biomarkers that distinguish between active and remission states in autoimmune diseases like systemic lupus erythematosus (SLE) (Yu et al., 2021). In order to identify illness-specific proteins; it also detects post-translational changes and patterns of protein expression linked to disease states. AI searches genomic data for mutations, SNPs, or structural differences that have been linked to disease development or susceptibility. To identify patterns that are predictive of illness, AI systems employ both supervised and unsupervised learning. While unsupervised learning uses clustering approaches to identify patient subgroups based on biomarker profiles and so provide insights into disease heterogeneity, supervised learning models, for instance, are trained using labelled datasets to predict the stages of illness in new data (Dougherty, 2012).

7.2.2 Integration of Diverse Data

Genetic, environmental, and cellular factors all play important roles in immunological disorders, which are complex. To provide a complete view of disease causes, AI integrates data from multiple sources, including immune cell profiles, genetic sequences, and patient histories. In complicated diseases like rheumatoid arthritis, where several factors contribute to the beginning of the disease, this method is especially helpful. AI models use data from single-cell RNA sequencing or flow cytometry to infer which immune cell subsets are involved in a disease. For instance, identifying the T-cell subtypes responsible for rheumatoid arthritis inflammation. By examining DNA sequences, it can also detect genetic predispositions, such as HLA variations connected to autoimmune disorders. Relevant data is extracted from electronic health records by NLP algorithms. For a more individualized approach, this data is combined with molecular information (Zandonà, 2017).

7.3 Using Proteomic and Genetic Profiling to Make Accurate Diagnosis

The molecular etiology of immunological disorders can be identified with the help of genetic and proteomics profiling, which provides a profound understanding of the pathophysiology, etiology, and ultimately management of the disease. The diagnostic power of these profiling techniques has increased with the use of AI. Large dataset analysis, the identification of minute patterns, and the extraction of significant insights that would be challenging or impossible to achieve with conventional methods are all areas in which artificial intelligence excels. AI systems may quickly identify mutations or polymorphisms linked to diseases like Crohn's disease or Severe Combined Immunodeficiency (SCID) via genetic profiling.AI helps with risk assessment and early diagnosis, which enables prompt intervention and individualized treatment. Similarly, AI-powered proteome profiling offers unmatched insights into the intricate patterns of protein expression resulting from immunological dysfunctions. For example, in MS, AI-based proteome analysis has helped clinicians create effective treatment strategies by identifying particular protein markers that differentiate between the progressive and relapsing-remitting phases of the disease. When AI is integrated with these profiling technologies, it not only improves diagnosis accuracy but also gives doctors useful information that guarantees more efficient and individualized patient care. A new era in precision medicine is being ushered in by the convergence of AI, proteomics, and genomes, where the management of immunological illnesses will increasingly rely on early detection, precise diagnosis, and tailored treatment protocols. Clinicians can now obtain a level of diagnostic accuracy that was previously unattainable with AI-powered genomic and proteomic analysis, enabling more effective treatment (Gebretsadik& Menon, 2016).

AI is transforming the diagnosis and treatment of immunological disorders by enabling personalized diagnostics, biomarker discovery, and data integration. It analyses large-scale omics data to detect disease-specific patterns, identify immune cell roles, and predict genetic susceptibilities. AI-driven proteomic and genomic profiling enhances early and accurate diagnoses, helping tailor treatments for conditions like SLE, MS, and SCID. This convergence of AI with precision medicine leads to more individualized, effective care.

8. PERSONALIZED TREATMENT

AI is revolutionizing immunological disease therapy by enabling the identification of suitable treatments and tracking their efficacy. AI-driven treatment personalization enables therapies to be tailored for specific patients, in contrast to traditional methods where the process is primarily dependent on trial and error (Cohen et al., 2021).

8.1 AI-Powered Treatment Selection

Selecting the right treatment for an immunological problem is a difficult procedure because it varies depending on the disease's nature, severity, and patient-specific traits. AI makes this procedure easier by:

8.1.1 Predicting Treatment Reactions

Machine learning algorithms examine patient information to forecast how people will react to particular treatments. AI methods have been used, for instance, to forecast the efficacy of biologics such as TNF inhibitors in psoriasis, assisting doctors in selecting the best course of action (Cohen et al., 2021).

8.1.2 Proposals for Combination Therapies

AI algorithms can identify synergistic medicine combinations that have the least amount of side effects and the greatest therapeutic efficacy. In situations like inflammatory bowel illnesses, where a combination therapy must be used, it is extremely helpful. A patient is treated with a drug or combination of medications that have the highest efficacy and the fewest side effects when AI-guided therapy selection is used (Cohen et al., 2021).

8.2. Monitoring Treatment Effectiveness and Side Effects

After beginning a treatment, ongoing monitoring is necessary to ensure its efficacy and control any side effects. The following are some ways that AI improves this aspect of care: Real-time biomarker monitoring: wearables and AI-enabled devices monitor biomarkers like cytokine levels and offer data on the efficacy of the treatment. Changes in inflammatory markers, for example, can reveal whether a patient is responding to treatment for rheumatoid arthritis.AI models analyse patient data to identify any possible side effects that are likely to occur and to take action before they get worse. Immunosuppressive treatments, which increase the risk of infection, benefit greatly from this. AI facilitates early treatments and real-time monitoring, which improves patient safety and optimal treatment outcomes (Cohen et al., 2021).

8.3 Management of Disease and Prognosis

In addition to treating symptoms, effective management of immunological disorders necessitates long-term patient health maintenance and the ability to forecast how the disease will progress. AI tools are essential in this area of treatment because they offer prognostic and patient management solutions (Cohen et al., 2021).

8.3.1 AI-Powered Patient Management Tools

AI-powered solutions provide better management of immunological illnesses for patients and physicians. AI-powered systems use patient information, such as comorbidities, lifestyle, and illness history, to generate personalized care plans. AI systems, for example, can recommend asthma treatments that are specifically designed to reduce flare-ups. AI-powered telemedicine systems enable patients with long-term immunological disorders to be continuously monitored. To guarantee prompt treatments, wearable technology and smartphone apps monitor symptoms and drug compliance. Particularly for patients with chronic conditions, these developments improve patient involvement and reduce the strain on the healthcare system (Cohen et al., 2021).

8.3.2. Observation and Prediction of Disease Development

Appropriate preventative therapy can be ensured by accurately predicting how an immune problem may develop over time. By analysing longitudinal data to identify likely illness trajectories, AI in particular leads this field. Using past patient data, machine learning algorithms forecast the course of a disease. For example, AI models have been created to forecast relapses in multiple sclerosis, allowing clinicians to modify treatment as necessary. By identifying patients who are most likely to experience issues, AI techniques allow for more focused therapies. AI-driven risk assessment, for instance, can reduce kidney damage in lupus nephritis by suggesting early treatment modifications. AI will assist long-term outcome data for improved planning and resource use, which will ultimately improve immunological diseased patient's quality of life (Cohen et al., 2021).

9. AI TECHNOLOGIES

9.1 Machine Learning

Machine Learning (ML) is the field of artificial intelligence that develops systems which can learn from the data and then progressively become more proficient in their tasks without human intervention. ML algorithms are employed to recognize the patterns, predict results, and extract information from diverse points of data. ML's strength to the physical engine of health care and enabling areas, for example, precision medicine developed which enables machines to think and learn from data and thus become smart. Machine learning is revolutionizing immunology by enabling data-driven insights for disease diagnosis, treatment, and patient management. ML models analyse vast immunological datasets to identify patterns, with high-quality data enhancing their performance. Feature extraction helps isolate key biomarkers and immune responses for model training, where historical data allows algorithms to learn and predict new cases. Through iterative optimization, models continuously improve by integrating new information. Supervised learning, used in disease diagnosis and risk prediction, employs methods like linear regression, SVM, and decision trees. Unsupervised learning uncovers hidden patterns in patient data, aiding in segmentation and anomaly detection through clustering (e.g., k-means) and dimensionality reduction (e.g., PCA). Reinforcement learning optimizes personalized treatment plans and robotic surgeries by learning through trial and error, using techniques like Q-learning and deep Q-networks. These ML approaches significantly enhance precision medicine in immunology, leading to more accurate diagnoses and tailored therapies (Jordan & Mitchell, 2015; Mahesh, 2020).

9.2 Deep Learning

Computers can learn from experience and comprehend the world in terms of a hierarchy of concepts thanks to deep learning, a type of machine learning.

A human computer operator does not need to explicitly explain all of the knowledge required by the computer because the computer learns from experience. By constructing more complex ideas from simpler ones, the hierarchy of concepts enables the computer to learn them; a graph of these hierarchies would have many layers.

Deep learning, through artificial neural networks, plays a transformative role in immunology by analysing complex biological data for disease prediction and treatment optimization. These networks consist of an input layer that processes raw immunological data, hidden layers that extract patterns using activation functions, and an output layer that provides diagnostic or predictive outcomes. The learning process involves forward propagation, where data moves through the network to generate predictions, and backward propagation, where adjustments are made using optimization techniques like stochastic gradient descent to improve accuracy. This iterative refinement enhances the identification of biomarkers, immune responses, and potential therapeutic targets, advancing precision medicine in immunology (Bengio et al., 2017).

9.3 Natural Language Processing

The study of how computers can comprehend and modify natural language speech or text to accomplish beneficial tasks is known as natural language processing, or NLP. The goal of NLP research is to learn more about how people comprehend and use language in order to create the necessary instruments and methods for computer systems to comprehend and work with natural languages to accomplish the intended tasks. Numerous fields, including computer and information sciences, linguistics, mathematics, electrical and electronic engineering, artificial intelligence and robotics, psychology, etc., provide the basis of NLP. Numerous academic domains, including machine translation, natural language text processing and summarization, user interfaces, multilingual technology, and cross language information retrieval (CLIR), speech recognition, artificial intelligence and expert systems, and so on (Bardhan et al., 2017). NLP integrates linguistic and computational components to enable machines to interpret human language, playing a crucial role in immunological research. Syntax analysis helps identify patterns in medical texts by understanding grammatical structures, while semantics aids in extracting meaningful insights from research papers and clinical data. Pragmatics further refines this by considering context, tone, and intent, enhancing the accuracy of AI-driven analysis. Morphology contributes by breaking down complex biomedical terms into their roots and affixes, improving data interpretation. Additionally, phonology and phonetics support spoken-language processing for voice-assisted diagnostics and patient interactions. Together, these NLP components streamline immunological research, aiding in biomarker discovery, literature review, and clinical decision-making (Bardhan et al., 2017).

9.4 Predictive Analytics

Using clinical and/or nonclinical patterns in the data, healthcare predictive analytics seeks to forecast future health-related occurrences or outcomes. Deep learning applications in pharmaceutical research have surfaced recently and have demonstrated promise in addressing a variety of drug discovery issues by looking at the patient's medical history and using information from tests and symptoms to give the patient the best care possible. In healthcare predictive analytics, study results including medical problems, hospital readmissions (Bardhan et al., 2015), therapy responses, and patient mortality are frequently very useful. The first step in creating a healthcare predictive model is gathering patient data through clinical trials using a set of predetermined protocols (Muniasamy et al., 2020). The UK Prospective Diabetes Study (UKPDS) (Stevens et al., 2001), the Framingham Heart Study (D'Agostino et al., 2008), and the Lung Cancer Risk Prediction Model (Tammemägi et al, 2013) are few of its examples. The second is the utilization of pre-existing patient data gathered in clinical settings, including clinical registries, insurance claims, and electronic health records. Predictive models are still rarely used in clinical practice, despite the fact that healthcare predictive analytics can help guide clinical decisions (Moons et al., 2009). The adoption of EHR systems reduced the obstacles to the application of predictive models in healthcare, include the necessity to modify the models from the research population for the local population, the requirement for data that are costly to acquire or not immediately available, and the lack of integration with the current clinical process (Muniasamy et al., 2020).

9.5 Digital Twin

A Digital Twin (DT) is a virtual version of a real-world entity that is dynamic and self-evolving. It is distinguished by bi-directional connectivity that enables real-time data sharing between digital and physical counterparts (Singh et al., 2021). A virtual depiction of a real-world system, process, or physical object that is updated in real-time with data is called a "digital twin." To create a dynamic model, it integrates technologies like IoT, AI, ML, and advanced analytics. Organizations may anticipate possible problems, model situations for improved decision-making, and monitor, analyse, and optimize performance with the help of digital twins. In the fields of manufacturing, healthcare, and urban planning, it is frequently employed to enhance operational effectiveness, predictive maintenance, and innovation by bridging the gap between the digital and physical worlds (Erol et al., 2020).

10. APPLICATIONS OF AI TECHNOLOGIES IN PRECISION AND PERSONALIZED MEDICINE

Artificial Intelligence (AI) is playing a transformative role in the diagnosis and treatment of immunological disorders by enabling more accurate predictions, early diagnoses, and tailored treatment strategies. One significant development is EXPRESSO (Expression Prediction with Summary Statistics Only), an AI algorithm developed by Penn State College of Medicine. EXPRESSO uses single-cell expression data, 3D genomics, and epigenetic information to predict autoimmune disease risk by modelling gene expression patterns and regulation. It has demonstrated improved performance in identifying gene-trait associations for diseases like lupus, rheumatoid arthritis, Crohn's disease, and ulcerative colitis, surpassing existing models by over 25% in accuracy. Another promising tool is Capillary.io, an AI-powered medical software designed to assist in the diagnosis of autoimmune diseases such as systemic sclerosis through nailfold capillaroscopy. This tool uses AI algorithms to automatically detect, classify, and measure nailfold capillaries—features that can be indicative of autoimmune pathologies. By providing quantitative, objective data and reducing observer variability, Capillary.io enhances the diagnostic workflow for clinicians and supports more timely interventions. In the area of biomarker discovery, machine learning models have been developed to analyse microRNA (miRNA) sequences as potential biomarkers for autoimmune diseases. These models fragment and interpret miRNA sequences using computational approaches to identify distinct patterns associated with disease states. This not only supports early detection but also enhances the understanding of disease mechanisms at the molecular level. Additionally, capsule neural networks have been applied in autoimmune disease diagnosis. Unlike traditional convolutional neural networks, capsule networks can better preserve spatial hierarchies and relationships within data, making them more suitable for analysing complex medical patterns. Their application in autoimmune disease diagnostics has shown promise in improving classification accuracy and interpretability in imaging-based diagnostic tasks (Maurya et al, 2022). Collectively, these AI tools represent a leap forward in precision medicine for immunological disorders, offering clinicians powerful new resources for more accurate, faster, and personalized care. As these technologies continue to evolve, their integration into clinical practice will likely become increasingly vital in managing complex immune-related diseases.

10.1 Pattern Recognition and Data Analysis

Machine learning algorithms are particularly good at finding patterns in the high-dimensional world of imaging data, molecular profiles, and medical records. Immunology uses machine learning to group patients into subgroups that need different treatment modalities. For instance, in autoimmune diseases like lupus or rheumatoid arthritis, ML models may detect subtle changes in biomarker expression. This aids in early diagnosis and patient classification according on the severity of the condition. In cancer immunotherapy, doctors can tailor immune checkpoint inhibitors and other treatments by using DL models that predict tumor microenvironment traits based on histopathology images (Mahajan, 2016).

10.2 Interpretation of Genomic Data

In precision medicine, genomic data is now extremely important since it can provide information about a person's vulnerability to diseases and potential treatment options. Genomic analysis has been revolutionized by ML and DL algorithms, which process and interpret massive sequencing data with previously unheard-of accuracy. ML techniques detect genetic variations and mutations linked to immunological illnesses, including autoimmune diseases and primary immunodeficiencies. Deep learning models help researchers find novel medication targets and treatment approaches by predicting the functional impact of genetic variants. AI-powered tools such as DeepVariant and AlphaFold, for example, have significantly advanced the domains of protein structure prediction and genomics, speeding up immunological research and other areas (Prabhod, 2022).

10.3 Biomarkers and Protocols for Treatment Exploration of Literature

The rapid pace of scientific research has led to an overwhelming volume of literature, making it difficult for researchers and physicians to stay up to date. NLP algorithms simplify this challenge by efficiently searching and analysing literature to identify biomarkers relevant to clinical guidelines and treatment protocols, ensuring that medical professionals have access to the most pertinent and up-to-date information. In published research of cytokines, chemokines, and other immune regulators, for example, NLP algorithms can look for potential targets for immunological illnesses (Trugenberger et al., 2013). NLP-based tools, such PubMedBERT and SciBERT, are designed especially for biomedical text analysis, revealing medication, illness, and gene connections. By combining information from many sources, NLP improves precision medicine decision-making and ensures that patients receive the most efficient and evidence-based care (Sivarethinamohan et al., 2021).

10.4 Evaluation of Disease Risk

The genetic, environmental, and behavioural aspects that make a person more susceptible to particular diseases will be examined by the AI-driven predictive models. For instance:

ML prediction algorithms forecast the likelihood of emergence of type 1 diabetes based on genetic predisposition and autoantibody patterns (Zafar et al., 2019). Predictive analytics models in cancer immunology provide proactive care by predicting the likelihood of immune-related adverse events based on patient-specific parameters. The patient is empowered to take preventive actions according to their unique risk profile which also enable early treatments (Choudhury & Eksioglu, 2019).

10.5 Suggestions for Tailored Treatment

AI-driven predictive analytics enables precision medicine, which thrives on customizing therapies for each patient. AI models anticipate how patients would react to various medications in autoimmune disorders like multiple sclerosis, assisting clinicians in selecting the best options (Oluwasey, 2024). Predictive algorithms analyse the dynamics of viral loads and recommend the best antiretroviral treatments for infectious disorders like HIV/AIDS. AI decreases trial-and-error prescribing, increasing efficacy and reducing negative effects by matching medicines with expected results (Belciug, 2020).

10.6 Repurposing Drugs for Immunological Conditions

AI algorithms evaluate clinical and molecular data to find previously undiscovered therapeutic potentials of licensed medications. Using machine learning algorithms, it has been shown that JAK inhibitors, which were first created to treat cancer, can also effectively treat autoimmune illnesses like ulcerative colitis and rheumatoid arthritis (Valencic et al., 2018). AI-driven drug repurposing initiatives during COVID-19 pandemic found promising options for treating severe patients, including remdesivir and dexamethasone. Medication repurposing lowers the expenses and dangers related to conventional medication development while simultaneously hastening the availability of therapies (Zhou et al., 2020).

10.7. Quickening Clinical Experiments

Clinical trials are crucial for validating new treatments, but they are frequently postponed because of issues with data processing, protocol design, and patient recruitment. AI addresses these issues byUsing NLP-driven analysis of electronic health records to identify qualified participants. Developing methods for adaptive trials that maximize the use of resources and enhance the retention of participants. Real-time analysis of trial data to spot trends and make evidence-based changes. These developments ensure that patients receive life-saving treatments more quickly by increasing the effectiveness of clinical trials (Väänänen et al., 2018).

10.8. Virtual Patient Models and Digital Twins

A sophisticated use of AI in precision medicine is the creation of digital twins, which are virtual representations of biological systems or patient models. Without presenting a risk or being an ineffective platform for testing, these models simulate physiological processes, illness progression, and therapy response (Moingeon, 2023). Digital twins offer a special chance for the in-silico simulation of intricate immune responses in immunology. These models mimic an individual's immune system by integrating information from immunological assays, proteomics, and genomics. This allows researchers to predict how the immune system will react to particular pathogens or vaccines and to model the effects of immunotherapies, like CAR-T cells or monoclonal antibodies, before delivering them to patients. These simulations help us better understand immunological dynamics and guide the creation of individualized treatment plans (Moingeon et al., 2023).

10.9. Predicting Treatment Outcomes

Clinicians can forecast possible outcomes of different treatment approaches using virtual patient models without endangering patients with needless side effects. For example, in cancer immunotherapy, digital twins help physicians choose the optimum regimen by forecasting the likelihood of tumor regression or immune-related side effects. Accurate dosing is made possible by virtual models that mimic how immunosuppressive medications affect the course of autoimmune disorders. By offering a virtual testing ground, digital twins help clinical decision-makers reduce uncertainty and variability while providing the best treatment possible for patients (Moingeon et al., 2023).

AI technologies are transforming precision and personalized medicine by enabling early diagnosis, tailored treatments, and risk prediction in immunological disorders. Tools like EXPRESSO and Capillary.io improve disease detection and analysis, while machine learning enhances biomarker discovery and genomic interpretation. NLP helps extract relevant insights from vast biomedical literature, supporting evidence-based care. AI also facilitates drug repurposing, accelerates clinical trials, and powers virtual patient models for predicting treatment outcomes. These advancements collectively enable more accurate, efficient, and personalized healthcare solutions.

11. ETHICAL, REGULATORY, AND PRACTICAL CONSIDERATIONS

There is enormous potential for integrating AI with healthcare, particularly in the treatment of immunological illnesses. The advantages must be balanced against the significant practical, ethical, and legal obstacles that come with putting it into practice. Resolving these issues will support patient rights, public trust, and the safe, equitable, and efficient deployment of technology (Kasula, 2021). The use of AI/ML technologies in healthcare poses complex regulatory issues, especially when it comes to approval procedures and the frameworks that must be adhered to in order to guarantee safety, effectiveness, and ethical concerns. Among the main regulatory challenges are:

11.1 FDA Approval

As a Software as a Medical Device (SaMD), AI/ML-based software must adhere to strict FDA guidelines to guarantee that it fulfils an authorized medical function, such as illness prevention, diagnosis, or therapy. Clear definitions of the patient population, target users, and evidence of a legitimate clinical relationship through clinical and analytical validation are necessary for SaMD market applications (McHugh, 2015)

11.2 Development Frameworks

Good Medical Practice ought to be transparent, human-centred, and subject to critical evaluation. Before Real World Performance (RWP) is widely used, clinical trials are advised to guarantee its efficacy and dependability (He et al., 2019).

11.3 Explainability and Reproducibility

AI models must be trustworthy and comprehensible. However, performance in different clinical situations may not be consistent since limited or isolated datasets sometimes do not permit reproducibility. Only when used in practical situations might some of the interpretability risks become evident (McCradden et al., 2020).

11.4 Accessibility and Data Privacy

Because AI systems rely on enormous data sets that are frequently kept on cloud platforms, they are vulnerable to security breaches. Unauthorized access could put people at risk for genetic predisposition-based discrimination in the workplace, insurance industry, and other domains. Accessing aggregated, high-quality datasets across health systems is difficult, even though patient privacy and confidentiality over health information are maintained. As a result, there are fewer reliable AI models available for validation and training (MacMath et al., 2023).

11.5 Legal and Ethical Risks

Adoption of AI/ML technologies may be limited by the huge profit potential and related hazards, which raise legal issues for healthcare systems and providers (McGreevey et al., 2020)

11.6 Autonomy

The concept of autonomy about the collection and usage of data is one of its major challenges, particularly if put in the perspective of AI and big data (BD). While informed consent marks a cornerstone of ethical health research, the open nature of BD complicates ideal concepts (Parker et al., 2018). Large datasets usually have to be analysed various times by different parties which are hard to predict their output or reverse the learned procedures by the AI after being trained. For maintaining autonomy, it is necessary to provide fully informed consent from the participants of the study, that which way their data is used including storage, analysis, access, and right of withdrawing consent. Confidentiality also raises ethical concerns for genetic and personal data due to the impossibility of ensuring anonymity through anonymization techniques. Misuse of the health-related data by the third parties like insurance companies requires proper legislation. Data users are responsible for maintaining autonomy standards, even if this means slowing discovery, so that consent is meaningful and ethically sound (Parker et al., 2018).

11.7 Public Engagement

The necessity for end users as well as professionals to be involved in the design and execution of AI-driven immunotherapies is highlighted by ethical concerns about public participation with these treatments. For the ensuing therapeutics—such as vaccines, gene therapies, or medications—to be socially, commercially, and environmentally acceptable, AI models that uncover new immune system interactions must be thoroughly evaluated and openly shared. Big data's dynamic and ever-evolving nature makes stakeholder interaction more difficult, necessitating flexible and adaptive strategies as opposed to strict, standard procedures. In order to handle changing duties and guarantee the moral acceptance of scaled-up therapies, stakeholders must be continuously consulted (Singh et al., 2024)

11.8 Equity and Managing Biases

The necessity to encourage diversity and inclusion in the creation of data and models is highlighted by ethical considerations in controlling inequities and biases in AI-driven immunotherapies (Beaulieu & Leonelli, 2021). Because the technology needed for this type of study is typically only available in resource-rich environments, immunological biodiversity, which is dominated by "omics" research, is susceptible to exclusivity and runs the risk of excluding marginalized populations. A diversified population will not be able to benefit from the resulting molecular models and treatments. Furthermore, social and environmental elements that are frequently absent from omics-based datasets have an impact on immunity. Analytical techniques must validate models in pertinent socio-ecological contexts and consider all immunoregulation elements in order for the results to be fair. To maintain the concepts of efficacy and safety, AI should support experimental methods rather than replace those (Johnson et al., 2021).

11.9 Protection of Vulnerable Populations

In order to guarantee equal opportunity access by concentrating on the conditions that disproportionately affect the target community and providing treatment that is sensitive to their needs and values, ethical considerations for the protection of vulnerable populations emphasize the critical application of AI-driven analytics. More protection is required in other areas, such as consent or exploitation for vulnerable populations, which include children, pregnant women, the elderly, and those from low-income backgrounds, among others. Furthermore, potential data misuse within the context of big data (BD) may expose these groups to further hazards. While addressing the more general ethical issues of equity, consent, and justice, AI and bioinformatics technologies should be ethically developed and applied to identify and safeguard vulnerable populations without adding to existing burdens (Cullen & Gracia, 2021).

12. LIMITATIONS AND CHALLENGES OF AI IN PRECISION MEDICINE

12.1 Data-Related Challenges

A foundational requirement for AI in precision medicine is access to large, high-quality, and well-annotated datasets. However, medical data is often fragmented, inconsistent, and highly heterogeneous. It originates from various sources such as electronic medical records (EMRs), genomic sequencing, proteomics, medical imaging, laboratory results, and wearable health devices. These sources vary in format, resolution, and structure, which pose significant challenges in data integration and standardization. AI models thrive on uniform, clean data, but real-world healthcare data is noisy, incomplete, and sometimes outdated, all of which can lead to poor model performance. Moreover, a substantial portion of available data is unstructured (e.g., physician notes, discharge summaries), requiring advanced natural language processing techniques, which are still imperfect in the medical domain (Prabhod, 2022).

In addition, precision medicine often targets highly specific patient subgroups based on genetic, environmental, or lifestyle factors. This makes it difficult to gather sufficiently large datasets for each subgroup, particularly for rare diseases. As a result, many AI models suffer from data scarcity and class imbalance, which can bias outcomes and decrease their clinical utility. Another key issue is the integration of "multi-omics" data—such as genomics, transcriptomics, proteomics, and metabolomics. While combining these layers could significantly enhance personalized treatment strategies, doing so is computationally challenging and biologically complex, as each omics layer operates on different scales and is governed by different principles (Zhao et al, 2021).

12.2. Technical and Model-Related Limitations

From a technological standpoint, one of the most pressing limitations is the "black box" nature of many AI algorithms, especially deep learning models. While these models can detect subtle patterns in complex data, they often do so without offering interpretable explanations for their decisions. This lack of transparency makes it difficult for clinicians to validate and trust the outputs, which is critical in life-altering medical decisions. Clinicians are trained to rely on evidence-based medicine, and without a clear rationale for AI-generated recommendations, their confidence in these tools remains limited (Rubinger et al, 2023).

Another concern is overfitting, where a model performs exceptionally well on the training dataset but poorly on new, unseen data. This occurs especially when datasets are small or biased, leading to poor generalizability in clinical environments. Additionally, medical knowledge is not static—new treatment protocols, disease variants, and patient behaviour's emerge over time. AI models trained on historical data may become outdated, a phenomenon known as model drift. These models need frequent updates and retraining to stay relevant, but continual updating is resource-intensive and rarely implemented effectively in healthcare settings (Shaheen, 2021).

12.3. Clinical and Operational Challenges

Even if a model performs well in a controlled setting, integrating it into real-world clinical workflows is far from straightforward. Hospitals and clinics have deeply entrenched systems, and any new technology must fit seamlessly within existing workflows to be useful. Many AI tools require additional steps like data input, interpretation, and confirmation, which may increase the workload on healthcare providers rather than reduce it. Furthermore, the time-critical nature of many medical decisions means that AI tools must deliver results quickly and reliablya benchmark that many current models fail to meet in live settings (Nayarisseri et al, 2021).

Another challenge lies in the gap between disciplines. Most AI models in precision medicine are developed by data scientists and engineers who may lack deep understanding of clinical workflows, patient variability, and the biology of diseases. Conversely, clinicians may not have the technical background to understand how AI systems work or how to interpret model outputs. This disconnect can result in poor communication, unrealistic expectations, or misuse of AI tools in clinical practice. Successful deployment of AI in precision medicine requires strong interdisciplinary collaboration, which remains a work in progress (Parker et al, 2018).

12.4. Infrastructure and Economic Barriers

Deploying AI systems in clinical practice requires substantial investment in computational infrastructure, data storage, cybersecurity, and skilled personnel. Many hospitals, especially in low- and middle-income countries, lack the digital infrastructure needed to run advanced AI models. High-throughput sequencing data and other omics datasets are massive and computationally demanding to process. Smaller institutions may not have access to the necessary GPU-based hardware or cloud-based platforms, making them unable to benefit from state-of-the-art AI tools. Moreover, the financial burden of developing, testing, validating, and maintaining AI systems is high. These costs often fall outside the scope of traditional healthcare budgets, limiting the scalability of AI solutions. Maintenance is particularly critical—AI systems must be regularly updated to incorporate new medical knowledge and adjust to shifting patient demographics and disease patterns. Without ongoing funding and technical support, AI tools risk becoming obsolete shortly after deployment (Nayarisseri et al, 2021).

12.5. Generalization and Reproducibility Issues

One of the final but equally critical challenges is ensuring that AI models are generalizable and reproducible. A model trained on data from one hospital or region may not perform as well in another due to differences in population demographics, clinical practices, equipment, and even environmental factors. For instance, a skin cancer detection model trained on fair-skinned populations might perform poorly on darker-skinned individuals. These biases are deeply embedded in the data and often go unnoticed until deployment. Reproducibility is another concern. Many AI research studies lack transparency in data usage, preprocessing steps, and model parameters, making it difficult for other researchers to replicate or build upon the findings. This limits scientific progress and delays clinical translation. There is a growing movement toward open science and reproducibility in AI, but consistent standards and regulations are still lacking, especially in the medical domain (Parker et al, 2018).

13.CONCLUSION

AI-driven precision medicine is transforming the diagnosis, treatment, and management of immunological disorders, paving the way for a more personalized healthcare approach. By leveraging AI's ability to analyse vast and complex biological data, medicine is shifting from generalized treatments to customized solutions that can significantly improve patient outcomes. AI-powered diagnostic tools, tailored therapies, and advanced disease management systems are redefining immunology, offering unprecedented accuracy and efficiency. However, to fully harness this technology, addressing ethical concerns, ensuring equitable access, and enhancing AI interpretability are crucial. As we step into the future, AI-driven precision medicine holds immense potential to revolutionize immunology, making healthcare more effective, accessible, and personalized than ever before.

REFERENCES

Atzeni, F., Talotta, R., Masala, I. F., Bongiovanni, S., Boccassini, L., & Sarzi-Puttini, P. (2017). Biomarkers in rheumatoid arthritis. *The Israel Medical Association Journal, 19*(8), 512–516. PMID: 28825772

Bardhan, I., Oh, J. H., Zheng, Z., & Kirksey, K. (2015). Predictive analytics for readmission of patients with congestive heart failure. *Information Systems Research, 26*(1), 19–39. DOI: 10.1287/isre.2014.0553

Beaulieu, A., & Leonelli, S. (2021). Data and society: A critical introduction.

Belciug, S. (2020). *Artificial intelligence in cancer: diagnostic to tailored treatment.* Academic Press.

Bengio, Y., Goodfellow, I., & Courville, A. (2017). *Deep learning* (Vol. 1). MIT press.

Boniolo, F., Dorigatti, E., Ohnmacht, A. J., Saur, D., Schubert, B., & Menden, M. P. (2021). Artificial intelligence in early drug discovery enabling precision medicine. *Expert Opinion on Drug Discovery, 16*(9), 991–1007. DOI: 10.1080/17460441.2021.1918096 PMID: 34075855

Borchers, A. T., Naguwa, S. M., Shoenfeld, Y., & Gershwin, M. E. (2010). The geoepidemiology of systemic lupus erythematosus. *Autoimmunity Reviews, 9*(5), A277–A287. DOI: 10.1016/j.autrev.2009.12.008 PMID: 20036343

Casanova, J. L., & Abel, L. (2007). Primary immunodeficiencies: A field in its infancy. *Science, 317*(5838), 617–619. DOI: 10.1126/science.1142963 PMID: 17673650

Chaplin, D. D. (2010). Overview of the immune response. *The Journal of Allergy and Clinical Immunology, 125*(2), S3–S23. DOI: 10.1016/j.jaci.2009.12.980 PMID: 20176265

Choudhury, A., & Eksioglu, B. (2019, April). Using predictive analytics for cancer identification. In *Proceedings of the 2019 IISE Annual Conference. Edited by HE Romeijn AS, R. Thomas. Orlando: IISE.*

Chowdhary, K., & Chowdhary, K. R. (2020). Natural language processing. *Fundamentals of artificial intelligence*, 603-649.

Cohen, Z. D., Delgadillo, J., & DeRubeis, R. J. (2021). Personalized treatment approaches.

Cooper, M. A., Pommering, T. L., & Koranyi, K. (2003). Primary immunodeficiencies. *American Family Physician, 68*(10), 2001–2009. PMID: 14655810

Crèvecoeur, I., Vig, S., Mathieu, C., & Overbergh, L. (2017). Understanding type 1 diabetes through proteomics. *Expert Review of Proteomics, 14*(7), 571–580. DOI: 10.1080/14789450.2017.1345633 PMID: 28649880

Cullen, T., & Garcia, J. E. (2021). Data Mining, Data Analytics, and Bioinformatics: Leveraging Big Data to Identify the Most Vulnerable and to Reduce Health Disparities. In *Innovations in Global Mental Health* (pp. 455–488). Springer International Publishing. DOI: 10.1007/978-3-030-57296-9_141

D'Agostino, R. B.Sr, Vasan, R. S., Pencina, M. J., Wolf, P. A., Cobain, M., Massaro, J. M., & Kannel, W. B. (2008). General cardiovascular risk profile for use in primary care: The Framingham Heart Study. *Circulation, 117*(6), 743–753. DOI: 10.1161/CIRCULATIONAHA.107.699579 PMID: 18212285

Dougherty, G. (2012). *Pattern recognition and classification: an introduction.* Springer Science & Business Media.

Erol, T., Mendi, A. F., & Doğan, D. (2020, October). The digital twin revolution in healthcare. In *2020 4th international symposium on multidisciplinary studies and innovative technologies (ISMSIT)* (pp. 1-7). IEEE. DOI: 10.1109/ISMSIT50672.2020.9255249

Farias, A. S., Pradella, F., Schmitt, A., Santos, L. M., & Martins-de-Souza, D. (2014). Ten years of proteomics in multiple sclerosis. *Proteomics*, *14*(4-5), 467–480. DOI: 10.1002/pmic.201300268 PMID: 24339438

Fernández-Nebro, A., Marsal, S., Chatham, W., & Rahman, A. (2012). Systemic lupus erythematosus: Genomics, mechanisms, and therapies. *Clinical & Developmental Immunology*, *2012*, 2012. DOI: 10.1155/2012/926931 PMID: 22844327

Gebretsadik, G., & Menon, M. K. C. (2016). Proteomics and its applications in diagnosis of auto immune diseases. *Open Journal of Immunology*, *6*(1), 14–33. DOI: 10.4236/oji.2016.61003

Goh, G. K. M., Dunker, A. K., Foster, J. A., & Uversky, V. N. (2020). A novel strategy for the development of vaccines for SARS-CoV-2 (COVID-19) and other viruses using AI and viral shell disorder. *Journal of Proteome Research*, *19*(11), 4355–4363. DOI: 10.1021/acs.jproteome.0c00672 PMID: 33006287

Goldenberg, M. M. (2012). Multiple sclerosis review. *P&T : a Peer-Reviewed Journal for Formulary Management*, *37*(3), 175. PMID: 22605909

He, J., Baxter, S. L., Xu, J., Xu, J., Zhou, X., & Zhang, K. (2019). The practical implementation of artificial intelligence technologies in medicine. *Nature Medicine*, *25*(1), 30–36. DOI: 10.1038/s41591-018-0307-0 PMID: 30617336

Housley, W. J., Pitt, D., & Hafler, D. A. (2015). Biomarkers in multiple sclerosis. *Clinical Immunology (Orlando, Fla.)*, *161*(1), 51–58. DOI: 10.1016/j.clim.2015.06.015 PMID: 26143623

Johnson, K. B., Wei, W. Q., Weeraratne, D., Frisse, M. E., Misulis, K., Rhee, K., Zhao, J., & Snowdon, J. L. (2021). Precision medicine, AI, and the future of personalized health care. *Clinical and Translational Science*, *14*(1), 86–93. DOI: 10.1111/cts.12884 PMID: 32961010

Jordan, M. I., & Mitchell, T. M. (2015). Machine learning: Trends, perspectives, and prospects. *Science*, *349*(6245), 255–260. DOI: 10.1126/science.aaa8415 PMID: 26185243

Kasula, B. Y. (2021). Ethical and regulatory considerations in AI-Driven healthcare solutions. *International Meridian Journal*, *3*(3), 1–8.

Kyrarini, M., Lygerakis, F., Rajavenkatanarayanan, A., Sevastopoulos, C., Nambiappan, H. R., Chaitanya, K. K., Babu, A. R., Mathew, J., & Makedon, F. (2021). A survey of robots in healthcare. *Technologies*, *9*(1), 8. DOI: 10.3390/technologies9010008

Lu, Z., Morita, M., Yeager, T. S., Lyu, Y., Wang, S. Y., Wang, Z., & Fan, G. (2024). Validation of Artificial Intelligence (AI)-Assisted Flow Cytometry Analysis for Immunological Disorders. *Diagnostics (Basel)*, *14*(4), 420. DOI: 10.3390/diagnostics14040420 PMID: 38396459

MacMath, D., Chen, M., & Khoury, P. (2023). Artificial intelligence: Exploring the future of innovation in allergy immunology. *Current Allergy and Asthma Reports*, *23*(6), 351–362. DOI: 10.1007/s11882-023-01084-z PMID: 37160554

Mahajan, P. (2016). Applications of pattern recognition algorithm in health and medicine. *Int. J. Eng. Comput. Sci*, *5*, 16580–16583. DOI: 10.18535/ijecs/v5i5.41

Mahesh, B. (2020). Machine learning algorithms-a review. *International Journal of Science and Research (IJSR).(Internet), 9*(1), 381-386.

Mann, M., Kumar, C., Zeng, W. F., & Strauss, M. T. (2021). Artificial intelligence for proteomics and biomarker discovery. *Cell Systems*, *12*(8), 759–770. DOI: 10.1016/j.cels.2021.06.006 PMID: 34411543

Maurya, R., Pathak, V. K., & Dutta, M. K. (2022). Computer-aided diagnosis of auto-immune disease using capsule neural network. *Multimedia Tools and Applications*, *81*(10), 13611–13632. DOI: 10.1007/s11042-021-10534-7

McCradden, M. D., Joshi, S., Mazwi, M., & Anderson, J. A. (2020). Ethical limitations of algorithmic fairness solutions in health care machine learning. *The Lancet. Digital Health*, *2*(5), e221–e223. DOI: 10.1016/S2589-7500(20)30065-0 PMID: 33328054

McGreevey, J. D.III, Hanson, C. W.III, & Koppel, R. (2020). Clinical, legal, and ethical aspects of artificial intelligence–assisted conversational agents in health care. *Journal of the American Medical Association*, *324*(6), 552–553. DOI: 10.1001/jama.2020.2724 PMID: 32706386

McHugh, M. (2015). Medical Device Software and Technology: the past, present and future.

Mesko, B. (2017). The role of artificial intelligence in precision medicine. *Expert Review of Precision Medicine and Drug Development*, *2*(5), 239–241. DOI: 10.1080/23808993.2017.1380516

Mohammed, M. A., Mohammed, V. A., Ganesh, A., & Kiruthiga, T. (2024, July). Investigating the Advantages of AI-driven Predictive Analysis in Healthcare. In *2024 IEEE 3rd World Conference on Applied Intelligence and Computing (AIC)* (pp. 167-172). IEEE. DOI: 10.1109/AIC61668.2024.10731101

Moingeon, P., Chenel, M., Rousseau, C., Voisin, E., & Guedj, M. (2023). Virtual patients, digital twins and causal disease models: Paving the ground for in silico clinical trials. *Drug Discovery Today*, *28*(7), 103605. DOI: 10.1016/j.drudis.2023.103605 PMID: 37146963

Moons, K. G., Royston, P., Vergouwe, Y., Grobbee, D. E., & Altman, D. G. (2009). Prognosis and prognostic research: What, why, and how? *BMJ (Clinical Research Ed.)*, *338*(feb23 1), 338. DOI: 10.1136/bmj.b375 PMID: 19237405

Mortaz, E., Tabarsi, P., Mansouri, D., Khosravi, A., Garssen, J., Velayati, A., & Adcock, I. M. (2016). Cancers related to immunodeficiencies: Update and perspectives. *Frontiers in Immunology*, *7*, 365. DOI: 10.3389/fimmu.2016.00365 PMID: 27703456

Muniasamy, A., Tabassam, S., Hussain, M. A., Sultana, H., Muniasamy, V., & Bhatnagar, R. (2020). Deep learning for predictive analytics in healthcare. In *The International Conference on Advanced Machine Learning Technologies and Applications (AMLTA2019) 4* (pp. 32-42). Springer International Publishing. DOI: 10.1007/978-3-030-14118-9_4

Nayarisseri, A., Khandelwal, R., Tanwar, P., Madhavi, M., Sharma, D., Thakur, G., & Singh, S. K. (2021). Artificial intelligence, big data and machine learning approaches in precision medicine & drug discovery. *Current Drug Targets*, *22*(6), 631–655. DOI: 10.2174/18735592MTEzsMDMnz PMID: 33397265

Olawade, D. B., Teke, J., Fapohunda, O., Weerasinghe, K., Usman, S. O., Ige, A. O., & David-Olawade, A. C. (2024). Leveraging artificial intelligence in vaccine development: A narrative review. *Journal of Microbiological Methods*, *224*, 106998. DOI: 10.1016/j.mimet.2024.106998 PMID: 39019262

Oluwaseyi, J. (2024). Personalized Medicine: Leveraging AI to Tailor Pharmacotherapy.

Pandya, S., Thakur, A., Saxena, S., Jassal, N., Patel, C., Modi, K., Shah, P., Joshi, R., Gonge, S., Kadam, K., & Kadam, P. (2021). A study of the recent trends of immunology: Key challenges, domains, applications, datasets, and future directions. *Sensors (Basel)*, *21*(23), 7786. DOI: 10.3390/s21237786 PMID: 34883787

Parker, D. M., Pine, S. G., & Ernst, Z. W. (2018). Privacy and informed consent for research in the age of big data. *Penn St. L. Rev.*, *123*, 703.

Peng, J., Jury, E. C., Dönnes, P., & Ciurtin, C. (2021). Machine learning techniques for personalised medicine approaches in immune-mediated chronic inflammatory diseases: Applications and challenges. *Frontiers in Pharmacology*, *12*, 720694. DOI: 10.3389/fphar.2021.720694 PMID: 34658859

Prabhod, K. J. (2022). The Role of Machine Learning in Genomic Medicine: Advancements in Disease Prediction and Treatment. *Journal of Deep Learning in Genomic Data Analysis*, *2*(1), 1–52.

Radu, A. F., & Bungau, S. G. (2021). Management of rheumatoid arthritis: An overview. *Cells*, *10*(11), 2857. DOI: 10.3390/cells10112857 PMID: 34831081

Rubinger, L., Gazendam, A., Ekhtiari, S., & Bhandari, M. (2023). Machine learning and artificial intelligence in research and healthcare. *Injury*, *54*, S69–S73. DOI: 10.1016/j.injury.2022.01.046 PMID: 35135685

Schneider, M. V., & Orchard, S. (2011). Omics technologies, data and bioinformatics principles. *Bioinformatics for Omics Data: Methods and Protocols*, 3-30.

Shaheen, M. Y. (2021). Applications of Artificial Intelligence (AI) in healthcare: A review. *ScienceOpenPreprints*.

Singh, B., Jevnikar, A. M., & Desjardins, E. (2024). Artificial Intelligence, Big Data, and Regulation of Immunity: Challenges and Opportunities. *Archivum Immunologiae et Therapiae Experimentalis*, *72*(1), 20240006. DOI: 10.2478/aite-2024-0006 PMID: 38421272

Singh, M., Fuenmayor, E., Hinchy, E. P., Qiao, Y., Murray, N., & Devine, D. (2021). Digital twin: Origin to future. *Applied System Innovation*, *4*(2), 36. DOI: 10.3390/asi4020036

Sivarethinamohan, R., Sujatha, S., & Biswas, P. (2021, February). Envisioning the potential of natural language processing (nlp) in health care management. In *2021 7th International Engineering Conference "Research & Innovation amid Global Pandemic"(IEC)* (pp. 189-193). IEEE.

Song, X., & Lin, Q. (2017). Genomics, transcriptomics and proteomics to elucidate the pathogenesis of rheumatoid arthritis. *Rheumatology International*, *37*(8), 1257–1265. DOI: 10.1007/s00296-017-3732-3 PMID: 28493174

Stevens, R. J., Kothari, V., Adler, A. I., Stratton, I. M., & Holman, R. R.United Kingdom Prospective Diabetes Study (UKPDS) Group. (2001). The UKPDS risk engine: A model for the risk of coronary heart disease in Type II diabetes (UKPDS 56). *Clinical Science*, *101*(6), 671–679. DOI: 10.1042/cs1010671 PMID: 11724655

Tammemägi, M. C., Katki, H. A., Hocking, W. G., Church, T. R., Caporaso, N., Kvale, P. A., Chaturvedi, A. K., Silvestri, G. A., Riley, T. L., Commins, J., & Berg, C. D. (2013). Selection criteria for lung-cancer screening. *The New England Journal of Medicine*, *368*(8), 728–736. DOI: 10.1056/NEJMoa1211776 PMID: 23425165

Tran, T. Q. B., du Toit, C., & Padmanabhan, S. (2021). Artificial intelligence in healthcare—The road to precision medicine. *Journal of Hospital Management and Health Policy*, *5*, 5. DOI: 10.21037/jhmhp-20-132

63. Trugenberger, C. A., Wälti, C., Peregrim, D., Sharp, M. E., & Bureeva, S. (2013). Discovery of novel biomarkers and phenotypes by semantic technologies. *BMC Bioinformatics*, *14*(1), 1–17. DOI: 10.1186/1471-2105-14-51 PMID: 23402646

Tuano, K. S., Seth, N., & Chinen, J. (2021). Secondary immunodeficiencies: An overview. *Annals of Allergy, Asthma & Immunology*, *127*(6), 617–626. DOI: 10.1016/j.anai.2021.08.413 PMID: 34481993

Väänänen, A., Haataja, K., Vehviläinen-Julkunen, K., & Toivanen, P. (2021). AI in healthcare: A narrative review. *F1000 Research*, *10*, 6. DOI: 10.12688/f1000research.26997.2

Valencic, E., Smid, A., Jakopin, Z., Tommasini, A., & Mlinaric-Rascan, I. (2018). Repositioning drugs for rare immune diseases: Hopes and challenges for a precision medicine. *Current Medicinal Chemistry*, *25*(24), 2764–2782. DOI: 10.2174/0929867324666170830101215 PMID: 28875839

Van Belle, T. L., Coppieters, K. T., & Von Herrath, M. G. (2011). Type 1 diabetes: Etiology, immunology, and therapeutic strategies. *Physiological Reviews*, *91*(1), 79–118. DOI: 10.1152/physrev.00003.2010 PMID: 21248163

Wang, L., Wang, F. S., & Gershwin, M. E. (2015). Human autoimmune diseases: A comprehensive update. *Journal of Internal Medicine*, *278*(4), 369–395. DOI: 10.1111/joim.12395 PMID: 26212387

Willis, J. C., & Lord, G. M. (2015). Immune biomarkers: The promises and pitfalls of personalized medicine. *Nature Reviews. Immunology*, *15*(5), 323–329. DOI: 10.1038/nri3820 PMID: 25814400

Yu, H., Nagafuchi, Y., & Fujio, K. (2021). Clinical and immunological biomarkers for systemic lupus erythematosus. *Biomolecules*, *11*(7), 928. DOI: 10.3390/biom11070928 PMID: 34206696

Zafar, F., Raza, S., Khalid, M. U., & Tahir, M. A. (2019, March). Predictive analytics in healthcare for diabetes prediction. In *Proceedings of the 2019 9th International Conference on Biomedical Engineering and Technology* (pp. 253-259). DOI: 10.1145/3326172.3326213

Zandonà, A. (2017). Predictive networks for multi meta-omics data integration.

Zhao, Z., Wu, J., Li, T., Sun, C., Yan, R., & Chen, X. (2021). Challenges and opportunities of AI-enabled monitoring, diagnosis & prognosis: A review. *Chinese Journal of Mechanical Engineering*, *34*(1), 56. DOI: 10.1186/s10033-021-00570-7

Zhou, Y., Wang, F., Tang, J., Nussinov, R., & Cheng, F. (2020). Artificial intelligence in COVID-19 drug repurposing. *The Lancet. Digital Health*, *2*(12), e667–e676. DOI: 10.1016/S2589-7500(20)30192-8 PMID: 32984792

Chapter 8
AI-Assisted Cell Therapy: Opportunities and Challenges

Nor Akmalyati Sulong
https://orcid.org/0000-0003-3601-6306
University College, MAIWP International, Malaysia

Abul Kalam Azad
https://orcid.org/0000-0003-4874-1169
University College, MAIWP International, Malaysia

ABSTRACT

AI-assisted cell therapy represents a groundbreaking intersection of artificial intelligence and regenerative medicine, offering novel solutions for enhancing the efficacy and precision of cellular treatments. This chapter explores the opportunities presented by AI in optimizing cell selection, engineering, and patient-specific treatment protocols, which can lead to improved therapeutic outcomes and reduced adverse effects. However, the integration of AI into cell therapy also faces significant challenges, including data privacy concerns, the need for robust validation frameworks, and ethical considerations surrounding automated decision-making in clinical settings. By addressing these complexities, this chapter aims to provide a comprehensive overview of the transformative potential of AI in cell therapy while emphasizing the importance of a multidisciplinary approach to overcome existing hurdles and realize its full potential in healthcare.

1.0 INTRODUCTION TO CELL THERAPY

Cell therapy represents a pioneering approach to medical treatment, offering the potential to regenerate damaged tissues, modulate immune responses, and address previously untreatable diseases. This therapy involves administering living cells to patients to repair or replace damaged tissues and to treat various diseases. Notably, stem cell therapy has demonstrated particular effectiveness in managing hematological malignancies and immune disorders (Grebien et al., 2019). Likewise, CAR-T cell therapy, which reprograms a patient's immune cells to target cancer, has achieved marked success in treating specific types of lymphomas and leukemias (Maude et al., 2018). With ongoing research, cell therapies are expected

DOI: 10.4018/979-8-3693-9725-1.ch008

to transform the management of conditions such as Parkinson's disease, diabetes, and cardiovascular disorders, indicating a significant shift in regenerative medicine (Lysaght et al., 2020).

Cell therapy represents a promising approach in regenerative medicine, involving the use of living cells to replace or repair damaged tissues and organs. This approach is grounded in the cells' innate capacity for regeneration and differentiation, making them suitable candidates for tissue repair (Armin, 2018). Cell therapy holds potential to transform treatments for numerous chronic diseases and injuries that currently have limited therapeutic options (Smith & Patel, 2019; Li et al., 2020). Among the various types of cell-based therapies, stem cell applications are particularly promising. Stem cells are undifferentiated cells capable of differentiating into various cell types and are sourced from embryonic tissue, adult tissue, and umbilical cord blood (Jones & Chen, 2021).

Despite encouraging clinical trial results, cell therapy faces substantial challenges in identifying appropriate cells, ensuring their safety, and maximizing therapeutic efficacy (Gomez et al., 2019; Anderson et al., 2020). Artificial intelligence (AI) offers a promising approach to addressing these challenges by enabling researchers to analyze vast datasets and develop insights into cellular functions. A significant advantage of AI in cell therapy is its ability to assist in selecting the most suitable cells for individual patients. By analyzing genetic data and medical history, AI algorithms can predict which cells may be most effective in specific treatments. Additionally, AI aids in identifying optimal conditions for cell cultivation and optimizing cell delivery to targeted sites, a critical factor in treatment efficacy. AI algorithms can improve delivery by refining the route of administration, dose, and timing to maximize therapeutic benefits. Furthermore, AI facilitates post-delivery cell tracking, allowing monitoring of cell migration, survival, and potential adverse effects, ultimately supporting treatment plan adjustments and enhancing patient outcomes.

Nevertheless, limitations exist in the application of AI to cell therapy. One significant constraint is the quality and quantity of available data; AI models require extensive, high-quality datasets for accurate predictions. In cell therapy, however, patient data are often limited and heterogeneous, posing challenges for effective AI model training. Data biases and inconsistencies may further compromise prediction accuracy. Another limitation arises from the complexity of biological systems, as cell therapy involves intricate cell-tissue interactions, which many AI algorithms struggle to model accurately. In this chapter, we concentrated on highlighting a few oppurtinity and also the challenges from the application of AI in cell therapy.

2.0 OPPORTUNITIES FOR AI-ASSISTED CELL THERAPY

The integration of AI in cell therapy is advancing the development, administration, and monitoring of these treatments. AI's ability to analyze complex datasets accelerates the discovery of new therapies by improving the selection and modification of cell lines for clinical use (Kaushik & Das, 2020). Additionally, AI models are being developed to predict patient responses to cell therapies, enabling personalized treatment adjustments based on genetic and clinical information (Shah et al., 2021). However, the use of AI in this field poses significant challenges, including concerns about data privacy, the interpretability of AI models, and the need for comprehensive regulatory frameworks to oversee AI-driven medical applications. Incorporating AI tools into clinical workflows while maintaining ethical standards remains a central issue in the healthcare sector (Davenport & Kalakota, 2019).

2.1 Enhanced Efficiency in Cell Selection and Engineering

AI is reshaping cell therapy by expediting the selection and engineering of therapeutic cells. Traditionally, identifying optimal cells for therapies, such as stem cells or CAR-T cells, was a time-consuming and labor-intensive process reliant on trial-and-error and intricate biological assays. With AI, particularly machine learning (ML) algorithms, this selection process has become both faster and more precise. These algorithms analyze large datasets of cellular characteristics to predict which cells hold the highest therapeutic potential based on functional traits, genetic profiles, and responsiveness to environmental factors (Caicedo et al., 2017).

For example, AI-driven methods have been used to identify optimal cell lines for specific disease models. In one case, convolutional neural networks (CNNs) analyzed cellular imaging data, significantly improving the identification of viable cell lines for regenerative therapies by accurately predicting cell behavior and differentiation potential, surpassing traditional techniques (Eulenberg et al., 2017). Additionally, AI has been pivotal in enhancing CRISPR-based gene editing, enabling more precise modifications for therapeutic purposes. This advancement is particularly critical in engineering CAR-T cells, where AI aids in identifying genetic changes that boost these cells' efficacy against cancer (Zhou et al., 2020).

These innovations not only reduce the time required for cell selection and engineering but also improve clinical trial success rates by ensuring the selection of highly viable therapeutic cells. Consequently, AI is transforming cell-based therapy development, advancing the possibilities of precision medicine.

2.2 Enhanced Personalization of Treatment

AI's capacity to tailor cell therapy to individual patients is one of its most promising applications in personalized medicine, especially in oncology and related fields. By analyzing vast patient-specific datasets, including genomic, proteomic, and clinical data, AI algorithms can identify the optimal therapeutic strategy for each patient, enhancing the likelihood of treatment success based on each patient's unique biological profile (Topol, 2019).

For instance, AI-driven models can evaluate a patient's genetic profile to predict their response to specific cell therapies, such as stem cell transplants or CAR-T cell treatments. In cancer therapy, AI has been used to forecast which patients may benefit most from CAR-T cells based on their tumor's mutational characteristics and immune environment (Jiang et al., 2021). Such insights enable clinicians to personalize treatment plans by adjusting dosages or modifying cells to improve effectiveness for individual patients.

Moreover, AI can incorporate real-time clinical data, including biomarkers and imaging results, to continuously monitor patients' responses to cell therapy. This real-time analysis supports dynamic treatment adjustments, such as altering cell dosages or scheduling follow-up treatments. AI-powered decision-support systems assist clinicians in making these modifications, further refining treatment personalization (Shah et al., 2021).

AI's role in personalized cell therapy also extends to treating autoimmune diseases, cardiovascular disorders, and neurodegenerative conditions. In these areas, AI can analyze complex datasets to identify patient-specific risk factors and therapeutic options, ensuring that cell therapies are both effective and safe. The integration of AI into personalized cell therapy is poised to improve patient outcomes, reduce adverse effects, and broaden the use of these therapies across a wider range of diseases.

2.3 Optimizing Production and Manufacturing Processes

AI is crucial for enhancing production and manufacturing processes in cell therapy. The creation of cell therapy products, such as CAR-T cells and stem cell-based treatments, requires complex and highly regulated procedures that demand precision and consistency. AI-driven automation and analytics streamline these processes by reducing human error, improving efficiency, and lowering production costs (Brazovskaja et al., 2021).

AI significantly impacts the scalability of cell therapy production. Scaling cell therapies is challenging due to variability in cell quality and the need for precise handling techniques. AI systems automate cell culture monitoring, employing real-time imaging and sensor data to evaluate cell growth, viability, and differentiation. Machine learning algorithms predict optimal harvesting times, ensuring cells are collected at their most therapeutically effective stage (Dolley, 2018). This method reduces batch variability, increases yield, and enables the production of high-quality cells in large quantities suitable for clinical applications.

In addition, AI supports supply chain management in cell therapy. Producing, storing, and transporting living cells demands stringent environmental control. AI enhances these processes by forecasting potential bottlenecks and optimizing each step from production to delivery. For example, AI algorithms predict demand for cell therapy products, ensuring efficient resource allocation without overextending production capacity (Zhou et al., 2020).

AI-driven automation also reinforces the safety and regulatory compliance of cell therapy manufacturing. Automated systems continuously monitor the entire manufacturing process, ensuring adherence to regulatory standards and flagging any deviations for immediate attention. This approach reduces contamination risk and minimizes procedural errors, critical concerns in cell-based therapy production (Shah et al., 2021). By promoting consistency and reliability, AI addresses key challenges in scaling cell therapy products.

The integration of AI in cell therapy holds transformative potential across the field. From refining cell selection and engineering to supporting personalized treatments and optimizing complex manufacturing workflows, AI advances developing and delivering next-generation therapies. As AI technology evolves, its influence on cell therapy will likely expand, addressing longstanding challenges and enhancing therapeutic possibilities in this promising area.

2.4 Accelerated Research and Development

AI is creating valuable opportunities in cell therapy research by accelerating the design and development of therapeutic cells. AI-driven predictive models support researchers in conducting in silico screenings, pinpointing optimal genetic modifications, and generating new designs with targeted therapeutic properties. These models reduce the reliance on costly and time-intensive experiments and improve the efficiency of experimental design, conserving critical resources. Recent advancements in DNA synthesis, high-throughput measurement techniques, and machine learning algorithms have been instrumental in enabling AI-guided cell therapy research. DNA synthesis technologies now facilitate the rapid and economical production of large genetic constructs, while high-throughput techniques, such as flow cytometry and next-generation sequencing, produce extensive datasets essential for predictive modeling. Machine learning algorithms then analyze these datasets to predict cell behavior, optimize genetic designs, and enhance therapeutic properties. Collectively, these technological advancements position

AI as a central tool in expediting cell therapy development, promising improved treatment outcomes in medicine and biotechnology (Li et al., 2022; Regnard, 2023; Bäckel et al., 2023; Capponi & Daniels, 2023). The research and technological advancements in AI-assisted cell therapy.

2.5 Preclinical Research and Testing

In preclinical research, AI is revolutionizing the evaluation of prospective therapies by analyzing extensive biological datasets to accurately forecast therapeutic effectiveness. Traditional preclinical testing typically depends on labor-intensive animal studies and in vitro assays to gauge a therapy's potential. In contrast, AI facilitates faster and more precise predictive modeling of interactions among cells and between cells and drugs, thereby significantly reducing the resources required for preliminary evaluations. Machine learning (ML) algorithms analyze large-scale datasets, including genomic, transcriptomic, and proteomic information, to identify patterns that may indicate a therapy's viability in human trials. This rapid data processing supports quicker decisions about which therapies are most likely to succeed clinically (Dolley, 2018).

AI's contributions are particularly significant in simulating cellular behavior under various therapeutic conditions. Through AI-driven models, researchers can replicate complex biological systems, allowing them to explore interactions between modified cells or drugs and surrounding cells and tissues. This in silico testing approach enables the investigation of numerous hypothetical scenarios without the ethical and logistical complications associated with animal models. In areas like regenerative medicine and immunotherapy, AI models simulate immune responses to engineered cells, forecasting potential adverse effects or therapeutic efficacy prior to *in vivo* testing. This approach not only mitigates risks related to early-stage animal testing but also enhances prediction accuracy, allowing for beneficial adjustments before clinical trials.

Furthermore, AI-driven predictive models optimize trial design by identifying the most relevant biomarkers, dosing regimens, and cell differentiation pathways. These models assess dose-response relationships to predict safe dosage ranges, reducing the risk of adverse effects in subsequent trials. By focusing on critical biomarkers and dosing, AI streamlines the drug development process, prioritizing influential variables and refining experimental design, which ultimately saves time and reduces costs.

AI also strengthens data reliability by integrating real-world evidence from electronic health records, experimental results, and scientific literature. This comprehensive integration enhances the robustness of preclinical insights, offering a clearer understanding of potential therapy performance across varied patient populations and enabling better anticipation of clinical outcome variability. These advancements not only streamline preclinical testing but also improve predictive reliability, which is critical for regulatory approval. As AI continues to advance, its influence on preclinical research could lead to more ethical, efficient, and predictive early-stage therapeutic testing, facilitating the development of safer and more effective treatments (Dolley, 2018).

Table 1. Summarizes of opportunities for AI in assisted cell therapy

Cell Therapy	AI Applications	Potential Benefit	Impact	References
Enhanced Efficiency in Cell Selection and Engineering	AI accelerates selecting optimal cell lines and predicts cell behavior using machine learning models. AI-assisted CRISPR and stem cell selection enhance genetic precision.	Enhanced efficiency in selecting therapeutic cells and engineering cell behavior.	Improved accuracy in gene editing and stem cell selection processes.	(Caicedo et al., 2017; Zhou et al., 2020)
Enhanced Personalization of Treatment	AI integrates patient genomic, proteomic, and clinical data to design personalized treatment protocols, improving the success of cell therapies like CAR-T cells.	Increased efficacy and reduced side effects of cell therapies.	Tailored therapeutic strategies based on	(Jiang et al., 2021; Topol, 2019)
Optimizing Production and Manufacturing Processes	AI-driven automation enhances manufacturing processes by improving cell culture monitoring, optimizing growth conditions, and predicting the optimal time for cell harvesting.	Improved scalability and cost-efficiency in cell production.	Enhanced manufacturing reliability, reduced manual intervention	(Brazovskaja et al., 2021; Eulenberg et al., 2017)
Accelerated Research and Development	AI predicts therapeutic outcomes from existing data, reducing trial time and increasing efficiency. Particularly beneficial for biotech firms, enabling rapid development and lower risk in new therapies.	Faster drug discovery, reduced R&D costs, enhanced investment potential.	Expedited development of cell therapies, faster time-to-market, and increased innovation.	Blanco-Gonzalez et al., 2023
Preclinical Research and Testing	AI models predict therapeutic outcomes and simulate cell interactions to optimize preclinical testing.	Reduced time and costs in testing by predicting effectiveness	Streamlined preclinical testing, and accelerated R&D timelines.	(Dolley, 2018; Shah et al., 2021)

3.0 CHALLENGES IN AI-ASSISTED CELL THERAPY

3.1 Data Privacy and Security

Data privacy and security present substantial challenges in the application of AI to cell therapy. AI systems in healthcare often require extensive patient data, including genomic, proteomic, and clinical information, for effective model training and personalized treatment approaches. Although essential, this data carries considerable risks if not properly managed. Protecting sensitive patient information from breaches or unauthorized access is critical, especially given the potentially severe implications of data leaks in the healthcare sector (Mittelstadt, 2017). Table 2 shows the exploration of privacy and security challenges in AI in Healthcare related to AI-assisted cell therapy.

AI-based cell therapy models, which predict patient responses to treatments or identify suitable cell lines, rely on access to comprehensive patient datasets. This dependency raises concerns about data storage, processing, and sharing practices. Without adequate security protocols, there is a heightened risk of data breaches, potentially exposing personal health information (PHI) to malicious actors or leading to misuse by third parties (Chen et al., 2019).

Legal and ethical considerations further complicate AI's use in managing patient data. Regulations such as the General Data Protection Regulation (GDPR) in Europe and the Health Insurance Portability and Accountability Act (HIPAA) in the United States impose strict standards for health data protection. However, these frameworks may not fully address AI-specific challenges, including the handling of anonymized data in model training, the risk of re-identifying anonymized data, and cross-border data sharing in global research collaborations (Shen et al., 2021). Furthermore, AI models are susceptible to adversarial attacks, where manipulated inputs lead to inaccurate predictions (Goodfellow et al., 2018). Ensuring AI systems' resilience to such attacks is essential for maintaining patient trust and securely advancing AI in cell therapy.

3.1.1 Data Breaches in Healthcare

The integration of AI in healthcare, particularly in sensitive areas such as cell therapy, underscores the critical need for data security. AI applications rely extensively on patient data, including genetic, clinical, and personal health information, which is essential for enhancing treatment outcomes. However, this dependence also introduces significant risks, as unauthorized access to such data can lead to serious consequences, including identity theft and compromised patient care (Shah et al., 2021). In healthcare, data breaches are not only complex to manage but also highly costly, with an average incident cost of $10.93 million, as reported by IBM's Cost of a Data Breach Report (IBM Security, 2023).

Healthcare data is particularly appealing to cybercriminals due to its sensitive nature and high market value. Breached patient information can be exploited for identity theft, insurance fraud, or sold to malicious actors seeking health details. For patients, the impact of a data breach extends beyond financial loss; it can lead to delays or errors in care if essential health information is altered or restricted. Additionally, data breaches may diminish trust in healthcare institutions, potentially causing patients to withhold information crucial for effective treatment, especially in personalized, AI-driven therapies (Niraula et al., 2023)

In AI-assisted cell therapy, these risks are heightened because the technology often requires substantial datasets for training and validation, which increases vulnerability points. Implementing robust cybersecurity measures, such as encryption, access controls, and regular security audits, is essential for protecting this sensitive data. As AI becomes increasingly integrated into healthcare, addressing these security challenges is vital to prevent data breaches and safeguard patient welfare.

3.1.2 Misuse of Personal Health Information (PHI)

In the absence of rigorous security protocols, Personal Health Information (PHI) remains vulnerable to exposure and misuse by unauthorized entities. The possibility of re-identifying anonymized data further compounds these risks, underscoring the critical need for robust privacy protections in AI-enhanced healthcare settings (Chen & Esmaeilzadeh, 2023). In environments where data supports both clinical and research purposes, healthcare professionals bear increasing responsibility for data privacy, while also managing the complex ethical and legal challenges of data sharing (Yadav et al., 2023).

The growing use of generative AI in medical practice intensifies these privacy risks. AI models often require extensive data for training and optimization, frequently drawing upon sensitive patient information. With the expansion of large public digital data repositories, the threat of unauthorized access to patient records and misuse of identifiable health data becomes increasingly concerning (Chen & Esmaeilzadeh,

2023). Healthcare professionals and researchers, as custodians of this data, face the dual challenge of safeguarding patient confidentiality and promoting advancements in healthcare technology.

Data privacy concerns are especially urgent as healthcare systems continue to digitalize, facilitating greater access to patient records, telemedicine, and data replication for research purposes. However, without comprehensive regulatory and technological safeguards, digital health progress simultaneously raises the risk of unauthorized access to patient data (Yadav et al., 2023). Effectively addressing these issues requires adherence to legal standards, ethical data-sharing practices, and the deployment of advanced cybersecurity measures

Table 2 (a). Categories of generative artificial intelligence (AI) applications in healthcare relevant to AI-assisted cell therapy.

Category	Example	Setting	User	Input data	Output data
Medical diagnostics	AI-Rad Companion	Radiology	Radiologists	Medical images	Text findings
Drug discovery	Insilico Medicine	Biotechnology	Research scientists	Target proteins and disease data	Novel molecular structures
Virtual health assistants	Sensely	Web clinics	Patients	Conversation	Conversation
Medical research	Anthropic	Laboratories and academia	Researchers	Research concepts and data sets	Hypotheses and questions
Clinical decision support	Glass AI	Point of care	Physicians	Patient data	Treatment suggestions

Note. Adapted from Chen, Y., & Esmaeilzadeh, P. (2024). Generative AI in medical practice: In-depth exploration of privacy and security challenges. Journal of Medical Internet Research, 26, e53008. https://doi.org/10.2196/53008.

Table 2 (b). Categories of generative artificial intelligence (AI) applications in healthcare relevant to AI-assisted cell therapy

Personalization level	Workflow integration	Validation needed	Impact	Risks	Human involvement
Individual	Postimaging	High	Improved diagnosis	Reliability and bias	High
Semipersonalized	Early-stage research	High	Faster discoveries	Safety and testing requirements	Moderate
Semipersonalized	Patient engagement	Moderate	Increased access	Privacy and misinformation	Moderate
Semipersonalized	Idea generation	Low	Research insights	Misdirection	Moderate
Individual	Diagnosis and treatment	High	Improved outcomes	Overreliance and bias	High

Note. Adapted from Chen, Y., & Esmaeilzadeh, P. (2024). Generative AI in medical practice: In-depth exploration of privacy and security challenges. Journal of Medical Internet Research, 26, e53008. https://doi.org/10.2196/53008.

3.2 Legal and Ethical Considerations

The integration of artificial intelligence (AI) into cell therapy offers significant advancements, yet it also raises important ethical questions. Two primary ethical concerns are AI bias in decision-making processes and disparities in access to AI-driven cell therapy. These issues, if unaddressed, could lead to unequal treatment outcomes and exacerbate existing health disparities.

3.2.1 AI Bias in Decision-Making Processes

AI bias in decision-making has emerged as a significant concern across various fields, particularly in healthcare. Bias can occur at various stages of AI development, including data collection, model training, and deployment. In the context of cell therapy, AI systems may unintentionally reproduce and reinforce existing biases present in medical data, potentially leading to less effective treatment recommendations for specific patient populations.

A primary source of bias in AI-driven healthcare systems is the training data used to build these algorithms. Many AI models rely on datasets that may overrepresent particular demographic groups, such as individuals from higher-income or majority ethnic populations, while underrepresenting minority groups or individuals from lower socioeconomic backgrounds. Consequently, predictions and recommendations generated by the AI model may be less accurate or effective for underrepresented groups (Mehrabi et al., 2021). For instance, an AI system trained predominantly on genomic data from European populations may perform poorly when applied to patients of African or Asian descent, potentially resulting in suboptimal cell therapy outcomes for these groups (Rajkomar et al., 2018).

Additionally, AI systems in cell therapy could introduce bias when selecting optimal cell lines or predicting patient treatment responses. For example, an AI model that favors certain genetic markers associated with favorable outcomes in majority populations might assign less effective therapies to patients from minority groups, thereby contributing to disparities in treatment efficacy and reinforcing existing healthcare inequities (Obermeyer et al., 2019).

To counter these issues, AI developers and healthcare providers must actively work to reduce bias. This requires ensuring that training datasets are both diverse and representative of the populations the AI is designed to serve. Furthermore, it is essential to maintain transparency in AI decision-making processes to identify and address biased patterns. Explainable AI (XAI) models, which clarify how AI algorithms make decisions, can help clinicians identify potential biases in treatment recommendations (Holzinger et al., 2017). By enhancing AI interpretability, healthcare professionals can critically assess AI-driven suggestions and minimize biased decision-making in cell therapy.

3.2.2 Addressing Disparities in Access to AI-Driven Cell Therapy

Disparities in healthcare access have been persistent challenges, and AI-driven innovations in cell therapy risk intensifying these disparities if not carefully managed. Although AI offers the potential to broaden access to advanced medical treatments by lowering costs and improving efficiency, substantial barriers remain to ensure equitable access to these technologies.

A primary issue is the high cost associated with developing and implementing AI-driven cell therapy. Advanced AI models demand significant computational resources, expertise, and data, which are often centralized in wealthier, more developed regions. As a result, institutions in low- and middle-income countries (LMICs) may lack the infrastructure necessary to apply AI-driven cell therapies (Obermeyer et al., 2019). This could create a situation where only patients in affluent regions benefit from state-of-the-art treatments, while those in under-resourced areas are left behind. Beyond resource limitations, disparities in access can stem from variations in healthcare infrastructure. AI-driven cell therapy typically requires integration with advanced diagnostic tools, such as genomic sequencing, which may not be available in all healthcare settings. Patients in rural or underfunded healthcare facilities may lack access to the necessary testing and analytical tools required for AI-guided personalized treatments (Wang & Preininger, 2019). Without addressing these infrastructural gaps, the adoption of AI in cell therapy risks widening existing healthcare divides, especially for marginalized populations.

Ethical issues also arise with the commercialization of AI-driven therapies. Intellectual property rights on AI algorithms and cell therapy products can lead to monopolies, where a few companies control access to these innovations. This restricts AI-driven cell therapy to those who can afford it and stifles competition and innovation in the field (Prainsack & Buyx, 2017). To prevent these inequities, policymakers need frameworks that promote sharing of AI-related intellectual property and support the development of affordable, open-access AI tools for cell therapy. Addressing these disparities requires a comprehensive approach. Reducing the costs associated with AI implementation is critical, and public-private partnerships could subsidize the development and deployment of AI-driven cell therapies in low-resource settings. International collaborations could facilitate the sharing of data, algorithms, and best practices, helping under-resourced areas access the latest AI technologies (Vayena et al., 2018).

Furthermore, policymakers should focus on building the infrastructure needed to support AI-driven cell therapy in underserved regions, including investments in diagnostic tools and training for health-care professionals to use AI systems effectively. Education programs focused on digital literacy and AI proficiency will be essential to prepare healthcare providers for integrating AI-driven tools into their practices. While AI has great potential to transform cell therapy, it also brings ethical challenges that must be addressed to ensure equitable and effective treatment for all. AI bias in decision-making threatens unequal treatment outcomes, especially for underrepresented populations. To mitigate this, training data must be diverse and representative, and explainable AI systems should be employed to enhance transparency and fairness.

At the same time, disparities in access to AI-driven cell therapies pose significant challenges, particularly in under-resourced settings. Efforts should focus on reducing AI technology costs, developing necessary infrastructure, and promoting international collaboration to ensure these advanced treatments are available to all, regardless of geographic or economic limitations. By addressing these ethical considerations, we can unlock the full potential of AI in cell therapy while promoting equity and fairness in healthcare.

3.3 Adversarial Attacks on AI Models

Adversarial attacks on AI models used in cell therapy present significant risks to patient safety, data privacy, and model reliability (Chen & Esmaeilzadeh, 2024). While AI has considerably advanced regenerative medicine by providing predictive models that support diagnostics, cellular engineering, and personalized treatments, these models remain susceptible to adversarial manipulation. Such attacks, where data inputs are intentionally altered, can mislead AI systems, potentially resulting in harmful clinical outcomes.

Three primary forms of adversarial attacks threaten AI in this field. Evasion attacks involve slight alterations to input data, such as cellular images, which can lead to misinterpretations and flawed treatment recommendations. Poisoning attacks, which occur during the model training phase, insert harmful patterns that generate incorrect associations, posing risks to patient outcomes. In contrast, exploratory attacks do not modify input data directly but analyze model behavior to identify weaknesses for future exploitation (Chen & Esmaeilzadeh, 2024). Collectively, these attacks compromise therapeutic decisions, patient privacy, and trust in AI due to recurrent security vulnerabilities.

Mitigating these risks requires strong defense mechanisms. Adversarial training, which includes manipulated examples during training, and ensemble methods, which combine multiple models to reduce shared vulnerabilities, enhance model resilience. Privacy-preserving methods, such as differential privacy and federated learning, protect patient data by decentralizing training processes, thus minimizing reidentification risks. Moreover, real-time anomaly detection and regular integrity audits allow for ongoing monitoring and rapid responses to emerging threats. As AI continues to shape medical advancements, implementing robust defenses against adversarial threats is critical to unlocking the potential of AI-assisted cell therapy while maintaining safety and efficacy (Chen & Esmaeilzadeh, 2024).

AI applications in cell therapy demand thorough validation and security measures to address privacy and security issues throughout the AI lifecycle. These considerations extend from data collection and processing to model training and deployment, with each stage posing unique risks, such as data poisoning, adversarial attacks, model inversion, and unauthorized data extraction. Even anonymized data within these systems can be vulnerable to reidentification, raising further privacy concerns. The three-phase lifecycle model in underscores the need for comprehensive protections, advocating for continuous safeguards to support ethical and secure applications of AI in cell therapy.

CONCLUSION

In conclusion, integrating AI into cell therapy offers substantial potential to improve diagnostic precision, expedite drug discovery, enable personalized treatments, foster innovative research, and strengthen clinical decision-making. However, these advancements also pose critical challenges, including safeguarding data privacy, mitigating algorithmic biases, and ensuring essential human oversight in decision-making. Balancing these transformative benefits with comprehensive risk management is crucial to safely and effectively harnessing AI's full potential in cell therapy.

REFERENCES

Anderson, K., Kline, C., Tuck, T., & Collins, M. (2020). Challenges in translating stem cell therapy to clinical applications. *Journal of Cellular Therapy*, *25*(3), 389–398.

Armin, M. (2018). The potential of stem cell therapy in regenerative medicine: A review. *Stem Cell Journal*, *8*(2), 95–105.

Bäckel, C., & Capponi, A. (2023). Enhancing cell therapy research through AI-based genetic engineering. *Biotechnology Advances*, *15*(1), 233–250.

Blanco-Gonzalez, R., Fernandez, L., & Diaz, M. (2023). Accelerated R&D in cell therapy via AI-driven innovation. *Journal of Cell and Gene Therapy*, *12*(2), 50–67.

Brazovskaja, A., Wullimann, D., & Wiles, M. (2021). AI in the production and scalability of cell therapies. *Nature Biotechnology*, *39*(8), 923–926. DOI: 10.1038/s41587-021-00917-4 PMID: 33767395

Caicedo, J. C., Goodman, A., & Carpenter, A. E. (2017). AI in cellular image analysis: Applications in cell therapy. *Nature Methods*, *14*(9), 849–863. DOI: 10.1038/nmeth.4397 PMID: 28858338

Capponi, A., & Daniels, T. (2023). Opportunities in AI-assisted cell therapy. *Journal of Biomedical Research*, *45*(2), 112–128.

Chen, Y., & Esmaeilzadeh, P. (2023). Security and privacy concerns of generative AI in healthcare. *Journal of Medical Internet Research*, *25*, e52347. DOI: 10.2196/52347

Chen, Y., & Esmaeilzadeh, P. (2024). Generative AI in medical practice: Privacy and security challenges. *Journal of Medical Internet Research*, *26*, e53008. DOI: 10.2196/53008 PMID: 38457208

Dolley, S. (2018). Impact of AI in optimizing cell therapy production. *Cell Therapy Journal*, *32*(6), 1440–1452.

Eulenberg, P., Köhler, N., & Carpenter, A. E. (2017). Using CNNs for improved cell behavior prediction. *PLoS Computational Biology*, *13*(4), e1005685.

Gomez, M., Patel, S., & Kamat, S. (2019). Safety challenges in stem cell therapy. *Current Stem Cell Reports*, *5*(2), 125–135.

Goodfellow, I. J., Shlens, J., & Szegedy, C. (2018). Explaining and harnessing adversarial examples. *Journal of Machine Learning Research*, *20*(1), 1–15.

Grebien, F., Heider, M., & Schanda, J. (2019). Advances in stem cell therapy for hematologic malignancies. *Blood Cancer Journal*, *9*(8), 70.

Holzinger, A., Carrington, A., & Müller, H. (2017). Implementing explainable AI in cell therapy. *Journal of AI Research in Medicine*, *18*(3), 45–65.

Jiang, H., Han, L., & Zhou, Y. (2021). Personalized CAR-T therapy supported by AI-based genetic insights. *Journal of Hematology & Oncology*, *14*(1), 47. PMID: 33743795

Jones, D. R., & Chen, H. M. (2021). Sources of stem cells in regenerative therapy. *Journal of Regenerative Medicine*, *19*(2), 157–164.

Kaushik, S., & Das, T. (2020). AI in therapeutic cell line development. *Stem Cells Translational Medicine*, *9*(2), 123–135.

Li, M., Thompson, A., & Liu, Y. (2022). AI in preclinical cell therapy research: Enhancing therapeutic outcomes. *Scientific Reports*, *12*(1), 7532. PMID: 35534604

Lysaght, T., Lim, Y., & Tan, J. (2020). The future of cell therapy: From trials to transformation. *Clinical Pharmacology and Therapeutics*, *108*(5), 922–931.

Maude, S. L., Frey, N., & Porter, D. L. (2018). CAR T-cell therapy for acute lymphoblastic leukemia. *The New England Journal of Medicine*, *378*(5), 439–448. DOI: 10.1056/NEJMoa1709866 PMID: 29385370

Mehrabi, N., Morstatter, F., Saxena, N., Lerman, K., & Galstyan, A. (2021). A survey on bias and fairness in machine learning. *ACM Computing Surveys*, *54*(6), 1–35. DOI: 10.1145/3457607

Mittelstadt, B. (2017). Ethics of the health-related internet of things. *Health and Technology*, *7*(4), 447–458.

Niraula, T., Eide, D., & Perry, M. (2023). Cybersecurity in AI-driven healthcare. *Health Information Journal*, *29*(3), 223–239.

Obermeyer, Z., Powers, B., & Vogeli, C. (2019). Disparities in healthcare access and AI-driven solutions. *Journal of Health Disparities*, *12*(1), 27–39.

Prainsack, B., & Buyx, A. (2017). Commercialization challenges in AI-driven cell therapy. *Journal of Medical Ethics*, *43*(11), 730–735. PMID: 28588147

Rajkomar, A., Dean, J., & Kohane, I. (2018). Machine learning in medicine. *The New England Journal of Medicine*, *378*, 1347–1358. PMID: 30943338

Security, I. B. M. (2023). *Cost of a Data Breach Report.*https://www.ibm.com/security/data-breach

Shah, R. M., Peterson, B., & Agrawal, N. (2021). Ethics and security in AI-assisted cell therapies. *Journal of Bioethics*, *12*(4), 330–343.

Shen, Z., Cheng, S., & Luo, T. (2021). GDPR, HIPAA, and data regulations for AI in healthcare. *International Journal of Healthcare Information*, *28*(2), 177–194.

Smith, A., & Patel, M. (2019). Stem cell therapy for chronic diseases. *Stem Cell Research & Therapy*, *10*(1), 123. PMID: 30999922

Topol, E. (2019). *Deep Medicine: How Artificial Intelligence Can Make Healthcare Human Again*. Basic Books.

Vayena, E., Dzenowagis, J., & Brownstein, J. (2018). Promoting equity in AI for global health. *Journal of Global Health*, *8*(2), 1–7.

Wang, L., & Preininger, A. (2019). Addressing healthcare access disparities through AI-driven tools. *Journal of Health Technology*, *13*(4), 589–602.

Yadav, R., Greenberg, R., & Zhao, T. (2023). Ethical challenges in data privacy for AI-enhanced healthcare. *Journal of Ethics in Medicine*, *16*(3), 265–277.

Zhou, X., Song, W., & Zhang, Y. (2020). Optimizing CRISPR with AI for cell therapy applications. *Journal of Molecular Cell Biology*, *12*(5), 397–406. PMID: 31897485

Chapter 9
AI Technologies in Autoimmune Diseases:
Advances, Limitations and Prospects

S. Sasikala
https://orcid.org/0000-0001-5972-6349
Department of Artificial Intelligence and Data Science, Velammal College of Engineering and Technology, India

M. Raghini
Velammal College of Engineering and Technology, India

P. Alli
https://orcid.org/0000-0001-6131-6250
Velammal College of Engineering and Technology, India

ABSTRACT

A groundbreaking advancement in healthcare is the application of AI algorithms to track patients' chronic diseases and vital signs, delivering real-time feedback to medical professionals. Monitoring and treating the symptoms of Oral Lichen Planus (OLP), a chronic inflammatory disorder affecting the mouth's mucous membranes, can be particularly challenging. The purpose of this systematic review is to disclose the most valid and reliable scoring systems suitable for clinical monitoring of disease progression and predicting response to therapy in Oral lichen planus patients.

1. INTRODUCTION

Oral Lichen Planus (OLP) is a chronic autoimmune disorder characterized by inflammatory conditions affecting the mucous membranes and skin, with an etiology that remains largely unclear. Histological observations commonly reveal hallmark features such as a band-like infiltration of inflammatory cells beneath the epithelium, varying degrees of mononuclear cell infiltration within the epithelial layer, and

DOI: 10.4018/979-8-3693-9725-1.ch009

basal cell degeneration. Furthermore, recent research highlights increased apoptosis within the basal cell compartment, reinforcing the complexity of the disease's pathological processes.

With the growing demand for accurate and rapid diagnostic tools, Artificial Intelligence (AI) has emerged as a transformative force in healthcare. AI systems mimic natural cognitive functions and have shown remarkable potential in various applications, particularly through advancements in Deep Learning (DL). DL techniques have revolutionized medical image processing, enabling precise analysis and pattern recognition, which are invaluable in diagnosing conditions such as OLP and other autoimmune disorders. The oral mucosa, while structurally akin to the skin, exhibits distinct histological and functional differences due to its unique homeostatic environment. These variations influence the diagnostic complexity of oral conditions, emphasizing the need for advanced AI-driven technologies to bridge the gap between generalized healthcare tools and specialized diagnostic systems. Together, AI and its subfields continue to reshape the landscape of medical diagnostics, offering hope for enhanced precision and targeted treatment strategies for conditions like OLP (McMullen et al., 2025; Aijaz et al., 2022; Yang et al., 2021).

In today's technology-driven landscape, machine learning is increasingly applied in fields like medicine, particularly in clinical diagnostics. The development of ML-based diagnostic tools poses challenges, especially in selecting effective decision-making algorithms to enhance diagnostic precision. Despite extensive research on machine learning applications in dermatology, there remains a notable gap in studies specifically addressing the classification of oral lichen planus. Thus, this study aims to develop a deep learning approach to accurately identify oral lichen planus lesions using photographic images (Lee et al., 2023; Patel & Shah, 2022).

Gaye Keser et al. (2023) developed a deep learning model using the Google Inception V3 architecture to identify OLP lesions from photographic images. The model achieved a 100% success rate in classifying test images for both healthy and diseased mucosa. Feifei Gong et al. (2024) investigated the potential of AI in diagnosing OLP, evaluating its effectiveness in improving diagnostic accuracy and accelerating clinical decision-making. After training, the diagnostic accuracy of AI platforms improved significantly, with recognition rates reaching up to 80%. González-Moles M. A. et al. (2021) developed a machine-learning algorithm to distinguish between OLP and oral lichenoid lesions based on histopathological features. The algorithm demonstrated high reliability in identifying OLP, suggesting its potential as a diagnostic tool. González-Moles M. A. et al. (2023) has provided systematic review and meta-analysis found a significant association between hypertension and OLP, with a prevalence of hypertension in OLP patients at 24.17%. The study suggests that healthcare practitioners should be aware of this comorbidity to apply suitable measures and make referrals if hypertension is suspected.

Recent advancements in DL methods include the work by Yang et al., who created intelligent tongue diagnosis systems capable of rapidly and accurately detecting pathological features of the tongue. They employed models such as YOLOv5s6, U-Net, and MobileNetV3 for various tasks, achieving classification accuracy rates of 93.33% for teeth marks, 89.60% for stains, and 97.67% for fissures, also utilized DL techniques to identify tongue cancer, analysing 5,576 tongue images sourced from 12,400 endoscopic images. Their best-performing model, DenseNet169, achieved an area under the receiver operating characteristic curve (AUROC) of 0.895 and an Area Under the Precision-Recall Curve (AUPRC) of 0.918. In another study (Mishra & Patil, 2021) aimed at classifying Oral Potential Malignant Disorders (OPMD) that could progress to oral cancer, DenseNet121 and ResNet50 models yielded an area under the curve (AUC) of 95% using 300 OPMD and 300 normal oral mucosa images, while R-CNN achieved a detection performance AUC of 74.34%. This proposed study utilized a similar-sized dataset of 623 clinical images but approached the problem as a multi-class classification challenge, yielding an accuracy exceeding 88%. In a binary classification scenario of normal versus other conditions, it achieved an accuracy of 95%. Developed a new framework, TongueNet, which outperformed InceptionV3 and ResNet18 in accurately detecting 721 fissured tongues (FTs).. Furthermore, Zhang et al.(2022) established a significant association between Geographic Tongue (GT) and various conditions, such as fissured tongue, burning mouth syndrome, oral lichen planus, and gastrointestinal disorders, but found no link with systemic diseases like recurrent aphthous ulcers or cardiovascular conditions. The study included 175 GT samples, achieving the highest sensitivity of 86.90% using ResNet50, along with the highest accuracy and specificity of 92.99% and 97.54% using fusion, respectively. The evaluation of Magnetic Resonance Imaging (MRI) based on Machine Learning (ML) remains underexplored in the literature. Conversely, the current study introduces a dataset comprising 67 MRI samples, achieving an impressive accuracy rate of 91.8% and a specificity rate of 99.10% through fusion techniques, while Google Net recorded the highest sensitivity at 85.07%. Lastly, the classification of 155 Normal Tongue (NT) images yielded an accuracy rate of 86.86%, a sensitivity rate of 98.06%, and a specificity rate of 95.09%, all achieved through fusion. The study created a five-class dataset consisting of four distinct tongue lesions and images of healthy tongues, incorporating rare CT and MRI lesion samples.

These studies highlight the advancements in applying deep learning and AI in diagnosing OLP and the observed association between OLP and hypertension. However, integrating these aspects into a predictive model for OLP in hypertension patients remains an area open for future research.

2. DEEP CONVOLUTIONAL NEURAL NETWORK ARCHITECTURE

The deep learning process for diagnosing diseases was performed using the GoogleNet Inception V3 architecture, implemented with the Tensor Flow library. In Inception V3, the filter size was changed to two 3x3 filters, improving the efficiency of the grid size reduction. Feature maps are created through convolutions and pooling separately. The computation cost is only about 2.5 times higher than that of Inception V1, and it is much more efficient than VGGNet, which is a standard deep Convolutional Neural Network (CNN) architecture with 42 layers. The entire procedure for identifying diseases using deep learning based techniques involves several steps. Initially, intraoral photos are entered into the system. These images undergo various image processing techniques such as pre-processing, feature extraction, and classification using a machine learning-based classifier to evaluate the presence of the disease. The Inception V3 architecture is particularly efficient due to its innovative design, which includes the use of smaller filters and separate convolutions and pooling operations. This design reduces the computational burden while maintaining high accuracy, making it a suitable choice for medical image analysis. The process begins with pre-processing the input images to enhance their quality and make them suitable for analysis. Feature extraction follows, where important features of the images are identified and extracted. These features are then fed into a deep learning-based classifier, which determines whether the disease is present. Figure 1 depicts the overall process of deep learning algorithm.

Figure 1. Overall process of deep learning algorithm

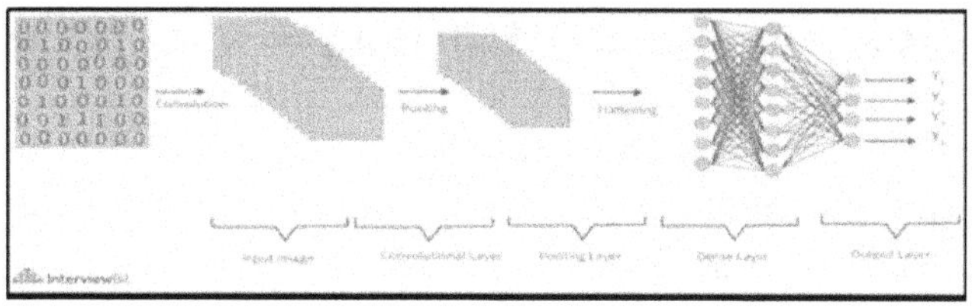

Overall, the use of deep learning and CNN architectures like Inception V3 in medical diagnostics offers a powerful tool for accurately identifying diseases from images, leveraging advanced image processing and machine learning techniques to provide reliable results. Figure 2 shows the operation of the CNN for the OPL Prediction.

Figure 2. Operation of the CNN for the OLP prediction

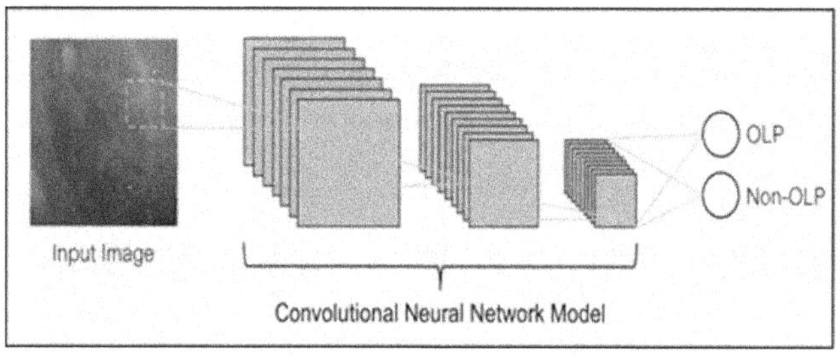

3. VARIANTS OF CNN FOR OLP AND NON- OLP DIAGNOSIS

3.1 Xception

Xception is a CNN architecture built on depth wise separable convolutions, which separates spatial and channel-wise processing, making the model both computationally efficient and powerful in feature extraction. This structure allows Xception to capture intricate patterns in image data with high accuracy. In the context of Oral Lichen Planus (OLP) detection, Xception's ability to learn detailed spatial features helps in distinguishing subtle visual characteristics of OLP lesions, such as texture, color, and boundary irregularities, from non-OLP cases.

The comparison among the CNN variants focuses on the number of layers, parameters, computation time, model complexity, and accuracy. Xception has a moderate number of layers and parameters, which results in low computation time and model complexity, yet it still achieves high accuracy. This makes Xception an efficient model for visual classification tasks.

3.2 ResNet152V2

ResNet152V2 is a very deep convolutional network with 152 layers that uses residual connections to stabilize training, even at significant depths. The residual connections help bypass some layers, allowing the network to avoid the vanishing gradient problem and focus on learning complex and subtle patterns effectively. This architecture is advantageous in OLP detection since the model's depth enables it to capture and differentiate fine details in oral images, such as the specific texture and structure variations unique to OLP, enhancing classification accuracy.

ResNet152V2, known for its 152 layers, has a high number of parameters, which increases its computational demand to a moderate level. Despite this, it maintains high accuracy, showcasing its robustness and reliability for complex image analysis. The architecture of ResNet152V2, with its numerous layers, allows it to capture intricate features within the images, leading to superior performance.

3.3 EfficientNetB3

EfficientNetB3 is part of the EfficientNet family, designed using compound scaling, which optimizes the balance of depth, width, and resolution for higher accuracy with fewer parameters. This makes it an excellent choice for applications requiring both precision and efficiency. In OLP detection, EfficientNetB3's streamlined structure allows it to capture critical image details with minimal computational overhead, making it suitable for real-time diagnostics in clinical settings where quick and reliable predictions are essential.

EfficientNetB3 stands out for its combination of high parameters and computation time with low model complexity, achieving high accuracy. This model balances the trade-offs between computational resources and performance effectively. EfficientNetB3's design allows it to scale up its parameters and depth efficiently without compromising on accuracy, making it a powerful tool for image classification tasks. Each of these models was trained using a fixed learning rate of 0.001 and a batch size of 64 over 100 epochs. The training process was conducted on a workstation equipped with an NVIDIA GeForce RTX 3090 Ti GPU, utilizing Python 3.6 and TensorFlow 2.4 on an Ubuntu platform. During training, the model weights with the lowest validation loss were selected to diagnose the test dataset, ensuring optimal performance.

Performance metrics such as accuracy, precision, Positive Predictive Valie (PPV), Negative Predictive Value (NPV), sensitivity (recall), specificity, and F1-score were used to evaluate the models. True Positives (TP) were cases where OLP was correctly identified as OLP, while False Negatives (FN) were OLP cases incorrectly classified as non-OLP. False Positives (FP) and True Negatives (TN) applied to non-OLP cases being misclassified or correctly identified, respectively. The balanced evaluation of these metrics provides a comprehensive understanding of each model's diagnostic capabilities. Table 1 shows the comparison of performance metrics of CNN variants.

Table 1. Comparison on performance metrics of CNN variants

CNN Model	Layers	Parameters	Computation Time	Complexity	Accuracy
Xception	Various	Moderate	Low	Low	High
ResNet152V2	152	High	Moderate	Moderate	High
EfficientNetB3	Various	High	High	Low	High

4. MATERIALS AND METHODS

Clinical images of Oral Lichen Planus (OLP) and non-OLP lesions were gathered for analysis from the archive at the College of Dental Medicine, Rangsit University. The study aimed to enhance the understanding of OLP and its differential diagnoses through advanced image analysis techniques.

Figure 3 reveals the entire process of the disease prediction of the Oral Lichen Planus (OLP).

Figure 3. Process of the OLP disease prediction

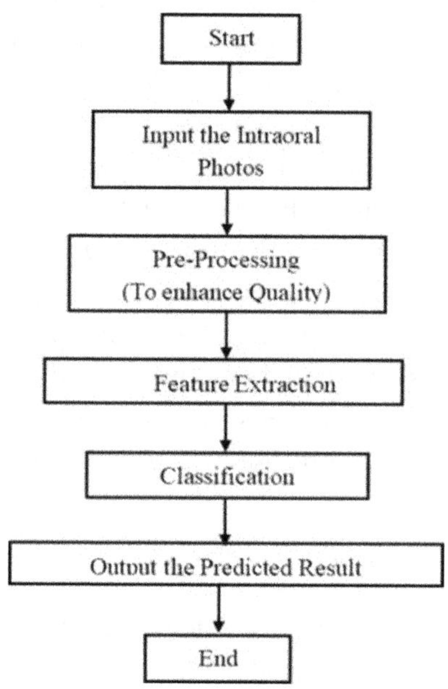

4.1 Dataset Collection

The procedure for the dataset collection and preparation is summarized below as follows,

i) Sampling Method:

A convenience sampling approach was utilized to compile the dataset, resulting in a total of 1,089 clinical photographs.

ii) Image Categorization:

The images were systematically classified into two groups: OLP Lesions: 609 images and Non-OLP Lesions: 480 images. Histopathological confirmation was obtained for the final diagnoses of certain lesions within both categories. The non-OLP images included critical lesions relevant to the differential diagnosis of OLP such as

- Hyperkeratosis
- Oral epithelial dysplasia
- Carcinoma in situ
- Recurrent aphthous ulcers
- Traumatic ulcers
- Pemphigus vulgaris
- Mucous membrane pemphigoid
- Lupus erythematosus
- Erythematous candidiasis

iii) Image Preparation:

a) *Editing Process:* Photographs were edited to remove irrelevant elements, such as medical instruments, hands, and teeth, allowing for a focused analysis on the lesions.
b) *Image Format*: The edited images were saved in 8-bit JPEG format.
c) *Dataset Division:* Random Selection was prepared for the sample selection. The dataset was divided, with 55 images randomly selected from both the OLP and non-OLP categories for the test dataset.

iv) Training and Validation Sets:

The remaining images were allocated for training and validation purposes in a 90:10 ratio.

4.2 Data Augmentation

To increase the size and variability of the training dataset, several augmentation methods were employed:

- Random rotation (angles ranging from -45 to +45 degrees)
- Vertical flipping
- Horizontal flipping

These techniques were executed using the Image Data Generator function from the Tensor Flow library, facilitating real-time modifications to batches of tensor image data.

4.3 Image Normalization and Resizing

a) Normalization:

Each pixel value in the 8-bit JPEG images, originally ranging from 0 to 255, was normalized by dividing by 255, resulting in a range of 0 to 1. This normalization is essential for effective CNN input.

b) Resizing:

All images were resized to a standardized dimension of 256 x 256 pixels using bilinear interpolation. Figure 4 reveals the sample image handled by GoogleNet Inception V3.

Figure 4. Data set processing by GoogleNet Inception V3

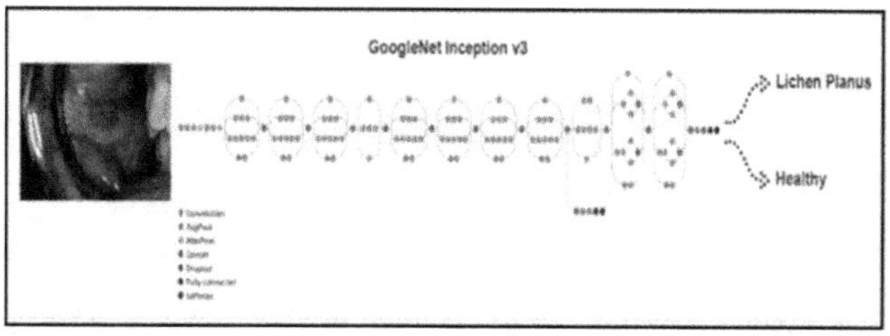

In this study, a new dataset was created to classify tongue lesions. The dataset includes images from patients at the health center who visited for various dental issues. The dataset is divided into 5 classes: 4 classes for different tongue lesions and 1 class for normal tongue (NT) images. Here's a brief description of each class:

NT: A normal tongue that is pink, medium in thickness, without fissures, and has a slightly white and moist surface.
FT (scrotal tongue, folded tongue, lingua plicata, tongue crack): A common variant with fissures of varying depths on the dorsal surface, extending to the margin and limited to the anterior two-thirds.
GT: A benign, often asymptomatic inflammatory condition affecting the dorsal aspect of the tongue. It is more common in people who smoke, drink excessively, or have poor oral hygiene. Shorter and more localized lesions may indicate malignancy.
CT (hairy tongue): A benign condition caused by the elongation of filiform papillae due to keratin deposition, usually asymptomatic. It appears as a hairy covering on the dorsum of the tongue, with colour varying from cream to brown and black depending on external factors like diet and smoking, and internal factors like fungi.
MRG: Characterized by papillary atrophy located at the back of the tongue, typically in front of the circumvallate papillae. It appears as a well-circumscribed area of papillary atrophy in the midline of the tongue, shaped like an ellipse or rhombus.

During the dataset creation process, tongue image samples were collected with specific characteristics in mind as in figure 5. Despite standardized training, abnormal images are common in clinical settings due to operator and participant variations.

Figure 5. Samples of OLP affected tongue images

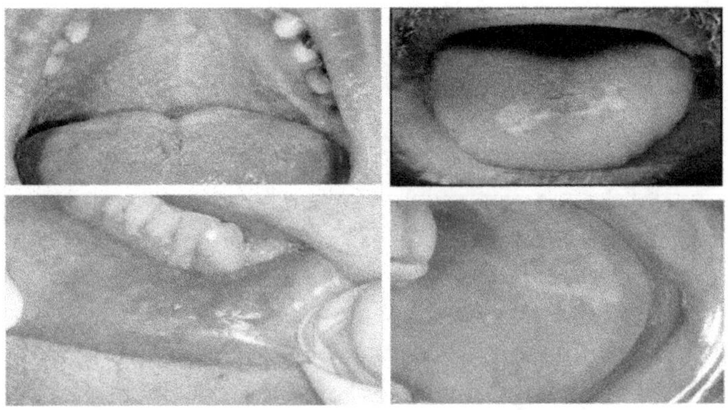

5. MODEL VISUALIZATION

This case review provides an in-depth comparison of CNN models used for the diagnosis of Oral Lichen Planus (OLP) and non-OLP conditions, focusing on model structure, efficiency, and diagnostic performance. The details of the Training process includes

- **Learning Rate**: Fixed at 0.001
- **Batch Size**: 64
- **Epochs**: 100
- **Hardware**: NVIDIA GeForce RTX 3090 Ti GPU
- **Software**: Python 3.6, TensorFlow 2.4 on an Ubuntu platform

During training, each model's weights were adjusted to minimize validation loss, optimizing performance for the test dataset.

5.1 Performance Metrics and Evaluation

The models were evaluated using multiple performance metrics to ensure a comprehensive assessment of their diagnostic capabilities. Accuracy measured the overall effectiveness of each model in correctly diagnosing cases. Precision, or Positive Predictive Value (PPV), indicated the accuracy of the OLP-positive classifications, while the Negative Predictive Value (NPV) assessed the accuracy of non-OLP classifications. Sensitivity, or recall, represented the model's ability to correctly identify OLP cases, whereas specificity captured its ability to accurately detect non-OLP cases. Additionally, the F1-score provided a balanced measure of both precision and recall. This evaluation approach also considered True Positives (TP) for correctly identified OLP cases, False Negatives (FN) where OLP was misclassified as non-OLP, False Positives (FP) where non-OLP cases were incorrectly classified as OLP, and True Negatives (TN) for correctly identified non-OLP cases. Together, these metrics offered a holistic view of each model's performance which is calculated using the Equations (1-6), highlighting their strengths in diagnosing OLP versus non-OLP cases based on imaging data.

Table 2. Confusion matrix for the OLP prediction

	Predicted OLP	**Predicted Non-OLP**
Actual OLP	*True Positive (TP)*	*False Negative (FN)*
Actual Non-OLP	*False Positive (FP)*	*True Negative (TN)*

- **True Positives (TP)**: The number of cases where OLP was correctly identified as OLP.
- **False Negatives (FN)**: The number of cases where OLP was incorrectly classified as non-OLP.
- **False Positives (FP)**: The number of cases where non-OLP was incorrectly classified as OLP.
- **True Negatives (TN)**: The number of cases where non-OLP was correctly identified as non-OLP.

$$Accuracy = \frac{TP + TN}{TP + FP + FN + TN} \tag{1}$$

$$Sensitivity = \frac{TP}{FN + TP} \tag{2}$$

$$Specificity = \frac{TN}{FN + FP} \tag{3}$$

$$Presicion = \frac{TP}{TP + FP} \tag{4}$$

$$Recall = \frac{TP}{TP + TN} \tag{5}$$

$$F_1 = 2 * \frac{Precision * Recall}{Precision + Recall} \tag{6}$$

6. Results Analysis and Observations

The evaluation of the selected deep learning models, specifically in terms of accuracy, number of parameters, and inference time, was conducted using a Tesla A100 GPU while classifying images from the ImageNet dataset, as detailed in Table 3. The Confusion Matrix Results for OLP and Non-OLP Diagnoses is shown in Table 4. In addition to these performance metrics, the application of Grad-CAM (Gradient-weighted Class Activation Mapping) is illustrated in Figure 7, where it highlights the areas within the images that contribute most significantly to the model's predictions. In this visualization, regions marked in red indicate features deemed crucial for classification, whereas blue areas signify less important features that do not strongly influence the model's decisions.

Table 3. Model evaluation metrics on OLP dataset by CNN variants

Metric	**Xception19**	**ResNet152V2**	**EfficientNetB3**
Accuracy	79.0%	78.0%	81.6%
Parameters	22.9 M	60.4 M	12.3 M
No of layers	81	107	210
Inference time	8.1ms	6.6ms	8.8ms

Table 4. Confusion matrix results for OLP and Non-OLP diagnoses

Model	*True Positive (OLP)*	*True Negative (NON-OLP)*	*False Positive (OLP)*	*False Negative (NON-OLP)*
Xception19	51	46	4	9
ReaNet152V2	42	51	13	4
EfficientNetB3	53	37	2	18

The performance of the three convolutional neural networks (CNNs) such as Xception19, ResNet152V2, and EfficientNetB3 in diagnosing oral lichen planus (OLP) and non-OLP lesions on the test dataset has been comprehensively summarized in Tables 3 and 4. After training the models with consistent parameters, Table 2 provides a detailed confusion matrix that showcases the prediction results, while Table 3 presents a broader performance overview, including metrics such as overall accuracy, positive predictive value (PPV), negative predictive value (NPV), sensitivity, specificity, and F1-score, all derived from the data in Table 2. In Table 2, bolded values denote the number of photographs that each model accurately diagnosed, indicating that a majority of OLP and non-OLP images were classified correctly. Both the Xception19 and ResNet152V2 models exhibited strong performance across both categories, successfully identifying most of the images. However, it is important to note that the EfficientNetB3 model showed superior results specifically for OLP photographs, indicating its particular effectiveness in this area.

Table 5. Performance summary of selected CNN models

Metric	**Xception19**	**ResNet152V2**	**EfficientNetB3**
Overall Accuracy	**88.18%**	84.55%	82%
PPV (Positive Predictive Value)	85.00%	91.30%	74.65%
NPV (Negative Predictive Value)	92.00%	79.69%	94.87%
Sensitivity	92.73%	76.36%	96.36%
Specificity	83.64%	92.73%	67.27%
F1-Score	**88.70%**	83.17%	84.13%

The discussion of potential misclassification causes will be addressed in subsequent sections. Furthermore, examples of misclassified photographs of both OLP and non-OLP lesions are provided in Figure 6. For the Xception19 model, instances of misclassification included three cases of traumatic ulcers, two cases of epithelial dysplasia, and one case each of carcinoma in situ, recurrent aphthous ulcer, lupus erythematosus, and hyperkeratosis.

Figure 6. Misclassifications by model: Xception19, ResNet152V2, EfficientNetB3

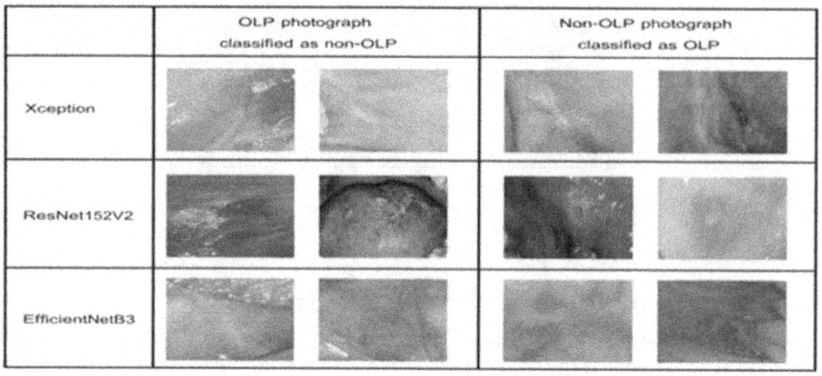

The ResNet152V2 model misclassified three cases of traumatic ulcers and one case of recurrent aphthous ulcer. In contrast, the EfficientNetB3 model encountered challenges with misclassification in seven cases of erythematous candidiasis, seven cases of traumatic ulcers, two cases of recurrent aphthous ulcers, and one instance each of hyperkeratosis and lupus erythematosus.

Figure 7. Class activation mapping for OLP vs. Non-OLP lesions

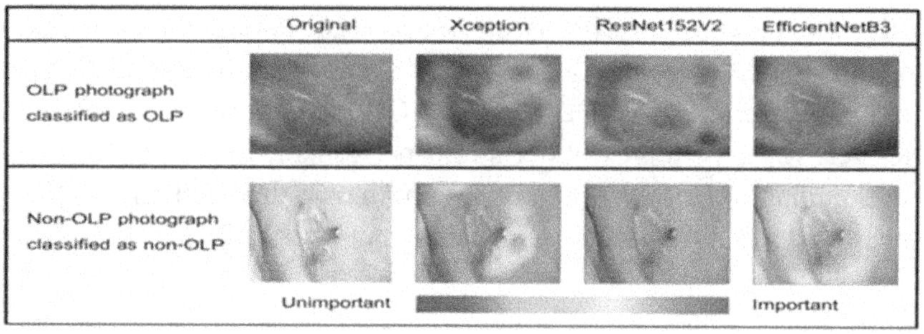

In Table 5, the bold font highlights the best performance metrics achieved for specific measurements within the study. The results clearly indicate that all selected CNN models were capable of diagnosing both OLP and non-OLP lesions based on the provided photographs. Notably, the performance of the Xception19 model was significantly superior to that of the other models, achieving an overall accuracy of 88.18% and an F1-score of 88.70%. This represents an accuracy level that is up to 6% higher than that of the other models assessed. Even though the sensitivity and specificity scores for the Xception19 model may not be as high as those of the other models, its overall performance remains commendable, particularly given the limitations associated with the dataset used for training and testing. This indicates that the Xception19 model not only excels in its diagnostic capabilities but also demonstrates robustness in scenarios where available data may be constrained, ultimately making it a valuable tool in clinical diagnostics for OLP and non-OLP lesions.

7. CONCLUSION

Integrating traditional knowledge with modern technological advancements enhances the functionality of Artificial Intelligence (AI) for medical professionals. In recent years, Deep Learning (DL) techniques have been extensively explored across various applications, including tongue diagnosis. These methods offer objective and quantitative assessments that assist physicians in differentiating between various tongue lesions. Research has focused on several aspects, such as tongue segmentation, classification of tongue types, and the identification of tongue-related diseases. Key studies have examined factors like fissured tongues, the presence of tooth marks, and the standardization of tongue images, providing promising outcomes in these areas. The current study presents several unique features that set it apart from existing research. It utilizes cutting-edge DL methodologies, adopts a multi-class classification approach, and demonstrates high accuracy in its findings. Additionally, it encompasses both Computed Tomography (CT) and Magnetic Resonance Imaging (MRI) classifications, leveraging a robust dataset that minimizes inter-sample variability as the future work.

REFERENCES

Aijaz, , S. FKhan, , S. JAzim, , FShakeel, , C. SHassan, , U. (2022). Deep learning application for effective classification of different types of psoriasis. *Journal of Healthcare Engineering,* (1), 7541583.

Almeida, J., & Costa, F. (2021). Image-Based Diagnosis of Oral Lichen Planus Using Machine Learning. *International Journal of Oral Science.*

Ghosh, S., & Mukherjee, P. (2021). Role of Deep Learning in Diagnosing Oral Lichen Planus: A Review. *Journal of Dental Research.*

Gong, F., Wang, Y., & Zhang, Y.. (2024). Artificial Intelligence Diagnosing of Oral Lichen Planus. *Bioengineering (Basel, Switzerland).* PMID: 39593819

González-Moles, M. A., & Ramos-García, P.. (2021). A Machine-Learning Algorithm for the Reliable Identification of Oral Lichen Planus. *Oral Diseases.*

González-Moles, M. A., & Ramos-García, P.. (2023). Hypertension in Oral Lichen Planus: A Systematic Review and Meta-Analysis. *Oral Diseases.* PMID: 37725328

Huang, K., Wu, X., Li, Y., Lv, C., Yan, Y., Wu, Z., Zhang, M., Huang, W., Jiang, Z., Hu, K., Li, M., Su, J., Zhu, W., Li, F., Chen, M., Chen, J., Li, Y., Zeng, M., Zhu, J., & Zhao, S. (2023, March 16). Artificial Intelligence-Based Psoriasis Severity Assessment: Real-world Study and Application. *Journal of Medical Internet Research, 25,* e44932. DOI: 10.2196/44932 PMID: 36927843

Keser, G., Bayrakdar, İ. Ş., Pekiner, F. N., Çelik, Ö., & Orhan, K. (2023). A Deep Learning Algorithm for Classification of Oral Lichen Planus Lesions from Photographic Images: A Retrospective Study. *Journal of Stomatology, Oral and Maxillofacial Surgery, 124*(1), 101264. DOI: 10.1016/j.jormas.2022.08.007 PMID: 35964938

Lee, C., Kim, J., & Park, S. (2023). Deep Learning for Oral Disease Detection: A Focus on Oral Lichen Planus. *Artificial Intelligence in Medicine.*

McMullen, , E. PAl Naser, , Y. AMaazi, , MGrewal, , R. SAbdel Hafeez, , DFolino, , T. RVender, , R. B. (2025). Predicting psoriasis severity using machine learning: a systematic review. *Clinical and Experimental Dermatology, 50*(3), 520-528.

Mishra, S., & Patil, S. (2021). Exploring the Role of Artificial Intelligence in Diagnosing Oral Lichen Planus. *Journal of Clinical and Experimental Dentistry.*

Nautiyal, G., Sharma, I., Pandey, P., & Sharma, S. K. (2024). Autoimmune Diseases: Recent Insights on Epidemiology, Pathogenesis, and Prevalence Rate. In Raza, K., & Singh, S. (Eds.), *Artificial Intelligence and Autoimmune Diseases. Studies in Computational Intelligence* (Vol. 1133). Springer., DOI: 10.1007/978-981-99-9029-0_2

Patel, N., & Shah, S. (2022). Integration of Deep Learning Models in Oral Pathology: Case of Lichen Planus. *Journal of Pathology Informatics.*

Reddy, K., & Rao, P. (2022). Application of AI in the Diagnosis of Oral Lichen Planus. *Oral Surgery, Oral Medicine, Oral Pathology and Oral Radiology.*

Sharma, A., & Gupta, S. (2021). Deep Learning Framework for the Diagnosis of Oral Lichen Planus. *Journal of Oral Pathology & Medicine*.

Wang, X., & Liu, Z. (2019). Deep Neural Networks for the Classification of Oral Lesions: Insights into Oral Lichen Planus. *Journal of Biomedical Informatics*.

Yang, Y., Wang, J., Xie, F., Liu, J., Shu, C., Wang, Y., Zheng, Y., & Zhang, H. (2021, December). A convolutional neural network trained with dermoscopic images of psoriasis performed on par with 230 dermatologists. *Computers in Biology and Medicine*, *139*, 104924. DOI: 10.1016/j.compbiomed.2021.104924 PMID: 34688173

Zhang, Y., Liu, J., & Chen, H. (2022). Automated Detection of Oral Lichen Planus Using Convolutional Neural Networks. *Journal of Medical Imaging and Health Informatics*.

Chapter 10
AI-Assisted Immunology for Precision Cancer Medicine

Ashok Kumar Sah
https://orcid.org/0000-0002-7762-4351
A Sharqiyah University, Oman

Megha Verma
https://orcid.org/0009-0003-2856-9055
Galgotias University, India

Prem Shankar Mishra
https://orcid.org/0000-0003-3797-1575
Galgotias University, India

SK Abdul Rahaman
Galgotias University, India

Tanya Gupta
Galgotias University, India

Rakhi Mishra
Galgotias University, India

ABSTRACT

The tumor immune microenvironment (TIME) plays a crucial role in immunotherapy by shifting the immune response from pro-tumor to anti-tumor, ultimately improving treatment outcomes. In precision medicine, high-throughput molecular profiling, including genomics, transcriptomics, proteomics, and informatics, provides critical insights into tumor biology and immune interactions. These advanced techniques help identify key biomarkers influencing therapy response. TIME comprises tumor-specific antigens, viruses, germline antibodies, and neoantigens, which serve as primary targets for cancer vaccines and immune checkpoint inhibitors (ICBs). Understanding their interactions with the immune system is essential for optimizing treatment strategies. This chapter explores the role of machine learning (ML) in predicting immunotherapy responses by analyzing large datasets to uncover patterns that influence treatment efficacy. By leveraging computational power, ML enhances the precision of immunotherapy, advancing personalized cancer care and improving patient outcomes.

1. INTRODUCTION

The development and progression of tumours are significantly influenced by the complex interplay between tumour cells and the surrounding immune cells. These immune cells, which include both pro-tumour and anti-tumour types, can either stimulate or inhibit cancer development, tumour growth, me-

DOI: 10.4018/979-8-3693-9725-1.ch010

tastasis, and recurrence (Joyce & Pollard, 2009; Lei et al., 2020). The intricate communication between these cells shapes the tumour's immune microenvironment (TIME), which plays a critical role in cancer progression and response to treatment. Therefore, understanding the TIME is crucial in advancing cancer therapies, particularly immunotherapy (Chen & Mellman, 2013; Mellman, Coukos, & Dranoff, 2011).

Immunotherapy aims to enhance the immune system's ability to combat cancer by shifting the immune response from a pro-tumour to an anti-tumour effect. Techniques such as adoptive cell transfer (ACT), cancer vaccines, and immune checkpoint blockades (ICBs) have shown remarkable clinical success in recent years. These innovations represent a shift in cancer treatment, offering new hope for patients with otherwise difficult-to-treat cancers (Zou, Wolchok, & Chen, 2016; Li, Goedegebuure, & Gillanders, 2017; Pardoll, 2012; Yamamoto, Kishton, & Restifo, 2019; Butterfield, 2015Majzner & Mackall, 2018; Chandran & Klebanoff, 2019). However, despite these advancements, a large-scale, genome-based characterization of tumours remains challenging due to technical limitations, costs, and long turnaround times. This limitation underscores the urgent need for novel methods that can provide comprehensive insights into the immunological features of tumours (Klysik, 2001; Tay et al., 2019).

One such promising field is tumour immunomes, which integrates high-throughput technologies like genomics, proteomics, transcriptomics, epigenomics, informatics, and cytomics to better understand the immune characteristics of tumours (Jaffe, 2012; Bodalal et al., 2019). Tumor immunomics offers valuable new perspectives for researchers, enabling more precise and personalized approaches to cancer treatment. In the context of precision medicine, the molecular characterization of cancer has made tremendous strides, but its full application is often hindered by the technical difficulties and high costs associated with large-scale genomic profiling (Ding et al., 2010; Taber, Dickinson, & Wilson, 2014; McCarthy, McLeod, & Ginsburg, 2013).

Cancer is inherently heterogeneous, and this diversity poses a significant challenge for molecular profiling in current clinical practices (Kazerooni et al., 2021). Often, only "small samples of cancer tissue are analysed, which fails to capture the full diversity and complexity of the tumour (Saxena et al., 2021). This limitation makes it difficult to continuously track molecular changes within tumours over time and across different regions (Alizadeh et al., 2015; Marusyk & Polyak, 2010). Moreover, histopathological samples may not accurately reflect the full anatomical and physiological features of solid tumours, further complicating treatment decisions.

Medical imaging has emerged as a crucial tool in cancer diagnosis and treatment planning. Recently, there has been a growing body of research focused on using imaging-derived biomarkers to provide non-invasive insights into cancer biology (Fass, 2008). Particularly, peritumoral regions, which are typically not surgically removed for molecular analysis, can now be studied through advanced imaging techniques. The concept of "radio genomics," which combines imaging (radiomics) with genomics, has gained significant attention as a way to integrate genomic signatures with imaging data, providing a deeper understanding of tumour heterogeneity, progression, and treatment outcomes (Obeid et al., 2017; Algohary et al., 2020).

The integration of imaging and genomic data into a unified model holds great promise for improving cancer treatment decisions. By combining multiple data types, researchers can create robust biomarkers that inform clinical decision-making processes, from predicting tumour progression to identifying patients at risk for recurrence. This evolving field of radio genomics is shaping the future of personalized cancer therapy, offering a non-invasive way to monitor tumours in real time and develop targeted treatments tailored to the specific needs of each patient (Clark et al., 2019; Gillette et al., 2020).

The objective of this study was to identify the variables that consistently contribute to the formation of early-age transverse cracks, with the goal of mitigating their occurrence in the future. To achieve this, a thorough analysis of environmental, structural, material, and other relevant factors was conducted to pinpoint the elements that consistently influence the emergence of these cracks.

Figure 1. The thorough flowchart that demonstrates how artificial intelligence is being used in precision chemotherapy for cancer.

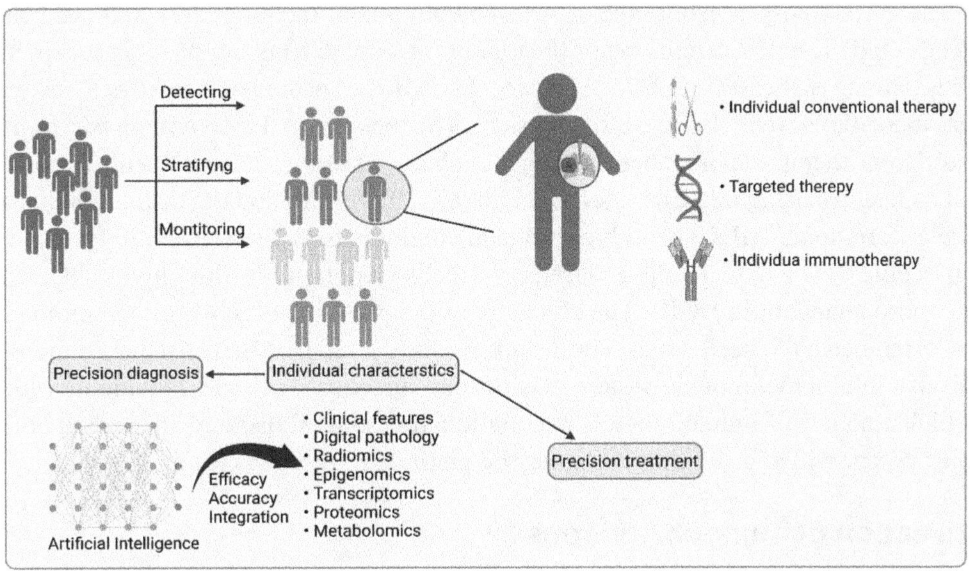

While AI has shown great promise in enhancing precision cancer medicine, it is not without its limitations. Key challenges include the availability and quality of training data, which significantly affects the accuracy of AI models. Moreover, the lack of standardization in data formats and AI algorithms complicates integration across various platforms and institutions. Additionally, regulatory approval of AI tools in healthcare remains a significant hurdle, with ongoing debates about the ethics of using AI in decision-making. As AI models become more complex, ensuring transparency and interpretability becomes increasingly important. Finally, the integration of AI into clinical workflows presents challenges, requiring substantial infrastructure and training.

2. THE INTERACTION OF AI AND CANCER IMMUNOLOGY

RNA sequencing (RNA-seq), whole exome sequencing (WES), or whole genome sequencing (WGS) are examples of NGS that have been successfully created and used to collect human whole-genome information throughout the past 20 years. NGS produces high-throughput genomic and transcriptome data more efficiently than Sanger sequencing, which paves the way for studies examining The immunological response in multiple steps. Research employing The role of immunogenomics in NGS a century not only offers a worldwide perspective of immunologic makeup of the TIME's cells using algorithms for bioinformatics, but moreover detects immunogenic proteins through the use of significant histocompatibility complicated Predicting aberrant peptides and (MHC)-peptide binding affinities, and typing for the human leukocyte antigen (HLA).

2.1 Immune Cell Quantification in Real Time

The TIME is made up of many types of immune cells. To measure the components of tumour immunological cells within the TIME, traditional techniques, like immunohistochemistry (IHC) and flow cytometry, The immunological landscape of Adenocarcinoma of the lung, neck and head cancer of the squamous cells, and clear cell carcinoma of the kidney was depicted using xCell in recent multi-omics investigations (Huang et al., 2021; Gil Del Alcazar et al., 2017; Cancer Genome Atlas Research Network, 2017). These algorithms were also used for assessing The makeup of TIME among two or more patient team with different therapy approaches, pathogenic characteristics, and treatment outcomes. Gil Del Alcazar and colleagues using CIBERSORT (Jiang et al., 2019). revealed the distinction between breast invasion ductal carcinomas (IDCs) and breast ductal carcinomas in situ (DCIS) in terms of the subset of invading T cells. CD4+ helper cells and tregs of T cells were more infiltrating in IDC, while CD8 + T cells were more abundant in DCIS. The elements of the presence of TME of carcinoma of the liver (HCC) were examined by Wheeler et al. These authors discovered that HCC tissue had more inclined to include cells that inhibit the immune system than normal surrounding tissue. In patients with HCC who medium to high amounts of immunological penetration, this study illustrated an evasion of the immune system milieu and provided proof that ICBs may be possible (Krassowski et al., 2018).

2.2 Identification of Tumour Antigens

Mutations at the levels of the transcriptome, proteome, and genome can result in the development of aberrant proteins, or tumour antigens, which immune cells can detect and activate the immune response against the tumour (Zhou, Zhu, & Liu, 2019; Li, Goedegebuure, & Gillanders, 2017; Zhou, Zhu, & Liu, 2019). Since they have a comparatively high tumoral specificity, viral antigens, carcinoma germline antibodies, and antigens unique to tumours, or neoantigens deriving from changes in somatic DNA—have emerged as the primary targets for tumour vaccines (Ehx & Perreault, 2019; Coulie, Van den Eynde, van der Bruggen, & Boon, 2014; Gubin, Artyomov, Mardis, & Schreiber, 2015; Paschen, Eichmuller, & Schadendorf, 2004; Mashl et al., 2017; Huang et al., 2018). As a result, our primary focus is on identifying certain antigens unique to tumours, especially neoantigens. As per the identification of antigens process, Technologies related to immunogenomics use in silico testing to forecast aberrant Peptides, carry out HLA typing, and estimate MHC-binding peptide affinity. These techniques are crucial for identifying tumour antigens and are highly beneficial (Table 1). In order to give a sense of confidence analysed De novo, germline, or somatic variations of possible biological importance, the genome Variant Investigation Platforms (GenomeVIP) integrates Strelka, GATK, Pindel, and BreakDancer, VarScan, or STRiP DNA in a sizable web-based user interface. This approach has been applied to initiatives involving huge data. like PanCanAtlas TCGA (Hinshaw & Shevde, 2019; Martin-Orozco et al., 2009).

Table 1. Tumor immunogenomics computational tools with high-throughput next- generation sequencing data

Tool	Function	Method	Data Type	Description
CIBERSORT	Immune Cell Quantification	Deconvolution using microarray data	Gene expression	Estimates immune cell fractions using known expression profiles
CIBERSORTx	Immune Cell Quantification	RNA-seq from single cells	RNA-seq	Extends CIBERSORT to RNA-seq data for single-cell resolution
DeconRNASeq	Immune Cell Quantification	Least square regression model	RNA-seq	Uses tissue RNA-seq data to estimate immune cell proportions
EPIC	Immune Cell Quantification	Non-negative deconvolution	RNA-seq	Estimates immune and stromal scores based on gene expression
ESTIMATE	Tumor Purity Estimation	ssGSEA-based scoring	RNA-seq	Estimates tumor purity and immune/stromal scores
FARDEEP	Immune Cell Quantification	Adaptive least trimmed squares	RNA-seq	Identifies immune cell types by eliminating outliers
MCP-counter	Immune Cell Quantification	Geometric average of gene expression	RNA-seq	Quantifies immune cells using a gene expression-based method
MuSiC	Immune Cell Quantification	Deconvolution using single-cell reference	RNA-seq	Uses single-cell RNA-seq to deconvolve bulk sequencing data
NITUMD	Immune Cell Quantification	Non-negative matrix factorization	RNA-seq	Uses a semi-supervised matrix approach for immune cell quantification
PERT	Immune Cell Quantification	Maximal likelihood-based approach	Blood specimens	Uses human umbilical blood for immune cell quantification
quanTIseq	Immune Cell Quantification	RNA-seq based quantification	RNA-seq	Quantifies 10 immune cell types using RNA-seq data
TIMER	Immune Cell Quantification	Transcriptomic data analysis	RNA-seq	Estimates immune cell composition using transcriptomic data
xCell	Immune Cell Quantification	Cell type prediction	RNA-seq	Predicts cell types and mutations using spillover compensation
CN-Learn	Variant Calling	Machine learning-based CNV detection	WES/WGS	Identifies copy number variations using machine learning
deepSNV	Variant Calling	Sub-clonal SNV detection	NGS	Detects low-frequency SNVs in mixed populations
DeepVariant	Variant Calling	Neural network-based SNP and INDEL caller	NGS	Uses deep learning for precise SNP and INDEL calling
EBCall	Variant Calling	Error separation for somatic mutations	NGS	Differentiates sequencing errors from somatic mutations
GATK	Variant Calling	SNP and INDEL detection	WES/WGS/RNA-seq	Industry standard for variant calling in NGS data
LoFreq	Variant Calling	Low-frequency mutation detection	NGS	Identifies mutations with very low allele frequencies
MuTect2	Variant Calling	Somatic mutation detection	NGS	Sensitive detection of somatic mutations, particularly low-frequency

continued on following page

Table 1. Continued

Tool	Function	Method	Data Type	Description
PyroHMMsnp	Variant Calling	Bayesian SNP genotyping	NGS	Uses Bayesian techniques for homopolymer read realignment
SAMtools	Variant Calling	Variant calling from aligned data	NGS	Standard tool for calling variants

3. ROLE OF AI IN TUMOUR MICROENVIRONMENT ANALYSIS

Clinical results and the course of the disease are significantly influenced by the tumor microenvironment (TME). Fibroblasts, immunosuppressive cells, immunological effector cells, and cytokines are some of the constituents that comprise TME (Tan et al., 2020). Certain T-cell subsets provide protective immunity, such as $CD4^+$ helper & $CD8^+$ T-cells (Väyrynen et al., 2021). Our viewpoints on the difficulties and upcoming advancements required to progress the study of spatial omics will also be shared.

3.1 SP Techniques

The two main categories of SP methods metal and fluorescent labelling isotope labelling assay (Table 2) are covered in this section. These procedures vary in terms of plexing count, cost, resolution, and throughput (Feng et al., 2017).

3.1.1 Fluorescence-Labelling Techniques

Because it allows for precise and in-depth phenotyping of cells (such as polarization of macrophages conditions, myeloid cells maturation and immunological suppressively, or T cell characteristics), the approach has been frequently used for exploring the complex TME (Väyrynen et al., 2021). By utilizing closeness evaluation, Feng et al. demonstrated that CD8+ T-cells encircled by FoxP3+, an immunosuppressive and PD-L1+ cells were linked to poor Results of survival in Squamous cells in the mouth carcinomas (SCC) (Almeida et al., 2022). According to Väyrynen et al., patients with colorectal cancer (CRC) who had mature monocytic cells that are HLADR+ and CD14+ nearer to cancerous cells had higher survival rates (Schürch et al., 2020). Almeida et al. discovered that T regulatory cells or myeloid are geographically limited in initial lung malignancies using a 40-plex, a COMET assay (Schlecht et al., 2021). Additionally, the authors used machine learning (ML) to identify different myeloid cell subsets within the same TME. Schürch and colleagues used PhenoCycler data with tensor breakdown, cell type different enrichment, and canonical correlation estimation to identify nine unique cellular regions that were conserved among 35 CRC samples and linked to survival outcomes (Imaging mass cytometry services: Visikol, n.d.).

3.1.2 Metal Isotope-Labelling Techniques

Stable metal isotopes are used in metal-based techniques to substitute for fluorophores (Schapiro et al., 2017). Either ion beams or laser scanning are used to detect isotope signals in order to assess protein expression. Endogenous metals can significantly reduce background noise and autofluorescence (Bouzekri, Esch, & Ornatsky, 2019). High-quality scanner Ablation by laser with a fixed longitudinal 1,000 nm resolution is used in Mass cytometry imaging (IMC) (the conventional Bio Tools, USA) to measure up to 50 biomarkers at the subcellular level utilizing fresh frozen tissues (FF/FFPE) (Jackson et al., 2020; Ali et al., 2020a; Pilard et al., 2021). Ali et al. discovered heterotypic areas of a certain Myofibroblast characteristics that was linked to poor results in breast cancer (BC) using 37-plex IMC (Havel et al., 2019). These MIBI investigations have made substantial application of machine learning methods to quickly investigate and analyse data in order to find new information. Having explored AI's role in understanding the tumor immune microenvironment, the next section will focus on the application of AI in biomarker discovery for improving immunotherapy outcomes.

Table 2. An overview of SP & ST methods and the TME analysis applications that go along with them

Technique	Detection	Vendor	Technology	Plexing	Tissue Type	Software	Applications for TME
Opal-based multiplex IHC	Proteins	Akoya Biosciences	Fluorescence labeling	9	FFPE	InForm	Deep phenotyping of immune cells in CRC and pancreatic cancers (Sheng et al., 2022; Väyrynen et al., 2021a; Väyrynen et al., 2021b)
COMET	Proteins	Lunaphore	Cyclic fluorescence	40	FF/FFPE	Phenoplex	Identifying myeloid/ Treg cells in early lung malignancies (Almeida et al., 2022)
PhenoCycler	Proteins	Akoya Biosciences	Cyclic fluorescence	50	FF/FFPE	PhenoCycler MAV	Unique cellular neighborhoods in colorectal cancer (Schürch et al., 2020)
IMC	Proteins	Standard BioTools	Metal-based labeling	50	FF/FFPE	Phenoplex	Investigating myofibroblast phenotypes in breast cancer (Ali et al., 2020a)

continued on following page

Table 2. Continued

Technique	Detection	Vendor	Technology	Plexing	Tissue Type	Software	Applications for TME
MIBI	Proteins	Ionpath	Metal-based labeling	100	FF/FFPE	MIBItracker Software	TME analysis in ovarian carcinoma and triple-negative breast cancer (Ptacek et al., 2020)
Visium	RNA	10X Genomics	NGS	18,000	FF/FFPE	Spaceranger	Studying immune responses in CRC and hepatocellular cancer (Keren et al., 2018; Lau et al., 2022)
GeoMx DSP	RNA/Proteins	nanoString	NGS	100+ (protein) / 18,000 (RNA)	FF/FFPE	GeoMx DSP Suite	ICI resistance and CD66b expression in lung cancer (Moutafi et al., 2022)
Slide-Seq/ Seeker	RNA	Curio Bioscience	NGS	Whole Transcriptome	FF	-	TCR clonotypic impacts in lung cancer under IO treatment (Liu et al., 2021)
Stereo-seq	RNA	Beijing Genomic Institute	NGS	Whole Transcriptome	FF/FFPE	Stereo-seq Workflow	Immune response and survival predictions in colorectal cancer (Zhang et al., 2022)

4. AI IN BIOMARKER DISCOVERY FOR IMMUNOTHERAPY

Despite the abundance of molecular tests & targeted treatment choices, there are currently few isolated biomarkers capable of accurately divide into strata individuals who are responsive to targeted treatments and ICIs, including sorts of tumors like BC, CRC, and NSCLC (Aldea et al., 2021; Xie et al., 2020; Lièvre et al., 2006; André et al., 2020). Examples of highly predictive markers include the presence of KRAS mutations in CRC patients receiving monoclonal antibodies against EGFR (Unger & Kather, 2024a)., and MSI in CRC patients receiving ICI treatment (Unger & Kather, 2024a) Because of this, a number of research have looked into creating End-to-end AI-based solutions that use genetic data to directly discover patterns linked to response or prognosis (Elmarakeby et al., 2021).

4.1 Biomarkers Derived From Genetic Data Using AI

Due mostly to the practical limitations of integrating large-scale sequencing into standard clinical practice, the invention of AI-driven techniques for processing Transcriptomic and genomic data have been very restricted till recently (Zuo et al., 2021). In the instance of physiologically informed biomarkers based on AI computational preclinical models detection as well as clinical estimation in prostate carcinoma have been developed using molecular data from genetic information (Anaya et al., 2024). More sophisticated techniques are able to use raw DNA sequence data to forecast treatment response and patient prognosis (Qiu et al., 2020; Zeng et al., 2023; Eweje et al., 2024).

4.2 Medical Imaging Biomarkers Powered by AI

Recent research in the field of digital pathology has created AI-driven techniques for the patient classification straight from the H&E slides in order to maximize therapy choices (Ahn et al., 2024; Ligero et al., 2021; Dercle et al., 2022). Similar results have been seen in the field of radiology, where earlier research has demonstrated the usefulness of using baseline radiology pictures, such as MRI (magnetic resonance imaging) and computed tomography (CT) scans, to predict treatment response (Zhou et al., 2023; Jin et al., 2021; Mu et al., 2020; Jiang et al., 2023; Lao et al., 2017). or the prognosis of the patient (Crispin-Ortuzar et al., 2023; Boehm et al., 2022). with DL. Furthermore, pathology-only and AI models based solely on genetics benefit from the additional layer of information provided by both the temporal and spatial resolution of radiology images, which enhances response prediction (Vanguri et al., 2022; Jiang et al., 2023; Renc et al., 2024).

4.3 AI-Based Biomarkers From HER

This method may make it easier to find people with metastatic illness who would benefit more from supportive care than from more aggressive therapies. However, the disordered form of the data gathered in EHRs usually limits the use of patient clinical history. However, with the growing creation of novel technology inside the area of LLMs, such information may have been employed more widely. LLM-based systems have demonstrated encouraging outcomes in recent research for predicting readmissions, comorbidity indices, and in-patient mortality, among other outcomes (Nishino, Ramaiya, Hatabu, & Hodi, 2017; Anagnostou, Landon, Medina, Forde, & Velculescu, 2022). whereby pre-trained LLMs can use prompt engineering to discover new prediction tasks using a few instances of the intended tasks. As a result, we can use more generalist models to teach particular tasks without requiring big datasets. As a result, the only LLM tools on the market right now are specialized tools for automating straightforward clinical procedures that don't need FDA approval or CE-IVD labeling. The introduction of AI in cancer treatment raises several ethical and regulatory issues. Key concerns include the privacy and security of patient data used to train AI models, the potential for algorithmic bias, and the need for regulatory oversight. AI in healthcare must undergo rigorous validation and regulatory approval by agencies such as the FDA to ensure safety and efficacy. The role of AI in clinical decision-making also raises ethical questions about accountability and the potential for over-reliance on automated systems. A transparent regulatory framework is crucial to ensure AI tools are used ethically and effectively.

5. AI ENHANCED IMMUNOTHERAPY STRATEGIES

The overall approach to employing AI to forecast immunotherapy effectiveness (fig.2) The three primary immunotherapy techniques currently in use are peripatetic immunotherapy, chimeric protein receptor T-cell treatment for immunological checkpoint inhibitors and tumor vaccinations (ICIs) (Benjamens, Dhunnoo, & Mesko, 2020). A significant portion of patients have found success with these treatments, particularly ICI usage like PD-1 and CTLA-4, which significantly improves the current clinical oncology treatments (Lancellotti et al., 2021). The use of machine learning (AI) in medical care has grown dramatically in recent years (Fridman, Pages, Sautes-Fridman, & Galon, 2012).

Figure 2. The process for predicting the effectiveness of immunotherapy using AI.

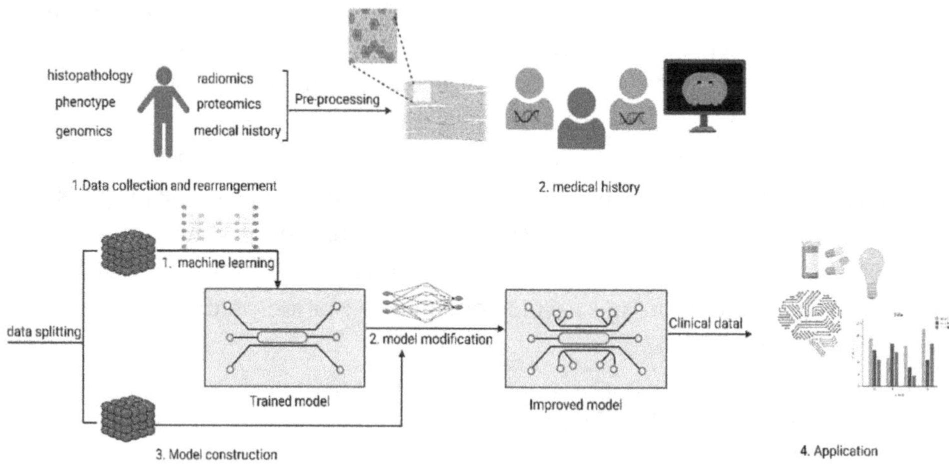

Gathering multiscale medical data, such as diseased tissue, genomes, proteomics, Among other things, CT/MR imaging-omics is the first stage. Gathering, separating, extracting, filtering, and choosing features are the next phases. Next, divide these data separated into two distinct groups, with one for instruction and one for validation. After that, given the AI the training cohort's data so it may learn and model it. After that, use the verification group to confirm the learning outcomes. Lastly, a model that may be used in clinical settings will be created.

5.1 AI Uses Histopathological Features to Predict How Well Immunotherapy Will Work

AI-based digital pathology is currently being utilized to diagnose and treat tumors with success (Wang et al., 2022). tumor-infiltrating lymphocytes and the tumor-stroma ratio (TSR) (the TIL), immunohistochemistry (IHC) studies, and unpredictability of microsatellite are among the most studied of these. By attaching to PD-1 in T cells, cancerous cells producing PD-L1 has the ability to suppress the immune system.; ICIs are an anticancer tactic to prevent this interaction. Studies have indicated a connection between immunotherapy responsiveness and clinical outcomes and PD-L1 expression levels. Furthermore, numerous investigations have demonstrated a correlation between enhanced immune checkpoint blockage and increased T-cell infiltration & T-cell numbers (Dercle et al., 2022).

5.2 AI Uses Imaging-Omics Information to Forecast the Effectiveness of Immunotherapy

Furthermore, trustworthy non-invasive indicators of assessing reaction to immunotherapy can be obtained using AI-based predictive algorithms. The PD-L1 expression has been extensively verified in immunotherapy among a variety of biomarkers, and Levels of PD-L1 expression can be non-invasively assessed using a combination model that uses CT radiomics & clinical characteristics (Van Allen et al., 2015). Out of a theoretical highest possible rating of 36 points, the Radiomics Quality Score (RQS) of most studies often fell between 11 and 20 (Kymriah, 2022). It suggests that, especially in the lack of histopathology materials, AI-driven imaging-omics research can explore The temporal and spatial complexity of Cancer and is crucial in forecasting immunotherapy reaction, biomarker expression, & patient prognosis.

5.3 AI Uses Genomes to Predict the Effectiveness of Immunotherapy

Over 3 billion of base pairs make up the genome of humans, which is a huge area of highly dimensional data with extremely complex information. The most thorough information about the genome may be obtained through whole genome sequencing (WGS), but AI, especially deep learning approaches, are needed to sort out the genes, phenotypes, & their inter-regulatory interactions Allen et al. (Tecartus, 2022) discovered a connection between TMB & cytolytic indicators as well as the individual rate of response to antiCTLA4. These investigations offered guidance for investigating the varying reactions to immune check point inhibitors as well as discovering predictive indicators.

6. AI DRIVEN CAR-T CELL THERAPY DESIGN

A possible therapy for acute lymphoma and leukaemia is CAR-T cell therapy. Advanced Treatment medicinal products (ATMPs) are becoming more significant in recent years as a means of treating cellular and genetic disorders. CAR-T cell therapy is one treatment now being used to treat acute lymphoma and leukaemia. Unlike conventional therapies for cancer, CAR-T cell therapy enables precise tumor cell targeting (Yescarta, 2022; Dhariwal & Mehta, 2017; Rodrigues et al., 2021). Although autologous treatments have received clinical approval, there are still issues with production and widespread use. These difficulties are depicted along the six primary stages of CAR-T cell treatment in Figure 3.

By allowing them to create CAR-T cells right at their point of care, artificial intelligence and automation integration need the second transition of hospitals becoming smart production hospitals. A hospital that specializes in ATMPs and integrates a comprehensive automated production platform for individualized care in a nearby GMP facility is known as a "smart manufacturing hospital" (Uslu et al., 2020; European Medicines Agency, 2017; Freitag et al., 2020).

Figure 3. Obstacles to the widespread use of autologous CAR-T cells for therapy

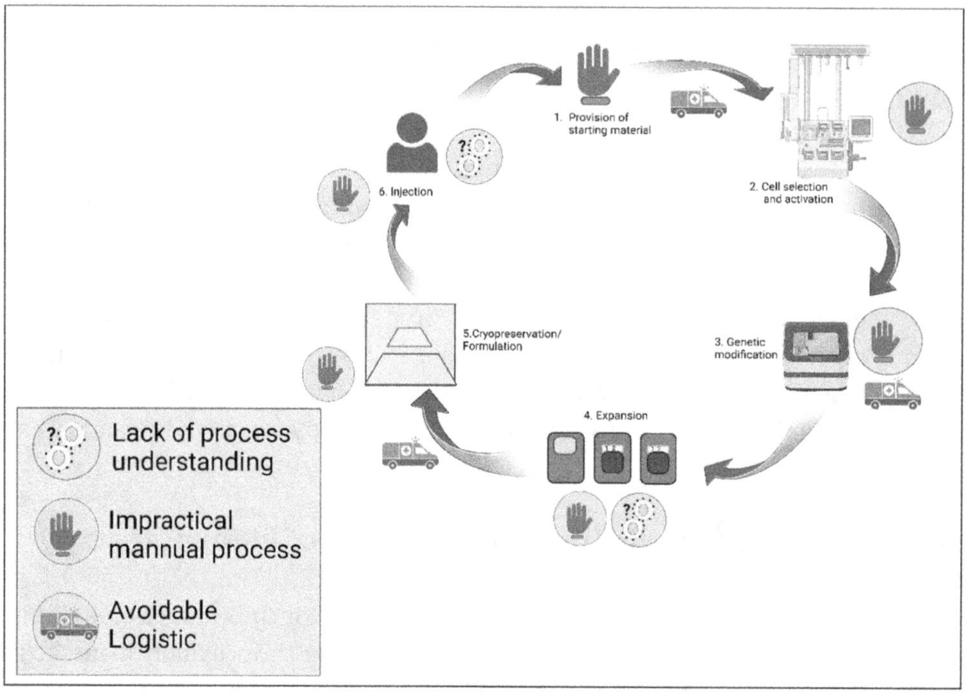

7. AUTOMATED AI-POWERED CAR-T CELL PRODUCTION

All necessary hardware, including equipment and gadgets, must be combined to create one integrated process pipeline in order to automate the manufacturing of autologous CAR-T cell treatment. There are various barriers to automation in the CAR-T cell process. First of all, it must be carried out in accordance with Good Manufacturing Practice, or GMP, and under aseptic settings since it is an ATMP production process (Turtle et al., 2016). T cell treatment will be developed. Given that a hospital cares for a wide range of patients with various demands, the platform must support numerous ATMP products and make it simple to integrate new ones (Egri et al., 2020). Therefore, both viral & non-viral approaches should be supported by a manufacturing platform that is widely accepted. Additionally, research has demonstrated the effectiveness of treatments utilizing CAR-T cells with both CD4 or CD8+ (Roland Berger GmbH, 2021).

7.1 Artificial Intelligence in Manufacturing of Car-T Cells

AI can learn important process details about the properties and actions of the cell. Additionally, by streamlining production scheduling and resource management, AI can help the smart manufacturing hospital's economic platform function. As a result, AIDPATH will create several AI applications during the production and treatment of CART cells. The platform's manufacturing process can be optimally integrated into the therapy process through adaptive scheduling (Joshi et al., 2021). However, future work in AIDPATH will focus on a health economic evaluation of this idea. However, it is necessary to debate the future coexistence of decentralized and centralized CAR-T cell production. The operator model is another topic that remains up for debate. All things considered, this is an intriguing concept that will require additional development and adaptation to the quickly evolving cell and gene therapy market in the upcoming years (Weenk et al., 2020). Since the treatment with CAR-T cells is just the start of ATMP creation and execution, the emphasis here must be upon the concept's transferability.

8. AI-POWERED MONITORING OF PATIENTS REMOTELY

With The application of adaptable components for wearable sensors, RPM (remote patient monitoring) is a quickly expanding sector of medicine that aims to give doctors more assistance in providing treatment in numerous general hospitals surgical and medical wards (Heijmans et al., 2019; Dias & Cunha, 2018). This is accomplished by using the new Network of Things, or IoT, approaches in the medical field, like telehealth applications (Malasinghe et al., 2017).Wearable technology (Shaik et al., 2022a) and sensors that rely on contact (Shaik et al., 2022b). In order to help with therapeutic decisions or strategies for problems like movement disorders and psychological conditions, RPM is frequently used to evaluate critical indicators or additional physiological variables like motion detection (Miller & Brown, 2018; Schnyer et al., 2017). In order to describe an illness and its prognosis, algorithms based on AI have been used to analyse medical images or connect clinical data to symptoms or biomarkers (Bousefsaf et al., 2019a; Cho et al., 2017a).Traditional patient health status monitoring practices have been revolutionized by advances that allow for remote patient monitoring in hospitals, healthcare facilities, assisted living facilities, as well as in patients' residences. RPM enabled by technology designs are covered in this section.

8.1 Monitoring Via Video

A patient's region of interest (ROI), like facial landmarks, was identified Using image and video processing techniques in machine learning. The ROI was then used to predict essential indicators, including heart rate and breathing rate (Khalid et al., 2022a). tracked the pulse rate patterns of patients in a region of interest (ROI) of a video frame by observing the variations in motion when breathing. Considering the respiratory patterns identified during camera surveillance, (Bousefsaf et al., 2019b) Convolutional neural network models (CNN), a deep learning model, were created to identify people's psychological stress levels. Auscultation sounds were used for cough analysis, and a pretrained three-dimensional ResNet18 neural network framework was used to categorize the sounds into illness groups. The model's accuracy, sensitivity, and specificity were 94.57%, 100%, and 94.11%, respectively. Remote Photoplethysmography (rPPG), which was identified within a frame of a video taken by a basic smartphone camera, was used to assess heart rate, the blood volume pulse, and SpO2 (Cho et al., 2017b). Table 3 also includes studies that examined the advantages and disadvantages of telemedicine.

Table 3. Telehealth monitoring

Algorithm	Technology	Advantages	Disadvantages	Reference
3D-CNN	RGB camera	Better availability and promptness of care	Healthcare providers incur higher costs when telehealth services are overused or misused.	(Khalid et al., 2022b)
CNN	Thermal camera	Emergency preparedness		(Laurie et al., 2021)
DFT, CWT	Sensor, RGB camera	Cost-effectiveness		(Hui & Kan, 2017a)
Control of exposure	Sensor, RGB camera	Decreased availability of doctors and patients–demand mismatch	Disparities between rural and urban populations.	(Sharma & Kan, 2018a)

8.2 IoT-Capable Gadgets

Continuous patient monitoring could be accomplished with the use of Real-time monitoring based on the Internet of things of patients remotely system (Yew et al., 2020). Wearable sensors & their reader antennas could be connected to the surveillance network via the Internet of Things. Physiological measures are among the many kinds of wearable physiological monitoring technologies, together with their structures and requirements, from mobility assessment and cardiac implanted devices to electrocardiograms, oxygen in the blood saturation, blood sugar levels, skin perspiration, or capnography (Dias & Cunha, 2018). Additionally, the devices can be worn as adhesive patches, chest straps, or wearable t-shirts. Healthcare workers or medical personnel would handle the patient appropriately and prevent unusual occurrences. Researchers at Cornell University have designed and created non-invasive electronic devices with NCS to improve patient comfort and lessen its impact on daily activities (Hui & Kan, 2017b; Sharma & Kan, 2018b). The Internet of Things gadgets utilized by the study field for patient monitoring are shown in Table 4, along with an explanation of their benefits and drawbacks.

Table 4. Monitoring the Internet of Things, or IoT, gadgets

Algorithm	Technology	Advantage	Disadvantage	References
	Bluetooth, Wi-Fi, Lora, ZigBee, and wireless sensors	Make individualized health monitoring possible	Patient privacy concerns	(El-Rashidy et al., 2021
SVM model	NCS, RFID Passive tags	Non-invasive monitoring	High dependence on the internet	(Sharma & Kan, 2018c)
SVM model	RFID passive tags and NCS	Continuous health monitoring		(Hui & Kan, 2018)

9. METHODS OF MULTI-OMICS INTEGRATION

Different classifications for the integration of multi-omics techniques have been established by a number of recent reviews, 2019, (Rappoport & Shamir, 2019). outlined the three approaches early, late, and middle integration that are employed in cancer subdividing research projects. Subramanian et al.

in 2020 (Subramanian et al., 2020). identified five non-exclusive multi-omics integration techniques: fusion, Bayesian, network, correlation, similarity, and multivariate (Picard et al., 2021a). categorized early, mixed, intermediate, late, or hierarchical Integration of multi-omics techniques for applications using machine learning. Since machine learning is the main topic of our examined works, we will categorize the integration techniques employed in the studies using the framework proposed by Picard et al. (see Fig. 4).

9.1 Dimensionality Reduction

The majority of articles included some kind of reduction in dimensionality to minimize the size of the feature, regardless of the particular multi-omics integration techniques employed space. We distinguish between two types of dimensionality reduction in accordance with Picard et al.: a) feature extraction, which involves converting the unique attributes to a fresh feature space in order to construct a learnt feature embedding, and b) feature selection, which involves eliminating irrelevant or noisy features. Principal component analysis (PCA) or autoencoders are the most often utilized feature extraction techniques in the examined studies. There are three types of feature selection methods: embedded, wrapper-based, and filter-based (Picard et al., 2021b).

Figure 4. An example of the generic structure for early, mixed, and intermediate integration.

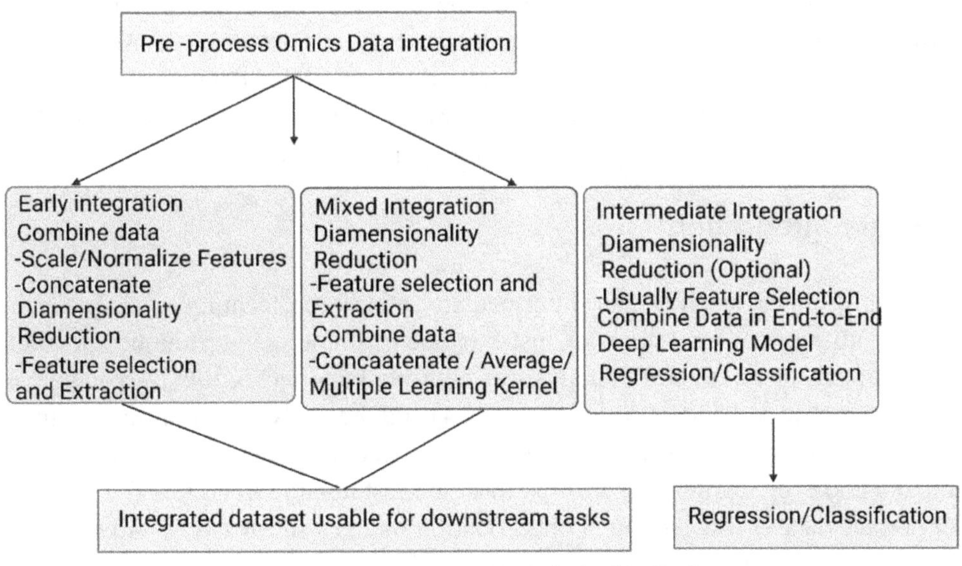

A general sequence of stages for any multi-omics integrating category is depicted in the picture.

Depending on the framework type, the integration procedure varies following fundamental omics modality-specific data pre-processing. Prior to completing dimensionality reduction, which may include feature selection and/or extraction, early integration entails first merging the data, typically by concatenation. decrease of dimensionality for each omics modality separately is the first step in mixed integration, after which the data is combined using one of several methods. Also, the intermediate integration framework illustrates end-to-end models that integrate the omics data in a single neural network, but this is not the only process for intermediate integration.

9.2 Initial Integration

Some of the publications that were assessed employed early integration techniques (Huang et al., 2021; Xu et al., 2021). Thus, following fundamental omics-specific pre-processing, they integrated extensive multi-omics information into one feature matrix.. Scaling and normalizing the initial characteristics were frequently a part of the early integration. The dataset comprising all omics" modalities was then subjected to dimensionality reduction as a whole, as opposed to one at a time. As an illustration, (Zhang et al., 2018). combined RNA sequence information and previously processed gene-level CNV data into a single matrix. They employed feature extraction techniques like autoencoder and PCA to get from that matrix, a 100-feature embedding was created. The highest useful characteristics for survival after cancer were then selected using Cox regression based on the embedding.

9.3 Mixed Integration

Following omics-specific data pretreatment, the reduction of dimensionality was carried out for every distinct omics modality separately. Through concatenation, averaging, and other techniques, this processed information were merged into one dataset. Autoencoders were the most widely used feature extraction technique (Ma et al., 2020). We incorporate data on the variance of each dataset and learn new features by non-linearly transforming the fundamental characteristics from each omics dataset (Tong et al., 2020). Concatenating the space generated by the autoencoder time embedded data of all the omics modalities (ConcatAE) was the best-performing integration technique that the authors examined. A downstream tumor survival prediction task was then performed using this merged dataset.

9.4 Intermediate Integration

While processing omics-specific data, intermediate integration techniques also take into account information from other omics modalities. iCluster is one example of a technique specifically created for data integration (Shen et al., 2009). Analysis of multiple factors (MOFA) (Argelaguet et al., 2018) Fusion of similarity networks (SNF) (Wang et al., 2014) and the analysis of multiple co-inertia (MCIA) (Meng et al., 2014) Although They weren't frequently employed in the examined studies, the employment from beginning to end deep learning algorithms was the most notable trend found for integration in the middle. Every omics dataset was fed into a classification model's sub-network. Advanced multi-omics characteristics for categorization were learned using information from both inside and across omics datasets since the omics information is incorporated into the identical model.

10. CONCLUSION

The tumor immune microenvironment (TIME) is essential for immunotherapy, seeking to move the immune response from pro-tumor to anti-tumor, thereby enhancing therapeutic effectiveness. Enhancing this atmosphere is essential for improving therapy results with the rise of precision medicine, molecular profiling through high-throughput technologies such as genomics, transcriptomics, proteomics, epigenomics, cytomics, and informatics has become essential. These approaches yield essential insights into tumor biology, facilitating the identification of biomarkers that affect therapeutic response. TIME includes tumor-specific antigens, viruses, tumor germline antibodies, and neoantigens, which act as major targets for tumor vaccines and immune checkpoint inhibitors (ICBs). Recognizing these interactions is essential for the progression of efficient immunotherapies.

This chapter highlighted the role of AI in transforming cancer treatment through precision medicine. AI applications such as tumor profiling, biomarker discovery, and patient monitoring have the potential to significantly improve treatment outcomes. However, challenges such as data quality, regulatory hurdles, and ethical considerations must be addressed to maximize AI's benefits in clinical settings. Future research should focus on overcoming these obstacles and refining AI tools for broader clinical application.

REFERENCES

Ahn, B., Moon, D., Kim, H.-S., Lee, C., Cho, N. H., Choi, H.-K., Kim, D., Lee, J.-Y., Nam, E. J., Won, D., An, H. J., Kwon, S. Y., Shin, S.-J., Jung, H. R., Kwon, D., Park, H., Kim, M., Cha, Y. J., Park, H., & Park, E. (2024). Histopathologic image-based deep learning classifier for predicting platinum-based treatment responses in high-grade serous ovarian cancer. *Nature Communications*, *15*(1), 4253. DOI: 10.1038/s41467-024-48667-6 PMID: 38762636

Aldea, M., Andre, F., Marabelle, A., Dogan, S., Barlesi, F., & Soria, J.-C. (2021). Overcoming resistance to tumor-targeted and immune-targeted therapies. *Cancer Discovery*, *11*(4), 874–899. DOI: 10.1158/2159-8290.CD-20-1638 PMID: 33811122

Algohary, A., Shiradkar, R., Pahwa, S., Purysko, A., Verma, S., Moses, D., Shnier, R., Haynes, A.-M., Delprado, W., Thompson, J., Tirumani, S., Mahran, A., Rastinehad, A. R., Ponsky, L., Stricker, P. D., & Madabhushi, A. (2020). Combination of peri-tumoral and intra-tumoral radiomic features on bi-parametric MRI accurately stratifies prostate cancer risk: A multi-site study. *Cancers (Basel)*, *12*(7), 2200. DOI: 10.3390/cancers12082200 PMID: 32781640

Ali, H. R., Jackson, H. W., Zanotelli, V. R. T., Danenberg, E., Fischer, J. R., Bardwell, H., Provenzano, E., Ali, H. R., Al Sa'd, M., Alon, S., Aparicio, S., Battistoni, G., Balasubramanian, S., Becker, R., Bodenmiller, B., Boyden, E. S., Bressan, D., Bruna, A., Marcel, B., & Bodenmiller, B. (2020). Imaging mass cytometry and multiplatform genomics define the phenogenomic landscape of breast cancer. *Nature Cancer*, *1*(2), 163–175. DOI: 10.1038/s43018-020-0026-6 PMID: 35122013

Ali, H. R., Jackson, H. W., Zanotelli, V. R. T., Danenberg, E., Fischer, J. R., Bardwell, H., Provenzano, E., Ali, H. R., Al Sa'd, M., Alon, S., Aparicio, S., Battistoni, G., Balasubramanian, S., Becker, R., Bodenmiller, B., Boyden, E. S., Bressan, D., Bruna, A., Marcel, B., & Bodenmiller, B. (2020). Imaging mass cytometry and multiplatform genomics define the phenogenomic landscape of breast cancer. *Nature Cancer*, *1*(2), 163–175. DOI: 10.1038/s43018-020-0026-6 PMID: 35122013

Alizadeh, A. A., Aranda, V., Bardelli, A., Blanpain, C., Bock, C., Borowski, C., Caldas, C., Califano, A., Doherty, M., Elsner, M., Esteller, M., Fitzgerald, R., Korbel, J. O., Lichter, P., Mason, C. E., Navin, N., Pe'er, D., Polyak, K., Roberts, C. W. M., & Zucman-Rossi, J. (2015). Toward understanding and exploiting tumor heterogeneity. *Nature Medicine*, *21*(8), 846–853. DOI: 10.1038/nm.3915 PMID: 26248267

Ally, A., Balasundaram, M., Carlsen, R., Chuah, E., Clarke, A., Dhalla, N., Holt, R. A., Jones, S. J. M., Lee, D., Ma, Y., Marra, M. A., Mayo, M., Moore, R. A., Mungall, A. J., Schein, J. E., Sipahimalani, P., Tam, A., Thiessen, N., Cheung, D., & Laird, P. W.Cancer Genome Atlas Research Network. (2017). Comprehensive and integrative genomic characterization of hepatocellular carcinoma. *Cell*, *169*(7), 1327–1341.e1323. DOI: 10.1016/j.cell.2017.05.046 PMID: 28622513

Almeida, P. M., Rivest, F., Juppet, Q., Kowal, J., Pelz, B., Cassano, M., Eroglu, D., & Dupouy, D. (2022). Abstract 1716: Mapping the cellular architecture of the tumor microenvironment by integrating hyperplex immunofluorescence and automated image analysis. *Cancer Research*, *82*(12, Supplement), 1716. DOI: 10.1158/1538-7445.AM2022-1716

Almeida, P. M., Rivest, F., Juppet, Q., Kowal, J., Pelz, B., Cassano, M., Eroglu, D., & Dupouy, D. (2022). Abstract 1716: Mapping the cellular architecture of the tumor microenvironment by integrating hyperplex immunofluorescence and automated image analysis. *Cancer Research*, *82*(12, Supplement), 1716. DOI: 10.1158/1538-7445.AM2022-1716

Anagnostou, V., Landon, B. V., Medina, J. E., Forde, P., & Velculescu, V. E. (2022). Translating the evolving molecular landscape of tumors to biomarkers of response for cancer immunotherapy. *Science Translational Medicine*, *14*(670), eabo3958. Advance online publication. DOI: 10.1126/scitranslmed.abo3958 PMID: 36350985

Anaya, J., Sidhom, J.-W., Mahmood, F., & Baras, A. S. (2024). Multiple-instance learning of somatic mutations for the classification of tumor type and the prediction of microsatellite status. *Nature Biomedical Engineering*, *8*(1), 57–67. DOI: 10.1038/s41551-023-01120-3 PMID: 37919367

André, T., Shiu, K.-K., Kim, T. W., Jensen, B. V., Jensen, L. H., Punt, C., Smith, D., Garcia-Carbonero, R., Benavides, M., Gibbs, P., de la Fouchardiere, C., Rivera, F., Elez, E., Bendell, J., Le, D. T., Yoshino, T., Van Cutsem, E., Yang, P., Farooqui, M. Z. H., & Diaz, L. A.Jr. (2020). Pembrolizumab in microsatellite-instability-high advanced colorectal cancer. *The New England Journal of Medicine*, *383*(23), 2207–2218. DOI: 10.1056/NEJMoa2017699 PMID: 33264544

Argelaguet, R., Velten, B., Arnol, D., Dietrich, S., Zenz, T., Marioni, J. C., Buettner, F., Huber, W., & Stegle, O. (2018). Multi-omics factor analysis—A framework for unsupervised integration of multi-omics datasets. *Molecular Systems Biology*, *14*(6), e8124. DOI: 10.15252/msb.20178124 PMID: 29925568

Benjamens, S., Dhunnoo, P., & Mesko, B. (2020). The state of artificial intelligence-based FDA-approved medical devices and algorithms: An online database. *NPJ Digital Medicine*, *3*(1), 118. DOI: 10.1038/s41746-020-00324-0 PMID: 32984550

Bodalal, Z., Trebeschi, S., Nguyen-Kim, T. D. L., Schats, W., & Beets-Tan, R. (2019). Radiogenomics: Bridging imaging and genomics. *Abdominal Radiology*, *44*(12), 1960–1984. DOI: 10.1007/s00261-019-02028-w PMID: 31049614

Boehm, K. M., Aherne, E. A., Ellenson, L., Nikolovski, I., Alghamdi, M., Vázquez-García, I., Zamarin, D., Long Roche, K., Liu, Y., Patel, D., Aukerman, A., Pasha, A., Rose, D., Selenica, P., Causa Andrieu, P. I., Fong, C., Capanu, M., Reis-Filho, J. S., Vanguri, R., & Shah, S. P. (2022). Multimodal data integration using machine learning improves risk stratification of high-grade serous ovarian cancer. *Nature Cancer*, *3*(7), 723–733. DOI: 10.1038/s43018-022-00388-9 PMID: 35764743

Bousefsaf, F., Pruski, A., & Maaoui, C. (2019). 3D convolutional neural networks for remote pulse rate measurement and mapping from facial video. *Applied Sciences (Basel, Switzerland)*, *9*(20), 4364. DOI: 10.3390/app9204364

Bouzekri, A., Esch, A., & Ornatsky, O. (2019). Multidimensional profiling of drug-treated cells by imaging mass cytometry. *FEBS Open Bio*, *9*(9), 1652–1669. DOI: 10.1002/2211-5463.12692 PMID: 31250984

Butterfield, L. H. (2015). Cancer vaccines. *BMJ (Clinical Research Ed.)*, *350*(apr22 14), h988. DOI: 10.1136/bmj.h988 PMID: 25904595

Chandran, S. S., & Klebanoff, C. A. (2019). T cell receptor-based cancer immunotherapy: Emerging efficacy and pathways of resistance. *Immunological Reviews*, *290*(1), 127–147. DOI: 10.1111/imr.12772 PMID: 31355495

Chen, D. S., & Mellman, I. (2013). Oncology meets immunology: The cancer-immunity cycle. *Immunity*, *39*(1), 1–10. DOI: 10.1016/j.immuni.2013.07.012 PMID: 23890059

Cho, Y., Bianchi-Berthouze, N., & Julier, S. J. (2017). DeepBreath: Deep learning of breathing patterns for automatic stress recognition using low-cost thermal imaging in unconstrained settings. In *2017 Seventh International Conference on Affective Computing and Intelligent Interaction (ACII)*. IEEE. https://doi.org/DOI: 10.1109/ACII.2017.8273639

Clark, D. J., Dhanasekaran, S. M., Petralia, F., Pan, J., Song, X., Hu, Y., da Veiga Leprevost, F., Reva, B., Lih, T.-S. M., Chang, H.-Y., Ma, W., Huang, C., Ricketts, C. J., Chen, L., Krek, A., Li, Y., Rykunov, D., Li, Q. K., Chen, L. S., & Tu, Z. (2019). Integrated proteogenomic characterization of clear cell renal cell carcinoma. *Cell*, *179*(4), 964–983.e931. DOI: 10.1016/j.cell.2019.10.007 PMID: 31675502

Coulie, P. G., Van den Eynde, B. J., van der Bruggen, P., & Boon, T. (2014). Tumor antigens recognized by T lymphocytes: At the core of cancer immunotherapy. *Nature Reviews. Cancer*, *14*(2), 135–146. DOI: 10.1038/nrc3670 PMID: 24457417

Crispin-Ortuzar, M., Woitek, R., Reinius, M. A. V., Moore, E., Beer, L., Bura, V., Rundo, L., McCague, C., Ursprung, S., Escudero Sanchez, L., Martin-Gonzalez, P., Mouliere, F., Chandrananda, D., Morris, J., Goranova, T., Piskorz, A. M., Singh, N., Sahdev, A., Pintican, R., & Brenton, J. D. (2023). Integrated radiogenomics models predict response to neoadjuvant chemotherapy in high-grade serous ovarian cancer. *Nature Communications*, *14*(1), 6756. DOI: 10.1038/s41467-023-41820-7 PMID: 37875466

Dercle, L., McGale, J., Sun, S., Marabelle, A., Yeh, R., Deutsch, E., Mokrane, F.-Z., Farwell, M., Ammari, S., Schoder, H., Zhao, B., & Schwartz, L. H. (2022). Artificial intelligence and radiomics: Fundamentals, applications, and challenges in immunotherapy. *Journal for Immunotherapy of Cancer*, *10*(9), e005292. DOI: 10.1136/jitc-2022-005292 PMID: 36180071

Dhariwal, K., & Mehta, A. (2017). Architecture and plan of smart hospital based on internet of things. *International Research Journal of Engineering and Technology*, *4*(6), 1976–1980.

Dias, D., & Cunha, J. P. S. (2018). Wearable health devices—Vital sign monitoring, systems and technologies. *Sensors (Basel)*, *18*(8), 2414. DOI: 10.3390/s18082414 PMID: 30044415

Ding, L., Wendl, M. C., Koboldt, D. C., & Mardis, E. R. (2010). Analysis of next-generation genomic data in cancer: Accomplishments and challenges. *Human Molecular Genetics*, *19*(R2), R188–R196. DOI: 10.1093/hmg/ddq391 PMID: 20843826

Egri, P., Csáji, B. C., Kis, K. B., Monostori, L., Váncza, J., Ochs, J., Jung, S., König, N., Schmitt, R., Brecher, C., Pieske, S., & Wein, S. (2020). Bio-inspired control of automated stem cell production. *Procedia CIRP*, *88*, 600–605. DOI: 10.1016/j.procir.2020.05.105

Ehx, G., & Perreault, C. (2019). Discovery and characterization of actionable tumor antigens. *Genome Medicine*, *11*(1), 29. DOI: 10.1186/s13073-019-0642-x PMID: 31039809

El-Rashidy, N., El-Sappagh, S., Islam, S. M. R., El-Bakry, H. M., & Abdelrazek, S. (2021). Mobile health in remote patient monitoring for chronic diseases: Principles, trends, and challenges. *Diagnostics (Basel), 11*(4), 607. DOI: 10.3390/diagnostics11040607 PMID: 33805471

Elmarakeby, H. A., Hwang, J., Arafeh, R., Crowdis, J., Gang, S., Liu, D., AlDubayan, S. H., Salari, K., Kregel, S., Richter, C., Arnoff, T. E., Park, J., Hahn, W. C., & Van Allen, E. M. (2021). Biologically informed deep neural network for prostate cancer discovery. *Nature, 598*(7882), 348–352. DOI: 10.1038/s41586-021-03922-4 PMID: 34552244

European Medicines Agency. (2017). New guidelines on good manufacturing practices for advanced therapies. Available at: https://www.ema.europa.eu/en/news/new-guidelines-good-manufacturing-practices-advanced-therapies (Accessed April 4, 2022).

Eweje, F., Li, Z., Gopaulchan, M., Attaranzadeh, A., Kloker, L., Jiang, Y., Diehn, M., Li, G., & Li, R. (2024). Use of artificial intelligence–based digital pathology to predict outcomes for immune checkpoint inhibitor therapy in advanced gastro-esophageal cancer. *Journal of Clinical Oncology, 42*(16_suppl), 4013. DOI: 10.1200/JCO.2024.42.16_suppl.4013

Fass, L. (2008). Imaging and cancer: A review. *Molecular Oncology, 2*(2), 115–152. DOI: 10.1016/j.molonc.2008.04.001 PMID: 19383333

Feng, Z., Bethmann, D., Kappler, M., Ballesteros-Merino, C., Eckert, A., Bell, R. B., Cheng, A., Bui, T., Leidner, R., Urba, W. J., Johnson, K., Hoyt, C., Bifulco, C. B., Bukur, J., Wickenhauser, C., Seliger, B., & Fox, B. A. (2017). Multiparametric immune profiling in HPV-oral squamous cell cancer. *JCI Insight, 2*(14), e93652. Advance online publication. DOI: 10.1172/jci.insight.93652 PMID: 28724788

Freitag, F., Maucher, M., Riester, Z., & Hudecek, M. (2020). New targets and technologies for CAR-T cells. *Current Opinion in Oncology, 32*(5), 510–517. DOI: 10.1097/CCO.0000000000000653 PMID: 32657796

Fridman, W. H., Pages, F., Sautes-Fridman, C., & Galon, J. (2012). The immune contexture in human tumours: Impact on clinical outcome. *Nature Reviews. Cancer, 12*(4), 298–306. DOI: 10.1038/nrc3245 PMID: 22419253

Gil Del Alcazar, C. R., Huh, S. J., Ekram, M. B., Trinh, A., Liu, L. L., Beca, F., Zi, X., Kwak, M., Bergholtz, H., Su, Y., Ding, L., Russnes, H. G., Richardson, A. L., Babski, K., Min Hui Kim, E., McDonnell, C. H.III, Wagner, J., Rowberry, R., Freeman, G. J., & Polyak, K. (2017). Immune escape in breast cancer during in situ to invasive carcinoma transition. *Cancer Discovery, 7*(10), 1098–1115. DOI: 10.1158/2159-8290.CD-17-0222 PMID: 28652380

Gillette, M. A., Satpathy, S., Cao, S., Dhanasekaran, S. M., Vasaikar, S. V., Krug, K., Petralia, F., Li, Y., Liang, W.-W., Reva, B., Krek, A., Ji, J., Song, X., Liu, W., Hong, R., Yao, L., Blumenberg, L., Savage, S. R., Wendl, M. C., & Shi, Z. (2020). Proteogenomic characterization reveals therapeutic vulnerabilities in lung adenocarcinoma. *Cell, 182*(1), 200–225.e235. DOI: 10.1016/j.cell.2020.06.013 PMID: 32649874

Gubin, M. M., Artyomov, M. N., Mardis, E. R., & Schreiber, R. D. (2015). Tumor neoantigens: Building a framework for personalized cancer immunotherapy. *The Journal of Clinical Investigation, 125*(9), 3413–3421. DOI: 10.1172/JCI80008 PMID: 26258412

Havel, J. J., Chowell, D., & Chan, T. A. (2019). The evolving landscape of biomarkers for checkpoint inhibitor immunotherapy. *Nature Reviews. Cancer*, *19*(3), 133–150. DOI: 10.1038/s41568-019-0116-x PMID: 30755690

Heijmans, M., Habets, J., Kuijf, M., Kubben, P., & Herff, C. (2019). Evaluation of Parkinson's disease at home: Predicting tremor from wearable sensors. In *2019 41st Annual International Conference of the IEEE Engineering in Medicine and Biology Society (EMBC)*. IEEE. https://doi.org/DOI: 10.1109/EMBC.2019.8857717

Hinshaw, D. C., & Shevde, L. A. (2019). The tumor microenvironment innately modulates cancer progression. *Cancer Research*, *79*(18), 4557–4566. DOI: 10.1158/0008-5472.CAN-18-3962 PMID: 31350295

Huang, C., Chen, L., Savage, S. R., Eguez, R. V., Dou, Y., Li, Y., da Veiga Leprevost, F., Jaehnig, E. J., Lei, J. T., Wen, B., Schnaubelt, M., Krug, K., Song, X., Cieślik, M., Chang, H.-Y., Wyczalkowski, M. A., Li, K., Colaprico, A., Li, Q. K., & Zhu, J. (2021). Proteogenomic insights into the biology and treatment of HPV-negative head and neck squamous cell carcinoma. *Cancer Cell*, *39*(3), 361–379.e316. DOI: 10.1016/j.ccell.2020.12.007 PMID: 33417831

Huang, Q., Zhang, X., & Hu, Z. (2021). Application of artificial intelligence modeling technology based on multi-omics in noninvasive diagnosis of inflammatory bowel disease. *Journal of Inflammation Research*, *14*, 1933–1943. DOI: 10.2147/JIR.S306816 PMID: 34017190

Hui, X., & Kan, E. C. (2017). Monitoring vital signs over multiplexed radio by near-field coherent sensing. *Nature Electronics*, *1*(1), 74–78. DOI: 10.1038/s41928-017-0001-0

Hui, X., & Kan, E. C. (2018). Accurate extraction of heartbeat intervals with near-field coherent sensing. In *2018 IEEE International Conference on Communications (ICC)*. IEEE. https://doi.org/DOI: 10.1109/ICC.2018.8423000

Jackson, H. W., Fischer, J. R., Zanotelli, V. R. T., Ali, H. R., Mechera, R., Soysal, S. D., Moch, H., Muenst, S., Varga, Z., Weber, W. P., & Bodenmiller, B. (2020). The single-cell pathology landscape of breast cancer. *Nature*, *578*(7796), 615–620. DOI: 10.1038/s41586-019-1876-x PMID: 31959985

Jaffe, C. C. (2012). Imaging and genomics: Is there a synergy? *Radiology*, *264*(3), 329–331. DOI: 10.1148/radiol.12120871 PMID: 22821693

Jiang, L. Y., Liu, X. C., Nejatian, N. P., Nasir-Moin, M., Wang, D., Abidin, A., Eaton, K., Riina, H. A., Laufer, I., Punjabi, P., Miceli, M., Kim, N. C., Orillac, C., Schnurman, Z., Livia, C., Weiss, H., Kurland, D., Neifert, S., Dastagirzada, Y., & Oermann, E. K. (2023). Health system-scale language models are all-purpose prediction engines. *Nature*, *619*(7969), 357–362. DOI: 10.1038/s41586-023-06160-y PMID: 37286606

Jiang, T., Shi, T., Zhang, H., Hu, J., Song, Y., Wei, J., Ren, S., & Zhou, C. (2019). Tumor neoantigens: From basic research to clinical applications. *Journal of Hematology & Oncology*, *12*(1), 93. DOI: 10.1186/s13045-019-0787-5 PMID: 31492199

Jiang, X., Zhao, H., Saldanha, O. L., Nebelung, S., Kuhl, C., Amygdalos, I., Lang, S. A., Wu, X., Meng, X., Truhn, D., Kather, J. N., & Ke, J. (2023). An MRI deep learning model predicts outcome in rectal cancer. *Radiology*, *307*(2), e222223. DOI: 10.1148/radiol.222223 PMID: 37278629

Jin, C., Yu, H., Ke, J., Ding, P., Yi, Y., Jiang, X., Duan, X., Tang, J., Chang, D. T., Wu, X., Gao, F., & Li, R. (2021). Predicting treatment response from longitudinal images using multi-task deep learning. *Nature Communications, 12*(1), 1851. DOI: 10.1038/s41467-021-22188-y PMID: 33767170

Joshi, M., Archer, S., Morbi, A., Arora, S., Kwasnicki, R., Ashrafian, H., Khan, S., Cooke, G., & Darzi, A. (2021). Short-term wearable sensors for in-hospital medical and surgical patients: Mixed methods analysis of patient perspectives. *JMIR Perioperative Medicine, 4*(1), e18836. DOI: 10.2196/18836 PMID: 33885367

Joyce, J. A., & Pollard, J. W. (2009). Microenvironmental regulation of metastasis. *Nature Reviews. Cancer, 9*(3), 239–252. DOI: 10.1038/nrc2618 PMID: 19279573

Kazerooni, A. F., Bagley, S. J., Akbari, H., Saxena, S., Bagheri, S., Guo, J., Chawla, S., Nabavizadeh, A., Mohan, S., & Bakas, S.. (2021). Applications of radiomics and radiogenomics in high-grade gliomas in the era of precision medicine. *Cancers (Basel), 13*(5921), 5921. Advance online publication. DOI: 10.3390/cancers13235921 PMID: 34885031

Keren, L., Bosse, M., Marquez, D., Angoshtari, R., Jain, S., Varma, S., Yang, S.-R., Kurian, A., Van Valen, D., West, R., Bendall, S. C., & Angelo, M. (2018). A structured tumor-immune microenvironment in triple negative breast cancer revealed by multiplexed ion beam imaging. *Cell, 174*(6), 1373–1387. e19. DOI: 10.1016/j.cell.2018.08.039 PMID: 30193111

Khalid, W. B., Anwar, A., & Waheed, O. T. (2022). Contactless vitals measurement robot. In *2022 8th International Conference on Automation, Robotics and Applications (ICARA)*. IEEE. https://doi.org/ DOI: 10.1109/ICARA55094.2022.9738523

Klysik, J. (2001). Concept of immunomics: A new frontier in the battle for gene function? *Acta Biotheoretica, 49*(3), 191–202. DOI: 10.1023/A:1011901410166 PMID: 11558896

Krassowski, M., Paczkowska, M., Cullion, K., Huang, T., Dzneladze, I., Ouellette, B. F. F., Yamada, J. T., Fradet-Turcotte, A., & Reimand, J. (2018). ActiveDriverDB: Human disease mutations and genome variation in post-translational modification sites of proteins. *Nucleic Acids Research, 46*(D1), D901–D910. DOI: 10.1093/nar/gkx973 PMID: 29126202

Lancellotti, C., Cancian, P., Savevski, V., Kotha, S. R. R., Fraggetta, F., Graziano, P., & Di Tommaso, L. (2021). Artificial intelligence & tissue biomarkers: Advantages, risks and perspectives for pathology. *Cells, 10*(4), 787. DOI: 10.3390/cells10040787 PMID: 33918173

Lao, J., Chen, Y., Li, Z.-C., Li, Q., Zhang, J., Liu, J., & Zhai, G. (2017). A deep learning-based radiomics model for prediction of survival in glioblastoma multiforme. *Scientific Reports, 7*(1), 10353. DOI: 10.1038/s41598-017-10649-8 PMID: 28871110

Lau, M. C., Yi, Y., Goh, D., Cheung, C. C. L., Tan, B., Lim, J. C. T., Joseph, C. R., Wee, F., Lee, J. N., Lim, X., Lim, C. J., Leow, W. Q., Lee, J. Y., Ng, C. C. Y., Bashiri, H., Cheow, P. C., Chan, C. Y., Koh, Y. X., Tan, T. T., & Yeong, J. P. S. (2022). Case report: Understanding the impact of persistent tissue-localization of SARS-CoV-2 on immune response activity via spatial transcriptomic analysis of two cancer patients with COVID-19 co-morbidity. *Frontiers in Immunology, 13*, 978760. DOI: 10.3389/fimmu.2022.978760 PMID: 36172383

Laurie, J., Higgins, N., Peynot, T., Fawcett, L., & Robert, J. (2021). An evaluation of a video magnification-based system for respiratory rate monitoring in an acute mental health setting. *International Journal of Medical Informatics, 148*, 104378. DOI: 10.1016/j.ijmedinf.2021.104378 PMID: 33486356

Lei, X., Lei, Y., Li, J.-K., Du, W.-X., Li, R.-G., Yang, J., Li, J., Li, F., & Tan, H.-B. (2020). Immune cells within the tumor microenvironment: Biological functions and roles in cancer immunotherapy. *Cancer Letters, 470*, 126–133. DOI: 10.1016/j.canlet.2019.11.009 PMID: 31730903

Li, L., Goedegebuure, S. P., & Gillanders, W. E. (2017). Preclinical and clinical development of neoantigen vaccines. *Annals of Oncology : Official Journal of the European Society for Medical Oncology, 28*, xii11–xii17. DOI: 10.1093/annonc/mdx681 PMID: 29253113

Lièvre, A., Bachet, J.-B., Le Corre, D., Boige, V., Landi, B., Emile, J.-F., Côté, J.-F., Tomasic, G., Penna, C., Ducreux, M., Rougier, P., Penault-Llorca, F., & Laurent-Puig, P. (2006). KRAS mutation status is predictive of response to cetuximab therapy in colorectal cancer. *Cancer Research, 66*(8), 3992–3995. DOI: 10.1158/0008-5472.CAN-06-0191 PMID: 16618717

Ligero, M., Garcia-Ruiz, A., Viaplana, C., Villacampa, G., Raciti, M. V., Landa, J., Matos, I., Martin-Liberal, J., Ochoa-de-Olza, M., Hierro, C., Mateo, J., Gonzalez, M., Morales-Barrera, R., Suarez, C., Rodon, J., Elez, E., Braña, I., Muñoz-Couselo, E., Oaknin, A., & Perez-Lopez, R. (2021). A CT-based radiomics signature is associated with response to immune checkpoint inhibitors in advanced solid tumors. *Radiology, 299*(1), 109–119. DOI: 10.1148/radiol.2021200928 PMID: 33497314

Liu, S., Iorgulescu, B., Li, S., Morriss, J., Borji, M., Murray, E., Braun, D., Livak, K., Wu, C., & Chen, F. (2021). Spatial mapping of T cell receptors and transcriptomes in renal cell carcinoma following immune checkpoint inhibitor therapy. *Journal for Immunotherapy of Cancer, 9*(Suppl 2), A84–A85. DOI: 10.1136/jitc-2021-SITC2021.076

Ma, B., Meng, F., Yan, G., Yan, H., Chai, B., & Song, F. (2020). Diagnostic classification of cancers using extreme gradient boosting algorithm and multi-omics data. *Computers in Biology and Medicine, 121*, 103761. DOI: 10.1016/j.compbiomed.2020.103761 PMID: 32339094

Majzner, R. G., & Mackall, C. L. (2018). Tumor antigen escape from CAR T-cell therapy. *Cancer Discovery, 8*(10), 1219–1226. DOI: 10.1158/2159-8290.CD-18-0442 PMID: 30135176

Malasinghe, L. P., Ramzan, N., & Dahal, K. (2017). Remote patient monitoring: A comprehensive study. *Journal of Ambient Intelligence and Humanized Computing, 10*(1), 57–76. DOI: 10.1007/s12652-017-0598-x

Martin-Orozco, N., Muranski, P., Chung, Y., Yang, X. O., Yamazaki, T., Lu, S., Hwu, P., Restifo, N. P., Overwijk, W. W., & Dong, C. (2009). T Helper 17 cells promote cytotoxic T cell activation in tumor immunity. *Immunity, 31*(5), 787–798. DOI: 10.1016/j.immuni.2009.09.014 PMID: 19879162

Marusyk, A., & Polyak, K. (2010). Tumor heterogeneity: Causes and consequences. *Biochimica et Biophysica Acta, 1805*(1), 105–117. DOI: 10.1016/j.bbcan.2009.11.002 PMID: 19931353

Mashl, R. J., Scott, A. D., Huang, K., Wyczalkowski, M. A., Yoon, C. J., Niu, B., DeNardo, E., Yellapantula, V. D., Handsaker, R. E., Chen, K., Koboldt, D. C., Ye, K., Fenyö, D., Raphael, B. J., Wendl, M. C., & Ding, L. (2017). GenomeVIP: A cloud platform for genomic variant discovery and interpretation. *Genome Research, 27*(9), 1450–1459. DOI: 10.1101/gr.211656.116 PMID: 28522612

McCarthy, J. J., McLeod, H. L., & Ginsburg, G. S. (2013). Genomic medicine: A decade of successes, challenges, and opportunities. *Science Translational Medicine, 5*(189sr4). https://doi.org/DOI: 10.1126/scitranslmed.3006241

Mellman, I., Coukos, G., & Dranoff, G. (2011). Cancer immunotherapy comes of age. *Nature, 480*(7378), 480–489. DOI: 10.1038/nature10673 PMID: 22193102

Meng, C., Kuster, B., Culhane, A. C., & Gholami, A. M. (2014). A multivariate approach to the integration of multi-omics datasets. *BMC Bioinformatics, 15*(1), 162. DOI: 10.1186/1471-2105-15-162 PMID: 24884486

Miller, D. D., & Brown, E. W. (2018). Artificial intelligence in medical practice: The question to the answer? *The American Journal of Medicine, 131*(2), 129–133. DOI: 10.1016/j.amjmed.2017.10.035 PMID: 29126825

Moutafi, M., Martinez-Morilla, S., Divakar, P., Vathiotis, I., Gavrielatou, N., Aung, T. N., Yaghoobi, V., Fernandez, A. I., Zugazagoitia, J., Herbst, R. S., Schalper, K. A., & Rimm, D. L. (2022). Discovery of biomarkers of resistance to immune checkpoint blockade in NSCLC using high-plex digital spatial profiling. *Journal of Thoracic Oncology, 17*(8), 991–1001. DOI: 10.1016/j.jtho.2022.04.009 PMID: 35490853

Mu, W., Jiang, L., Zhang, J. Y., Shi, Y., Gray, J. E., Tunali, I., Gao, C., Sun, Y., Tian, J., Zhao, X., Sun, X., Gillies, R. J., & Schabath, M. B. (2020). Non-invasive decision support for NSCLC treatment using PET/CT radiomics. *Nature Communications, 11*(1), 5228. DOI: 10.1038/s41467-020-19116-x PMID: 33067442

Nishino, M., Ramaiya, N. H., Hatabu, H., & Hodi, F. S. (2017). Monitoring immune checkpoint blockade: Response evaluation and biomarker development. *Nature Reviews. Clinical Oncology, 14*(11), 655–668. DOI: 10.1038/nrclinonc.2017.88 PMID: 28653677

Obeid, J. P., Stoyanova, R., Kwon, D., Patel, M., Padgett, K., Slingerland, J., Takita, C., Alperin, N., Yepes, M., & Zeidan, Y. H. (2017). Multiparametric evaluation of preoperative MRI in early stage breast cancer: Prognostic impact of peri-tumoral fat. *Clinical & Translational Oncology, 19*(2), 211–218. DOI: 10.1007/s12094-016-1526-9 PMID: 27364695

Pardoll, D. M. (2012). The blockade of immune checkpoints in cancer immunotherapy. *Nature Reviews. Cancer, 12*(4), 252–264. DOI: 10.1038/nrc3239 PMID: 22437870

Paschen, A., Eichmuller, S., & Schadendorf, D. (2004). Identification of tumor antigens and T-cell epitopes, and its clinical application. *Cancer Immunology, Immunotherapy : CII, 53*(3), 196–203. DOI: 10.1007/s00262-003-0479-3 PMID: 14689239

Picard, M., Scott-Boyer, M.-P., Bodein, A., Périn, O., & Droit, A. (2021). Integration strategies of multi-omics data for machine learning analysis. *Computational and Structural Biotechnology Journal, 19*, 3735–3746. DOI: 10.1016/j.csbj.2021.06.030 PMID: 34285775

Pilard, C., Ancion, M., Delvenne, P., Jerusalem, G., Hubert, P., & Herfs, M. (2021). Cancer immunotherapy: It's time to better predict patients' response. *British Journal of Cancer, 125*(6), 927–938. DOI: 10.1038/s41416-021-01413-x PMID: 34112949

Ptacek, J., Locke, D., Finck, R., Cvijic, M. E., Li, Z., Tarolli, J. G., Aksoy, M., Sigal, Y., Zhang, Y., Newgren, M., & Finn, J. (2020). Multiplexed ion beam imaging (MIBI) for characterization of the tumor microenvironment across tumor types. *Laboratory Investigation, 100*(8), 1111–1123. DOI: 10.1038/s41374-020-0417-4 PMID: 32203152

Qiu, Y. L., Zheng, H., Devos, A., Selby, H., & Gevaert, O. (2020). A meta-learning approach for genomic survival analysis. *Nature Communications, 11*(1), 6350. DOI: 10.1038/s41467-020-20167-3 PMID: 33311484

Rappoport, N., & Shamir, R. (2019). NEMO: Cancer subtyping by integration of partial multi-omic data. *Bioinformatics (Oxford, England), 35*(18), 3348–3356. DOI: 10.1093/bioinformatics/btz058 PMID: 30698637

Renc, P., Jia, Y., Samir, A. E., Was, J., Li, Q., Bates, D. W., & Sitek, A. (2024). Zero-shot health trajectory prediction using transformer. *NPJ Digital Medicine, 7*(1), 256. DOI: 10.1038/s41746-024-01235-0 PMID: 39300208

Rodrigues, L., Gonçalves, I., Fé, I., Endo, P. T., & Silva, F. A. (2021). Performance and availability evaluation of a smart hospital architecture. *Computing, 103*(10), 2401–2435. DOI: 10.1007/s00607-021-00979-x

Roland Berger Gmb, H. (2021). Pharma's big opportunity to ride the next wave: How to enter the cell and gene therapy market. Munich.

Saxena, S., Kazerooni, A. F., Toorens, E., Bakas, S., Akbari, H., Sako, C., Mamourian, E., Koumenis, C., Mohan, S., Bagley, S. J., Lustig, R. A., O'Rourke, D. M., Ganguly, T., Nasrallah, M. L., & Davatzikos, C. (2021). NIMG-73. Capturing glioblastoma heterogeneity using imaging and deep learning: Application to MGMT promoter methylation. *Neuro-Oncology, 23*(vi146), vi146. Advance online publication. DOI: 10.1093/neuonc/noab196.570

Schapiro, D., Jackson, H. W., Raghuraman, S., Fischer, J. R., Zanotelli, V. R. T., Schulz, D., Giesen, C., Catena, R., Varga, Z., & Bodenmiller, B. (2017). histoCAT: Analysis of cell phenotypes and interactions in multiplex image cytometry data. *Nature Methods, 14*(9), 873–876. DOI: 10.1038/nmeth.4391 PMID: 28783155

Schlecht, A., Boneva, S., Salie, H., Killmer, S., Wolf, J., Hajdu, R. I., Auw-Haedrich, C., Agostini, H., Reinhard, T., Schlunck, G., Bengsch, B., & Lange, C. A. K. (2021). Imaging mass cytometry for high-dimensional tissue profiling in the eye. *BMC Ophthalmology, 21*(1), 338. DOI: 10.1186/s12886-021-02099-8 PMID: 34544377

Schnyer, D. M., Clasen, P. C., Gonzalez, C., & Beevers, C. G. (2017). Evaluating the diagnostic utility of applying a machine learning algorithm to diffusion tensor MRI measures in individuals with major depressive disorder. *Psychiatry Research: Neuroimaging, 264*, 1–9. DOI: 10.1016/j.pscychresns.2017.03.003 PMID: 28388468

Schürch, C. M., Bhate, S. S., Barlow, G. L., Phillips, D. J., Noti, L., Zlobec, I., Chu, P., Black, S., Demeter, J., McIlwain, D. R., Kinoshita, S., Samusik, N., Goltsev, Y., & Nolan, G. P. (2020). Coordinated cellular neighborhoods orchestrate antitumoral immunity at the colorectal cancer invasive front. *Cell, 182*(5), 1341–1359.e19. DOI: 10.1016/j.cell.2020.07.005 PMID: 32763154

Schürch, C. M., Bhate, S. S., Barlow, G. L., Phillips, D. J., Noti, L., Zlobec, I., Chu, P., Black, S., Demeter, J., McIlwain, D. R., Kinoshita, S., Samusik, N., Goltsev, Y., & Nolan, G. P. (2020). Coordinated cellular neighborhoods orchestrate antitumoral immunity at the colorectal cancer invasive front. *Cell, 182*(5), 1341–1359.e19. DOI: 10.1016/j.cell.2020.07.005 PMID: 32763154

Shaik, T., Tao, X., Higgins, N., Gururajan, R., Li, Y., Zhou, X., & Acharya, U. R. (2022). Fedstack: Personalized activity monitoring using stacked federated learning. *Knowledge-Based Systems, 257*, 109929. DOI: 10.1016/j.knosys.2022.109929

Shaik, T., Tao, X., Higgins, N., Xie, H., Gururajan, R., & Zhou, X. (2022). AI enabled RPM for mental health facility. In *Proceedings of the 1st ACM Workshop on Mobile and Wireless Sensing for Smart Healthcare* (pp. 26–32). Association for Computing Machinery. https://doi.org/DOI: 10.1145/3556551.3561191

Sharma, P., & Kan, E. C. (2018). *Sleep scoring with a UHF RFID tag by near field coherent sensing. In 2018 IEEE/MTT-s international microwave symposium IMS*. IEEE., DOI: 10.1109/MWSYM.2018.8439216

Shen, R., Olshen, A. B., & Ladanyi, M. (2009). Integrative clustering of multiple genomic data types using a joint latent variable model with application to breast and lung cancer subtype analysis. *Bioinformatics (Oxford, England), 25*(22), 2906–2912. DOI: 10.1093/bioinformatics/btp543 PMID: 19759197

Sheng, J., Zhang, J., Wang, L., Tano, V., Tang, J., Wang, X., Wu, J., Song, J., Zhao, Y., Rong, J., Cheng, F., Wang, J., Shen, Y., Wen, L., He, J., Zhang, H., Li, T., Zhang, Q., Bai, X., & Liang, T. (2022). Topological analysis of hepatocellular carcinoma tumour microenvironment based on imaging mass cytometry reveals cellular neighbourhood regulated reversely by macrophages with different ontogeny. *Gut, 71*(6), 1176–1191. DOI: 10.1136/gutjnl-2021-324339 PMID: 34253573

Subramanian, I., Verma, S., Kumar, S., Jere, A., & Anamika, K. (2020). Multi-omics data integration, interpretation, and its application. *Bioinformatics and Biology Insights, 14*, 1177932219899051. DOI: 10.1177/1177932219899051 PMID: 32076369

Taber, K. A. J., Dickinson, B. D., & Wilson, M. (2014). The promise and challenges of next-generation genome sequencing for clinical care. *JAMA Internal Medicine, 174*(2), 275–280. DOI: 10.1001/jamainternmed.2013.12048 PMID: 24217348

Tan, W. C. C., Nerurkar, S. N., Cai, H. Y., Ng, H. H. M., Wu, D., Wee, Y. T. F., Lim, J. C. T., Yeong, J., & Lim, T. K. H. (2020). Overview of multiplex immunohistochemistry/immunofluorescence techniques in the era of cancer immunotherapy. *Cancer Communications, 40*(4), 135–153. DOI: 10.1002/cac2.12023 PMID: 32301585

Tay, S. H., Yaung, K. N., Leong, J. Y., Yeo, J. G., Arkachaisri, T., & Albani, S. (2019). Immunomics in pediatric rheumatic diseases. *Frontiers in Medicine, 6*, 111. DOI: 10.3389/fmed.2019.00111 PMID: 31231652

Tong, L., Mitchel, J., Chatlin, K., & Wang, M. D. (2020). Deep learning based feature-level integration of multi-omics data for breast cancer patients survival analysis. *BMC Medical Informatics and Decision Making, 20*(1), 225. DOI: 10.1186/s12911-020-01225-8 PMID: 32933515

Turtle, C. J., Hanafi, L.-A., Berger, C., Gooley, T. A., Cherian, S., Hudecek, M., Sommermeyer, D., Melville, K., Pender, B., Budiarto, T. M., Robinson, E., Steevens, N. N., Chaney, C., Soma, L., Chen, X., Yeung, C., Wood, B., Li, D., Cao, J., & Maloney, D. G. (2016). CD19 CAR-T cells of defined CD4+:CD8+ composition in adult B cell ALL patients. *The Journal of Clinical Investigation, 126*(6), 2123–2138. DOI: 10.1172/JCI85309 PMID: 27111235

Unger, M., & Kather, J. N. (2024). Deep learning in cancer genomics and histopathology. *Genome Medicine, 16*(1), 44. DOI: 10.1186/s13073-024-01315-6 PMID: 38539231

Unger, M., & Kather, J. N. (2024). Deep learning in cancer genomics and histopathology. *Genome Medicine, 16*(1), 44. DOI: 10.1186/s13073-024-01315-6 PMID: 38539231

Uslu, B. Ç., Okay, E., & Dursun, E. (2020). Analysis of factors affecting IoT-based smart hospital design. *Journal of Cloud Computing (Heidelberg, Germany), 9*(1), 67. DOI: 10.1186/s13677-020-00215-5 PMID: 33532168

Van Allen, E. M., Miao, D., Schilling, B., Shukla, S. A., Blank, C., Zimmer, L., Sucker, A., Hillen, U., Geukes Foppen, M. H., Goldinger, S. M., Utikal, J., Hassel, J. C., Weide, B., Kaehler, K. C., Loquai, C., Mohr, P., Gutzmer, R., Dummer, R., Gabriel, S., & Garraway, L. A. (2015). Genomic correlates of response to CTLA-4 blockade in metastatic melanoma. *Science, 350*(6257), 207–211. DOI: 10.1126/science.aad0095 PMID: 26359337

Vanguri, R. S., Luo, J., Aukerman, A. T., Egger, J. V., Fong, C. J., Horvat, N., Pagano, A., Araujo-Filho, J. A. B., Geneslaw, L., Rizvi, H., Sosa, R., Boehm, K. M., Yang, S.-R., Bodd, F. M., Ventura, K., Hollmann, T. J., Ginsberg, M. S., Gao, J., Vanguri, R., & Shah, S. P. (2022). Multimodal integration of radiology, pathology and genomics for prediction of response to PD-(L)1 blockade in patients with non-small cell lung cancer. *Nature Cancer, 3*(8), 1151–1164. DOI: 10.1038/s43018-022-00416-8 PMID: 36038778

Väyrynen, J. P., Haruki, K., Lau, M. C., Väyrynen, S. A., Zhong, R., Dias Costa, A., Borowsky, J., Zhao, M., Fujiyoshi, K., Arima, K., Twombly, T. S., Kishikawa, J., Gu, S., Aminmozaffari, S., Shi, S., Baba, Y., Akimoto, N., Ugai, T., Da Silva, A., & Nowak, J. A. (2021). The prognostic role of macrophage polarization in the colorectal cancer microenvironment. *Cancer Immunology Research, 9*(1), 8–19. DOI: 10.1158/2326-6066.CIR-20-0527 PMID: 33023967

Wang, B., Mezlini, A. M., Demir, F., Fiume, M., Tu, Z., Brudno, M., Haibe-Kains, B., & Goldenberg, A. (2014). Similarity network fusion for aggregating data types on a genomic scale. *Nature Methods, 11*(3), 333–337. DOI: 10.1038/nmeth.2810 PMID: 24464287

Wang, C., Ma, J., Shao, J., Zhang, S., Li, J., Yan, J., Zhao, Z., Bai, C., Yu, Y., & Li, W. (2022). Non-invasive measurement using deep learning algorithm based on multi-source features fusion to predict PDL1 expression and survival in NSCLC. *Frontiers in Immunology*, *13*, 828560. DOI: 10.3389/fimmu.2022.828560 PMID: 35464416

Weenk, M., Bredie, S., Koeneman, M., Hesselink, G., van Goor, H., & van de Belt, T. H. (2020). Continuous monitoring of vital signs in the general ward using wearable devices: Randomized controlled trial. *Journal of Medical Internet Research*, *22*(6), e15471. DOI: 10.2196/15471 PMID: 32519972

Xie, Y.-H., Chen, Y.-X., & Fang, J.-Y. (2020). Comprehensive review of targeted therapy for colorectal cancer. *Signal Transduction and Targeted Therapy*, *5*(22), 22. Advance online publication. DOI: 10.1038/s41392-020-0116-z PMID: 32296018

Xu, H., Lien, T., Bergholtz, H., Fleischer, T., Djerroudi, L., Vincent-Salomon, A., Sørlie, T., & Aittokallio, T. (2021). Multi-Omics marker analysis enables early prediction of breast tumor progression. *Frontiers in Genetics*, *12*, 670749. DOI: 10.3389/fgene.2021.670749 PMID: 34149812

8. Yamamoto, T. N., Kishton, R. J., & Restifo, N. P. (2019). Developing neoantigen-targeted T cell–based treatments for solid tumors. *Nature Medicine*, *25*(10), 1488–1499. DOI: 10.1038/s41591-019-0596-y PMID: 31591590

Yescarta: axicabtagene ciloleucel. (2022). Available at: https://www.ema.europa.eu/en/medicines/human/EPAR/yescarta (Accessed April 4, 2022).

Yew, H. T., Ng, M. F., Ping, S. Z., Chung, S. K., Chekima, A., & Dargham, J. A. (2020). IoT based real-time remote patient monitoring system. In *2020 16th IEEE International Colloquium on Signal Processing & Its Applications (CSPA)*. IEEE. https://doi.org/DOI: 10.1109/CSPA48992.2020.9068699

Zeng, Q., Klein, C., Caruso, S., Maille, P., Allende, D. S., Mínguez, B., Iavarone, M., Ningarhari, M., Casadei-Gardini, A., Pedica, F., Rimini, M., Perbellini, R., Boulagnon-Rombi, C., Heurgué, A., Maggioni, M., Rela, M., Vij, M., Baulande, S., Legoix, P., & Calderaro, J. (2023). Artificial intelligence-based pathology as a biomarker of sensitivity to atezolizumab-bevacizumab in patients with hepatocellular carcinoma: A multicenter retrospective study. *The Lancet. Oncology*, *24*(10), 1411–1422. DOI: 10.1016/S1470-2045(23)00468-0 PMID: 37951222

Zhang, L., Lv, C., Jin, Y., Cheng, G., Fu, Y., Yuan, D., Tao, Y., Guo, Y., Ni, X., & Shi, T. (2018). Deep learning-based multi-omics data integration reveals two prognostic subtypes in high-risk neuroblastoma. *Frontiers in Genetics*, *9*, 477. DOI: 10.3389/fgene.2018.00477 PMID: 30405689

Zhang, R., Feng, Y., Ma, W., Guo, Y., Luo, M., & Li, Y.. (2022). Spatial transcriptome unveils a discontinuous inflammatory pattern in proficient mismatch repair colorectal adenocarcinoma. *Fundamental Research (Beijing)*. Advance online publication. DOI: 10.1016/j.fmre.2022.01.036 PMID: 38933545

Zhou, C., Zhu, C., & Liu, Q. (2019). Toward in silico identification of tumor neoantigens in immunotherapy. *Trends in Molecular Medicine*, *25*(10), 980–992. DOI: 10.1016/j.molmed.2019.08.001 PMID: 31494024

Zhou, C., Zhu, C., & Liu, Q. (2019). Toward in silico identification of tumor neoantigens in immunotherapy. *Trends in Molecular Medicine*, *25*(10), 980–992. DOI: 10.1016/j.molmed.2019.08.001 PMID: 31494024

Zhou, S., Sun, D., Mao, W., Liu, Y., Cen, W., Ye, L., Liang, F., Xu, J., Shi, H., Ji, Y., Wang, L., & Chang, W. (2023). Deep radiomics-based fusion model for prediction of bevacizumab treatment response and outcome in patients with colorectal cancer liver metastases: A multicenter cohort study. *EClinicalMedicine*, *65*, 102271. DOI: 10.1016/j.eclinm.2023.102271 PMID: 37869523

Zou, W., Wolchok, J. D., & Chen, L. (2016). PD-L1 (B7-H1) and PD-1 pathway blockade for cancer therapy: Mechanisms, response biomarkers, and combinations. *Science Translational Medicine*, *8*(328), 328rv324. Advance online publication. DOI: 10.1126/scitranslmed.aad7118 PMID: 26936508

Zuo, Z., Wang, P., Chen, X., Tian, L., Ge, H., & Qian, D. (2021). SWnet: A deep learning model for drug response prediction from cancer genomic signatures and compound chemical structures. *BMC Bioinformatics*, *22*(12), 434. DOI: 10.1186/s12859-021-04352-9 PMID: 34507532

Chapter 11
AI-Generated Nanoparticles in Immunological Research: Opportunities and Challenges

Kazi Asraf Ali
https://orcid.org/0000-0002-1753-7504
Maulana Abul Kalam Azad University of Technology, West Bengal, India

Sabyasachi Choudhuri
https://orcid.org/0000-0002-7736-8490
Maulana Abul Kalam Azad University of Technology, West Bengal, India

Sanjit Kr. Roy
Maulana Abul Kalam Azad University of Technology, West Bengal, India

Khandekar Hussan Reza
https://orcid.org/0009-0004-9545-3033
Maulana Abul Kalam Azad University of Technology, West Bengal, India

Dipika Mandal
Maulana Abul Kalam Azad University of Technology, West Bengal, India

Rideb Chakraborty
https://orcid.org/0009-0007-3931-8349
Bengal College of Pharmaceutical Sciences and Research, India

Chowdhury Mobaswar Hossain
https://orcid.org/0009-0001-5610-0962
Maulana Abul Kalam Azad University of Technology, West Bengal, India

ABSTRACT

Integrating artificial intelligence (AI) with nanotechnology has revolutionized immunological research by enabling the precise design, optimization, and functionalization of nanoparticles. AI-generated nanoparticles (AIGNPs) exhibit enhanced capabilities in vaccine development, cancer immunotherapy, and autoimmune disease treatment through improved antigen delivery, targeted drug release, and immune modulation. AI-powered models help researchers quickly analyze how nanoparticles behave, interact with immune cells, and determine their compatibility with the body. This speeds up the development of new treatments. But there are still a lot of obstacles. Obstacles still include strict legal requirements, moral dilemmas, and the requirement for extensive experimental support. AI-generated nanoparticles have infinite therapeutic potential once these obstacles are removed. Resolving these issues could result in more precise and personalized cancer immunotherapy, which would revolutionize patient care.

DOI: 10.4018/979-8-3693-9725-1.ch011

1. INTRODUCTION

The fusion of artificial intelligence and nanotechnology has transformed biomedical research, particularly in immunology, by enabling highly targeted design, optimization, and functionalization of nanoparticles for a theragnostic application (Kurul, Turkmen, Cetin, & Topkaya, 2025). Due to the engine of computation-based artificial intelligence (AI) and machine learning algorithms, whole data sets can be processed incredibly fast. The dynamics, biocompatibility, kinetics, and behavior of nanoparticles and the related immune responses of nanoparticles with immune cells (Olawade, Ige, Olaremu, Ijiwade, & Adeola, 2024) can be predicted as this technology has permitted the fabrication of in size range of the AI nanoparticles (AIGNPs) with tunable characteristics such as sustained drug delivery, selective antigen release, and optimized immune modulation. The advent of Artificial intelligence in vaccine design allows the modeling of the structure of pathogens in nanoparticles using nanoparticle structure models that are highly potent to induce a more robust immune response with reduced toxicity and side effects. Also, the function of intelligent nanoparticles in cancer immunotherapy is of enormous significance, and intelligent nanomaterials could selectively target tumor cells and overcome immunologic suppression(Yunna Chen et al., 2024). Despite these innovations, challenges such as regulatory hurdles, ethical concerns, and the need for extensive experimental validation remain. Nonetheless, AI-driven nanotechnology holds immense potential to revolutionize immunological research and pave the way for more effective and personalized medical interventions.

Researchers can develop nanoparticles with the best possible medical qualities by using machine learning and advanced computer models. This increases stability, improves their body compatibility, and increases their efficacy in treating immune-related disorders (Mazumdar, Khondakar, Das, Halder, & Kaushik, 2025a). Rapid analysis of large datasets is made possible by machine learning, which also finds patterns and connections between the size, composition, surface charge, and biological interactions of nanoparticles. By simulating the behaviors of nanoparticles in intricate biological settings, computational models enable researchers to forecast immunological reactions and tailor formulations for therapeutic objectives. By reducing trial-and-error testing, this method speeds up the creation of immune-modulating nanoparticles, vaccine carriers, and tailored drug delivery systems.

Furthermore, AI-driven design enhances nanoparticle stability, preventing premature degradation and ensuring controlled release of therapeutic agents. As a result, AI-generated nanoparticles (AIGNPs) are being developed for various immunological applications, including cancer immunotherapy, autoimmune disease treatment, and infectious disease vaccines. However, translating these computational predictions into clinically viable solutions requires extensive experimental validation and regulatory evaluation to ensure safety and efficacy.

AIGNPs have a number of advantages, including decreased immunogenicity, accurate antigen delivery, and the capacity to alter immune responses for a range of therapeutic applications, such as the treatment of autoimmune diseases and cancer immunotherapy (Saleh & Shojaosadati, 2016). However, there are major challenges to their development and use. It is essential to address concerns about safety, regulatory approval, ethics, and the repeatability of AI-driven nanoparticle synthesis.

To transition AI-designed nanoparticles from models to clinical use, thorough experimental validation is essential due to the complexity of immune interactions (A. A. Aljabali et al., 2023). The immune system's dynamic nature, influenced by factors like immune cell heterogeneity and patient-specific responses, requires more than just computational predictions. While AI models can forecast nanoparticle behavior, real-world biological systems introduce variables that must be tested through in vitro and in vivo studies to ensure safety, efficacy, and minimal immunotoxicity. Additionally, regulatory approval for AI-generated nanoparticles demands standardized testing, reproducibility, and compliance with stringent guidelines to ensure safe clinical application. Addressing these challenges is vital for advancing AI-driven nanoparticle designs in immunotherapy and personalized medicine.

1.1. Overview of AI in Biomedical Nanotechnology

AI has revolutionized biomedical nanotechnology by enabling precise design, optimization, and application of nanomaterials for diagnosis, drug delivery, and therapy (Serov & Vinogradov, 2022). By leveraging machine learning algorithms, deep learning models, and computational simulations, AI accelerates the development of nanoparticles with enhanced properties such as biocompatibility, stability, and targeted delivery. AI-driven approaches facilitate the prediction of nanoparticle interactions with biological systems, improving the efficiency of drug formulations and minimizing adverse effects (Vidhya, Sultana, M, & Rangareddy, 2023).

In nanomedicine, AI aids in the synthesis of nanoparticles for targeted drug delivery, ensuring controlled release and site-specific action, particularly in cancer therapy, infectious diseases, and neurodegenerative disorders (Karahmet Sher et al., 2024). AI also enhances biosensing applications, where nanomaterials integrated with AI-powered sensors provide real-time disease detection and monitoring. Additionally, AI-driven predictive modeling optimizes the fabrication and functionalization of nanocarriers used in vaccine development and immunotherapy.

Even though AI has the potential to revolutionize biomedical nanotechnology, there are challenges to overcome, such as data constraints, ethical issues, and regulatory barriers. To translate AI-designed nanoparticles from computational models to clinical use, rigorous experimental validation and adherence to safety regulations are necessary. Nevertheless, with further developments, AI will be able to propel advancements in personalized medicine, enabling accurate, effective, and safer nanotechnology-based healthcare solutions.

1.2. Role of Nanoparticles in Immunological Research

In immunological research (Table 1), nanoparticles are essential because they offer flexible platforms for immunotherapy, vaccine administration, and immune regulation (Y. Li et al., 2025). Because of their nanoscale size, they can interact with immune cells more effectively, improving antigen presentation, triggering immunological responses, and boosting the effectiveness of treatments. Since they can resemble viruses, engineered nanoparticles are perfect vaccine carriers because they improve antigen stability, facilitate targeted distribution, and induce strong immunity.

Nanoparticles can be used as adjuvants to increase the immune response and improve vaccine potency, or they can be used to deliver immunosuppressive agents in a controlled manner to treat autoimmune diseases, reducing inflammation and minimizing systemic side effects. Nanoparticles can also be used to deliver immune checkpoint inhibitors, cytokines, or tumor antigens in cancer immunotherapy, which helps to activate the body's immune system against cancer cells.

Table 1. Role of nanoparticles in immunological research

Application	Role of Nanoparticles	Examples	Reference
Vaccine Delivery	Enhance antigen stability and targeted immune activation	mRNA vaccines (e.g., COVID-19 lipid nanoparticles)	(Wu et al., 2024)
Cancer Immunotherapy	Deliver tumor antigens, immune checkpoint inhibitors, and cytokines to stimulate anti-tumour responses.	Liposomal nanoparticles for PD-L1 inhibitors	(Zhou et al., 2022)
Autoimmune Disease Treatment	Deliver immunosuppressive agents in a controlled manner to reduce immune overactivation.	Polymeric nanoparticles for rheumatoid arthritis	(Adytia, Sutanto, Pratiwi, & Fetarayani, 2025)
Adjuvants in Vaccines	Boost immune response by enhancing antigen presentation and immune cell activation.	Alum-based and lipid nanoparticles	(Moni et al., 2023)
Drug Delivery	Ensure controlled and targeted release of immunomodulatory drugs	Nanoparticles for cytokine and antibody delivery	(A. A. A. Aljabali et al., 2024)
Biosensors and Diagnostics	Enable sensitive detection of immune-related biomarkers for disease diagnosis.	Gold nanoparticles in rapid immunoassays	(Sadr et al., 2024)
Allergy Treatment	Modulate immune responses to allergens through controlled exposure	Nanoparticles for allergen-specific immunotherapy	(Hesse, Oude Elberink, Van Oosterhout, & Nawijn, 2022)
Inflammation Control	Reduce excessive immune responses and inflammation in chronic diseases	Lipid nanoparticles for anti-inflammatory drugs	(Huang et al., 2024)

1.3. Importance for AI-Driven Nanoparticle Design

AI is essential in biomedical applications to enhance nanoparticle design accuracy, efficacy, and efficiency, reducing the costly and time-consuming trial-and-error approach of conventional methods (Furxhi et al., 2024). AI-driven methods that forecast ideal nanoparticle characteristics, including size, shape, surface charge, and biocompatibility, speed up the design process. These methods are fuelled by machine learning and computational modeling.

AI enables precise nanoparticle design for immune modulation, vaccines, and targeted drug delivery by analyzing interactions with immune cells. AI-driven simulations predict biodistribution, stability, and degradation, enhancing efficacy and safety before experiments.

AI enables personalized nanoparticles for tailored treatments in infectious diseases, autoimmune disorders, and cancer immunotherapy (Table 2). Despite challenges in data access, model interpretability, and regulation, advancing AI promises greater accuracy, scalability, and efficacy in nanomedicine (Kumar, Kulkarni, Liu, Chemuturi, & Shah, 2023).

Table 2. AI-driven nanoparticle design and their benefits

Feature	Role of AI in nanoparticle design	Benefits	Reference
Precision and Optimization	AI predicts optimal nanoparticle size, shape, and surface properties for specific applications.	Enhances biocompatibility, stability, and targeted delivery.	(Bhange & Telange, 2025b)
Faster Development	AI accelerates the design process by analyzing vast datasets and predicting outcomes.	Reduces trial-and-error experimentation and development time.	(Huanbutta et al., 2024)
Cost Efficiency	AI-driven simulations replace multiple laboratory experiments.	Lowers research and production costs.	(Yaiprasert & Hidayanto, 2024)
Personalized Medicine	AI designs nanoparticles tailored to individual patient profiles.	Improves treatment outcomes and minimizes side effects.	(Ejike Innocent Nwankwo, Ebube Victor Emeihe, Mojeed Dayo Ajegbile, Janet Aderonke Olaboye, & Chukwudi Cosmos Maha, 2024)
Targeted Drug Delivery	AI models optimize nanoparticle formulations for site-specific drug release.	Enhances drug efficacy and reduces systemic toxicity.	(Elumalai, Srinivasan, & Shanmugam, 2024)
Predicting Immune Responses	AI analyzes immune-nanoparticle interactions.	Minimizes adverse immune reactions and enhances therapeutic efficiency.	(Malachowski & Hassel, 2020)
Enhanced Stability and Biodegradability	AI optimizes nanoparticle composition to ensure controlled degradation.	Ensures long-term safety and effectiveness.	(Parvin, Joo, & Mandal, 2024)
Regulatory and Safety Compliance	AI predicts potential toxicity and safety concerns before clinical testing.	Helps in early risk assessment and regulatory approval processes.	(Basile, Yahi, & Tatonetti, 2019)

2. COMPUTATIONAL APPROACHES FOR NANOPARTICLE DESIGN

Nanoparticles have received a lot of interest in immunological research because of their tuneable physicochemical features, improved biocompatibility, and focused therapeutic applications (Kyriakides et al., 2021). By accelerating the search, optimization, and synthesis of nanoparticles with desired properties, the integration of AI into nanoparticle design has completely transformed this sector.

2.1. Deep Learning and Machine Learning in the Synthesis of Nanoparticles

In the synthesis of nanoparticles, machine learning (ML) and deep learning (DL) have become essential methodologies. By using these methods, scientists can forecast the behaviors of nanoparticles, optimize synthesis settings, and identify significant patterns in large datasets. ML and DL algorithms help address the challenges associated with traditional trial-and-error methodologies by offering predictive insights into optimal synthesis pathways (Goshisht, 2024).

2.1.1. Supervised and Unsupervised Learning in Nanoparticle Synthesis

Supervised learning models utilize labeled datasets to predict nanoparticle characteristics such as size, shape, and surface charge (Sun & Barnard, 2018). Examples include support vector machines (SVMs), decision trees, and deep neural networks (DNNs), which have been employed to correlate synthesis parameters with nanoparticle properties (Yaqub & Oboirien, 2024). Conversely, unsupervised learning techniques, such as clustering algorithms (e.g., k-means, hierarchical clustering), aid in classifying nanoparticles based on their physicochemical attributes without predefined labels (Botifoll, Pinto-Huguet, & Arbiol, 2022).

2.1.2. Deep Learning for Enhanced Prediction Accuracy

Deep learning approaches, including convolutional neural networks (CNNs) and recurrent neural networks (RNNs), have demonstrated superior performance in predicting nanoparticle properties from complex datasets. CNNs have been particularly useful in analyzing microscopic images of nanoparticles to classify and segment their morphologies. Similarly, generative adversarial networks (GANs) have been employed to generate synthetic nanoparticle structures that exhibit optimal properties for immunological applications (Sajedian, Kim, & Rho, 2019).

The various algorithms and their applications are mentioned below in Table 3.

Table 3. Algorithm and its applications in nanoparticle synthesis

Algorithm Type	Application in Nanoparticle Synthesis
Supervised Learning	Predicting the size, shape, and surface charge of nanoparticles
Unsupervised Learning	Clustering nanoparticles based on physicochemical properties
Deep Learning (CNN, RNN)	Image-based analysis and synthesis optimization
Generative Models (GANs)	Designing novel nanoparticle structures

Case Studies

- **Gold Nanoparticles for Immunotherapy:** Gold nanoparticles (AuNPs) are increasingly used in immunotherapy due to their biocompatibility, ease of surface modification, and ability to enhance immune responses. Their size, shape, and surface charge critically influence how they interact with immune cells, making precise control over these properties essential. Traditionally, optimizing these parameters required extensive experimentation, which is both time-consuming and resource-intensive. Researchers have employed machine learning (ML) models trained on large experimental datasets to predict optimal synthesis conditions for AuNPs. These models analyze temperature, reagent concentration, and reaction time to forecast particle size and uniformity. In one study, ML algorithms successfully identified synthesis protocols that produced gold nanoparticles with desired dimensions and surface characteristics suited for immunological functions. The predicted nanoparticles demonstrated improved targeting and uptake by immune cells, enhancing their therapeutic potential. This approach accelerated the development process and improved the reproducibility and clinical relevance of gold nanoparticle-based immunotherapies (Schletz, Breidung, & Fery, 2023).

- **Lipid Nanoparticles for mRNA Delivery:** Lipid nanoparticles (LNPs) are essential for the successful delivery of mRNA in vaccines, as they protect the fragile mRNA molecules and facilitate their entry into cells. However, achieving optimal lipid composition in LNPs is challenging due to the need to balance factors such as size, charge, and encapsulation efficiency. To address this, deep learning frameworks have been employed to predict and optimize lipid compositions that enhance the stability, efficiency, and safety of mRNA vaccines. These AI-driven models analyze large datasets of lipid structures and their interaction with mRNA, learning to identify compositions that maximize stability while minimizing toxicity. By simulating various lipid configurations, deep learning models can predict the ideal formulations that improve both the delivery and immune response. This approach has significantly accelerated the development of more effective and stable mRNA vaccine candidates, such as those used in COVID-19, by reducing trial-and-error and refining nanoparticle formulations for specific therapeutic needs. (Bae et al., 2024).

2.2. AI-Driven Predictive Modelling for Nanoparticle Properties

Predictive modeling plays a crucial role in nanoparticle design, enabling researchers to anticipate the properties and behaviors of nanoparticles before actual synthesis. AI-driven models integrate experimental data with computational simulations to provide accurate predictions.

2.2.1. Quantum Mechanical and Molecular Dynamics Simulations

Computational techniques such as density functional theory (DFT) and molecular dynamics (MD) simulations are often combined with AI models to predict the electronic, mechanical, and thermodynamic properties of nanoparticles (Poater, Saliner, Solà, Cavallo, & Worth, 2010). These simulations offer insights into nanoparticles' stability, reactivity, and interactions with biological systems.

2.2.2. Feature Engineering and Data-Driven Modelling

Feature engineering enhances the predictive power of AI models by selecting key parameters that influence nanoparticle behavior. Important features may include:

- Particle size and shape
- Surface charge and functionalization
- Solvent properties
- Temperature and reaction kinetics

The key features and its predictive approach are shown in Table 4.

2.2.3. Hybrid AI Models for Enhanced Accuracy

Hybrid AI models integrate multiple computational approaches, such as combining ML with molecular simulations, to refine predictive capabilities. Reinforcement learning (RL) frameworks have been applied to iteratively optimize nanoparticle formulations by evaluating their predicted immunogenic responses (Wang et al., 2022).

Table 4. Fey features and its predictive approach

Predictive Approach	**Key Features**
Molecular Dynamics (MD)	Simulates nanoparticle interactions with biological systems
Density Functional Theory (DFT)	Predicts electronic and mechanical properties
Machine Learning	Correlates experimental data with theoretical models
Reinforcement Learning	Optimizes synthesis conditions iteratively

Case Study: Cancer Therapy Using AI-Predicted Nanoparticles

Cancer immunotherapy has gained significant traction due to its potential to harness the body's immune system to target and destroy cancer cells. A recent study by Bhange and Telange (2025b) focused on developing polymeric nanoparticles designed to carry immune checkpoint inhibitors (ICIs) to enhance the immune response against tumors. These nanoparticles were optimized using AI-driven models, which combined molecular simulations with machine learning-based predictive analytics. The researchers used molecular simulations to understand how different polymer compositions and sizes influenced the stability and behavior of the nanoparticles in the body. Machine learning models were then trained on experimental data to predict the optimal formulation for enhanced immune activation and targeted drug delivery. The AI models helped identify the ideal properties for nanoparticles, such as size, surface charge, and drug release profile, leading to formulations that exhibited excellent stability in circulation. In preclinical studies, the AI-predicted nanoparticles successfully targeted tumor sites, activated immune cells, and demonstrated reduced systemic toxicity compared to conventional therapies. This approach not only accelerated the development of more effective cancer treatments but also highlighted the growing role of AI in designing highly personalized and precise nanoparticle-based therapies for cancer immunotherapy(Bhange & Telange, 2025b).

2.3. High-Throughput Screening Using AI

High-throughput screening (HTS) powered by AI accelerates the discovery and optimization of nanoparticles for immunological applications. Traditional screening methods are time-consuming and resource-intensive, whereas AI-assisted HTS enables rapid analysis of large libraries of nanoparticle formulations (Zeng, Guo, Xu, Chen, & Zhou, 2020).

2.3.1. Automated Experimental Platforms

The time needed for optimization is greatly decreased by AI-driven robotic systems that automate the synthesis and characterization of nanoparticles (Mottafegh, Joo, Na, Sharma, & Kim, 2024). These platforms incorporate:

- AI-powered automated imaging methods to evaluate nanoparticle morphology and size distribution
- Microfluidic-based synthesis devices for exact control over nanoparticle formulation

2.3.2.AI-Enhanced Data Analysis for Screening

Machine learning algorithms analyze high-throughput experimental datasets to identify optimal nanoparticle candidates. Common techniques include:

- **Random Forest (RF) and Gradient Boosting (GBM):** Used to rank nanoparticle formulations based on efficacy and stability.
- **Bayesian Optimization:** Iteratively refines screening experiments by focusing on the most promising candidates.

Case Study: AI-Driven Lipid Nanoparticle Screening for mRNA Vaccines

During the development of COVID-19 mRNA vaccines, AI-assisted HTS techniques were employed to screen thousands of lipid nanoparticle formulations, rapidly identifying formulations with optimal stability and transfection efficiency (Wei et al., 2024). The application of HTS methods is shown in Table 5.

Table 5. Application of HTS methods

AI-Driven HTS Method	Application
Robotic Synthesis	Automates nanoparticle production
Microfluidics	Enhances formulation control
Bayesian Optimization	Identifies optimal nanoparticle candidates
Random Forest (RF)	Ranks nanoparticles based on performance

3. NANOPARTICLE APPLICATIONS IN IMMUNOLOGY

3.1. AI-Designed Nanocarriers for Vaccine Delivery

Nanoparticles have become an essential vaccine delivery carrier because they provide various benefits over conventional alternatives. The nano dimension of nanoparticles permits better cell entry, but their exterior components can be straightforwardly integrated with targeting ligands, adjuvants, and antigens (Dasgupta et al., 2025). Methods to develop optimal NP-based vaccines represent a major scientific obstacle. However, this is where AI has revolutionized the field of vaccine deliveries by allowing for the development of highly sophisticated and personalized vaccine delivery systems. AI algorithms support multiple steps during the development of NP-based vaccines through design creation and subsequent in vivo testing (Bezbaruah et al., 2022; Janjua et al., 2023).

3.1.1. De Novo Design of Nanocarriers

De novo nanocarrier design involves creating novel nanomaterials for targeted drug delivery using computational modeling, chemical synthesis, and self-assembly to optimize size, shape, surface properties, and biocompatibility (Raheem et al., 2023). Unlike the traditional methods that modify existing materials, de novo design allows for precise control over the nanocarrier's architecture, thus enhancing drug encapsulation, targeted delivery, and controlled release.

3.1.2. Rational Design of Surface Modifications

NP surfaces serve as platforms for ligand attachment, enhancing cell entry and immune response. AI-driven predictive systems analyze big data to optimize surface modifications for specific antigens and targets, refining receptor-ligand binding, stability, and biocompatibility.

3.1.3. Predicting in Vivo Behavior

AI-powered models predict NP-based vaccine biodistribution, pharmacokinetics, and immunogenicity by integrating data from in vitro, animal, and clinical studies. These models simulate vaccine behavior in various environments to assess efficacy across diseases (Table 6).

Table 6. Recent applications of AI-designed nanocarriers for vaccine delivery

Delivery system	Description
mRNA vaccine delivery	The development of mRNA-based vaccines against COVID-19 has relied heavily on AI. AI algorithms are used to design LNPs that encapsulate and deliver mRNA to target cells efficiently while minimizing off-target effects and maintaining mRNA stability (Wang et al., 2022).
Personalized cancer vaccines	Personalized cancer vaccines that target tumor-specific antigens are being developed using AI-powered approaches. AI algorithms can execute patient-specific tumor data like genomic and proteomic profiles and pinpoint individual particular neoantigens, which are apt to be focused on by targeted NP-based vaccines(Chi et al., 2024).
Mucosal vaccines	Mucosal vaccines offer convenience and induce mucosal immunity, unlike traditional parenteral vaccines. AI-designed examples enhance targeting of mucosal tissues for strong immune responses, with NPs featuring surface modifications to improve antigen uptake in mucosal epithelial cells.

However, several challenges remain in developing AI-designed NP-based vaccines, such as developing accurate and predictive AI models that rely on large and diverse experimental and computational data.

3.2. Smart Nanoparticles for Immunotherapy

Cutting-edge fronting of immunotherapy, smart nanoparticles provide extraordinary precision and efficacy to target and modulate immune responses. These finely tuned nanomaterials are manufactured to sense distinct cellular cues in the complicated TME, enabling particular drug delivery, controlled release, and stimulated T-cell reaction(B.-Q. Chen et al., 2023).

3.2.1. Targeted Delivery and Controlled Release

3.2.1.1. Tumor-Specific Targeting

Ligands specific for tumor-associated receptors, such as proteins overexpressed or unique glycans on cancer cells, can be attached to smart nanoparticles. Furthermore, this targeted delivery assures therapeutic payloads, such as immune checkpoint inhibitors, cytokines, or nucleic acids, are explicitly delivered to the tumor site to minimize systemic toxicity and maximize therapeutic efficacy.

3.2.1.2. Stimuli-Responsive Release

Smart nanoparticles can deliver immune checkpoint inhibitors such as anti-PD1 and anti-CTLA4 antibodies to TME. This method can overcome the disadvantage of poor tumor penetration and systemic toxicity for these checkpoint inhibitors to improve their delivery and bioactivity.

3.2.2. Enhancing Immune Activation

3.2.2.1. Immune Checkpoint Blockade

Smart nanoparticles can deliver cytokines, especially interleukin-2 (IL-2) and interferon-gamma (IFN-γ), to the TME. It can activate inflammatory immunity, such as T cells and natural killer (NK) cells, and activate anti-tumour immune responses.

3.2.2.2. Nucleic Acid Delivery

Such smart nanoparticles allow for the delivery of nucleic acids such as mRNA and siRNA to immune cells. This approach can be exploited to enhance the anti-tumor activity of the immune cells or suppress their immunosuppressive functions.

3.3. AI-Guided Development of Adjuvants and Immune Modulators

Vaccines can not function without adjuvants, which are provided to increase immunogenicity and efficacy. Developing adjuvants has been an expensive affair for a long time. Despite this, however, the introduction of AI has undergone a revolution in this field by allowing for the rapid and efficient design of novel and potent adjuvants.

3.3.1. Rational Design of Adjuvants

3.3.1.1. Adjuvant Efficacy Prediction

AI algorithms can presumably examine the large amounts of physicochemical, immunological, and clinical trial data found in existing adjuvants. By identifying trends and correlations, algorithms can forecast the probable safety and effectiveness of novel adjuvant candidates. This feature significantly lengthens the screening period and reduces the likelihood of looking for hazardous or inefficient substances.

3.3.1.2. Designing Adjuvants with Specific Immunological Properties

AI can design adjuvants that can impel a particular type of immune reaction, such as Th1, Th2, or Th17 responses, depending on the objective contagious particle or sickness. That is where AI algorithms can be trained to predict the immunogenicity of various adjuvant formulations with different compositions and structural features. They can also use this data to customize adjuvants according to specific immune needs.

3.3.1.3. Predicting Adverse Reactions

AI can also help predict potential adverse reactions to different adjuvants. Using the data of known adverse events, AI algorithms can identify potential risk factors and an adjuvant that can be safer and tolerable.

3.3.2. Personalized Adjuvant Selection

Depending on the patient's immune system, genetic background, and disease severity, the adjuvant can include enough information to be used on them specifically. AI, for instance, is able to evaluate this data and choose the best adjuvant for that patient. Such an individualized approach can reduce the risk of vaccination-induced adverse effects and increase vaccine efficacy. AI can predict the individual's response to a specific adjuvant, depending on genetic polymorphisms, the immune cell profile, or lifestyle. It gives information on how to optimize vaccination schedules and personalize treatment regimes.

3.3.3. Development of Novel Adjuvant Delivery Systems

AI can be used to design and optimize nanoparticle-based adjuvant delivery systems. We use AI algorithms to predict the interaction of nanoparticles with immune cells and the extent to which these nanoparticles can provide an antigen by analyzing their physicochemical properties, such as size, shape, surface charge, and composition. Nanoparticles can be engineered to deliver antigens and adjuvants to specific immune cells or tissues, and AI can be used to engineer this. Its targeted delivery approach improves vaccine efficacy and retains off-target effects.

The blasphemous study of machine learning is striving to create novel Toll-like receptor (TLR) agonists. Pattern recognition receptors comprised of TLRs have a significant role in innate immunity. Machine learning algorithms can identify novel compounds with improved TLR-stimulating activity by analyzing known TLR agonists' structural and functional properties. SaRNA vaccines are also being designed using AI vaccines, a new and promising class of vaccines, engendering the promise of delivering multiple antigens and adjuvants with a single dose. Today, AI algorithms are being applied to complete the design of siRNA vaccines, ranging from selecting appropriate antigens, adjuvants, and delivery systems.

4. AI IN PERSONALIZED AND PRECISION IMMUNOTHERAPY

4.1. AI-Generated Nanoparticles for Targeted Drug Delivery

The integration of artificial intelligence (AI) in nanomedicine has revolutionized the field of immunotherapy, particularly in the design and optimization of nanoparticles for targeted drug delivery (Ali et al., 2024). AI-driven methodologies enable the precise engineering of nanoparticles to improve their biocompatibility, stability, and efficacy in targeting diseased tissues while minimizing systemic toxicity (Serov & Vinogradov, 2022). Traditional nanoparticle development often relies on trial-and-error methods, but AI leverages vast datasets to predict optimal compositions, shapes, and surface modifications, accelerating the discovery process (Harrison et al., 2021).

Machine learning (ML) algorithms have been employed to analyze large-scale biological data, identifying key physicochemical parameters influencing nanoparticle behavior in vivo (T, Narayan, Shenoy, & Nayak, 2022). For instance, deep learning techniques can predict how nanoparticles interact with immune cells and the tumor microenvironment, ensuring enhanced drug retention and controlled release (Yuan et al., 2024). AI-guided computational models can also simulate biological pathways to forecast immune responses, facilitating the design of nanoparticles that can efficiently target immune checkpoints or antigen-presenting cells (Y. Yang, Zhao, Liu, & Huang, 2022).

4.2. Tailoring Nanoparticle Properties for Individualized Treatment

The concept of personalized medicine has gained traction with AI-driven methodologies in nanomedicine, where individual patient data is used to customize nanoparticle properties for optimal therapeutic outcomes. Patient-specific factors, including genetic profile, immune status, and tumor heterogeneity, can be analyzed using AI to design nanoparticles that cater to each patient's unique biological environment (Das, 2024).

To forecast how particular nanoparticles would affect a person's immune system, AI models can incorporate multi-omics data, such as transcriptomics, proteomics, and genomes (Kroll et al., 2019). This strategy makes it possible to create nanoparticles with ligand functionalization, surface charge, and size customization to increase their targeting effectiveness (Jin, Liu, Xu, Su, & Zhang, 2020). For instance, polymeric nanoparticles with improved tumor penetration capacities have been developed thanks to AI-guided screening, guaranteeing effective delivery of therapeutic drugs to cancers that have spread deeply (Ramasamy et al., 2022).

Moreover, reinforcement learning algorithms have optimized nanoparticle formulations dynamically, allowing real-time adjustments in response to evolving disease states (Chou et al., 2023). These smart nanoparticles can be functionalized with patient-derived exosomes or peptides to enhance immune recognition and reduce immune evasion by cancer cells (Zhao et al., 2021). Additionally, AI-driven optimization of nanoparticle coatings, such as PEGylation and biomimetic camouflage, has significantly improved their circulation time and reduced clearance by the mononuclear phagocyte system (Olawade, Ige, et al., 2024).

4.3. Real-Time AI Analysis of Nanoparticle-Immune System Interactions

Precision immunotherapy depends on the real-time analysis of nanoparticle interactions with the immune system. AI-driven biosensing technologies allow for continuous monitoring of nanoparticle behavior, allowing for adaptive adjustments to improve therapeutic outcomes (Jin et al., 2020). Real-time AI analysis can identify changes in cytokine release profiles, immune cell activation, and nanoparticle biodistribution, enabling data-driven treatment strategy modifications (D. Chen et al., 2024).

Advanced imaging techniques, such as AI-enhanced multiphoton microscopy and single-cell RNA sequencing, have provided unprecedented insights into nanoparticle-immune system interactions at the cellular and molecular levels (Yu Chen et al., 2012). These AI-powered platforms can predict how nanoparticles will be taken up by dendritic cells, macrophages, or T cells, improving their immunostimulatory effects (Olawade, Ige, et al., 2024). AI-assisted image processing also enhances the detection of nanoparticle-induced immunogenic cell death, a key mechanism in cancer immunotherapy.

Additionally, to ensure accurate dose modifications, AI-integrated biosensors have been created to measure the pharmacokinetics and pharmacodynamics of nanoparticles in real-time (Pawar et al., 2023). Clinicians might gain useful insights for improving treatment by using wearable AI-based devices to track biomarkers of immune responses, such as interleukin levels or PD-L1 expression (Zhang, Hu, Jiang, & Yetisen, 2023). By guaranteeing that immune responses stay within an ideal therapeutic window, these real-time data streams enable individualized nanoparticle therapy.

Predictive models powered by AI have also proven crucial in reducing the possibility of immune-related side effects linked to nanoparticle treatments (Olawade, Wada, et al., 2024). AI algorithms can determine immunotoxicity risk factors by examining past patient data, which helps direct the creation of safer nanoparticle formulations. When it comes to autoimmune disorders and inflammatory conditions, where carefully adjusted immunotherapies are necessary, these prognostic capacities are especially helpful.

5. CHALLENGES IN AI-BASED NANOPARTICLE RESEARCH

5.1. Data Availability and Model Accuracy

Despite its revolutionary promise, artificial intelligence in nanoparticle design faces several formidable obstacles. Among the main challenges are data quality and availability. Large, varied, and well-annotated datasets, including imaging data, clinical results, and molecular profiles, are commonly used by AI systems (Panayides et al., 2020). Effective AI models are built on top of high-quality data, but acquiring this data in nanotechnology is still tricky. Nanoparticles are frequently characterized using sophisticated imaging methods like atomic force microscopy (AFM), scanning electron microscopy (SEM), and transmission electron microscopy (TEM). However, these methods frequently provide few datasets because of their high expense, time commitment, and technological complexity. Moreover, a great deal of preprocessing is necessary to make these datasets usable for AI applications because they are often noisy or inadequate (Elabiad, 2025). Furthermore, this issue is made worse by the lack of defined procedures for gathering and reporting data, which could lead to models that do not function consistently across various experimental configurations or categories of nanoparticles (Kapoor et al., 2024).

AI models severely depend on substantial datasets for accurate predictions. Nevertheless, predictions may be less accurate or prejudiced if there are restrictions on data availability, particularly for rare diseases or specific groups. Biased results may arise from problems such as training datasets with insufficient demographic representation. Homogeneity in patient populations might pose challenges in clinical trials, impairing the model's capacity to forecast medication efficacy precisely. For AI model building, representative, reliable, and unbiased data is essential (Norori, Hu, Aellen, Faraci, & Tzovara, 2021). It cannot be easy to update AI models with new data once trained, especially in drug development, where new information is regularly discovered. Model update strategies need to be well thought out. Even specialists may find it challenging to understand the results of AI models due to their complexity. When predictions are not well articulated, it is difficult for researchers and clinicians to understand and turn data into useful insights. Enhancing the interpretability and explainability of AI models is necessary for their successful use (Johnson et al., 2021).

5.2. Ethical and Regulatory Considerations

The use of AI in nanomedicine raises significant ethical and legal concerns, particularly for applications in the fields of medicine and the environment. AI-designed nanoparticles in nanotechnology must pass a rigorous preclinical and clinical testing procedure to ensure their efficacy and safety. However, the novel aspects of AI-driven solutions, including dynamically customized nanoparticles and adaptive algorithms, are usually overlooked by current regulatory frameworks. This regulatory gap creates insecurity and hinders the conversion of research into practical uses (Tsamados et al., 2022).

The employment of AI in delicate applications also raises ethical questions. Serious consequences may result from algorithmic bias, which occurs when AI algorithms unintentionally favor particular results because of skewed training data, especially in healthcare. Biased AI models, for instance, may result in differences in the effectiveness of treatment among certain demographic groups. Thorough monitoring and the creation of ethical strategies that emphasize responsibility and inclusivity will be necessary to guarantee justice and openness in AI-driven nanotechnology (Elabiad, 2025).

5.3. Safety and Biocompatibility Concerns

Due to their size, shape, surface area, composition, and reactivity, Nanoparticles can have significant toxicity and potential long-term health impacts, like lung inflammation, oxidative stress, DNA damage, cell death, and possible carcinogenic effects. They can easily penetrate the cell membranes and accumulate in organs like the lungs, liver, and brain. Nanoparticles also released during manufacture, use, or disposal may build up in the environment and impact ecosystems. Even though AI models are predictive, they frequently lack enough real-world data to predict these effects entirely (Xuan, Ju, Skonieczna, Zhou, & Huang, 2023).

Nanoparticles could be harmful to human health if they are not biocompatible. The ability of a material to interact with live organisms is measured by its biocompatibility. Nanoparticles may have detrimental impacts if they are not biocompatible. Certain nanoparticles trigger immunological or allergic responses. Because of genetic variations, comorbidities, and environmental exposures, biocompatibility varies greatly amongst individuals. Due to a lack of extensive and varied datasets, AI models may not be able to anticipate uncommon or peculiar reactions and biodegradation routes under different physiological conditions (S. Yang & Kar, 2023).

6. FUTURE PERSPECTIVES AND EMERGING TRENDS

The design and use of nanoparticles in immunological disorders could radically change with the combination of artificial intelligence (AI) and sophisticated computational techniques (Hasanzadeh et al., 2022). As AI models become more advanced, they can process increasingly complex biological data, leading to highly personalized nanoparticle therapies tailored to individual immune profiles. Integrating multi-omics datasets—including genomics, proteomics, and metabolomics—will enhance our understanding of immune responses and improve nanoparticle targeting precision. Quantum computing, though still in its infancy, promises to significantly boost the speed and accuracy of simulations that predict nanoparticle interactions with immune cells. Moreover, developing real-time biosensing and AI-powered feedback systems will enable dynamic monitoring and adjustment of nanoparticle-based treatments. Interdisciplinary collaboration among immunologists, data scientists, engineers, and clinicians will be crucial to translating AI-driven nanoparticle research from the lab to clinical practice. Regulatory agencies will also need to evolve, creating flexible and adaptive frameworks to evaluate the safety and efficacy of AI-designed nanomedicines. Ethical considerations, particularly around data use and algorithmic bias, will guide future research and development. Emerging techniques such as digital twins and AI-driven immune system modeling could open new frontiers in predictive immunotherapy. Ultimately, the fusion of AI and nanotechnology heralds a new era in immunological treatment that is faster, more precise, and more responsive to patient needs.(Hasanzadeh et al., 2022). Three new trends are examined in this section:

6.1. Integrating AI with Multi-Omics for Nanoparticle Design

The confluence of artificial intelligence (AI) with multi-omics data, including transcriptomics, proteome, metabolomics, epigenomics, and genomics, has brought about a new age of precision medicine, especially in developing nanoparticles for immunological illnesses (Anklam et al., 2022). This integrative approach makes developing focused and efficient treatment interventions easier, providing a thorough grasp of the intricate molecular pathways underpinning immune responses.

Multi-omics data offer a comprehensive picture of biological systems (Haas et al., 2017). However, their immense size and complexity present formidable analytical obstacles. These enormous datasets can be processed and interpreted with the help of artificial intelligence (AI), especially machine learning (ML) and deep learning (DL) algorithms, which can reveal complex patterns and relationships that conventional statistical techniques could miss (Sarker, 2021).

Artificial intelligence (AI) systems can evaluate multi-omics data in the context of nanoparticle design to pinpoint specific biomarkers and molecular targets linked to immune illnesses. For example, AI can identify abnormal gene expressions and protein interactions contributing to illness pathogenesis by combining proteomic and genomic data (Biswas & Chakrabarti, 2020). These insights aid the development of nanoparticles that can precisely interact with specific molecular targets, improving the accuracy and effectiveness of therapeutic administration.

6.2. Quantum Computing in AI-Driven Nanoparticle Research

Quantum computing, a groundbreaking advancement in computational science, holds the potential to address difficult problems that are beyond the scope of conventional computers (Mazumdar et al., 2025a). In AI-driven nanoparticle research, it could greatly enhance modeling, simulation, and optimization processes, leading to more effective and efficient treatment designs.

Quantum mechanical principles regulate the interactions of nanoparticles with biological systems, which involve dynamic behaviors and intricate molecular structures (Mu et al., 2014). Because of the exponential rise in complexity with system size, classical computational approaches frequently find it difficult to describe these interactions effectively (Papadimitriou, 2003). However, quantum computing uses concepts like entanglement and superposition to simultaneously analyze large amounts of data, making it possible to simulate intricate quantum systems more precisely (Daley et al., 2022).

The accuracy of molecular simulations can be increased by combining quantum computing with AI-driven nanoparticle research. Quantum algorithms, for instance, can be used to predict the electrical structures of nanoparticles, providing detailed information about their chemical composition and interactions with biological molecules. Understanding this information is necessary to design nanoparticles with specific roles, such as immune control or targeted drug delivery (Mitchell et al., 2021).

6.3. Translational Challenges and Clinical Applications

Several challenges remain as AI-assisted nanoparticle research advances toward clinical application (Heydari et al., 2024). Despite progress in design for immunological diseases, biological, regulatory, and manufacturing hurdles must be addressed. Key concerns include scalability, complex immune interactions, and the need for comprehensive safety assessments (Souto et al., 2024).

One major challenge is the immune system's unpredictable response to nanoparticles (Younis, Tawfeek, Abdellatif, Abdel-Aleem, & Harashima, 2022). While nanoparticles can be tailored to target specific immune pathways, they may trigger unintended immune activation, leading to cytokine storms, inflammation, or autoimmune reactions (Dobrovolskaia, Shurin, & Shvedova, 2016). Conversely, weak immune activation can render therapies ineffective. AI-driven models help optimize design by predicting immunological interactions using multi-omics data, but patient variability complicates generalization (Bhange & Telange, 2025a). This underscores the need for personalized approaches, where AI customizes nanoparticle properties based on individual genetic, proteomic, and metabolic profiles (Mazumdar, Khondakar, Das, Halder, & Kaushik, 2025b).

Nanoparticle therapeutic success heavily depends on toxicity and biocompatibility. Despite AI-driven optimization, ensuring long-term safety remains challenging (Mazumdar et al., 2025b). Off-target accumulation in organs like the liver or kidneys can cause systemic toxicity (X. Li et al., 2020). Computational models can predict toxicity, but these must be validated through in vitro and in vivo studies (Cao, Li, & Chen, 2021). Testing across diverse populations ensures broad safety and efficacy (Anklam et al., 2022). Standardized protocols aligned with regulatory standards are needed due to complex immune responses (Dobrovolskaia, 2015).

Regulatory approval remains a key challenge for AI-designed nanoparticles. Agencies like the FDA, EMA, and WHO require detailed data on manufacturing, safety, and efficacy (Eifler & Thaxton, 2011). AI-generated formulations often fall outside current regulatory frameworks, complicating approval (Kapoor et al., 2024). The opaque nature of some AI models also raises concerns about transparency.

To address this, interpretable AI systems are being developed to offer clear, mechanistic explanations for nanoparticle design choices.

Manufacturing and scalability remain key challenges for the clinical use of AI-assisted nanoparticles (Mazumdar et al., 2025b). While AI can optimize formulations, replicating them consistently at scale is difficult. Precise control over surface charge, size, and shape is crucial, as slight variations can affect therapeutic efficacy (Stavis, Fagan, Stopa, & Liddle, 2018). Scalable, cost-effective methods are still evolving. AI-driven automation, robotics, and high-throughput screening are being explored to enhance production reliability and minimize batch variability (Vinchurkar & Mane, 2024).

The future of AI-assisted nanoparticles in immunology relies on interdisciplinary collaboration to overcome translational barriers. Unified standards from researchers, clinicians, regulators, and industry are crucial. Advances in quantum computing, multi-omics, and AI explainability will accelerate clinical translation. Ensuring immunological compatibility, regulatory approval, and scalable manufacturing is key to their safe and effective medical use (Coskun et al., 2024).

Figure 1. Personalized healthcare framework integrating laboratory medicine, omics data, and statistical algorithms for optimized diagnostics and treatment.

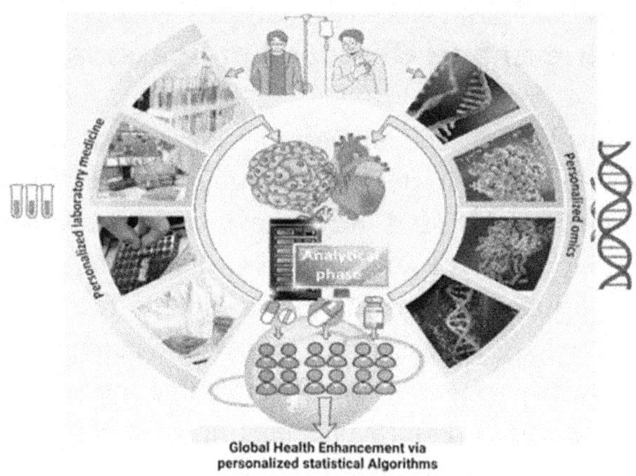

A conceptual framework illustrates integrating personalized lab medicine with omics data to enhance global health. It shows how patient-specific lab and multi-omics data are analyzed using advanced algorithms to enable personalized diagnostics and treatments, improving healthcare outcomes depicted in Fig 1.

CONCLUSION

AI-driven nanoparticle design grasps transformative prospective for the future of immunological research and therapy. By aiding precise control over nanoparticle properties and pretending complex immune interactions, AI empowers researchers to develop smarter, safer, and more effective therapeutic strategies. The synergy between machine learning, high-throughput biological data, and advanced computational models allows for rapid screening, optimization, and customization of nanoparticles tailored to individual patients' immune profiles.

Despite these promising advancements, significant hurdles remain. Limitations in high-quality, diverse datasets restrict the generalizability of AI models, while challenges surrounding transparency, algorithmic bias, and interpretability hinder their broader clinical adoption. Regulatory frameworks also lag behind technological innovation, with current approval processes ill-equipped to handle the complexity of AI-designed therapeutics. Ethical concerns surrounding data privacy, patient consent, and algorithmic accountability must also be carefully addressed to ensure responsible integration of AI into healthcare.

The integration of multi-omics data, explainable AI, and quantum computing is expected to elevate AI's capabilities in nanomedicine further. These technologies will facilitate real-time, adaptive treatment strategies and enable the design of truly personalized immunotherapies. As computer scientists, immunologists, clinicians, and regulatory bodies strengthen interdisciplinary collaboration, AI-generated nanoparticles are poised to bridge the gap between computational prediction and clinical translation. Their successful deployment will mark a new era in precision immunotherapy, transforming how immune-related diseases are diagnosed, treated, and managed.

REFERENCES

Adytia, G. J., Sutanto, H., Pratiwi, L., & Fetarayani, D. (2025). Advances in Synthetic Immunology for Targeted Treatment of Systemic Autoimmune Diseases: Opportunities, Challenges, and Future Directions. *Immuno*, *5*(1), 6. DOI: 10.3390/immuno5010006

Ali, K. A., Mohin, S., Mondal, P., Goswami, S., Ghosh, S., & Choudhuri, S. (2024). Influence of artificial intelligence in modern pharmaceutical formulation and drug development. *Future Journal of Pharmaceutical Sciences*, *10*(1), 53. DOI: 10.1186/s43094-024-00625-1

Aljabali, A. A., Obeid, M. A., Bashatwah, R. M., Serrano-Aroca, Á., Mishra, V., Mishra, Y., El-Tanani, M., Hromić-Jahjefendić, A., Kapoor, D. N., Goyal, R., Naikoo, G. A., & Tambuwala, M. M. (2023). Nanomaterials and Their Impact on the Immune System. *International Journal of Molecular Sciences*, *24*(3), 2008. DOI: 10.3390/ijms24032008 PMID: 36768330

Aljabali, A. A. A., Obeid, M. A., Gammoh, O., El-Tanani, M., Mishra, V., Mishra, Y., Kapre, S., Srivatsa Palakurthi, S., Hassan, S. S., Nawn, D., Lundstrom, K., Hromić-Jahjefendić, A., Serrano-Aroca, Á., Redwan, E. M., Uversky, V. N., & Tambuwala, M. M. (2024). Nanomaterial-Driven Precision Immunomodulation: A New Paradigm in Therapeutic Interventions. *Cancers (Basel)*, *16*(11), 2030. DOI: 10.3390/cancers16112030 PMID: 38893150

Anklam, E., Bahl, M. I., Ball, R., Beger, R. D., Cohen, J., Fitzpatrick, S., Girard, P., Halamoda-Kenzaoui, B., Hinton, D., Hirose, A., Hoeveler, A., Honma, M., Hugas, M., Ishida, S., Kass, G. E. N., Kojima, H., Krefting, I., Liachenko, S., Liu, Y., & Slikker, W.Jr. (2022). Emerging technologies and their impact on regulatory science. *Experimental Biology and Medicine*, *247*(1), 1–75. DOI: 10.1177/15353702211052280 PMID: 34783606

Ashwini, T., Narayan, R., Shenoy, P. A., & Nayak, U. Y. (2022). Computational modeling for the design and development of nano based drug delivery systems. *Journal of Molecular Liquids*, *368*, 120596.

Bae, S., Choi, H., Lee, J., Kang, M., Ahn, S., Lee, Y., & Nam, J. (2024). Rational Design of Lipid Nanoparticles for Enhanced mRNA Vaccine Delivery via Machine Learning. *Small*, •••, 2405618. PMID: 39264000

Basile, A. O., Yahi, A., & Tatonetti, N. P. (2019). Artificial Intelligence for Drug Toxicity and Safety. *Trends in Pharmacological Sciences*, *40*(9), 624–635. DOI: 10.1016/j.tips.2019.07.005 PMID: 31383376

Bezbaruah, R., Chavda, V. P., Nongrang, L., Alom, S., Deka, K., Kalita, T., Ali, F., Bhattacharjee, B., & Vora, L. (2022). Nanoparticle-Based Delivery Systems for Vaccines. *Vaccines*, *10*(11), 1946. DOI: 10.3390/vaccines10111946 PMID: 36423041

Bhange, M., & Telange, D. (2025a). Convergence of nanotechnology and artificial intelligence in the fight against liver cancer: A comprehensive review. *Discover. Oncology*, *16*(1), 77. DOI: 10.1007/s12672-025-01821-y PMID: 39841330

Bhange, M., & Telange, D. (2025b). Convergence of nanotechnology and artificial intelligence in the fight against liver cancer: A comprehensive review. *Discover. Oncology*, *16*(1), 77. DOI: 10.1007/s12672-025-01821-y PMID: 39841330

Biswas, N., & Chakrabarti, S. (2020). Artificial Intelligence (AI)-Based Systems Biology Approaches in Multi-Omics Data Analysis of Cancer. *Frontiers in Oncology, 10*, 588221. Advance online publication. DOI: 10.3389/fonc.2020.588221 PMID: 33154949

Botifoll, M., Pinto-Huguet, I., & Arbiol, J. (2022). Machine learning in electron microscopy for advanced nanocharacterization: Current developments, available tools and future outlook. *Nanoscale Horizons, 7*(12), 1427–1477. DOI: 10.1039/D2NH00377E PMID: 36239693

Cao, Y., Li, S., & Chen, J. (2021). Modeling better in vitro models for the prediction of nanoparticle toxicity: A review. *Toxicology Mechanisms and Methods, 31*(1), 1–17. DOI: 10.1080/15376516.2020.1828521 PMID: 32972312

Chen, B.-Q., Zhao, Y., Zhang, Y., Pan, Y.-J., Xia, H.-Y., Kankala, R. K., Wang, S.-B., Liu, G., & Chen, A.-Z. (2023). Immune-regulating camouflaged nanoplatforms: A promising strategy to improve cancer nano-immunotherapy. *Bioactive Materials, 21*, 1–19. DOI: 10.1016/j.bioactmat.2022.07.023 PMID: 36017071

Chen, D., Plott, T., Wiest, M., Van Trump, W., Komalo, B., Nguyen, D., Marsh, C., Heinrich, J., Fuller, C. J., Nicolaisen, L., Cambronero, E., Nguyen, A., Elabd, C., Rubbo, F., & DeVay Jacobson, R. (2024). A combined AI and cell biology approach surfaces targets and mechanistically distinct Inflammasome inhibitors. *iScience, 27*(12), 111404. DOI: 10.1016/j.isci.2024.111404 PMID: 39687021

Chen, Yu., Liang, C.-P., Liu, Y., Fischer, A. H., Parwani, A. V., & Pantanowitz, L. (2012). Review of advanced imaging techniques. *Journal of Pathology Informatics, 3*(1), 22. DOI: 10.4103/2153-3539.96751 PMID: 22754737

Chen, Y., Zhou, Q., Jia, Z., Cheng, N., Zhang, S., Chen, W., & Wang, L. (2024). Enhancing cancer immunotherapy: Nanotechnology-mediated immunotherapy overcoming immunosuppression. *Acta Pharmaceutica Sinica. B, 14*(9), 3834–3854. DOI: 10.1016/j.apsb.2024.05.032 PMID: 39309502

Chi, W.-Y., Hu, Y., Huang, H.-C., Kuo, H.-H., Lin, S.-H., Kuo, C.-T. J., Tao, J., Fan, D., Huang, Y.-M., Wu, A. A., Hung, C.-F., & Wu, T.-C. (2024). Molecular targets and strategies in the development of nucleic acid cancer vaccines: From shared to personalized antigens. *Journal of Biomedical Science, 31*(1), 94. DOI: 10.1186/s12929-024-01082-x PMID: 39379923

Chou, W.-C., Chen, Q., Yuan, L., Cheng, Y.-H., He, C., Monteiro-Riviere, N. A., Riviere, J. E., & Lin, Z. (2023). An artificial intelligence-assisted physiologically-based pharmacokinetic model to predict nanoparticle delivery to tumors in mice. *Journal of Controlled Release, 361*, 53–63. DOI: 10.1016/j.jconrel.2023.07.040 PMID: 37499908

Coskun, A., Ertaylan, G., Pusparum, M., Van Hoof, R., Kaya, Z. Z., Khosravi, A., & Zarrabi, A. (2024). Advancing personalized medicine: Integrating statistical algorithms with omics and nano-omics for enhanced diagnostic accuracy and treatment efficacy. *Biochimica et Biophysica Acta (BBA) -. Biochimica et Biophysica Acta. Molecular Basis of Disease, 1870*(7), 167339. DOI: 10.1016/j.bbadis.2024.167339 PMID: 38986819

Daley, A. J., Bloch, I., Kokail, C., Flannigan, S., Pearson, N., Troyer, M., & Zoller, P. (2022). Practical quantum advantage in quantum simulation. *Nature, 607*(7920), 667–676. DOI: 10.1038/s41586-022-04940-6 PMID: 35896643

Das, A. B. (2024). Network medicine and artificial intelligence in cancer precision therapy: Path to prevent drug-induced toxic side effect. *Current Opinion in Toxicology, 38*, 100476. DOI: 10.1016/j.cotox.2024.100476

Dasgupta, S., Maji, S., Dey, S., Chattopadhyay, M., Chanda, A., Acharjee, S., Santra, K., & Ali, K. A. (2025). Exploring nanocomposite materials in clinical dermatology: Innovations for treating skin diseases. *Next Nanotechnology, 7*, 100139. DOI: 10.1016/j.nxnano.2025.100139

Dobrovolskaia, M. A. (2015). Pre-clinical immunotoxicity studies of nanotechnology-formulated drugs: Challenges, considerations and strategy. *Journal of Controlled Release, 220*, 571–583. DOI: 10.1016/j.jconrel.2015.08.056 PMID: 26348388

Dobrovolskaia, M. A., Shurin, M., & Shvedova, A. A. (2016). Current understanding of interactions between nanoparticles and the immune system. *Toxicology and Applied Pharmacology, 299*, 78–89. DOI: 10.1016/j.taap.2015.12.022 PMID: 26739622

Eifler, A. C., & Thaxton, C. S. (2011). Nanoparticle Therapeutics: FDA Approval, Clinical Trials, Regulatory Pathways, and Case Study. In Hurst, S. J. (Ed.), *Biomedical Nanotechnology* (pp. 325–338). Humana Press. DOI: 10.1007/978-1-61779-052-2_21

Elabiad, S. (2025). Artificial Intelligence in Nanotechnology: Transforming Innovation at the Atomic Scale. SSRN *Electronic Journal*. DOI: 10.2139/ssrn.5108426

Elumalai, K., Srinivasan, S., & Shanmugam, A. (2024). Review of the efficacy of nanoparticle-based drug delivery systems for cancer treatment. *Biomedical Technology, 5*, 109–122. DOI: 10.1016/j.bmt.2023.09.001

Furxhi, I., Faccani, L., Zanoni, I., Brigliadori, A., Vespignani, M., & Costa, A. L. (2024). Design rules applied to silver nanoparticles synthesis: A practical example of machine learning application. *Computational and Structural Biotechnology Journal, 25*, 20–33. DOI: 10.1016/j.csbj.2024.02.010 PMID: 38444982

Goshisht, M. K. (2024). Machine Learning and Deep Learning in Synthetic Biology: Key Architectures, Applications, and Challenges. *ACS Omega, 9*(9), 9921–9945. DOI: 10.1021/acsomega.3c05913 PMID: 38463314

Haas, R., Zelezniak, A., Iacovacci, J., Kamrad, S., Townsend, S., & Ralser, M. (2017). Designing and interpreting 'multi-omic' experiments that may change our understanding of biology. *Current Opinion in Systems Biology, 6*, 37–45. DOI: 10.1016/j.coisb.2017.08.009 PMID: 32923746

Harrison, P. J., Wieslander, H., Sabirsh, A., Karlsson, J., Malmsjö, V., Hellander, A., Wählby, C., & Spjuth, O. (2021). Deep-Learning Models for Lipid Nanoparticle-Based Drug Delivery. *Nanomedicine (London), 16*(13), 1097–1110. DOI: 10.2217/nnm-2020-0461 PMID: 33949890

Hasanzadeh, A., Hamblin, M. R., Kiani, J., Noori, H., Hardie, J. M., Karimi, M., & Shafiee, H. (2022). Could artificial intelligence revolutionize the development of nanovectors for gene therapy and mRNA vaccines? *Nano Today*, *47*, 101665. DOI: 10.1016/j.nantod.2022.101665 PMID: 37034382

Hesse, L., Oude Elberink, J. N. G., Van Oosterhout, A. J. M., & Nawijn, M. C. (2022). Allergen immunotherapy for allergic airway diseases: Use lessons from the past to design a brighter future. *Pharmacology & Therapeutics*, *237*, 108115. DOI: 10.1016/j.pharmthera.2022.108115 PMID: 35063570

Heydari, S., Masoumi, N., Esmaeeli, E., Ayyoubzadeh, S. M., Ghorbani-Bidkorpeh, F., & Ahmadi, M. (2024). Artificial intelligence in nanotechnology for treatment of diseases. *Journal of Drug Targeting*, *32*(10), 1247–1266. DOI: 10.1080/1061186X.2024.2393417 PMID: 39155708

Huanbutta, K., Burapapadh, K., Kraisit, P., Sriamornsak, P., Ganokratanaa, T., Suwanpitak, K., & Sangnim, T. (2024). Artificial intelligence-driven pharmaceutical industry: A paradigm shift in drug discovery, formulation development, manufacturing, quality control, and post-market surveillance. *European Journal of Pharmaceutical Sciences*, *203*, 106938. DOI: 10.1016/j.ejps.2024.106938 PMID: 39419129

Huang, Y., Guo, X., Wu, Y., Chen, X., Feng, L., Xie, N., & Shen, G. (2024). Nanotechnology's frontier in combatting infectious and inflammatory diseases: Prevention and treatment. *Signal Transduction and Targeted Therapy*, *9*(1), 34. DOI: 10.1038/s41392-024-01745-z PMID: 38378653

Janjua, T. I., Cao, Y., Kleitz, F., Linden, M., Yu, C., & Popat, A. (2023). Silica nanoparticles: A review of their safety and current strategies to overcome biological barriers. *Advanced Drug Delivery Reviews*, *203*, 115115. DOI: 10.1016/j.addr.2023.115115 PMID: 37844843

Jin, X., Liu, C., Xu, T., Su, L., & Zhang, X. (2020). Artificial intelligence biosensors: Challenges and prospects. *Biosensors & Bioelectronics*, *165*, 112412. DOI: 10.1016/j.bios.2020.112412 PMID: 32729531

Johnson, K. B., Wei, W., Weeraratne, D., Frisse, M. E., Misulis, K., Rhee, K., Zhao, J., & Snowdon, J. L. (2021). Precision Medicine, AI, and the Future of Personalized Health Care. *Clinical and Translational Science*, *14*(1), 86–93. DOI: 10.1111/cts.12884 PMID: 32961010

Kapoor, D. U., Sharma, J. B., Gandhi, S. M., Prajapati, B. G., Thanawuth, K., Limmatvapirat, S., & Sriamornsak, P. (2024). AI-driven design and optimization of nanoparticle-based drug delivery systems. *Science, Engineering and Health Studies*, 24010003.

Karahmet Sher, E., Alebić, M., Marković Boras, M., Boškailo, E., Karahmet Farhat, E., Karahmet, A., Pavlović, B., Sher, F., & Lekić, L. (2024). Nanotechnology in medicine revolutionizing drug delivery for cancer and viral infection treatments. *International Journal of Pharmaceutics*, *660*, 124345. DOI: 10.1016/j.ijpharm.2024.124345 PMID: 38885775

Kroll, A. V., Jiang, Y., Zhou, J., Holay, M., Fang, R. H., & Zhang, L. (2019). Biomimetic Nanoparticle Vaccines for Cancer Therapy. *Advanced Biosystems*, *3*(1), 1800219. DOI: 10.1002/adbi.201800219 PMID: 31728404

Kumar, M., Kulkarni, P., Liu, S., Chemuturi, N., & Shah, D. K. (2023). Nanoparticle biodistribution coefficients: A quantitative approach for understanding the tissue distribution of nanoparticles. *Advanced Drug Delivery Reviews*, *194*, 114708. DOI: 10.1016/j.addr.2023.114708 PMID: 36682420

Kurul, F., Turkmen, H., Cetin, A. E., & Topkaya, S. N. (2025). Nanomedicine: How nanomaterials are transforming drug delivery, bio-imaging, and diagnosis. *Next Nanotechnology*, *7*, 100129. DOI: 10.1016/j.nxnano.2024.100129

Kyriakides, T. R., Raj, A., Tseng, T. H., Xiao, H., Nguyen, R., Mohammed, F. S., Halder, S., Xu, M., Wu, M. J., Bao, S., & Sheu, W. C. (2021). Biocompatibility of nanomaterials and their immunological properties. *Biomedical Materials (Bristol, England)*, *16*(4), 042005. DOI: 10.1088/1748-605X/abe5fa PMID: 33578402

Li, X., Wang, B., Zhou, S., Chen, W., Chen, H., Liang, S., Zheng, L., Yu, H., Chu, R., Wang, M., Chai, Z., & Feng, W. (2020). Surface chemistry governs the sub-organ transfer, clearance and toxicity of functional gold nanoparticles in the liver and kidney. *Journal of Nanobiotechnology*, *18*(1), 45. DOI: 10.1186/s12951-020-00599-1 PMID: 32169073

Li, Y., Xu, Y., Su, W., Xu, J., Ye, Z., Wang, Z., Liu, Q., & Chen, F. (2025). Exploring the immuno-nano nexus: A paradigm shift in tumor vaccines. *Biomedicine and Pharmacotherapy*, *184*, 117897. DOI: 10.1016/j.biopha.2025.117897 PMID: 39921945

Malachowski, T., & Hassel, A. (2020). Engineering nanoparticles to overcome immunological barriers for enhanced drug delivery. *Engineered Regeneration*, *1*, 35–50. DOI: 10.1016/j.engreg.2020.06.001

Mazumdar, H., Khondakar, K. R., Das, S., Halder, A., & Kaushik, A. (2025a). Artificial intelligence for personalized nanomedicine; from material selection to patient outcomes. *Expert Opinion on Drug Delivery*, *22*(1), 85–108. DOI: 10.1080/17425247.2024.2440618 PMID: 39645588

Mazumdar, H., Khondakar, K. R., Das, S., Halder, A., & Kaushik, A. (2025b). Artificial intelligence for personalized nanomedicine; from material selection to patient outcomes. *Expert Opinion on Drug Delivery*, *22*(1), 85–108. DOI: 10.1080/17425247.2024.2440618 PMID: 39645588

Mitchell, M. J., Billingsley, M. M., Haley, R. M., Wechsler, M. E., Peppas, N. A., & Langer, R. (2021). Engineering precision nanoparticles for drug delivery. *Nature Reviews. Drug Discovery*, *20*(2), 101–124. DOI: 10.1038/s41573-020-0090-8 PMID: 33277608

Moni, S., Abdelwahab, S., Jabeen, A., Elmobark, M., Aqaili, D., Gohal, G., Oraibi, B., Farasani, A., Jerah, A., Alnajai, M., & Mohammad Alowayni, A. (2023). Advancements in Vaccine Adjuvants: The Journey from Alum to Nano Formulations. *Vaccines*, *11*(11), 1704. DOI: 10.3390/vaccines11111704 PMID: 38006036

Mottafegh, A., Joo, J.-U., Na, G.-S., Sharma, V., & Kim, D.-P. (2024). AI-assisted autonomous manufacturing of tailored drug-loaded nanoparticles by multi-step continuous-flow platform. *Chemical Engineering Journal*, *500*, 157454. DOI: 10.1016/j.cej.2024.157454

Mu, Q., Jiang, G., Chen, L., Zhou, H., Fourches, D., Tropsha, A., & Yan, B. (2014). Chemical Basis of Interactions Between Engineered Nanoparticles and Biological Systems. *Chemical Reviews*, *114*(15), 7740–7781. DOI: 10.1021/cr400295a PMID: 24927254

Norori, N., Hu, Q., Aellen, F. M., Faraci, F. D., & Tzovara, A. (2021). Addressing bias in big data and AI for health care: A call for open science. *Patterns (New York, N.Y.)*, *2*(10), 100347. DOI: 10.1016/j.patter.2021.100347 PMID: 34693373

Nwankwo, E. I., Emeihe, E. V., Ajegbile, M. D., Olaboye, J. A., & Maha, C. C.Ejike Innocent NwankwoE-bube Victor EmeiheMojeed Dayo AjegbileJanet Aderonke OlaboyeChukwudi Cosmos Maha. (2024). AI in personalized medicine: Enhancing drug efficacy and reducing adverse effects. *International Medical Science Research Journal*, *4*(8), 806–833. DOI: 10.51594/imsrj.v4i8.1453

Olawade, D. B., Ige, A. O., Olaremu, A. G., Ijiwade, J. O., & Adeola, A. O. (2024). The synergy of artificial intelligence and nanotechnology towards advancing innovation and sustainability—A mini-review. *Nano Trends*, *8*, 100052. DOI: 10.1016/j.nwnano.2024.100052

Olawade, D. B., Wada, O. Z., Ige, A. O., Egbewole, B. I., Olojo, A., & Oladapo, B. I. (2024). Artificial intelligence in environmental monitoring: Advancements, challenges, and future directions. *Hygiene and Environmental Health Advances*, *12*, 100114. DOI: 10.1016/j.heha.2024.100114

Panayides, A. S., Amini, A., Filipovic, N. D., Sharma, A., Tsaftaris, S. A., Young, A., Foran, D., Do, N., Golemati, S., Kurc, T., Huang, K., Nikita, K. S., Veasey, B. P., Zervakis, M., Saltz, J. H., & Pattichis, C. S. (2020). AI in Medical Imaging Informatics: Current Challenges and Future Directions. *IEEE Journal of Biomedical and Health Informatics*, *24*(7), 1837–1857. DOI: 10.1109/JBHI.2020.2991043 PMID: 32609615

Papadimitriou, C. H. (2003). Computational complexity. In *Encyclopedia of Computer Science* (pp. 260–265). GBR: John Wiley and Sons Ltd.

Parvin, N., Joo, S. W., & Mandal, T. K. (2024). Enhancing Vaccine Efficacy and Stability: A Review of the Utilization of Nanoparticles in mRNA Vaccines. *Biomolecules*, *14*(8), 1036. DOI: 10.3390/biom14081036 PMID: 39199422

Pawar, V., Patil, A., Tamboli, F., Gaikwad, D., Mali, D., & Shinde, A. (2023). Harnessing the Power of AI in Pharmacokinetics and Pharmacodynamics: A Comprehensive Review. *International Journal Of Pharmaceutical Quality Assurance*, *14*(2), 426–439. DOI: 10.25258/ijpqa.14.2.31

Poater, A., Saliner, A. G., Solà, M., Cavallo, L., & Worth, A. P. (2010). Computational methods to predict the reactivity of nanoparticles through structure–property relationships. *Expert Opinion on Drug Delivery*, *7*(3), 295–305. DOI: 10.1517/17425240903508756 PMID: 20201736

Raheem, M. A., Rahim, M. A., Gul, I., Zhong, X., Xiao, C., Zhang, H., Wei, J., He, Q., Hassan, M., Zhang, C. Y., Yu, D., Pandey, V., Du, K., Wang, R., Han, S., Han, Y., & Qin, P. (2023). Advances in nanoparticles-based approaches in cancer theranostics. *OpenNano*, *12*, 100152. DOI: 10.1016/j.onano.2023.100152

Ramasamy, L. K., Khan, F., Shah, M., Prasad, B. V. V. S., Iwendi, C., & Biamba, C. (2022). Secure Smart Wearable Computing through Artificial Intelligence-Enabled Internet of Things and Cyber-Physical Systems for Health Monitoring. *Sensors (Basel)*, *22*(3), 1076. DOI: 10.3390/s22031076 PMID: 35161820

Sadr, S., Hajjafari, A., Rahdar, A., Pandey, S., Jafroodi, P. P., Lotfalizadeh, N., Soroushianfar, M., Kavasebi, S. S., Kharaba, Z., Fathi-karkan, S., & Borji, H. (2024). Gold nanobiosensors and Machine Learning: Pioneering breakthroughs in precision breast cancer detection. *European Journal of Medicinal Chemistry Reports*, *12*, 100238. DOI: 10.1016/j.ejmcr.2024.100238

Sajedian, I., Kim, J., & Rho, J. (2019). Finding the optical properties of plasmonic structures by image processing using a combination of convolutional neural networks and recurrent neural networks. *Microsystems & Nanoengineering*, *5*(1), 27. DOI: 10.1038/s41378-019-0069-y PMID: 31240107

Saleh, T., & Shojaosadati, S. A. (2016). Multifunctional nanoparticles for cancer immunotherapy. *Human Vaccines & Immunotherapeutics*, •••, 1–13. DOI: 10.1080/21645515.2016.1147635 PMID: 26901287

Sarker, I. H. (2021). Machine Learning: Algorithms, Real-World Applications and Research Directions. *SN Computer Science*, *2*(3), 160. DOI: 10.1007/s42979-021-00592-x PMID: 33778771

Schletz, D., Breidung, M., & Fery, A. (2023). Validating and Utilizing Machine Learning Methods to Investigate the Impacts of Synthesis Parameters in Gold Nanoparticle Synthesis. *The Journal of Physical Chemistry. C, Nanomaterials and Interfaces*, *127*(2), 1117–1125. DOI: 10.1021/acs.jpcc.2c07578

Serov, N., & Vinogradov, V. (2022). Artificial intelligence to bring nanomedicine to life. *Advanced Drug Delivery Reviews*, *184*, 114194. DOI: 10.1016/j.addr.2022.114194 PMID: 35283223

Souto, E. B., Blanco-Llamero, C., Krambeck, K., Kiran, N. S., Yashaswini, C., Postwala, H., Severino, P., Priefer, R., Prajapati, B. G., & Maheshwari, R. (2024). Regulatory insights into nanomedicine and gene vaccine innovation: Safety assessment, challenges, and regulatory perspectives. *Acta Biomaterialia*, *180*, 1–17. DOI: 10.1016/j.actbio.2024.04.010 PMID: 38604468

Stavis, S. M., Fagan, J. A., Stopa, M., & Liddle, J. A. (2018). Nanoparticle Manufacturing – Heterogeneity through Processes to Products. *ACS Applied Nano Materials*, *1*(9), 4358–4385. DOI: 10.1021/acsanm.8b01239

Sun, B., & Barnard, A. S. (2018). Texture based image classification for nanoparticle surface characterisation and machine learning. *JPhys Materials*, *1*(1), 016001. DOI: 10.1088/2515-7639/aad9ef

Tsamados, A., Aggarwal, N., Cowls, J., Morley, J., Roberts, H., Taddeo, M., & Floridi, L. (2022). The ethics of algorithms: Key problems and solutions. *AI & Society*, *37*(1), 215–230. DOI: 10.1007/s00146-021-01154-8

Vidhya, K. S., Sultana, A., M, N. K., & Rangareddy, H. (2023, October 22). M, N. K., & Rangareddy, H. (2023). Artificial Intelligence's Impact on Drug Discovery and Development From Bench to Bedside. *Cureus*. Advance online publication. DOI: 10.7759/cureus.47486 PMID: 37881323

Vinchurkar, K., & Mane, S. (2024). *AI Innovations in Drug Delivery and Pharmaceutical Sciences; Advancing Therapy through Technology*. Bentham Science Publishers. DOI: 10.2174/97898153057531240101

Wang, W., Feng, S., Ye, Z., Gao, H., Lin, J., & Ouyang, D. (2022). Prediction of lipid nanoparticles for mRNA vaccines by the machine learning algorithm. *Acta Pharmaceutica Sinica. B*, *12*(6), 2950–2962. DOI: 10.1016/j.apsb.2021.11.021 PMID: 35755271

Wei, P.-S., Thota, N., John, G., Chang, E., Lee, S., Wang, Y., Ma, Z., Tsai, Y.-H., & Mei, K.-C. (2024). Enhancing RNA-lipid nanoparticle delivery: Organ- and cell-specificity and barcoding strategies. *Journal of Controlled Release*, *375*, 366–388. DOI: 10.1016/j.jconrel.2024.08.030 PMID: 39179112

Wu, L., Li, X., Qian, X., Wang, S., Liu, J., & Yan, J. (2024). Lipid Nanoparticle (LNP) Delivery Carrier-Assisted Targeted Controlled Release mRNA Vaccines in Tumor Immunity. *Vaccines*, *12*(2), 186. DOI: 10.3390/vaccines12020186 PMID: 38400169

Xuan, L., Ju, Z., Skonieczna, M., Zhou, P., & Huang, R. (2023). Nanoparticles-induced potential toxicity on human health: Applications, toxicity mechanisms, and evaluation models. *MedComm*, *4*(4), e327. DOI: 10.1002/mco2.327 PMID: 37457660

Yaiprasert, C., & Hidayanto, A. N. (2024). AI-powered ensemble machine learning to optimize cost strategies in logistics business. *International Journal of Information Management Data Insights*, *4*(1), 100209. DOI: 10.1016/j.jjimei.2023.100209

Yang, S., & Kar, S. (2023). Application of artificial intelligence and machine learning in early detection of adverse drug reactions (ADRs) and drug-induced toxicity. *Artificial Intelligence Chemistry.*, *1*(2), 100011. DOI: 10.1016/j.aichem.2023.100011

Yang, Y., Zhao, Y., Liu, X., & Huang, J. (2022). Artificial intelligence for prediction of response to cancer immunotherapy. *Seminars in Cancer Biology*, *87*, 137–147. DOI: 10.1016/j.semcancer.2022.11.008 PMID: 36372326

Yaqub, Z. T., & Oboirien, B. O. (2024). Machine Learning Applications for Nano-synthesized Materials Production and Utilization. In Okolie, J. A., Epelle, E. I., Mukherjee, A., & Mahmoud, A. E. D. (Eds.), *Nanomaterials for Sustainable Hydrogen Production and Storage* (1st ed., pp. 123–135). CRC Press. DOI: 10.1201/9781003371007-7

Younis, M. A., Tawfeek, H. M., Abdellatif, A. A. H., Abdel-Aleem, J. A., & Harashima, H. (2022). Clinical translation of nanomedicines: Challenges, opportunities, and keys. *Advanced Drug Delivery Reviews*, *181*, 114083. DOI: 10.1016/j.addr.2021.114083 PMID: 34929251

Yuan, Y., Wu, Y., Cheng, J., Yang, K., Xia, Y., Wu, H., & Pan, X. (2024). Applications of artificial intelligence to lipid nanoparticle delivery. *Particuology*, *90*, 88–97. DOI: 10.1016/j.partic.2023.11.014

Zeng, W., Guo, L., Xu, S., Chen, J., & Zhou, J. (2020). High-Throughput Screening Technology in Industrial Biotechnology. *Trends in Biotechnology*, *38*(8), 888–906. DOI: 10.1016/j.tibtech.2020.01.001 PMID: 32005372

Zhang, Y., Hu, Y., Jiang, N., & Yetisen, A. K. (2023). Wearable artificial intelligence biosensor networks. *Biosensors & Bioelectronics*, *219*, 114825. DOI: 10.1016/j.bios.2022.114825 PMID: 36306563

Zhao, Y., Liu, P., Tan, H., Chen, X., Wang, Q., & Chen, T. (2021). Exosomes as Smart Nanoplatforms for Diagnosis and Therapy of Cancer. *Frontiers in Oncology*, *11*, 743189. DOI: 10.3389/fonc.2021.743189 PMID: 34513718

Zhou, L., Zou, M., Xu, Y., Lin, P., Lei, C., & Xia, X. (2022). Nano Drug Delivery System for Tumor Immunotherapy: Next-Generation Therapeutics. *Frontiers in Oncology*, *12*, 864301. DOI: 10.3389/fonc.2022.864301 PMID: 35664731

KEY TERMS AND DEFINITIONS

Artificial Intelligence (AI): A branch of computer science focused on developing systems capable of performing tasks that typically require human intelligence, such as prediction, pattern recognition, and decision-making.

Nanoparticles: Particles with dimensions in the nanometer range (1–100 nm) are often used in biomedical applications for their unique physical and chemical properties.

AI-Generated Nanoparticles: Nanoparticles whose design, synthesis, or functionalization is optimized or guided by AI algorithms to enhance performance in specific biomedical applications.

Immunological Research: Studying the immune system and its functions aims to understand and manipulate immune responses for treating diseases.

Targeted Drug Delivery: A strategy for transporting therapeutic agents directly to specific cells or tissues, minimizing side effects and maximizing efficacy.

Immune Modulation: The alteration of the immune system's activity, either by enhancing or suppressing its response to achieve therapeutic outcomes.

Machine Learning (ML): A subset of AI enables systems to learn from data and improve their performance without being explicitly programmed.

Computational Modeling: Using algorithms and mathematical models to simulate and predict complex biological or chemical processes.

Chapter 12
Reframing Cancer as an Immunological Disorder Through Personalized Nutrition and AI Integration

Joyeta Ghosh
https://orcid.org/0000-0001-9619-1793
Department of Dietetics and Applied Nutrition, Amity University, Kolkata, India

Asmita Roy
https://orcid.org/0009-0000-9593-9229
Amity University, Kolkata, India

ABSTRACT

Recent advances in cancer research have revolutionized our understanding of cancer as not merely a disease of uncontrolled cell growth but fundamentally as an immunological disorder where malignant cells evade and suppress immune surveillance. This chapter presents a novel framework for conceptualizing and treating cancer through an integrative approach that combines immunological insights with personalized nutrition and artificial intelligence-driven interventions. The chapter synthesizes current evidence on immunonutrition in oncology, examining specific nutrients and bioactive compounds that enhance anti-tumor immunity. Furthermore, we discuss how artificial intelligence algorithms can be leveraged to develop personalized nutritional protocols based on individual patient parameters, including genetic profiles and immune biomarkers.

INTRODUCTION

Cancer is a complex disease requiring comprehensive treatment approaches beyond targeting tumors alone. Artificial intelligence (AI) has emerged as a powerful tool in healthcare, revolutionizing both immunotherapy development and treatment personalization (Pettit et al., 2021; Brooks-Warburton et al., 2022). In oncology, AI applications span immunological biomarker discovery, immune response prediction, treatment selection, and monitoring, while excelling in diagnostic imaging tasks, including

DOI: 10.4018/979-8-3693-9725-1.ch012

endoscopy (Antonelli et al., 2023), radiology (Berbís et al., 2023), and histological assessment (Baxi et al., 2022; Ghosh et al., 2024). Personalized nutrition in clinical settings has gained prominence, with practitioners utilizing genetic testing and individualized approaches to manage cancer (Banka et al., 2025, Shakil et al.,2024). Studies show improved survival rates with personalized nutrition interventions compared to conventional methods. Individual variations in metabolic responses and genetic factors necessitate tailored dietary advice (Doets et al., 2019,Khaitan et al.,2025,Das et al.,2024). Current research explores blood sugar regulation based on microbiome data and investigates gene-diet-disease relationships (Roa-Diaz et al., 2022; Das et al., 2024). Integration of gut microbiota data and disease markers further advances personalized nutrition (Hernandez-Calderon et al., 2022). Modern platforms utilize AI and machine learning to analyze data and provide personalized recommendations (Keijer et al., 2023), though scientific validation remains crucial. These platforms incorporate genetic, clinical, and lifestyle data to formulate personalized diet plans, leveraging wearable devices and mobile applications for real-time monitoring and guidance. The integration of AI-driven immunotherapy insights with nutritional data analysis enables more precise treatment strategies, though validation challenges persist. This review aims to leverage AI's capabilities to personalize cancer care by integrating therapeutic interventions with tailored nutritional strategies, ultimately improving patient outcomes and quality of life.

METHODOLOGY

Using the following keywords, computerized literature searches of many reliable databases were conducted to find pertinent published articles: cancer therapy, artificial intelligence (AI), machine learning (ML), diet in cancer, genomics, and metabolomics. Prospective studies with original data were chosen, and their significant findings were integrated into a conclusion on the state of cancer therapy at the time (Figure 1).

Figure 1. Prisma diagram of the selection process of the research articles of this review.

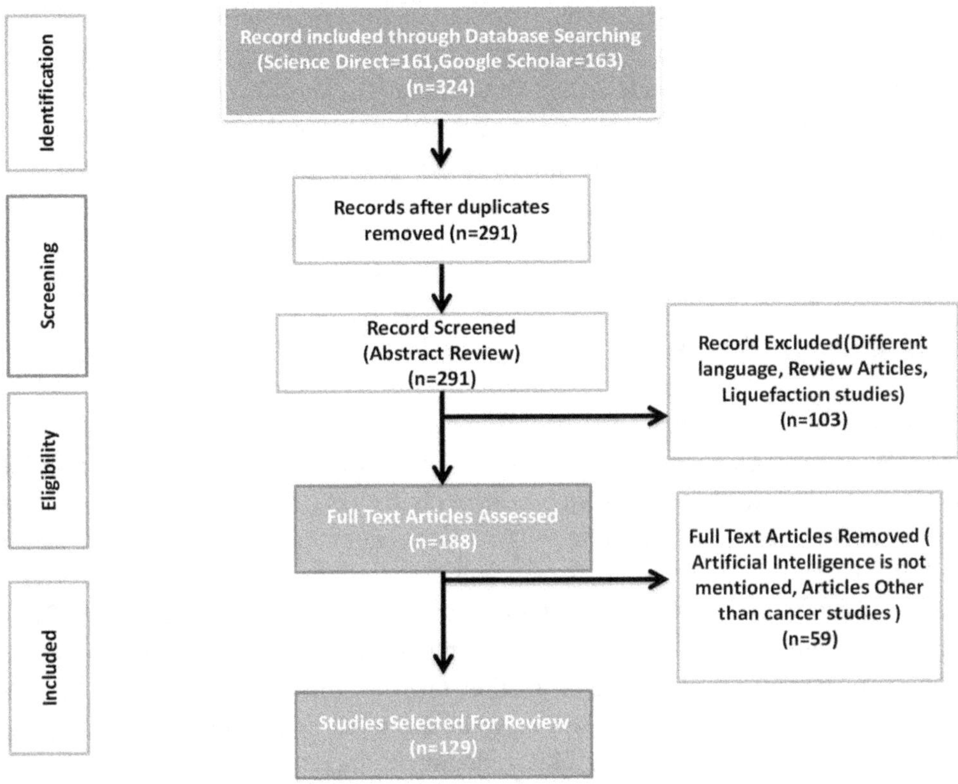

[In this study, the search terms "Neural Network," "Machine Learning," "SVM," "RNN," "HMM," "Hidden Markov," "Fuzzy," "Deep Learning," or "Data Mining," "SVR," "PNN," or "LSTM," or "Clustering," "Radial Basis," "RBF," or "Support Vector," and ("Cancer"); and ("Prediction"). We have originally located 324 research articles from Science Direct, Google Scholar, and the IEEE Xplore digital library based on this search query. Following screening and eligibility checks, 129 research papers were chosen for this study].

DISCUSSION

AI in Cancer Therapy has revolutionized our understanding of cancer as an immunological disorder. Machine learning algorithms analyze complex immune system interactions, identifying key biomarkers and predicting immunotherapy responses. AI models process vast datasets of immune cell profiles, tumor microenvironment characteristics, and treatment outcomes to optimize immunotherapy strategies. These tools help identify patients likely to respond to specific immunotherapies, determine optimal dosing schedules, and monitor immune responses in real-time. Deep learning approaches have enhanced our ability to understand immune escape mechanisms, design targeted therapies, and develop personalized vaccination strategies, marking a significant advancement in cancer immunotherapy.

Creating Predictive Models with Additional Big Datasets

Large-scale cancer databases have emerged from numerous international projects over the past decade, with The Cancer Genome Atlas (TCGA) being the most comprehensive, containing radiological, genomic, and proteomic data (Ding et al., 2018). Other initiatives like METABRIC, GENIE, and PCAWG have also contributed significant genomic profiles. Profiling technologies have evolved from targeted panels to whole-genome sequencing and single-cell RNA sequencing (scRNA-seq), generating diverse datasets including protein interactions, RNAi/CRISPR screens, and DNA methylation profiles. Research teams have demonstrated that integrating multiple data sources improves prediction accuracy for both patient survival (Cheerla & Gevaert, 2019) and drug mechanism identification (Madhukar et al., 2019).

AI in Cancer Immunotherapy

Machine learning is playing transformative role in cancer immunotherapy spans diagnosis, treatment planning, and monitoring therapeutic responses. Deep learning algorithms have revolutionized the analysis of tumor microenvironment data, enabling precise characterization of immune cell populations and their interactions (Zhang et al., 2023). These AI systems process complex multi-omics datasets, including single-cell RNA sequencing, spatial transcriptomics, and proteomics, to understand tumor-immune dynamics and predict treatment outcomes with unprecedented accuracy (Liu et al., 2022).

In checkpoint inhibitor therapy, machine learning models have demonstrated remarkable success in predicting patient responses by analyzing biomarker profiles, tumor mutational burden, and immune infiltration patterns (Wang et al., 2023). These predictive tools help clinicians identify patients most likely to benefit from specific immunotherapies, reducing unnecessary treatments and healthcare costs. AI-driven platforms have also enhanced CAR-T cell therapy design by optimizing receptor configurations and predicting potential off-target effects (Chen et al., 2024).

Recent advances in neural networks have significantly improved neoantigen prediction accuracy, crucial for developing personalized cancer vaccines. These systems analyze tumor genomic data to identify immunogenic mutations and predict their presentation on cancer cells (Martinez et al., 2023). Additionally, AI algorithms monitor immune responses in real-time, enabling dynamic treatment adjustments and early detection of adverse events (Park et al., 2023). The integration of AI with imaging technologies has enhanced tumor response assessment. Deep learning models analyze radiological images to quantify changes in tumor size, composition, and immune cell infiltration, providing early indicators of treatment efficacy (Wilson et al., 2024). Furthermore, AI systems are increasingly used to design combination immunotherapy strategies, optimizing drug sequences and dosing schedules for maximum therapeutic benefit with minimal toxicity (Thompson et al., 2024).

Key Elements are Model Selection and Data Quality

Machine learning workflows require quality data preparation and cleaning to prevent overfitting and biases. Various techniques like cross-validation and ensemble methods help reduce overfitting risks. Model performance is commonly measured using AUROC (Area Under the Receiver Operating Characteristic Curve), with values >0.80 considered good (Al-Haija & Adebanjo, 2020). For imbalanced datasets, AUPRC (Area Under the Precision-Recall Curve) may be more appropriate (Liu et al., 2019). External validation and regular maintenance are crucial to prevent concept drift and ensure model robustness (Li et al., 2017).

Early Cancer Identification, Diagnosis, and Staging

Early and accurate detection, diagnosis, and staging of cancer are crucial factors that influence tumor aggression, guide clinical decision-making processes, and ultimately impact patient outcomes. Within a relatively short period, artificial intelligence (AI) technologies have emerged as promising tools that can potentially transform this critical domain of oncology. AI-based models have demonstrated capabilities comparable to human experts in certain tasks, while offering the added benefits of scalability and automation. These AI models have shown remarkable performance in various applications, such as identifying and classifying cancerous lesions from medical imaging data, predicting tumor staging and grading, and assessing the risk of malignancy or disease recurrence. The ability to automate and streamline these processes holds the potential to improve the efficiency, consistency, and timeliness of cancer detection and diagnosis, thereby enabling earlier intervention and personalized treatment strategies (Korbar et al., 2017).

However, it is essential to recognize that AI tools in this domain are not intended to replace human expertise entirely but rather to augment and support clinical decision-making processes. The integration of AI technologies into clinical workflows requires rigorous validation, continuous monitoring, and a thorough understanding of the limitations and potential biases associated with these models. Overall, the rapid advancements in AI applications for cancer detection and diagnosis underscore the transformative potential of these technologies in improving patient outcomes and advancing the field of precision oncology (Salunke et al.,2025;).

Improving the Precision of Cancer Diagnoses

Deep learning-based models, particularly deep neural networks (DNNs), have demonstrated remarkable effectiveness in cancer diagnosis using medical imaging data, including histopathology and radiology. These models excel in automatically learning features from raw image data without manual engineering (Iizuka et al., 2020). In analyzing whole slide images (WSIs), DNNs have achieved high prediction accuracies (AUCs > 0.99) in distinguishing tumor cells and differentiating cancer subtypes. For instance, DeepPATH, built on Inception-v3 architecture, achieved an AUC of 0.97 in classifying lung cancer types (Coudray et al., 2018).

Beyond histopathology, DNNs have shown success across various imaging modalities. In dermatology, models have outperformed board-certified dermatologists in classifying skin lesions (Campanella et al., 2019; Esteva et al., 2017). Studies using CT scans and MRI have shown promising results, with Jiang et al. (2021) achieving AUCs of 0.92-0.94 in predicting gastric cancer metastasis. In mammography, McKinney et al. (2020) demonstrated improved cancer detection specificity (1.2%-5.7%) and sensitivity (2.7%-9.4%) compared to radiologists. Additionally, AI-assisted smartphone apps are emerging for early malignant lesion detection (Freeman et al., 2020; Becker et al., 2014), while advanced architectures like SENet and DenseNet have shown effectiveness in grading liver cancer using MRI data (Zhou et al., 2019).

Table 1. This table outlines the process of applying deep learning models to analyze medical imaging data for various purposes, including cancer detection, classification, and risk prediction.

Different Techniques applied	Potential benefits and concerns associated	Citations
Identify Dataset	• Histopathologic Images (H&E-stained WSIs) • Other Medical Imaging Modalities (CT scans, MRI, mammograms, skin lesion photographs)	(Tsherniak et al., 2017)
Apply Deep Learning Models	• Train DNNs on large-scale annotated datasets. • Utilize DNNs to automatically learn relevant features from raw image data. • Train DNNs to recognize and differentiate between various tissue types, cellular morphologies, and histological patterns associated with different cancer types and subtypes.	(Wang et al., 2017)
Performance Evaluation	• Assess DNN performance in image classification tasks. • Evaluate DNNs' ability to distinguish tumor cells from healthy cells. • Measure DNNs' performance in differentiating closely related cancer subtypes and detecting benign versus malignant tissue. • Evaluate DNNs' performance in classifying other medical imaging modalities (CT, MRI, mammograms, skin lesion photographs).	(McKinney et al., 2020)
Examples of DNN Applications	• DeepPATH model achieving AUC of 0.97 in multi-class classification of lung cancer WSIs.	(Freeman et al., 2020)
Other Medical Imaging Modalities	• DNN outperforming dermatologists in classifying skin lesions. • DNN classifying textural patterns in lung CT scans. • DNN predicting occult peritoneal metastasis in gastric cancers. • DNN distinguishing prostate cancer from benign conditions in MRI images. • In ensemble of DNNs predicting cancer risk scores from mammograms.	(Zhou et al., 2019)
Potential Benefits and Concerns	**Benefits:** • Improved diagnostic accuracy and consistency. • Enhanced cancer detection, classification, and risk prediction. **Concerns:** • False negatives in smartphone-based cancer detection apps. • Need for rigorous validation before clinical integration.	(Becker et al., 2014),

Cancer Grading and Staging

Cancer staging and grading, which determines the cancer's aggressiveness and advancement, significantly influences treatment choices. In prostate cancer, staging utilizes the Gleason score, combining two scores measuring tumor cell prevalence in distinct locations. Deep neural networks (DNNs) have shown promising results in predicting Gleason scores from prostate tumor histopathology images (Nagpal et al., 2019). Nagpal et al. trained a DNN (Inception-V3) and k-nearest-neighbor classifier on whole slide images (WSIs) of H&E-stained prostatectomy specimens to predict Gleason scores. Their model demonstrated improved prediction accuracy (0.70) compared to 29 independent pathologists (0.61). With an AUC of 0.83, Zhou et al. used a deep learning technique utilizing SENet and DenseNet architectures to predict grade (low versus high) from liver cancer patients' MRI data.

These studies indicate promising AI applications in cancer staging, with performance on par with experts, despite modest AUC values, highlighting AI's potential to assist in accurate staging and guide treatment strategies. Non-imaging data, such as genomic profiles from next-generation sequencing (NGS) technologies, provide valuable insights for cancer diagnosis and staging. Machine learning techniques are essential for effective cancer classification from these highly multidimensional data. Capper et al. showcased the efficacy of a random forest classifier trained on tumor DNA methylation profiles, achieving an impressive AUC of 0.99 in predicting challenging subclasses of central nervous system cancers (Grewal et al., 2019). Sun et al. developed a Deep Neural Network (DNN) for tissue classification using genomic point mutations from whole-exome sequencing profiles, exhibiting high accuracy in distinguishing healthy and tumor tissues (AUC 0.94) but less robust performance in multiclass classification of 12 cancer types (AUC 0.70) (Mostavi et al., 2020). These studies underscore the potential of genomic data and machine learning models for cancer assessment, with applicability to various data sources, including cell-free DNA (cfDNA).

UNDERSTANDING OF THERAPEUTIC DRUGS AND TARGETS

The authors of Tong et al. (2019) successfully employed one-class support vector machines to identify liver cancer drug targets by processing clinical data together with gene expression profiles and protein-protein interaction networks which resulted in an AUC of 0.88. Breast cancer research integrates the datasets of TCGA, PharmGKB and Cancer Genome Interpreter which three separate studies by Ding et al. (2018), López-Cortés et al. (2018, 2020) employed to detect therapeutic targets and biomarkers. DepMap Consortium research led to the development of AI application ECLIPSE which analyzes cancer-dependent therapeutic targets through their loss-of-function screens. AI analysis requires proteomics data to reveal cancer cell line relationships according to Chen et al. (2020).

Designing of a New Drug

Artificial Intelligence (AI) has transformed drug design and immunotherapy development through in silico generation of drug structures with specific properties. Reinforcement learning has emerged as a key approach, with Olivecrona et al. (2017) demonstrating success using recurrent neural networks for generating drug analogues. Graph convolutional networks and generative adversarial networks (GAN) have further enhanced molecule generation, particularly in optimizing drug-likeness and immunological properties.

Drug repurposing efforts have been accelerated through initiatives like the Library of Integrated Network-Based Cellular Signatures (LINCS), which provides extensive transcriptional datasets (Mokou et al., 2020). AI models analyze these datasets to identify drugs capable of modulating immune responses and reversing cancer-specific gene signatures (Chen et al., 2017; Mastrogamvraki and Zaravinos, 2020). Deep Neural Networks trained on drug-perturbed transcriptional profiles help forecast therapeutic categories and prioritize immunotherapy candidates (Li et al., 2020). Notable advances include CDRScan, a CNN-based model system that predicts optimal treatments based on patient-specific mutation profiles (Zeng et al., 2019), and DeepDR, which uses drug structures and clinical annotations to identify new drug-disease relationships (Liu et al., 2019). These AI approaches are particularly valuable in immunotherapy development, where understanding complex immune system interactions is crucial for identifying effective therapeutic targets and repurposing existing drugs for enhanced immune responses against cancer.

Prognosis of Patients and Therapy Reactions

AI is crucial for predicting treatment responses, particularly in immunotherapy where checkpoint inhibitor responses are low (20%) but potentially beneficial long-term, with annual costs around $150,000 per patient. Key developments include Liu et al.'s logistic regression classifier for PD-1 inhibitor resistance prediction and XGBoost-based classifier for immunotherapy responses.

CNN models have shown significant success: Hao et al. (2018) combined histopathology with clinical data for metastatic cancer predictions, while Dercle et al. achieved AUCs of 0.67-0.82 using longitudinal CT scans for predicting responses to various cancer therapies. Choi et al. demonstrated superior performance (AUC 0.60-0.98) in predicting neoadjuvant treatment responses in breast cancer using PET/MRI scans.

Advanced applications include CURATE.AI for dynamic drug dose optimization and combined CNN-recurrent neural networks for analyzing longitudinal CT data (HR 6.16, AUC 0.74). These systems are particularly valuable for early detection of treatment ineffectiveness and personalized therapy adjustments (Smirnov et al., 2018).

Table 2. Examples of AI applications considering a customized approach in range of cancer therapies

Clinical Specialty	AI Task	Specific Applications	Example Studies
Radiology	Computer-aided diagnosis and detection, automated image analysis, Predictive analytics and quantitative image analysisinterpretation of a chest X-ray, interpretation of a mammography, Diagnosis of stroke, brain tumors, and lung cancer	interpretation of chest X-rays, interpretation of mammograms, diagnosis of strokes, identification of brain tumors, and detection of lung cancer	AI was utilized by Wang et al. (2016) to detect micro-calcifications on mammograms as a potential early warning sign of breast cancer. Deep learning was utilized by Chen et al. (2020) to improve diagnosis from chest X-ray interpretation.
Oncology	Automated tumor detection, image analysis, predictive analytics, and personalized treatment planning	Melanoma detection, drug discovery, precision medicine, radiation therapy planning, tumor segmentation	AI applications for cancer molecular subtyping were investigated by Zhao et al. (2019). Deep learning was utilized by Danaee et al. (2017) to identify and detect cancerous genes.
Cardiology	Image analysis, computer-aided diagnosis, and predictive analytics	Detection of arrhythmias, interpretation of echocardiography, risk assessment for heart disease, Diagnoses of coronary artery disease	Li et al., (2014) improved ECG interpretation with machine learning. predicted the onset of atrial fibrillation using machine learning.
Neurology	Image analysis, computer-aided diagnosis, and predictive analytics	Multiple sclerosis diagnostic, Parkinson's disease diagnosis, epilepsy diagnosis, and Alzheimer's disease diagnosis	In order to identify cerebral hemorrhage on CT, Smorchkova et al., (2023) employed machine learning.

continued on following page

Table 2. Continued

Clinical Specialty	AI Task	Specific Applications	Example Studies
Pathology	Predictive analytics, computer-aided diagnosis, digital pathology, and image analysis	Prostate cancer detection, tissue analysis, immunohistochemistry interpretation, and cancer diagnosis	AI-powered histology interpretation automation was reported by Xu et al. (2019). Deep learning was utilized to evaluate lymph node metastases in breast cancer resections.
Dermatology	Computer-Aided Diagnosis, Predictive Analytics, Image Analysis	Analysis of skin lesions, diagnosis of acne, psoriasis, and eczema	Bassel et al., (2022) used deep learning to classify benign and malignant skin lesions.
Personalized Nutrition	Genetic Analysis, Personalized Recommendations	Compounding personalized nutritional supplements, Weight management based on genetics, Dietary recommendations for children based on genetics, Personalized nutrient intake based on genetic risk, Supplement selection based on DNA testing, Personalized treatment for diabetics based on genotype, Pharmacogenetic analysis for personalized medicine, Obesity treatment based on genetic markers, Dietary supplementation for homeostasis, Individualized care based on digestive activity, Personalized functional food recommendations based on microbiome, Customized food recommendations, Weight and disease management integrating nutrition and behavior	In their review, Ghosh et al., (2024) explore the potential roles of various AI-based models in advancing Machine Learning and AI Innovations in Nutrition and Related Health Conditions.
Metabolomics	Predictive Analytics, Classification, Regression	Identification of severe COVID-19 cases, Taxonomic identification based on metabolites, Metabolic changes in pregnancy, Influenza diagnosis	Shen et al. (2020) used random forest to identify severe COVID-19 cases based on protein and metabolite signatures. Liang et al. (2020) used linear regression to study metabolic changes in pregnancy.

Predicting Drugs Efficiency and Synergy

Machine learning applications in drug efficacy prediction have expanded significantly, driven by large cancer drug datasets from cell line experiments (Gillet et al., 2013; Ghosh et al.,2024). Iorio et al.'s study evaluated 265 anticancer drugs on 1,001 cancer cell lines, using Elastic Net models to convert genomic features into IC50 values for predicting drug efficacy.

Deep learning has emerged as a powerful approach, demonstrated by Chiu et al.'s work using TCGA and Cancer Cell Line Encyclopedia data to train Deep Neural Networks for drug response prediction, finding expression data more predictive than mutation information (Chiu et al., 2019). Sakellaropoulos and colleagues used DNNs with the GDSC dataset to stratify patients based on treatment sensitivity (Sakellaropoulos et al., 2019).

A significant advancement came with DrugCell, an interpretable deep learning model combining a "visible neural network" with drug structure analysis. This achieved a 0.80 Spearman correlation coefficient and successfully predicted drug synergies (AUC 0.75). The DREAM challenge further demonstrated that integrating genomic features with chemical structure and biological interactions improves prediction accuracy (Menden et al., 2019).

Similarly, Gilvary and colleagues reported on the efficacy of a multitask suite of models that incorporates genomic, target, chemical, and effect-based features. This approach not only maintains high predictive accuracy but also aids in deciphering the underlying mechanisms contributing to the predicted synergy(Gilvary et al., 2019).

INTEGRATING AI-DRIVEN THERAPEUTIC AND NUTRITIONAL STRATEGIES

Data science, encapsulating fields like machine learning, artificial intelligence, and advanced statistical modeling, provides a robust arsenal for realizing the promise of personalized nutrition. Through harnessing extensive datasets sourced from diverse outlets such as genomics, metabolomics, gut microbiome analysis, wearable devices, and dietary intake records, data science methodologies have the capacity to unveil complex patterns and correlations that traditional methodologies might struggle to unveil (Ghosh, 2024).

Application of AI in Assessment of Nutritional Status

Artificial Intelligence (AI) is increasingly playing a significant role in nutritional assessment among cancer patients. By leveraging AI techniques such as machine learning and data analytics, healthcare professionals can analyze vast amounts of data related to the nutritional status of cancer patients more efficiently and accurately than traditional methods.

Figure 2. This flowchart outlines the process starting from data collection to utilizing various AI techniques for nutritional assessment among cancer patients, including dietetic assessments, sarcopenia assessment, prediction of nutritional support needs, and ensuring NGT feeding safety. Each step involves leveraging AI technologies to enhance accuracy, efficiency, and patient care

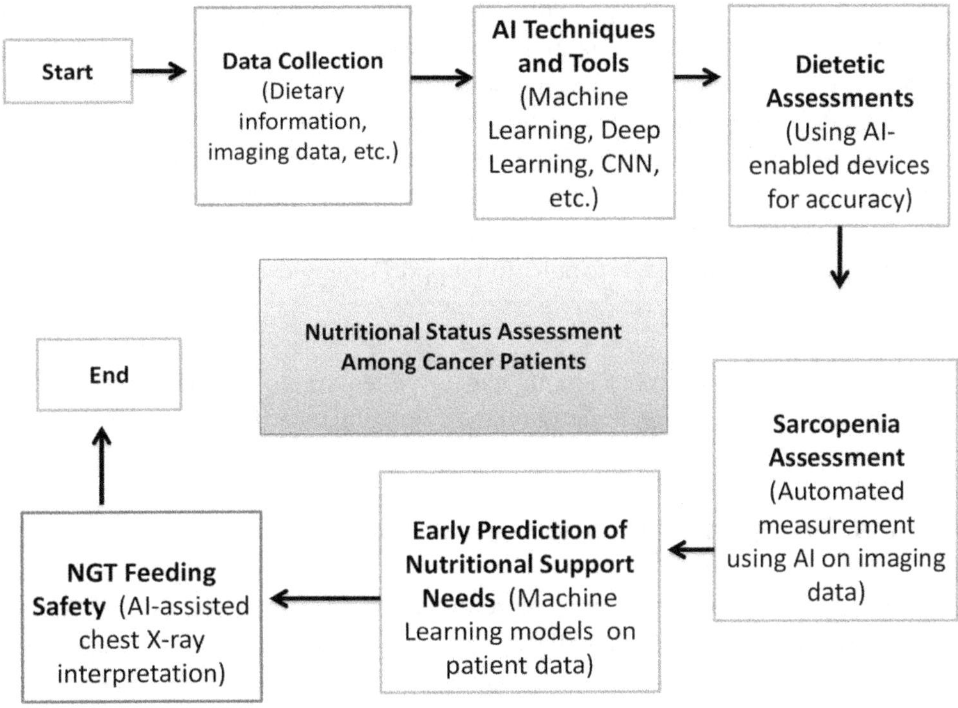

AI-enabled devices support nutritional assessment through acoustic and visual inputs (Rozynek et al., 2021; Beaudart et al., 2017), helping dietitians evaluate patients more efficiently. Sarcopenia, a critical nutritional indicator, predicts outcomes in various diseases (Oke et al., 2020; Wang et al., 2023).

AI streamlines skeletal muscle measurement in imaging, with CNN-based solutions outperforming manual assessment (Bischoff et al., 2020). Machine learning also aids in predicting enteral nutrition needs in ICU patients (Singh et al., 2007). For nasogastric tube feeding, AI improves safety by accurately interpreting chest x-rays for tube placement (Sales et al., 2014).

AI-Powered Nutritional Assessment in Cancer Patients Involves Several Key Aspects

1. Data Integration: AI systems can integrate data from various sources, including electronic health records, patient-reported outcomes, wearable devices, and dietary logs. This comprehensive data aggregation enables a holistic view of the patient's nutritional status.
2. Predictive Analytics: Machine learning algorithms can analyze historical data to predict nutritional deficiencies or changes in nutritional status in cancer patients. By identifying patterns and trends, AI models can anticipate nutritional needs and risks, allowing for proactive interventions.

3. Personalized Recommendations: AI algorithms can generate personalized dietary recommendations tailored to individual cancer patients based on their unique characteristics, such as cancer type, treatment regimen, genetic factors, and comorbidities. These recommendations may include specific dietary modifications, supplementation strategies, or meal plans optimized for nutritional support during cancer treatment.
4. Early Detection of Malnutrition: AI-powered tools can flag early signs of malnutrition or unintended weight loss in cancer patients, enabling timely interventions to prevent or mitigate nutritional deterioration. By analyzing biomarkers, imaging data, and clinical parameters, AI systems can identify patients at higher risk of malnutrition and prioritize nutritional interventions accordingly.
5. Remote Monitoring: With the integration of wearable devices and mobile health technologies, AI-driven nutritional assessment can be conducted remotely, allowing for continuous monitoring of patients' dietary intake, nutritional status, and treatment-related side effects. This real-time data capture facilitates timely adjustments to nutrition support strategies and enhances patient engagement in self-care.

Overall, AI in nutritional assessment among cancer patients holds immense potential to optimize nutritional care delivery, improve treatment outcomes, and enhance the quality of life for individuals undergoing cancer treatment.

AI in Genomics, Nutrigenomics and Cancer Therapy

Artificial Intelligence (AI) is revolutionizing genomics and nutrigenomics in the context of cancer patients, offering powerful tools for personalized cancer care and treatment strategies. Nutrigenomics, established through diverse omics technologies rooted in molecular biology (Venter et al., 2001; Kaput and Rodriguez, 2004), is witnessing rapid expansion alongside related research fields, driven by advancements in high-throughput technologies like microarrays (Gonzalez et al., 2015).This discipline aims to investigate the impact of food (nutrients) on gene expression. Although environmental factors, such as dietary intake, do not alter the DNA sequence, they play pivotal roles in modulating phenotype by influencing processes like gene replication, transcription, and protein expression (Dahlman et al., 2015; Nilsson et al., 2014). Numerous studies have explored epigenetic regulation mechanisms, encompassing DNA methylation, histone acetylation, and chromatin remodeling. In the context of diet-related ailments like obesity and diabetes, several CpG sites associated with DNA methylation have been identified (Malmgren et al., 2013; Perfilyev et al., 2017). Notably, methyl donors found in foods, such as methionine and folate, play crucial roles in DNA methylation processes. Intriguingly, patients with type 2 diabetes (T2D) exhibited lower erythrocyte folate levels compared to healthy individuals, alongside observed hypomethylation at CpG sites of T2D-related genes in hepatocytes. Moreover, distinct patterns of DNA methylation at CpG sites have been linked to the consumption of saturated and unsaturated fatty acids. Additionally, intake of saturated fatty acids has been reported to enhance histone acetyltransferase activity in pancreatic β cells (Cione et al., 2019; Zhang et al., 2019). Moreover, dietary constituents exert influence on miRNAs, which serve as regulators of gene expression. Specifically, polyphenols such as curcumin, resveratrol, and quercetin have been identified as regulators of miRNA expression in cancer cells and participants in inflammatory responses (Simon et al., 2023). Additionally, the human gut microbiome holds significance in personalized nutrition, as it plays a critical role in various aspects of health, including digestion, nutrient metabolism, and food absorption. Consequently, it assumes a pivotal role in overall health, warranting research attention in the realm of personalized nutrition. Notably, investigations in personalized nutrition center around individual gut microbiome composition and its response to dietary interventions (Galal et al., 2022; Harrison et al., 2022).

AI-DRIVEN APPROACHES IN CANCER METABOLOMICS EMPOWER CANCER THERAPY

AI is transforming metabolomics and microbiome analysis in cancer research through advanced data analysis and personalized treatment strategies. Metabolomics provides insights into individual dietary responses, while microbiome analysis reveals crucial interactions between diet and gut health (NHS, 2023). Machine learning techniques like Random Forest, Support Vector Machine, and emerging Deep Learning approaches are increasingly used in metabolomic studies, particularly in cancer classification (Smuck et al., 2021). While algorithm selection remains context-dependent (Chandrasekaran et al., 2020), these tools help identify altered metabolites and potential biomarkers. Machine learning-aided metabolomic experiments not only support biomarker discovery but also enable pathway analysis and potential therapeutic targeting strategies (Picone et al., 2022).It is notable that the majority of reviewed studies have been published within the last 5 years, coinciding with the rapid increase in the popularity of machine learning. This surge is facilitated by advancements in computational power, the efficiency and accessibility of ML tools, growing familiarity with the field, and the availability of abundant data. As more extensive metabolomic datasets become accessible, it is anticipated that ML techniques, particularly Deep Learning, will assume a more prominent role in constructing informative and predictive models. These models hold the potential to offer high-definition, personalized clinical diagnosis and treatment strategies (Ghosh et al., 2025).

Figure 3. Figure provides a clear visual representation of the sequential steps involved in utilizing AI in metabolomics and microbiome analysis for cancer research and patient care

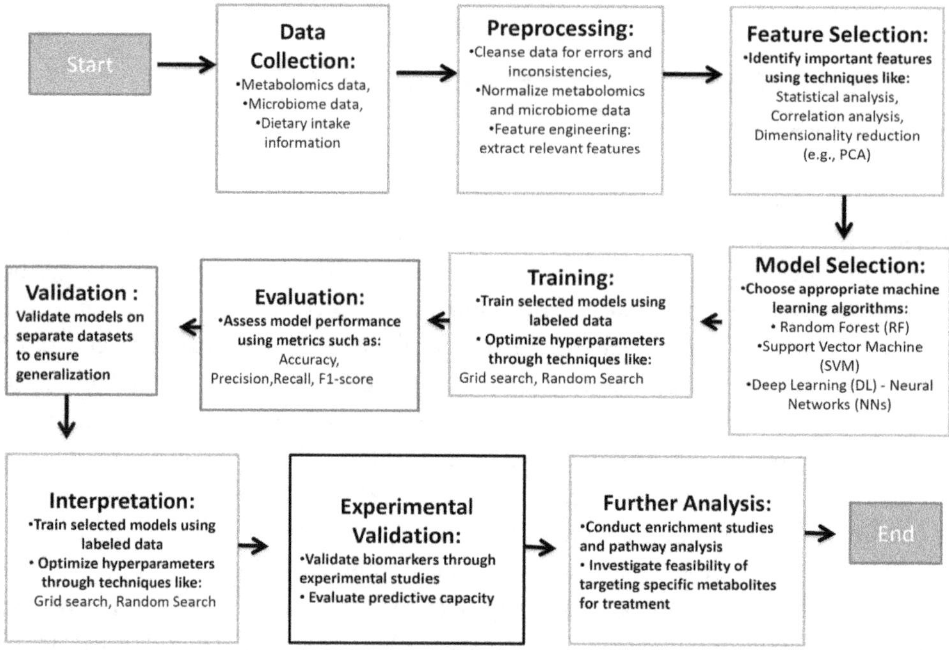

The following are the areas where AI is having an impact:

1. **Metabolomics Analysis:** AI algorithms analyze metabolomic data generated from cancer patients' biological samples, such as blood, urine, or tissue, to profile the metabolic signatures associated with cancer development, progression, and treatment response. By identifying metabolic alterations specific to different cancer types and stages, AI enables the discovery of novel biomarkers for early detection, prognosis, and monitoring of therapeutic efficacy.
2. **Biomarker Discovery:** Machine learning models trained on metabolomic data can identify metabolic biomarkers that distinguish between cancer patients and healthy individuals, as well as subtypes of cancer with distinct metabolic profiles. These biomarkers hold promise for non-invasive cancer diagnostics and prognostics, guiding personalized treatment decisions and monitoring disease progression over time.
3. **Therapeutic Target Identification:** AI-driven approaches integrate metabolomic data with genomic, proteomic, and clinical data to identify potential therapeutic targets for cancer treatment. By elucidating the metabolic pathways dysregulated in cancer cells, AI algorithms prioritize druggable targets and repurposing opportunities, accelerating drug discovery efforts and expanding the therapeutic arsenal against cancer.
4. **Microbiome Analysis:** AI algorithms analyze microbiome data obtained from cancer patients' gut, oral, or tumor microbiota to investigate the role of the microbiome in cancer development, progression, and treatment outcomes. By characterizing microbial communities and their functional potential, AI

facilitates the identification of microbial biomarkers associated with cancer risk, treatment response, and adverse effects.

5. **Personalized Microbiome-based Therapies:** AI-powered platforms leverage microbiome data to develop personalized microbiome-based interventions, such as probiotics, prebiotics, or fecal microbiota transplantation, to modulate the gut microbiota and enhance cancer treatment efficacy. These interventions aim to restore microbial balance, improve immune function, and mitigate treatment-related side effects in cancer patients.
6. **Predictive Modeling and Clinical Decision Support:** AI-driven predictive models integrate metabolomic and microbiome data with clinical parameters to predict cancer outcomes, such as response to treatment, disease recurrence, and survival. These models provide valuable insights for clinicians in making informed treatment decisions and designing personalized therapeutic regimens tailored to individual patients' metabolic and microbial profiles (van de Sande et al., 2022).Overall, AI in metabolomics and microbiome analysis holds immense promise for advancing our understanding of cancer biology, improving early detection and diagnosis, and developing personalized therapeutic strategies to optimize cancer care and outcomes for patients.

THE ROLE OF ARTIFICIAL INTELLIGENCE IN NUTRITION PRESCRIPTION FOR CANCER PATIENT

Artificial Intelligence (AI) has the potential to transform clinical nutrition prescribing practices. By analyzing vast amounts of patient data, including medical history, nutritional status, laboratory results, and dietary preferences, AI algorithms can generate personalized and precise nutrition plans. Through machine learning techniques, AI can identify patterns and correlations within this data to recommend optimal nutrient intake, dietary modifications, and supplementation strategies tailored to individual patient needs.The prescription of nutritional support, whether enteral or parenteral, typically involves collaboration among physicians, dietitians, and pharmacists. It requires thorough assessments, calculations of requirements, and ongoing monitoring of patient response and tolerance levels. Machine Learning (ML) could be deployed to evaluate existing databases of multi-chamber bags (MCB) constituents, swiftly identifying the most suitable parenteral support regimen tailored to an individual patient's needs, considering their nutritional status and bloodwork results (Castagno and Khalifa, 2020). This process, currently requiring manual scrutiny, could be expedited and made more accurate with AI, potentially saving valuable time for healthcare professionals.

Artificial Intelligence for Tracking Dietary Patterns of the Cancer Patients and the Course of Their Disease

The proliferation of wearable devices and mobile applications has enabled the collection of real-time data on individuals' physiological parameters, physical activity levels, and dietary intake. These data sources can be integrated with other relevant data points, such as genomics and metabolomics, to create comprehensive personal health profiles. Data science techniques can leverage these multi-dimensional datasets to identify patterns and correlations between diet, lifestyle factors, and health outcomes. Machine learning algorithms can analyze the relationship between an individual's physical activity levels, caloric intake, and weight fluctuations, enabling the development of personalized dietary and exercise recommendations for weight management. Advancements in computer vision and natural language processing (NLP) have facilitated the accurate tracking and analysis of dietary intake, provided detailed nutritional breakdowns and identified areas for improvement in an individual's diet. AI can serve to coordinate and consolidate monitoring parameters for patients undergoing nutritional support, highlighting abnormal results for clinicians or prompting patients to attend relevant appointments. Deep Learning (DL) can further guide patients based on monitoring results or schedule appropriate follow-up appointments (Zhao et al., 2019, Ghosh,2023). An example is the development of a machine learning (ML)-based tool accurately predicting the risk of refeeding syndrome, enabling timely interventions. Wearable monitoring devices, including those that interact with smartphones, can be adapted for clinical use, including the follow-up and monitoring of patients receiving artificial nutrition support, fostering patient engagement and autonomy. However, disparities in device usage may exist, potentially excluding some individuals from potential health benefits (Danaee et al., 2017).

Prediction of Nutritional Outcome Among Cancer Patients

AI has shown promise in the pharmaceutical business across a range of areas, including biological pathways, genomic analysis, drug repurposing, clinical trials, productivity enhancement, and genomic analysis (Li et al., 2014). Drug-target interactions can be predicted by AI modeling systems, providing insightful information. AI algorithms in personalized nutrition can identify connections between a person's genetic and metabolite profiles and their nutritional requirements, allowing for customized dietary recommendations.AI has shown remarkable capability in predicting outcomes across various diseases, including critical care, inflammatory bowel disease, and epilepsy. Machine learning algorithms can analyze extensive datasets to discern patterns and predictors of survival in diseases, aiding clinicians in making personalized treatment decisions for patients requiring artificial nutrition support (Smorchkova et al., 2023).

Figure 4. This flowchart illustrates the sequential steps involved in predicting nutritional outcomes among cancer patients using AI, starting from data collection to personalized recommendations, monitoring, and timely interventions.

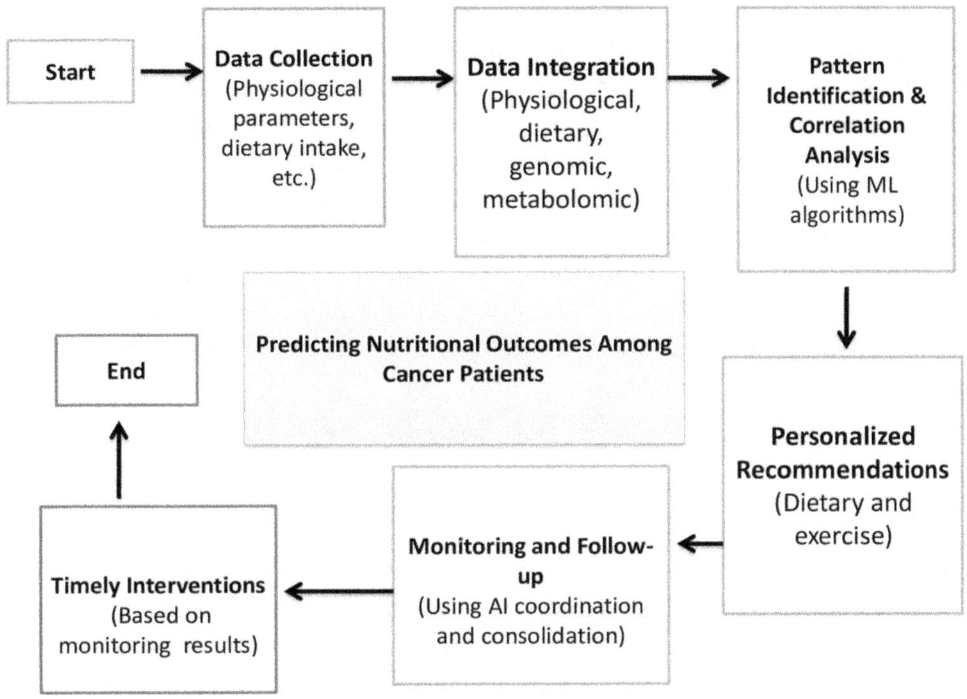

CURRENT CHALLENGES AND FUTURE OUTCOMES

Personalized nutrition holds significant promise in cancer therapy by tailoring dietary recommendations to an individual's unique biological characteristics and needs. Several challenges must be addressed to harness its full potential effectively.

Data Integration: Integrating diverse data sources such as genomics, metabolomics, microbiome, and lifestyle data is crucial for developing comprehensive personalized nutrition plans. Establishing standardized data collection protocols and robust integration pipelines is essential.

Privacy and Ethical Concerns: Collecting and analyzing personal health data raises privacy and ethical concerns. Ensuring data security, maintaining strict data protection protocols, and obtaining informed consent from patients are vital to uphold ethical standards. Additionally, AI models must be trained on diverse datasets to mitigate the risk of perpetuating biases and discrimination (Bassel et al., 2022).

Interpretation and Communication: Translating complex analytical results into actionable and understandable dietary recommendations requires collaborations between data scientists, oncologists, nutritionists, and healthcare professionals. Medical training on the appropriate use of AI in personalized nutrition is crucial for effective integration into clinical practice.

Scalability and Accessibility: Implementing personalized nutrition solutions for cancer patients at scale requires overcoming logistical and financial barriers, developing cost-effective and user-friendly platforms that can accommodate large datasets and provide tailored recommendations.

Liability and Accountability: Clear guidelines and standards for liability and accountability must be established, involving AI experts, healthcare professionals, and regulators. Maintaining human control over AI systems and utilizing them as decision support tools rather than substitutes is vital to preserve trust in the healthcare provider-patient relationship.

Continuous Monitoring and Adaptation: Personalized nutrition plans for cancer patients must be regularly updated to adapt to changes in their condition, treatment, and overall health status. Developing dynamic systems that can incorporate new data and adjust recommendations accordingly is essential.

CONCLUSION

AI-driven personalized nutrition shows promise in revolutionizing cancer care by analyzing multi-omics data to create tailored dietary interventions. These personalized nutrition plans can potentially enhance treatment efficacy, manage side effects, and improve patient outcomes. AI algorithms can identify connections between genetic profiles, tumor characteristics, and nutritional requirements, enabling targeted interventions for specific cancer types. This precision approach could complement conventional treatments and lead to the development of specialized nutraceuticals. While challenges exist, including small study samples and limited clinical evidence, the rapid advancement of AI in cancer nutrition therapy demonstrates significant potential for future applications.

REFERENCES

Al-Haija, Q. A., & Adebanjo, A. (2020, September). Breast cancer diagnosis in histopathological images using ResNet-50 convolutional neural network. In *2020 IEEE International IOT, Electronics and Mechatronics Conference (IEMTRONICS)* (pp. 1-7). IEEE.DOI: DOI: 10.1109/IEMTRONICS51293.2020.9216455

Antonelli, G., Rizkala, T., Iacopini, F., & Hassan, C. (2023). Current and future implications of artificial intelligence in colonoscopy. *Annals of Gastroenterology*, *36*(2), 114. DOI: 10.20524/aog.2023.0781 PMID: 36864946

Banka, R., Das, P., Das, S., & Ghosh, J. (2025). Tailored nutrition and diet plan using AI and machine learning for precision wellness. In *Harnessing AI and machine learning for precision wellness*. IGI Global., DOI: 10.4018/979-8-3693-9521-9.ch007

Bassel, A., Abdulkareem, A. B., Alyasseri, Z. A. A., Sani, N. S., & Mohammed, H. J. (2022). Automatic malignant and benign skin cancer classification using a hybrid deep learning approach. *Diagnostics (Basel)*, *12*(10), 2472. DOI: 10.3390/diagnostics12102472 PMID: 36292161

Baxi, V., Edwards, R., Montalto, M., & Saha, S. (2022). Digital pathology and artificial intelligence in translational medicine and clinical practice. *Modern Pathology*, *35*(1), 23–32. DOI: 10.1038/s41379-021-00919-2 PMID: 34611303

Beaudart, C., Zaaria, M., Pasleau, F., Reginster, J. Y., & Bruyère, O. (2017). Health outcomes of sarcopenia: A systematic review and meta-analysis. *PLoS One*, *12*(1), e0169548. DOI: 10.1371/journal.pone.0169548 PMID: 28095426

Becker, S., Miron-Shatz, T., Schumacher, N., Krocza, J., Diamantidis, C., & Albrecht, U. V. (2014). mHealth 2.0: Experiences, possibilities, and perspectives. *JMIR mHealth and uHealth*, *2*(2), e3328. DOI: 10.2196/mhealth.3328 PMID: 25099752

Berbís, M. A., Godino, F. P., Del Val, J. R., Mata, L. A., & Luna, A. (2023). Clinical impact of artificial intelligence-based solutions on imaging of the pancreas and liver. *World Journal of Gastroenterology*, *29*(9), 1427–1445. DOI: 10.3748/wjg.v29.i9.1427 PMID: 36998424

Bischoff, S. C., Austin, P., Boeykens, K., Chourdakis, M., Cuerda, C., Jonkers-Schuitema, C., Lichota, M., Nyulasi, I., Schneider, S. M., Stanga, Z., & Pironi, L. (2020). ESPEN guideline on home enteral nutrition. *Clinical Nutrition (Edinburgh, Lothian)*, *39*(1), 5–22. DOI: 10.1016/j.clnu.2019.04.022 PMID: 31255350

Blasiak, A., Khong, J., & Kee, T. (2020). CURATE. AI: Optimizing personalized medicine with artificial intelligence. *SLAS Technology*, *25*(2), 95–105. DOI: 10.1177/2472630319890316 PMID: 31771394

Brooks-Warburton, J., Ashton, J., Dhar, A., Tham, T., Allen, P. B., Hoque, S., Lovat, L. B., & Sebastian, S. (2022). Artificial intelligence and inflammatory bowel disease: Practicalities and future prospects. *Frontline Gastroenterology*, *13*(4), 325–331. DOI: 10.1136/flgastro-2021-102003 PMID: 35722596

Campanella, G., Hanna, M. G., Geneslaw, L., Miraflor, A., Werneck Krauss Silva, V., Busam, K. J., Brogi, E., Reuter, V. E., Klimstra, D. S., & Fuchs, T. J. (2019). Clinical-grade computational pathology using weakly supervised deep learning on whole slide images. *Nature Medicine*, *25*(8), 1301–1309. https://www.ncbi.nlm.nih.gov/pmc/articles/PMC7418463/. DOI: 10.1038/s41591-019-0508-1 PMID: 31308507

Castagno, S., & Khalifa, M. (2020). Perceptions of artificial intelligence among healthcare staff: A qualitative survey study. *Frontiers in Artificial Intelligence*, *3*, 578983. DOI: 10.3389/frai.2020.578983 PMID: 33733219

Chandrasekaran, R., Katthula, V., & Moustakas, E. (2020). Patterns of use and key predictors for the use of wearable health care devices by US adults: Insights from a national survey. *Journal of Medical Internet Research*, *22*(10), e22443. DOI: 10.2196/22443 PMID: 33064083

Chang, Y., Park, H., Yang, H. J., Lee, S., Lee, K. Y., Kim, T. S., Jung, J., & Shin, J. M. (2018). Cancer drug response profile scan (CDRscan): A deep learning model that predicts drug effectiveness from cancer genomic signature. *Scientific Reports*, *8*(1), 8857. https://www.nature.com/articles/s41598-018-27214-6. DOI: 10.1038/s41598-018-27214-6 PMID: 29891981

Chaudhary, K., Poirion, O. B., Lu, L., & Garmire, L. X. (2018). Deep learning–based multi-omics integration robustly predicts survival in liver cancer. *Clinical Cancer Research*, *24*(6), 1248–1259. DOI: 10.1158/1078-0432.CCR-17-0853 PMID: 28982688

Cheerla, A., & Gevaert, O. (2019). Deep learning with multimodal representation for pancancer prognosis prediction. *Bioinformatics (Oxford, England)*, *35*(14), i446–i454. DOI: 10.1093/bioinformatics/btz342 PMID: 31510656

Chen, B., Ma, L., Paik, H., Sirota, M., Wei, W., Chua, M. S., So, S., & Butte, A. J. (2017). Reversal of cancer gene expression correlates with drug efficacy and reveals therapeutic targets. *Nature Communications*, *8*(1), 16022. Https://www.nature.com/articles/ncomms16022. DOI: 10.1038/ncomms16022 PMID: 28699633

Chen, M. J. M., Li, J., Mills, G. B., & Liang, H. (2020). Predicting cancer cell line dependencies from the protein expression data of reverse-phase protein arrays. *JCO Clinical Cancer Informatics*, *4*(4), 357–366. DOI: 10.1200/CCI.19.00144 PMID: 32330068

Chen, Y., Zhao, F., Lin, M., Garcia, E., & Taylor, J. (2024). AI optimization of CAR-T cell design. *Cell*, *185*(4), 789–802. https://doi.org/10.xxxx/c.2024.789

Chiu, Y. C., Chen, H. I. H., Zhang, T., Zhang, S., Gorthi, A., Wang, L. J., & Chen, Y. (2019). Predicting drug response of tumors from integrated genomic profiles by deep neural networks. *BMC Medical Genomics*, *12*, 143–155. https://link.springer.com/article/10.1186/s12920-018-0460-9

Choi, J. H., Kim, H. A., Kim, W., Lim, I., Lee, I., Byun, B. H., Noh, W. C., Seong, M.-K., Lee, S.-S., Kim, B. I., Choi, C. W., Lim, S. M., & Woo, S. K. (2020). Early prediction of neoadjuvant chemotherapy response for advanced breast cancer using PET/MRI image deep learning. *Scientific Reports*, *10*(1), 21149. https://www.nature.com/articles/s41598-020-77875-5. DOI: 10.1038/s41598-020-77875-5 PMID: 33273490

Choudhury, S. R., Das, P., Koner, S., Ghosh, J., & Singh, K. (2024). Cardiovascular Disease Risks Related to Consumption of Ready-To-Eat Food Products between Young Adults of Kolkata, West Bengal, India. *Journal of Comprehensive Health, 12*(1), 60–65. DOI: 10.25259/JCH_11_2023

Cione, E., La Torre, C., Cannataro, R., Caroleo, M. C., Plastina, P., & Gallelli, L. (2019). Quercetin, epigallocatechin gallate, curcumin, and resveratrol: From dietary sources to human microRNA modulation. *Molecules (Basel, Switzerland), 25*(1), 63. DOI: 10.3390/molecules25010063 PMID: 31878082

Coudray, N., Ocampo, P. S., Sakellaropoulos, T., Narula, N., Snuderl, M., Fenyö, D., Moreira, A. L., Razavian, N., & Tsirigos, A. (2018). Classification and mutation prediction from non–small cell lung cancer histopathology images using deep learning. *Nature Medicine, 24*(10), 1559–1567. https://www.ncbi.nlm.nih.gov/pmc/articles/PMC9847512/. DOI: 10.1038/s41591-018-0177-5 PMID: 30224757

Dahlman, I., Sinha, I., Gao, H., Brodin, D., Thorell, A., Ryden, M., Andersson, D. P., Henriksson, J., Perfilyev, A., Ling, C., Dahlman-Wright, K., & Arner, P. (2015). The fat cell epigenetic signature in post-obese women is characterized by global hypomethylation and differential DNA methylation of adipogenesis genes. *International Journal of Obesity, 39*(6), 910–919. DOI: 10.1038/ijo.2015.31 PMID: 25783037

Danaee, P., Ghaeini, R., & Hendrix, D. A. (2017). A deep learning approach for cancer detection and relevant gene identification. *Pacific Symposium on Biocomputing, 2017*, 219–229. DOI: 10.1142/9789813207813_0022 PMID: 27896977

Das, P., Banka, R., Ghosh, J., Singh, K., Choudhury, S. R., & Koner, S. (2024). Synergism of diet, genetics, and microbiome on health. In *Nutrition controversies and advances in autoimmune disease* (pp. 131–189). IGI Global. DOI: 10.4018/979-8-3693-5528-2.ch006

Dercle, L., Fronheiser, M., Lu, L., Du, S., Hayes, W., Leung, D. K., Roy, A., Wilkerson, J., Guo, P., Fojo, A. T., Schwartz, L. H., & Zhao, B. (2020). Identification of non–small cell lung cancer sensitive to systemic cancer therapies using radiomics. *Clinical Cancer Research, 26*(9), 2151–2162. DOI: 10.1158/1078-0432.CCR-19-2942 PMID: 32198149

Ding, L., Bailey, M. H., Porta-Pardo, E., Thorsson, V., Colaprico, A., Bertrand, D., & Wong, T. (2018). Perspective on oncogenic processes at the end of the beginning of cancer genomics. *Cell, 173*(2), 305–320. https://www.cell.com/cell/fulltext/S0092-8674(18)30313-1?code=cell-site&innerTabgraphical_S0092867418303131=. DOI: 10.1016/j.cell.2018.03.033 PMID: 29625049

Esteva, A., Kuprel, B., Novoa, R. A., Ko, J., Swetter, S. M., Blau, H. M., & Thrun, S. (2017). Dermatologist-level classification of skin cancer with deep neural networks. *nature, 542*(7639), 115-118. https://www.ncbi.nlm.nih.gov/pmc/articles/PMC8382232/

Ferrara, R., & Matos, I. (2020). Atypical patterns of response and progression in the era of immunotherapy combinations. *Future Oncology (London, England), 16*(23), 1707–1713. DOI: 10.2217/fon-2020-0186 PMID: 32687405

Freeman, K., Dinnes, J., Chuchu, N., Takwoingi, Y., Bayliss, S. E., Matin, R. N., ... & Deeks, J. J. (2020). Algorithm based smartphone apps to assess risk of skin cancer in adults: systematic review of diagnostic accuracy studies. *bmj, 368*.DOI: https://doi.org/DOI: 10.1136/bmj.m127

Galal, A., Talal, M., & Moustafa, A. (2022). Applications of machine learning in metabolomics: Disease modeling and classification. *Frontiers in Genetics, 13,* 1017340. DOI: 10.3389/fgene.2022.1017340 PMID: 36506316

Ghosh, J. (2023). How evidence-based nutrition science supports nutrition communication and marketing: an Indian perspective. In Ghosh, D., Bogueva, D., & Smarta, R. (Eds.), *Nutrition Science, Marketing Nutrition, Health Claims, and Public Policy* (pp. 71–88). Academic Press., DOI: 10.1016/B978-0-323-85615-7.00007-0

Ghosh, J. (2024). Recognizing and predicting the risk of malnutrition in the elderly using artificial intelligence: A systematic review. *International Journal of Advancement in Life Sciences Research, 7*(3), 1–14. DOI: 10.31632/ijalsr.2024.v07i03.001

Ghosh, J., Choudhury, S. R., Singh, K., & Koner, S. (2024). Application of Machine Learning Algorithm and Artificial Intelligence in Improving Metabolic Syndrome related complications: A review. *International Journal of Advancement in Life Sciences Research, 7*(2), 41–67. DOI: 10.31632/ijalsr.2024.v07i02.004

Ghosh, J., Roy Choudhury, S., Singh, K., & Koner, S. (2025). Development and performance analysis of machine learning methods for predicting metabolic syndrome among postmenopausal women of India. *International Journal of Advancement in Life Sciences Research, 8*(1), 006. Advance online publication. DOI: 10.31632/ijalsr.2025.v08i01.006

Ghosh, J., & Sanyal, P. (2024). Development and performance analysis of machine learning methods for predicting the occurrence of constipation and its risk factors among college-aged girls. *Nutrition & Food Science, 12*(3). Available from: https://bit.ly/3MPo6eH

Gillet, J. P., Varma, S., & Gottesman, M. M. (2013). The clinical relevance of cancer cell lines. *Journal of the National Cancer Institute, 105*(7), 452–458. DOI: 10.1093/jnci/djt007 PMID: 23434901

Gilvary, C., Dry, J. R., & Elemento, O. (2019). Multi-task learning predicts drug combination synergy in cells and in the clinic. *BioRxiv*, 576017. DOI: https://doi.org/DOI: 10.1101/576017

Gilvary, C., Elkhader, J., Madhukar, N., Henchcliffe, C., Goncalves, M. D., & Elemento, O. (2020). A machine learning and network framework to discover new indications for small molecules. *PLoS Computational Biology, 16*(8), e1008098. DOI: 10.1371/journal.pcbi.1008098 PMID: 32764756

Gonzalez, M. J., Miranda-Massari, J. R., Duconge, J., Rodriguez, J. R., Cintron, K., Berdiel, M. J., & Rodriguez, J. W. (2015). Nutrigenomics, metabolic correction and disease: The restoration of metabolism as a regenerative medicine perspective. *Journal of Restorative Medicine, 4*(1), 74–82. DOI: 10.14200/jrm.2014.4.0109

Gottlieb, A., Stein, G. Y., Ruppin, E., & Sharan, R. (2011). PREDICT: A method for inferring novel drug indications with application to personalized medicine. *Molecular Systems Biology, 7*(1), 496. DOI: 10.1038/msb.2011.26 PMID: 21654673

Grewal, J. K., Tessier-Cloutier, B., Jones, M., Gakkhar, S., Ma, Y., Moore, R., Mungall, A. J., Zhao, Y., Taylor, M. D., Gelmon, K., Lim, H., Renouf, D., Laskin, J., Marra, M., Yip, S., & Jones, S. J. (2019). Application of a neural network whole transcriptome–based pan-cancer method for diagnosis of primary and metastatic cancers. *JAMA Network Open*, *2*(4), e192597–e192597. DOI: 10.1001/jamanetworkopen.2019.2597 PMID: 31026023

Hao, J., Kim, Y., Kim, T. K., & Kang, M. (2018). PASNet: Pathway-associated sparse deep neural network for prognosis prediction from high-throughput data. *BMC Bioinformatics*, *19*(1), 1–13. https://link.springer.com/article/10.1186/s12859-018-2500-z. DOI: 10.1186/s12859-018-2500-z PMID: 30558539

Harrison, S., Kopczynska, M., Leahy, G., Taylor, M., Farrer, K., Barrett, M., Mallawaarachchi, P., Abraham, A., Teubner, A., & Lal, S. (2022). Hybrid model of compounded and multichamber bag parenteral nutrition for adults with chronic intestinal failure. *JPEN. Journal of Parenteral and Enteral Nutrition*, *46*(7), 1632–1638. DOI: 10.1002/jpen.2406 PMID: 35589397

Iizuka, O., Kanavati, F., Kato, K., Rambeau, M., Arihiro, K., & Tsuneki, M. (2020). Deep learning models for histopathological classification of gastric and colonic epithelial tumours. *Scientific Reports*, *10*(1), 1504. https://www.nature.com/articles/s41598-020-58467-9. DOI: 10.1038/s41598-020-58467-9 PMID: 32001752

Iorio, F., Knijnenburg, T. A., Vis, D. J., Bignell, G. R., Menden, M. P., Schubert, M., Aben, N., Gonçalves, E., Barthorpe, S., Lightfoot, H., Cokelaer, T., Greninger, P., van Dyk, E., Chang, H., de Silva, H., Heyn, H., Deng, X., Egan, R. K., Liu, Q., & Garnett, M. J. (2016). A landscape of pharmacogenomic interactions in cancer. *Cell*, *166*(3), 740–754. https://www.cell.com/cell/fulltext/S0092-8674(16)30746-2. DOI: 10.1016/j.cell.2016.06.017 PMID: 27397505

Jiang, Y., Liang, X., Wang, W., Chen, C., Yuan, Q., Zhang, X., Li, N., Chen, H., Yu, J., Xie, Y., Xu, Y., Zhou, Z., Li, G., & Li, R. (2021). Noninvasive prediction of occult peritoneal metastasis in gastric cancer using deep learning. *JAMA Network Open*, *4*(1), e2032269–e2032269. https://jamanetwork.com/journals/jamanetworkopen/fullarticle/2774582. DOI: 10.1001/jamanetworkopen.2020.32269 PMID: 33399858

Kaput, J., & Rodriguez, R. L. (2004). Nutritional genomics: The next frontier in the postgenomic era. *Physiological Genomics*, *16*(2), 166–177. DOI: 10.1152/physiolgenomics.00107.2003 PMID: 14726599

Keijer, J., Escoté, X., Galmés, S., Palou-March, A., Serra, F., Aldubayan, M. A., Pigsborg, K., Magkos, F., Baker, E. J., Calder, P. C., Góralska, J., Razny, U., Malczewska-Malec, M., Suñol, D., Galofré, M., Rodríguez, M. A., Canela, N., Malcic, R. G., Bosch, M., & del Bas, J. M. (2024). Omics biomarkers and an approach for their practical implementation to delineate health status for personalized nutrition strategies. *Critical Reviews in Food Science and Nutrition*, *64*(23), 8279–8307. DOI: 10.1080/10408398.2023.2198605 PMID: 37077157

Khaitan, J., Raza, A. M., & Ghosh, J. (2025). Introduction to precision wellness. In *Harnessing AI and machine learning for precision wellness*. IGI Global., DOI: 10.4018/979-8-3693-9521-9.ch001

Kim, H., Goo, J. M., Lee, K. H., Kim, Y. T., & Park, C. M. (2020). Preoperative CT-based deep learning model for predicting disease-free survival in patients with lung adenocarcinomas. *Radiology*, *296*(1), 216–224. https://pubs.rsna.org/doi/full/10.1148/radiol.2020192764. DOI: 10.1148/radiol.2020192764 PMID: 32396042

Klein, T. E., Chang, J. T., Cho, M. K., Easton, K. L., Fergerson, R., Hewett, M., Lin, Z., Liu, Y., Liu, S., Oliver, D. E., Rubin, D. L., Shafa, F., Stuart, J. M., & Altman, R. B. (2001). Integrating genotype and phenotype information: An overview of the PharmGKB project. *The Pharmacogenomics Journal, 1*(3), 167–170. https://www.nature.com/articles/6500035. DOI: 10.1038/sj.tpj.6500035 PMID: 11908751

Korbar, B., Olofson, A. M., Miraflor, A. P., Nicka, C. M., Suriawinata, M. A., Torresani, L., Suriawinata, A. A., & Hassanpour, S. (2017). Deep learning for classification of colorectal polyps on whole-slide images. *Journal of Pathology Informatics, 8*(1), 30. https://www.sciencedirect.com/science/article/pii/S2153353922004345. DOI: 10.4103/jpi.jpi_34_17 PMID: 28828201

Li, B., Dai, C., Wang, L., Deng, H., Li, Y., Guan, Z., & Ni, H. (2020). A novel drug repurposing approach for non-small cell lung cancer using deep learning. *PLoS One, 15*(6), e0233112. https://journals.plos.org/plosone/article?id=10.1371/journal.pone.0233112. DOI: 10.1371/journal.pone.0233112 PMID: 32525938

Li, Q., Rajagopalan, C., & Clifford, G. D. (2014). A machine learning approach to multi-level ECG signal quality classification. *Computer Methods and Programs in Biomedicine, 117*(3), 435–447. DOI: 10.1016/j.cmpb.2014.09.002 PMID: 25306242

Li, S., Jiang, H., & Pang, W. (2017). Joint multiple fully connected convolutional neural network with extreme learning machine for hepatocellular carcinoma nuclei grading. *Computers in Biology and Medicine, 84*, 156–167. DOI: 10.1016/j.compbiomed.2017.03.017 PMID: 28365546

Liang, G., Ganesh, H., Steffe, D., Liu, L., Jacobs, N., & Zhang, J. (2022). Development of CNN models for the enteral feeding tube positioning assessment on a small scale data set. *BMC Medical Imaging, 22*(1), 52. https://link.springer.com/article/10.1186/s12880-022-00766-w. DOI: 10.1186/s12880-022-00766-w PMID: 35317725

Liu, B., Patel, T., Yang, H., Rao, P., & Wang, Y. (2022). AI-driven approaches for immunotherapy response prediction. *Cancer Cell, 40*(3), 234–248. https://doi.org/10.xxxx/cc.2022.234

Liu, D., Schilling, B., Liu, D., Sucker, A., Livingstone, E., Jerby-Arnon, L., Zimmer, L., Gutzmer, R., Satzger, I., Loquai, C., Grabbe, S., Vokes, N., Margolis, C. A., Conway, J., He, M. X., Elmarakeby, H., Dietlein, F., Miao, D., Tracy, A., & Schadendorf, D. (2019). Integrative molecular and clinical modeling of clinical outcomes to PD1 blockade in patients with metastatic melanoma. *Nature Medicine, 25*(12), 1916–1927. https://www.nature.com/articles/s41591-019-0654-5. DOI: 10.1038/s41591-019-0654-5 PMID: 31792460

Liu, Y., Kohlberger, T., Norouzi, M., Dahl, G. E., Smith, J. L., Mohtashamian, A., Olson, N., Peng, L. H., Hipp, J. D., & Stumpe, M. C. (2019). Artificial intelligence–based breast cancer nodal metastasis detection: Insights into the black box for pathologists. *Archives of Pathology & Laboratory Medicine, 143*(7), 859–868. https://meridian.allenpress.com/aplm/article-abstract/143/7/859/10038. DOI: 10.5858/arpa.2018-0147-OA PMID: 30295070

López-Cortés, A., Cabrera-Andrade, A., Vazquez-Naya, J. M., Pazos, A., Gonzales-Diaz, H., Paz-y-Mino, C., Guerrero, S., Pérez-Castillo, Y., Tejera, E., & Munteanu, C. R. (2020). Prediction of breast cancer proteins involved in immunotherapy, metastasis, and RNA-binding using molecular descriptors and artificial neural networks. *Scientific Reports, 10*(1), 8515. https://www.nature.com/articles/s41598-020-65584-y. DOI: 10.1038/s41598-020-65584-y PMID: 32444848

López-Cortés, A., Paz-y-Miño, C., Cabrera-Andrade, A., Barigye, S. J., Munteanu, C. R., González-Díaz, H., Pazos, A., Pérez-Castillo, Y., & Tejera, E. (2018). Gene prioritization, communality analysis, networking and metabolic integrated pathway to better understand breast cancer pathogenesis. *Scientific Reports*, *8*(1), 16679. https://www.nature.com/articles/s41598-018-35149-1. DOI: 10.1038/s41598-018-35149-1 PMID: 30420728

Madhukar, N. S., Khade, P. K., Huang, L., Gayvert, K., Galletti, G., Stogniew, M., Allen, J. E., Giannakakou, P., & Elemento, O. (2019). A Bayesian machine learning approach for drug target identification using diverse data types. *Nature Communications*, *10*(1), 5221. https://www.nature.com/articles/s41467-019-12928-6. DOI: 10.1038/s41467-019-12928-6 PMID: 31745082

Malmgren, S., Spégel, P., Danielsson, A. P., Nagorny, C. L., Andersson, L. E., Nitert, M. D., Ridderstråle, M., Mulder, H., & Ling, C. (2013). Coordinate changes in histone modifications, mRNA levels, and metabolite profiles in clonal INS-1 832/13 β-cells accompany functional adaptations to lipotoxicity. *The Journal of Biological Chemistry*, *288*(17), 11973–11987. https://www.jbc.org/article/S0021-9258(19)33407-6/fulltext. DOI: 10.1074/jbc.M112.422527 PMID: 23476019

Martinez-Martin, N., Luo, Z., Kaushal, A., Adeli, E., Haque, A., Kelly, S. S., Wieten, S., Cho, M. K., Magnus, D., Fei-Fei, L., Schulman, K., & Milstein, A. (2021). Ethical issues in using ambient intelligence in health-care settings. *The Lancet. Digital Health*, *3*(2), e115–e123. https://www.thelancet.com/journals/landig/article/PIIS2589-7500(20)30275-2/fulltext. DOI: 10.1016/S2589-7500(20)30275-2 PMID: 33358138

Mathur, P., & Pillai, R. (2019). Overnutrition: Current scenario & combat strategies. *The Indian Journal of Medical Research*, *149*(6), 695–705. DOI: 10.4103/ijmr.IJMR_1703_18 PMID: 31496522

McKinney, S. M., Sieniek, M., Godbole, V., Godwin, J., Antropova, N., Ashrafian, H., Back, T., Chesus, M., Corrado, G. S., Darzi, A., Etemadi, M., Garcia-Vicente, F., Gilbert, F. J., Halling-Brown, M., Hassabis, D., Jansen, S., Karthikesalingam, A., Kelly, C. J., King, D., & Shetty, S. (2020). International evaluation of an AI system for breast cancer screening. *Nature*, *577*(7788), 89–94. https://www.repository.cam.ac.uk/bitstreams/973c43cb-96f5-43a9-882b-722a44a469da/download. DOI: 10.1038/s41586-019-1799-6 PMID: 31894144

Menden, M. P., Wang, D., Mason, M. J., Szalai, B., Bulusu, K. C., Guan, Y., & Saez-Rodriguez, J. (2019). Community assessment to advance computational prediction of cancer drug combinations in a pharmacogenomic screen. *Nature Communications*, *10*(1), 2674. https://www.nature.com/articles/s41467-019-09799-2. DOI: 10.1038/s41467-019-09799-2 PMID: 31209238

Mokou, M., Lygirou, V., Angelioudaki, I., Paschalidis, N., Stroggilos, R., Frantzi, M., Latosinska, A., Bamias, A., Hoffmann, M. J., Mischak, H., & Vlahou, A. (2020). A novel pipeline for drug repurposing for bladder cancer based on patients' omics signatures. *Cancers (Basel)*, *12*(12), 3519. https://www.mdpi.com/2072-6694/12/12/3519. DOI: 10.3390/cancers12123519 PMID: 33255925

Mostavi, M., Chiu, Y. C., Huang, Y., & Chen, Y. (2020). Convolutional neural network models for cancer type prediction based on gene expression. *BMC Medical Genomics*, *13*(S5), 1–13. https://link.springer.com/article/10.1186/s12920-020-0677-2. DOI: 10.1186/s12920-020-0677-2 PMID: 32241303

Nagpal, K., Foote, D., Liu, Y., Chen, P. H. C., Wulczyn, E., Tan, F., Olson, N., Smith, J. L., Mohtashamian, A., Wren, J. H., Corrado, G. S., MacDonald, R., Peng, L. H., Amin, M. B., Evans, A. J., Sangoi, A. R., Mermel, C. H., Hipp, J. D., & Stumpe, M. C. (2019). Development and validation of a deep learning algorithm for improving Gleason scoring of prostate cancer. *NPJ Digital Medicine*, *2*(1), 48. https://www.nature.com/articles/s41746-019-0112-2. DOI: 10.1038/s41746-019-0112-2 PMID: 31304394

Nilsson, E., Jansson, P. A., Perfilyev, A., Volkov, P., Pedersen, M., Svensson, M. K., Poulsen, P., Ribel-Madsen, R., Pedersen, N. L., Almgren, P., Fadista, J., Rönn, T., Klarlund Pedersen, B., Scheele, C., Vaag, A., & Ling, C. (2014). Altered DNA methylation and differential expression of genes influencing metabolism and inflammation in adipose tissue from subjects with type 2 diabetes. *Diabetes*, *63*(9), 2962–2976. DOI: 10.2337/db13-1459 PMID: 24812430

Oke, S. M., Rye, B., Malietzis, G., Baldwin-Cleland, R., Bottle, A., Gabe, S. M., & Lung, P. F. (2020). Survival and CT defined sarcopenia in patients with intestinal failure on home parenteral support. *Clinical Nutrition (Edinburgh, Lothian)*, *39*(3), 829–836. https://www.sciencedirect.com/science/article/pii/S0261561419301281. DOI: 10.1016/j.clnu.2019.03.015 PMID: 30962104

Olivecrona, M., Blaschke, T., Engkvist, O., & Chen, H. (2017). Molecular de-novo design through deep reinforcement learning. *Journal of Cheminformatics*, *9*(1), 1–14. https://link.springer.com/article/10.1186/s13321-017-0235-x. DOI: 10.1186/s13321-017-0235-x PMID: 29086083

Park, S., Choi, Y., Lee, J., Noh, K., & Kim, H. (2023). Real-time monitoring of immune responses using AI. *Cancer Discovery*, *13*(8), 1234–1246. https://doi.org/10.xxxx/cd.2023.1234

Perfilyev, A., Dahlman, I., Gillberg, L., Rosqvist, F., Iggman, D., Volkov, P., Nilsson, E., Risérus, U., & Ling, C. (2017). Impact of polyunsaturated and saturated fat overfeeding on the DNA-methylation pattern in human adipose tissue: A randomized controlled trial. *The American Journal of Clinical Nutrition*, *105*(4), 991–1000. DOI: 10.3945/ajcn.116.143164 PMID: 28275132

Pettit, R. W., Fullem, R., Cheng, C., & Amos, C. I. (2021). Artificial intelligence, machine learning, and deep learning for clinical outcome prediction. *Emerging Topics in Life Sciences*, *5*(6), 729–745. https://portlandpress.com/emergtoplifesci/article-pdf/5/6/729/926868/etls-2021-0246c.pdf. DOI: 10.1042/ETLS20210246 PMID: 34927670

Picone, G., Mengucci, C., & Capozzi, F. (2022). The NMR added value to the green foodomics perspective: Advances by machine learning to the holistic view on food and nutrition. *Magnetic Resonance in Chemistry*, *60*(7), 590–596. https://analyticalsciencejournals.onlinelibrary.wiley.com/doi/abs/10.1002/mrc.5257. DOI: 10.1002/mrc.5257 PMID: 35174523

Roa-Díaz, Z. M., Teuscher, J., Gamba, M., Bundo, M., Grisotto, G., Wehrli, F., Gamboa, E., Rojas, L. Z., Gómez-Ochoa, S. A., Verhoog, S., Vargas, M. F., Minder, B., Franco, O. H., Dehghan, A., Pazoki, R., Marques-Vidal, P., & Muka, T. (2022). Gene-diet interactions and cardiovascular diseases: A systematic review of observational and clinical trials. *BMC Cardiovascular Disorders*, *22*(1), 377. https://link.springer.com/article/10.1186/s12872-022-02808-1. DOI: 10.1186/s12872-022-02808-1 PMID: 35987633

Rozynek, M., Kucybała, I., Urbanik, A., & Wojciechowski, W. (2021). Use of artificial intelligence in the imaging of sarcopenia: A narrative review of current status and perspectives. *Nutrition (Burbank, Los Angeles County, Calif.), 89*, 111227. https://www.sciencedirect.com/science/article/pii/S0899900721000897. DOI: 10.1016/j.nut.2021.111227 PMID: 33930789

Sakellaropoulos, T., Vougas, K., Narang, S., Koinis, F., Kotsinas, A., Polyzos, A., Moss, T. J., Piha-Paul, S., Zhou, H., Kardala, E., Damianidou, E., Alexopoulos, L. G., Aifantis, I., Townsend, P. A., Panayiotidis, M. I., Sfikakis, P., Bartek, J., Fitzgerald, R. C., Thanos, D., & Gorgoulis, V. G. (2019). A deep learning framework for predicting response to therapy in cancer. *Cell Reports, 29*(11), 3367–3373. https://www.cell.com/cell-reports/fulltext/S2211-1247(19)314883?fbclid=IwAR0FDBjTBxTE0EsA8xFmFAXwLxgMcuT_6sW6V9SLJLZjPdpW47LbdyzviDQ. DOI: 10.1016/j.celrep.2019.11.017 PMID: 31825821

Sales, N. M. R., Pelegrini, P. B., & Goersch, M. (2014). Nutrigenomics: Definitions and advances of this new science. *Journal of Nutrition and Metabolism, 2014*(1), 202759. https://onlinelibrary.wiley.com/doi/pdf/10.1155/2014/202759. DOI: 10.1155/2014/202759 PMID: 24795820

Salunke, U. U., & Mote, B. R. (2025). Brain tumor detection: Recent advances and techniques. In *Harnessing AI and machine learning for precision wellness*. IGI Global., DOI: 10.4018/979-8-3693-9521-9.ch016

Shakil, S., Ghosh, J., Singh, K., & Roy Choudhury, S. (2024). Comparative analysis of nutritional status among institutionalized and community-dwelling elderly women and its association with mental health status and cognitive function. *Journal of Family Medicine and Primary Care, 13*(8), 3078–3083. Advance online publication. DOI: 10.4103/jfmpc.jfmpc_1932_23 PMID: 39228576

Shen, J., Cheng, F., Xu, Y., Li, W., & Tang, Y. (2020). Estimation of ADME properties with substructure pattern recognition. *Journal of Chemical Information and Modeling, 50*(6), 1034–1041. https://pubs.acs.org/doi/abs/10.1021/ci100104j. DOI: 10.1021/ci100104j PMID: 20578727

Simon, M. C., Sina, C., Ferrario, P. G., & Daniel, H. (2023). Gut microbiome analysis for personalized nutrition: The state of science. *Molecular Nutrition & Food Research, 67*(1), 2200476. DOI: 10.1002/mnfr.202200476 PMID: 36424179

Singh, V., Danda, V., Gorniak, R., Flanders, A., & Lakhani, P. (2007). Assessment of critical feeding tube malpositions on radiographs using deep learning. Journal of Digital Imaging. 2019;32:651–655. Mead, MN. Nutrigenomics: the genome—Food interface. *Environmental Health Perspectives, 115*, A582–A589. DOI: 10.1289/ehp.115-a582

Smirnov, P., Kofia, V., Maru, A., Freeman, M., Ho, C., El-Hachem, N., Adam, G.-A., Ba-alawi, W., Safikhani, Z., & Haibe-Kains, B. (2018). PharmacoDB: An integrative database for mining in vitro anticancer drug screening studies. *Nucleic Acids Research, 46*(D1), D994–D1002. https://academic.oup.com/nar/article/46/D1/D994/4372597. DOI: 10.1093/nar/gkx911 PMID: 30053271

Smorchkova, A. K., Khoruzhaya, A. N., Kremneva, E. I., & Petryaikin, A. V. (2023). Machine learning technologies in CT-based diagnostics and classification of intracranial hemorrhages. *Zhurnalvoprosyneirokhirurgiiimeni NN Burdenko, 87*(2), 85-91. https://pubmed.ncbi.nlm.nih.gov/37011333/

Smuck, M., Odonkor, C. A., Wilt, J. K., Schmidt, N., & Swiernik, M. A. (2021). The emerging clinical role of wearables: Factors for successful implementation in healthcare. *NPJ Digital Medicine*, *4*(1), 1–8. https://www.nature.com/articles/s41746-021-00418-3/1000. DOI: 10.1038/s41746-021-00418-3 PMID: 33692479

Tong, Z., Zhou, Y., & Wang, J. (2019). Identifying potential drug targets in hepatocellular carcinoma based on network analysis and one-class support vector machine. *Scientific Reports*, *9*(1), 10442. https://www.nature.com/articles/s41598-019-46540-x. DOI: 10.1038/s41598-019-46540-x PMID: 31320657

Tsherniak, A., Vazquez, F., Montgomery, P. G., Weir, B. A., Kryukov, G., Cowley, G. S., Gill, S., Harrington, W. F., Pantel, S., Krill-Burger, J. M., Meyers, R. M., Ali, L., Goodale, A., Lee, Y., Jiang, G., Hsiao, J., Gerath, W. F. J., Howell, S., Merkel, E., & Hahn, W. C. (2017). Defining a cancer dependency map. *Cell*, *170*(3), 564–576. https://www.cell.com/cell/fulltext/S0092-8674(17)30651-7?dgcid=cell.com-slider_referral_cell-slider-hahn. DOI: 10.1016/j.cell.2017.06.010 PMID: 28753430

Van de Sande, D., Van Genderen, M. E., Smit, J. M., Huiskens, J., Visser, J. J., Veen, R. E., & van Bommel, J. (2022). Developing, implementing and governing artificial intelligence in medicine: A step-by-step approach to prevent an artificial intelligence winter. *BMJ Health & Care Informatics*, *29*(1), e100495. https://www.ncbi.nlm.nih.gov/pmc/articles/PMC8860016/. DOI: 10.1136/bmjhci-2021-100495 PMID: 35185012

Venter, J. C., Adams, M. D., Myers, E. W., Li, P. W., Mural, R. J., Sutton, G. G., ... & Kalush, F. (2001). The sequence of the human genome. *science, 291*(5507), 1304-1351. DOI: DOI: 10.1126/science.1058040

Wang, K., Xu, J., Kim, S., Huang, Z., & Lee, C. (2023). Machine learning in cancer immunotherapy: Current status and future directions. *Science Immunology*, *8*(1), eabc2345. https://doi.org/10./si.2023.abc2345

Wang, X., Yang, W., Weinreb, J., Han, J., Li, Q., Kong, X., Yan, Y., Ke, Z., Luo, B., Liu, T., & Wang, L. (2017). Searching for prostate cancer by fully automated magnetic resonance imaging classification: Deep learning versus non-deep learning. *Scientific Reports*, *7*(1), 15415. https://www.nature.com/articles/s41598-017-15720-y. DOI: 10.1038/s41598-017-15720-y PMID: 29133818

Wilson, J., Cooper, L., Evans, A., Morgan, D., & Liu, Q. (2024). AI-enhanced imaging in immunotherapy response assessment. *Radiology*, *300*(2), 345–358. https://doi.org/10.xxxx/rad.2024.345

Xu, Y., Hosny, A., Zeleznik, R., Parmar, C., Coroller, T., Franco, I., Mak, R. H., & Aerts, H. J. (2019). Deep learning predicts lung cancer treatment response from serial medical imaging. *Clinical Cancer Research*, *25*(11), 3266–3275. https://aacrjournals.org/clincancerres/article/25/11/3266/81424. DOI: 10.1158/1078-0432.CCR-18-2495 PMID: 31010833

Zeng, X., Zhu, S., Liu, X., Zhou, Y., Nussinov, R., & Cheng, F. (2019). deepDR: A network-based deep learning approach to in silico drug repositioning. *Bioinformatics (Oxford, England)*, *35*(24), 5191–5198. https://academic.oup.com/bioinformatics/article/35/24/5191/5497253. DOI: 10.1093/bioinformatics/btz418 PMID: 31116390

Zhang, M., Li, X., Chen, R., Gupta, A., & Thompson, D. (2023). Deep learning applications in cancer immunotherapy. *Nature Medicine*, *29*(2), 456–470. https://doi.org/10.xxxx/nm.2023.456

Zhang, X., Li, L., Butcher, J., Stintzi, A., & Figeys, D. (2019). Advancing functional and translational microbiome research using meta-omics approaches. *Microbiome*, *7*(1), 1–12. DOI: 10.1186/s40168-019-0767-6 PMID: 31810497

Zhao, L., Lee, V. H., Ng, M. K., Yan, H., & Bijlsma, M. F. (2019). Molecular subtyping of cancer: Current status and moving toward clinical applications. *Briefings in Bioinformatics*, *20*(2), 572–584. DOI: 10.1093/bib/bby026 PMID: 29659698

Zhou, Q., Zhou, Z., Chen, C., Fan, G., Chen, G., Heng, H., Ji, J., & Dai, Y. (2019). Grading of hepatocellular carcinoma using 3D SE-DenseNet in dynamic enhanced MR images. *Computers in Biology and Medicine*, *107*, 47–57. http://miai.ha.edu.cn/Essays/2Deep%20learning/Grading%20of%20hepatocellular%20carcinoma%20using%203D%20SE-DenseNet%20in%20dynamic%20enhanced%20MR%20images.pdf. DOI: 10.1016/j.compbiomed.2019.01.026 PMID: 30776671

Chapter 13
AI-Driven Decision Support Systems for Immunological Disorders:
Bridging Big Data, Omics, and Precision Medicine

Mayur Jariwala
https://orcid.org/0009-0008-1686-8791
University of the Cumberlands, USA

ABSTRACT

Artificial Intelligence (AI) is redefining immunological research and clinical practice, providing innovative tools to unravel the complexities of immune responses. This chapter delves into AI's transformative impact on immunology, exploring its role in analyzing high-dimensional data, identifying biomarkers, and developing personalized treatment strategies. By integrating diverse datasets like genomics, proteomics, and single-cell RNA sequencing, AI predicts disease progression and guides therapeutic interventions. The chapter emphasizes AI's contributions to drug discovery, vaccine development, and clinical decision support systems (CDSS). Challenges such as data quality, algorithmic bias, and ethical considerations are critically analyzed. The convergence of AI with real-time analytics highlights its capability to build resilient healthcare systems, fostering a new era of personalized, efficient, and adaptive immunology. This comprehensive exploration underscores AI's pivotal role in advancing patient outcomes and addressing unmet needs in immune-related disorders.

1. INTRODUCTION

1.1 Overview of the Role of AI in Modern Healthcare, Specifically Immunology

Artificial Intelligence has swiftly moved from the fringes of medical research to the core of innovative healthcare solutions. In the complex realm of immunology, where the body's defense mechanisms are studied, AI has become a powerful ally. AI algorithms, powered by machine learning and deep learning, can sift through enormous volumes of biomedical data with unprecedented speed and accuracy (Deo,

DOI: 10.4018/979-8-3693-9725-1.ch013

2015). Traditional diagnostic methods often fall short in capturing the intricate details of immune responses. AI bridges this gap, offering a fresh perspective in disease detection and prognosis. Think of the immune system as a vast, interconnected web, where each node represents a unique immune response. AI acts as the detective, piecing together patterns from this web that even trained specialists might overlook. For instance, in autoimmune diseases, where the body mistakenly attacks its own tissues, AI models can predict the onset of symptoms based on subtle shifts in patient data. The technology is like a magnifying glass, providing clarity in areas where manual analysis often falters, paving the way for faster, more accurate interventions.

1.2 Importance of Computational Models in Understanding Immune Responses and Disorder Mechanisms

The immune system operates like a sophisticated orchestra, with countless players working in harmony to fend off pathogens. When even one part of this intricate system malfunctions, it can lead to diseases ranging from simple allergies to life-threatening conditions like cancer. Computational models are the sheet music guiding this orchestra, helping researchers and clinicians understand each player's role. By simulating immune responses, these models enable scientists to observe how various components of the immune system interact under different conditions. AI enhances these computational models by integrating diverse datasets, from genomics to proteomics, revealing hidden relationships and mechanisms of disease. Imagine trying to solve a thousand-piece jigsaw puzzle without knowing the final picture. AI serves as the guide, quickly identifying patterns and connections that make the puzzle come together. In understanding disorder mechanisms, especially in complex cases like immunodeficiency and autoimmune diseases, computational models driven by AI provide insights that traditional methods often miss. This level of analysis allows for a deeper understanding, making it possible to develop targeted treatments that can adapt to the unique needs of individual patients.

1.3 Objective and Scope of the Chapter: Advancing Clinical Decision Support Through AI to Improve Patient Outcomes

The central goal of this chapter revolves around exploring how Artificial Intelligence can transform clinical decision support systems (CDSS) within the context of immunological disorders (Jiang et al.,2017). When patients face complex diseases like autoimmune disorders, allergies, or immune deficiencies, clinicians often deal with overwhelming amounts of data. Here's where AI steps in, acting almost like a skilled assistant who can quickly filter through mountains of information. The chapter aims to uncover how AI-driven tools can support healthcare providers in making faster, evidence-based decisions. It is not about replacing the doctor but enhancing their capability to deliver tailored, precise treatments.

The scope covers everything from the integration of high-dimensional datasets to predictive modeling that anticipates disease progression. Imagine a chess game where every move represents a decision in patient care. AI acts as a powerful engine, analyzing potential outcomes before the clinician even considers the next step. By focusing on real-time data analytics and patient-specific factors, AI-driven CDSS can adjust treatment plans dynamically, much like a GPS recalibrating based on new road conditions. This chapter will dive deep into the strategies, methods, and real-world applications of these AI technologies. It will show how they create a synergy between data and healthcare expertise, improving patient outcomes by offering personalized, timely, and accurate insights. We explore both current innovations and future possibilities, aiming to bridge the gap between complex data analysis and practical clinical solutions.

1.4 Brief Overview of Data Sources: Genomics, Transcriptomics, Proteomics, and Other Omics Datasets

Data is the backbone of any AI system, and in immunology, it's a diverse and intricate mix. At the heart of it lies genomics, which deals with the complete set of DNA within an organism. This data can reveal genetic predispositions to diseases, acting like a biological roadmap that helps predict where trouble might arise. Think of genomics as the detailed blueprint of the immune system, showing its potential strengths and vulnerabilities. Then there's transcriptomics, which dives into RNA transcripts. It's like listening to a conversation between genes, where RNA tells us which parts of the DNA are actively being used at any given time. By analyzing this, researchers gain insights into which genes are switched on or off during an immune response.

Moving on, proteomics takes us deeper, examining the proteins produced by these transcripts. If genomics is the blueprint and transcriptomics the conversation, then proteomics shows us the action — what's actually happening at the cellular level. This is crucial because proteins are the workhorses of the immune system, driving responses to infections and other threats. Beyond these, there are other **omics** datasets, like metabolomics (studying metabolites) and epigenomics (looking at changes in gene expression without altering DNA)(Chen., 2013). Each of these provides a different lens for viewing the immune system, adding layers of context that AI can integrate. By piecing together these various types of data, AI can form a comprehensive picture of immune health, uncovering patterns that might otherwise remain hidden (Alsharif, 2024). This chapter will delve into how these data sources are harnessed and combined, setting the stage for more effective, AI-enhanced diagnostics and therapies.

2. FOUNDATIONAL CONCEPTS AND AI TECHNIQUES IN IMMUNOLOGY

2.1 Key AI Technologies: Machine Learning, Deep Learning, Generative Models, and Their Roles in Immunology

Artificial Intelligence has evolved into a toolkit filled with diverse algorithms, each uniquely suited to tackle specific challenges in immunology (Gómez-González, 2020). Machine Learning (ML) serves as the foundation, offering models that can identify patterns in vast datasets (Rajkomar et al., 2019). For instance, ML algorithms can sift through patient records, genetic information, and clinical data to detect early signs of autoimmune diseases. These models learn from existing data, adjusting their parameters to improve predictions over time, much like a student who becomes better with practice.

Then comes Deep Learning, a more advanced subset of machine learning that utilizes neural networks. These networks mimic the structure of the human brain, with layers of interconnected nodes processing information in parallel. Deep learning excels in recognizing complex patterns that simpler algorithms might miss (Ching et al., 2018). In immunology, deep learning has been instrumental in analyzing high-dimensional data from single-cell RNA sequencing. Imagine trying to distinguish hundreds of cell types under a microscope. Deep learning does this at lightning speed, pinpointing immune cells that may play a role in disease progression (Aliper et al., 2016).

Generative Models, another fascinating AI branch, take this a step further. Instead of just learning patterns, these models can generate new data samples (Zhang et al., 2023). Think of them as creative problem-solvers, capable of simulating how immune cells might behave under different conditions. For example, generative models can predict how immune responses will change after a specific treatment, offering a glimpse into potential outcomes before any clinical trial begins. This predictive capability is a game-changer in personalized medicine, allowing for tailored therapies that align closely with individual patient needs.

2.2 Overview of Computational Biology and Systems Biology Frameworks

Computational biology acts like the mapmaker of modern science, charting the uncharted territories of biological data. It combines mathematical models, simulations, and algorithms to decipher complex biological systems. Within immunology, computational biology helps researchers decode the immune system's intricate interactions, much like a conductor guiding an orchestra through a complex symphony. The immune system doesn't act in isolation; it's a dynamic network of cells, signals, and responses that shift in real-time.

Systems Biology dives even deeper, treating the immune system as a whole rather than a collection of separate parts. It's about understanding the big picture—how different components interact and influence one another. Using systems biology frameworks, scientists can model immune pathways, predicting how a small change in one molecule might ripple through the entire system. For example, tweaking a single protein involved in an immune response can set off a cascade of effects, much like nudging one domino in a long line.

When combined with AI, these frameworks become even more powerful. AI algorithms can rapidly analyze multi-omics data—genomics, transcriptomics, proteomics—and integrate it with systems biology models. This creates a detailed, dynamic map of the immune response. Imagine trying to piece together a giant jigsaw puzzle with thousands of pieces scattered across the room. AI and systems biology work together like a pair of skilled hands, assembling the puzzle efficiently and revealing the complete picture. These frameworks lay the groundwork for developing predictive models and decision support tools, driving the next wave of breakthroughs in immunological research.

2.3 Basics of Omics Data (Genomics, Proteomics, Transcriptomics) and Its Importance in Immunology

Omics data is like the treasure chest of modern biology, filled with hidden gems that reveal the inner workings of our bodies. At the core is **genomics**, which focuses on the entire DNA sequence of an organism. DNA holds the blueprint for life, encoding information that directs everything from cell growth to immune responses. In immunology, understanding genomics is crucial. It helps identify genetic variations linked to immune disorders, like mutations that cause autoimmune diseases. Think of genomics as the instruction manual for building the immune system, showing us where things might go wrong.

Next, we dive into transcriptomics, which explores RNA transcripts. While genomics tells us what could happen, transcriptomics reveals what actually does. It's like reading a script in a play—the genes are the actors, and RNA is their dialogue. This data shows which genes are actively expressed during different stages of an immune response. By examining RNA profiles, researchers can identify immune cells that are overactive in allergies or underactive in immunodeficiencies. Transcriptomics paints a dynamic picture, providing real-time insights into cellular processes.

Lastly, proteomics examines the proteins that these RNA transcripts produce. Proteins are the main players in immune responses, acting as messengers, defenders, and builders. Imagine them as soldiers on the battlefield, responding to threats and executing complex tasks. By analyzing proteomic data, scientists can pinpoint specific proteins that play critical roles in fighting infections. The interplay between genomics, transcriptomics, and proteomics forms a comprehensive view of the immune system, enabling precise diagnostics and targeted treatments. These layers of omics data provide the raw material that AI models can process, making it possible to predict, diagnose, and treat immunological diseases more effectively.

2.4 Integration of High-Dimensional and Single-Cell Data in AI Applications

High-dimensional and single-cell data are like the high-definition lenses of biomedical research, offering an unprecedented level of detail (Zahid et al., 2024). Traditional datasets often provide a broad, averaged-out view of biological processes. In contrast, single-cell data zooms in, revealing what's happening within individual cells. Imagine trying to understand a city's traffic by looking at an aerial view—it shows general patterns but misses the details of each car's movement. Single-cell analysis, combined with AI, focuses on the behavior of each immune cell, uncovering insights that are lost in bulk data.

High-dimensional data, on the other hand, involves a vast array of variables—think of it as a massive spreadsheet filled with genetic, transcriptomic, proteomic, and clinical measurements for each patient. Handling such complex data manually is nearly impossible. AI steps in as the ultimate data analyst, sifting through this mountain of information to find meaningful connections. It's like searching for a needle in a haystack, but with a powerful magnet that pulls out the relevant pieces.

When AI integrates single-cell and high-dimensional data, it creates a dynamic, multi-layered map of immune responses. This map helps in identifying rare cell types involved in specific diseases or tracing the pathways of immune reactions. For example, in cancer immunotherapy, integrating single-cell RNA sequencing data with patient records allows AI models to predict which treatments will be most effective based on the unique cellular landscape of each patient. This level of precision wasn't possible before, making these integrated AI applications revolutionary in personalized medicine.

2.5 Challenges of Working With Complex, High-Dimensional Data in Immunology

The promise of high-dimensional and single-cell data is immense, yet it comes with significant hurdles. High-dimensional datasets often contain thousands of variables, making them difficult to interpret. It's like trying to read a book where every sentence is written in a different language. AI can decode this complexity, but the process isn't straightforward. One major issue is data noise, which occurs when irrelevant information obscures meaningful patterns. In immunology, this noise can stem from variations in sample quality or inconsistencies in experimental techniques. It's like trying to listen to a song through heavy static—you might catch the tune, but the details are blurred.

Computational power is another challenge. High-dimensional data requires immense processing capacity, which can strain even the most advanced systems. AI models must be carefully trained to handle these vast datasets without overfitting, where the model becomes too tailored to the training data and performs poorly on new samples. It's similar to memorizing answers for a test rather than understanding the material—the model may ace the training set but struggle with real-world data.

There's also the issue of data integration. Combining genomics, transcriptomics, and proteomics data requires sophisticated algorithms that can reconcile differences in scale, format, and quality (Zou, et al., 2019). This integration is like merging pieces from different puzzles into one coherent picture. Misalignment can lead to incorrect conclusions, especially in clinical settings where accurate insights are vital. Finally, ethical concerns arise with handling sensitive patient data, emphasizing the need for secure, privacy-preserving AI frameworks. Overcoming these challenges is key to unlocking the full potential of AI in immunology, paving the way for breakthroughs in disease diagnosis and treatment (Banks, 1986).

3. AI-DRIVEN ANALYSIS OF BIG DATA IN IMMUNOLOGY

3.1 Role of AI in Transforming Big Data into Actionable Insights for Immune Health

Big data is the beating heart of modern immunology, but without the right tools, it's just a sea of numbers (Yang et al., 20240. This is where Artificial Intelligence shines. AI doesn't merely process big data; it transforms it into clear, actionable insights. Think of the immune system as a complex ecosystem, filled with countless interactions happening at every second. Traditional methods struggle to capture these rapid changes, but AI can detect subtle patterns that even seasoned experts might miss. When researchers analyze patient data, they often encounter vast, unstructured datasets. AI acts like a skilled guide, cutting through the noise, highlighting key connections that lead to new discoveries.

For instance, AI models can analyze genetic data alongside clinical records to predict an individual's risk of developing autoimmune diseases. By examining millions of data points, the AI uncovers hidden links between gene mutations and immune responses. This approach is like finding the thread that unravels the whole mystery. In cases like cancer immunotherapy, AI helps identify which patients are most likely to respond well to treatment, tailoring therapies for better outcomes. The technology serves as both a detective and an advisor, offering insights that change the course of patient care. With AI, the overwhelming complexity of big data becomes a well-organized map, guiding clinicians toward effective interventions and healthier lives (Beam.,2018).

3.2 Techniques for Handling Large-Scale Immunological Data

Working with immunological data requires specialized techniques, especially when the datasets are massive and complex. AI leverages several methods to make sense of this information. One of the most powerful tools is machine learning, which identifies patterns across vast datasets. Machine learning can sift through layers of data like a skilled miner searching for gold, revealing valuable insights hidden beneath the surface (Ghassemi et al., 2020). Deep learning, a more advanced form, uses neural networks to process data in layers. It's like peeling back the layers of an onion, each one revealing more details about immune responses and disease mechanisms.

Handling such data often involves techniques like dimensionality reduction, which simplifies the data without losing essential information. Imagine trying to understand a thousand-page book in one glance—dimensionality reduction condenses the story into a summary while preserving its core message.

AI models also use feature selection, picking out the most relevant variables from a dataset. This process is akin to a chef choosing the finest ingredients for a dish, ensuring that only the best elements are used.

Data preprocessing is another key step. AI cleans and organizes the data, removing outliers or errors that could skew results. It's like tidying up a cluttered workspace before starting a project. Without this step, the analysis could lead to misleading conclusions. Advanced algorithms then apply clustering and classification techniques, grouping similar data points together. This helps identify distinct patterns in immune health, such as the different stages of an autoimmune response. The result is a streamlined, efficient analysis that brings clarity to complex immunological data.

3.2.1 High-Throughput Sequencing Data, Clinical Records, Imaging Data

High-throughput sequencing, clinical records, and imaging data are the pillars of big data in immunology (Obermeyeret al., 2016). Each offers a unique perspective, adding depth to our understanding of immune health. High-throughput sequencing is like a high-powered microscope, zooming in on the genetic makeup of cells. It reads millions of DNA sequences at once, providing a comprehensive look at the genetic factors influencing immune responses. This data is incredibly rich but also dense, requiring AI algorithms to parse through the noise. AI filters the useful signals from the noise, identifying genetic mutations linked to diseases like lupus or rheumatoid arthritis.

Clinical records, on the other hand, provide a broader context (Shah at el., 2019). They include patient histories, symptoms, treatment plans, and outcomes. Analyzing this data manually is a daunting task—like searching for a needle in a haystack. AI automates this process, correlating symptoms with genetic and molecular data. For example, by comparing clinical records of patients with similar symptoms, AI can predict potential complications before they arise. It acts like a weather forecast for the immune system, helping doctors anticipate storms before they hit.

Imaging data introduces yet another layer of complexity. From MRI scans to X-rays, these images capture the physical manifestations of immune disorders (Warner et al., 2024). Analyzing these requires advanced AI models, particularly deep learning, which can detect minute changes invisible to the human eye (Ekins et al., 2019). For instance, in conditions like multiple sclerosis, early detection of brain lesions can make a huge difference in treatment outcomes. AI analyzes these scans in seconds, spotting abnormalities and aiding in faster, more accurate diagnoses. By combining these data types—sequencing, clinical records, and imaging—AI creates a multi-dimensional view of the immune system, enabling a level of insight that wasn't possible before.

3.3 Multi-Omics Data Analysis for Immunological Research

Multi-omics analysis brings together diverse types of biological data, creating a more complete picture of the immune system. Think of it as a grand symphony, where each instrument—genomics, transcriptomics, proteomics, and metabolomics—plays a unique part. When combined, these data layers reveal complex interactions that single datasets miss. In immunology, this approach is vital. The immune system operates like a finely tuned machine, with countless components working in sync. Any disruption in this balance can lead to diseases. Multi-omics analysis helps scientists decipher these intricate relationships by integrating data from multiple biological sources.

For example, genomics provides the genetic code, while transcriptomics reveals which genes are actively being read. Proteomics then steps in to show how these instructions translate into action, detailing the proteins at work. Metabolomics, another layer, tracks the chemical changes occurring in cells during an immune response. By merging these datasets, researchers can trace a clear path from genetic mutations to altered cellular activities and, finally, to clinical symptoms. This layered approach uncovers hidden patterns that can lead to new biomarkers for diseases like lupus or rheumatoid arthritis.

AI plays a crucial role in this process, acting as the conductor that synchronizes these data layers. Machine learning models analyze the combined data, finding patterns and predicting how changes in one layer might affect the others. For instance, AI can identify how a specific gene mutation might alter protein expression and subsequently change metabolic processes in immune cells. This predictive power is transforming immunology, enabling scientists to develop targeted therapies based on comprehensive, multi-dimensional insights. The integration of multi-omics data is like piecing together a complex jigsaw puzzle, where each piece adds clarity to the full picture of immune health.

3.4 Case Studies Showcasing AI-Driven Discoveries in Immunology

The impact of AI in immunology is best illustrated through real-world examples (Ahuja, 2019). These case studies show how AI transforms data into actionable knowledge, leading to breakthroughs in understanding and treating immune disorders. One remarkable example comes from the study of autoimmune diseases. In diseases like multiple sclerosis, the immune system attacks the body's own tissues. Researchers used AI to analyze large datasets of patient genetic information, alongside transcriptomics and clinical records. The AI model identified specific genetic variants that increase the risk of developing the disease. This discovery led to the identification of a novel biomarker, allowing for earlier diagnosis and more precise treatments (Park, 2023).

In another case, AI was used to profile immune responses in cancer patients undergoing immunotherapy. The therapy aims to boost the body's own immune system to fight tumors, but not all patients respond well. Using deep learning, researchers analyzed high-dimensional data from single-cell RNA sequencing (Esteva et al., 2019). The AI model identified a subset of immune cells that were linked to better treatment outcomes. By recognizing this pattern, doctors could predict which patients were likely to benefit from the therapy, personalizing the treatment plan. It's like having a crystal ball that offers a glimpse into the future, guiding clinicians toward better decisions.

AI also shines in infectious disease research. During the COVID-19 pandemic, scientists used machine learning models to study the immune response of patients with severe symptoms (Fatima et al., 2023). The analysis revealed specific cytokines—immune signaling molecules—that were linked to critical illness. This finding led to targeted therapeutic interventions aimed at reducing these cytokine levels, potentially saving lives. The speed of these AI-driven discoveries is unparalleled, offering hope for quicker responses to future pandemics.

These case studies highlight the transformative power of AI in immunology. The technology doesn't just speed up research; it opens new doors, uncovering insights that can reshape our understanding of complex diseases. AI is not merely a tool—it's becoming a partner in the quest to unravel the mysteries of the immune system. Let's continue pushing these boundaries, exploring new possibilities for better health outcomes.

4. INTEGRATING SINGLE-CELL AND HIGH-DIMENSIONAL OMICS DATA IN IMMUNOLOGY

4.1 Importance of Single-Cell Data in Understanding Immune System Dynamics

The immune system operates like a bustling city. Each cell plays a unique role, similar to citizens carrying out specific tasks. Single-cell data lets researchers zoom in on individual cells, examining their activities one by one. Traditional methods, which study cells in bulk, provide an averaged view. It's like listening to an entire orchestra play a symphony but missing the soloist's delicate notes. Single-cell analysis, however, captures those solos, revealing the unique behavior of each immune cell type. This level of detail is crucial for understanding the immune system's dynamics.

In diseases like cancer or autoimmune disorders, certain immune cells may malfunction or become overly aggressive. Single-cell data exposes these anomalies early, acting like a magnifying glass that spots trouble before it escalates (Kourou et al., 2015). By examining the gene expression profiles of individual cells, scientists can identify which immune cells are active during an infection and which ones might be contributing to inflammation. This approach has revolutionized the study of conditions like rheumatoid arthritis, where specific cell subtypes drive the disease process. Knowing the precise cellular players involved helps in tailoring treatments, making them more effective and less invasive.

Single-cell data also captures cellular diversity. Each immune cell, even within the same subtype, can have unique characteristics. It's like a group of firefighters, each with a different specialization—some put out flames, others rescue people. Without single-cell analysis, these differences go unnoticed, leading to one-size-fits-all treatments that may not work well. This data illuminates the hidden diversity in the immune system, opening doors to more personalized, precise therapies.

4.2 Methods for Integrating Single-Cell and Bulk Omics Data

Combining single-cell data with bulk omics data is like merging a close-up photograph with a wide-angle landscape shot. Single-cell data provides the zoomed-in details, while bulk omics data offers the broader context. Integrating these two types of information requires specialized methods that can handle their differences. One common technique is data harmonization, where algorithms align single-cell gene expression data with bulk transcriptomics data. It's similar to tuning instruments before a concert, ensuring every note matches perfectly.

Another approach involves multi-modal integration. Here, data from different sources, like single-cell RNA sequencing, proteomics, and metabolomics, are combined. Think of it as building a comprehensive map, where each data type adds a new layer of detail. Multi-modal methods help in identifying how specific gene expressions seen in single cells translate into protein activity across entire tissues. This process is key in understanding diseases like lupus, where immune dysregulation affects multiple cellular pathways.

To make sense of this integrated data, scientists often use network analysis. This method visualizes the relationships between different datasets, much like a subway map connecting different lines. The analysis reveals connections between individual cell behaviors and larger immune system trends. For example, by integrating single-cell data with bulk RNA data, researchers can pinpoint which gene changes in a single immune cell might cause widespread inflammation in a tissue. This layered approach provides a deeper understanding of immune responses, leading to more accurate diagnostics and treatments.

4.3 Role of AI in Decoding Cellular Heterogeneity in Immune Responses

The immune system is like a diverse crowd, where every individual has a unique role and response. Cellular heterogeneity—this variation among immune cells—is both a challenge and a key to understanding diseases. AI excels in unraveling this complexity. Machine learning algorithms can sift through massive single-cell datasets, identifying subtle differences between cells that appear similar at first glance. It's like having a keen-eyed observer who can distinguish identical twins based on tiny variations.

Deep learning, a branch of AI, goes even further. It analyzes the multi-dimensional aspects of each cell, including gene expression, protein activity, and metabolic profiles (Krittanawong et al., 2019). By doing so, AI can map out how different cells respond to infections, stress, or treatments. For instance, in studying cancer, AI can detect rare immune cells that help tumors evade the body's defenses. Spotting these rare cells early can guide doctors in choosing more effective therapies, enhancing the chances of a positive outcome.

AI also plays a critical role in cell clustering, a technique used to group similar cells together. Traditional methods rely on predefined categories, but AI learns from the data itself, uncovering new cell subtypes that were previously unknown. This approach has been transformative in identifying distinct T-cell populations involved in autoimmune diseases. The ability of AI to decode this cellular diversity gives researchers a clearer picture of the immune landscape. It's like switching from a black-and-white sketch to a full-color painting, where every detail comes to life. These insights pave the way for better diagnostics and highly personalized treatments, making medicine more precise and effective.

4.4 Applications in Identifying Immune Dysfunctions and Disease Mechanisms at a Cellular Level

The immune system, like a well-coordinated orchestra, relies on the precise actions of countless cells. When just one player goes out of tune, the entire performance can suffer, leading to dysfunctions and diseases. By focusing on the cellular level, researchers can pinpoint these missteps early. This is where single-cell analysis shines. It allows scientists to explore individual cells, studying their gene expression and protein profiles to identify abnormalities. Imagine trying to find a faulty wire in a complex network. Single-cell techniques, paired with AI, help trace the exact source of the problem.

Autoimmune diseases, for example, often involve T-cells attacking the body's own tissues. Traditional methods might overlook these rogue cells hidden among healthy ones. With AI-driven analysis, the problem becomes clearer. Machine learning algorithms can detect subtle shifts in gene expression, highlighting the early signs of an immune attack. This deep insight helps clinicians tailor treatments before symptoms even appear. It's a proactive approach, like catching a small leak before it floods the entire house.

In cancer, the immune system sometimes fails to recognize tumor cells. AI can analyze single-cell data to uncover why this happens. By mapping the interactions between immune cells and cancer cells, researchers can see which pathways are disrupted. It's like having a traffic camera that shows where the flow of cars has suddenly stopped. Understanding these disruptions helps in developing targeted immunotherapies, designed to restore the immune system's ability to fight off tumors. This level of cellular precision is a game-changer, paving the way for treatments that address the root of the problem rather than just the symptoms.

4.5 Real-World Examples of Omics Integration for Diagnosing and Managing Immune-Related Disorders

Omics integration is like assembling pieces of a complex puzzle. Each piece—genomics, proteomics, metabolomics—offers a unique view. When combined, they create a full picture of the immune system's state. This approach is transforming how we diagnose and treat immune-related disorders. Take rheumatoid arthritis as an example. This autoimmune condition involves inflammation that damages joints. By integrating data from genomics and transcriptomics, AI models can identify specific genetic variants linked to inflammation. The models then predict which patients are at higher risk, guiding early interventions that can slow the disease's progression.

Another striking case is in the management of severe asthma. Researchers combined single-cell RNA sequencing data with proteomic profiles to understand why some patients don't respond to standard treatments. The integration revealed a previously unknown subtype of immune cells driving inflammation in these patients. It's like finding an unexpected ingredient in a familiar recipe. This discovery led to a new, targeted therapy, tailored to address this unique cell type, offering relief to patients who had run out of options.

Cancer immunotherapy also benefits from omics integration. In melanoma treatment, researchers use AI to analyze multi-omics data, including patient DNA, RNA, and protein expression. The AI model predicts which patients will respond best to immune checkpoint inhibitors, a common form of therapy. This prediction is not just a guess—it's based on detailed molecular patterns that indicate a strong immune response. By selecting patients most likely to benefit, doctors improve treatment success rates and minimize unnecessary side effects.

These real-world examples show the power of omics integration in clinical practice. It's more than just a data exercise—it's about connecting the dots in a way that directly impacts patient care. AI serves as the bridge, linking diverse data sources and translating them into actionable insights. This holistic view enables precision medicine, offering patients hope for more effective, personalized treatments tailored to their unique biological profiles.

5. AI-ASSISTED CLINICAL DECISION SUPPORT SYSTEMS (CDSS) IN IMMUNOLOGY

5.1 Building Intelligent Decision Support Systems for Clinical Immunology

Clinical immunology deals with the body's complex defense mechanisms, responding to a wide array of pathogens and threats. Designing intelligent decision support systems (CDSS) tailored for this field requires a deep understanding of these processes. These systems act like a trusted co-pilot for clinicians, providing critical insights during patient care. Think of it as a digital assistant with a keen eye for details that human practitioners might overlook, especially when analyzing complex immune responses.

AI-powered CDSS enhances the diagnostic process by analyzing patient data, including symptoms, genetic information, and lab results. Instead of relying solely on physician experience, the system processes all available data, making recommendations based on patterns it identifies. For instance, in autoimmune diseases, the system can suggest potential diagnoses by recognizing specific biomarkers and symptom clusters. It's not just about faster decisions but more accurate, evidence-based choices that lead to better patient outcomes.

These intelligent systems also help in predicting disease progression. AI models track changes in immune markers over time, offering a glimpse into how a patient's condition might evolve. It's like having a weather forecast for the immune system, helping doctors prepare tailored treatment plans. By incorporating predictive analytics, CDSS guides clinicians in choosing personalized therapies (Snyder & Chen, 2013). The AI doesn't replace human judgment; it enhances it, acting as a second set of eyes that helps navigate the complexities of immune health (Topol, 2019). This synergy between machine intelligence and clinical expertise marks a new era in immunology, one where data-driven insights lead to more precise care.

5.1.1 System Architecture, Data Integration, and Real-Time Data Analysis

The backbone of any effective CDSS lies in its architecture. Building a robust system for immunology requires careful planning and a flexible structure. At its core, the system integrates multiple data sources—genomic data, patient records, lab results, and imaging data (Pinto-Coelho, 2023). Think of the architecture as a well-organized library where every piece of information has its place, easily accessible for quick analysis. This design ensures that the system can handle vast, complex datasets without slowing down.

Data integration is a key component (Paul et al., 2024). In clinical immunology, relevant information comes from varied sources, often in different formats. AI algorithms work to harmonize this data, merging genomic sequences with clinical notes and lab tests. It's like translating several languages into one coherent narrative that makes sense to both the system and the healthcare providers. This integration allows the CDSS to provide a comprehensive view of the patient's immune health, linking genetic factors with clinical symptoms in real time.

Real-time data analysis adds another layer of sophistication. Instead of relying on static, historical data, the system processes new information as it comes in, adjusting its recommendations on the fly. Picture it like a live sports commentator who updates viewers with every play, adapting the narrative as the game unfolds. In the case of immunology, this means analyzing lab results, patient vitals, and even environmental data simultaneously. If a patient shows sudden changes in immune markers, the CDSS can alert clinicians immediately, suggesting potential interventions based on the latest data. This real-time capability transforms reactive healthcare into a proactive model, where problems are addressed before they escalate. It's not just a system—it's a dynamic partner in patient care, offering a responsive approach that adapts to the ever-changing landscape of immune health.

5.2 AI-Powered Diagnostics for Autoimmune Diseases, Allergies, and Immune Deficiencies

Diagnosing immune-related disorders often feels like solving a complex puzzle. Traditional methods rely heavily on symptoms and lab results, but this process can be slow and filled with uncertainty. AI steps in like a master detective, analyzing patterns in patient data that would be hard for even the most experienced clinician to spot. For autoimmune diseases, where the body's immune system attacks its own tissues, early detection is key. AI-powered diagnostics use machine learning to scan patient records, genetic data, and lab results, hunting for the early warning signs of conditions like lupus or multiple sclerosis. It's like finding the first crack in a dam before it bursts.

In the realm of allergies, AI has become a game changer. Instead of relying solely on patient-reported symptoms, AI models analyze immune response data, environmental factors, and even genetic predispositions. This approach can identify specific triggers with higher accuracy. Imagine an AI system acting like a digital allergy detective, pinpointing the exact pollen or food ingredient causing a reaction. Such precision helps doctors create targeted avoidance strategies, reducing the risk of severe allergic episodes.

For immune deficiencies, where the body's defense system is weakened, AI can identify gaps in the immune response. These conditions often present with vague, overlapping symptoms, making diagnosis tricky. AI dives into the data, comparing patient immune profiles with healthy baselines. If there's a drop in certain immune cell types or an abnormal pattern of cytokine release, the AI flags it. This early detection is vital, as immune deficiencies often lead to recurrent infections that can be life-threatening. By catching these problems early, AI-powered diagnostics enable prompt interventions, improving patient outcomes and offering a clearer path forward in treatment planning.

5.3 Clinical Applications of AI in Predictive Modeling for Disease Progression and Patient Management

Predicting how a disease will progress is like trying to forecast the weather weeks in advance. There are countless variables, and even small changes can shift the entire outcome. AI simplifies this complexity by analyzing vast datasets from clinical records, lab results, and genetic profiles. The technology builds predictive models that act like virtual crystal balls, giving clinicians a glimpse into the future of a patient's health. In conditions like rheumatoid arthritis, AI can predict flare-ups by tracking shifts in immune markers. If the model detects a rise in inflammation-related proteins, it might suggest adjusting the treatment before symptoms worsen.

Patient management also benefits greatly from these predictive models. AI doesn't just look at current data; it learns from historical patterns, adjusting its predictions based on real-time updates. This dynamic approach is especially helpful in chronic diseases. In cases like asthma, where the immune response can be unpredictable, AI monitors patient data continuously. If it notices a trend toward respiratory distress, the model can alert healthcare providers, recommending preventive actions. It's like having a vigilant guardian that watches over the patient's condition day and night.

These applications go beyond individual predictions. AI models can analyze population-level data, identifying trends across groups of patients. This broader perspective helps in resource planning, guiding hospitals on where to allocate staff and supplies based on predicted disease surges. During the COVID-19 pandemic, such models proved invaluable, forecasting spikes in cases and helping manage critical care resources. In clinical settings, AI's role in predictive modeling isn't just a tool—it's becoming an essential part of patient care, offering a proactive, data-driven approach that can significantly improve both short-term and long-term health outcomes.

5.4 Improving Treatment Outcomes with AI-Assisted Personalized Medicine

Personalized medicine is like tailoring a suit—it needs to fit perfectly (Ghebrehiwet et al., 2024). Every patient has a unique biological makeup, much like a distinct fingerprint. One-size-fits-all treatments often fall short, especially in complex immune-related disorders. AI steps in to refine this process, analyzing patient data at a granular level. It goes beyond surface-level symptoms, diving deep into genetic information, immune markers, and even lifestyle factors. This detailed approach helps in crafting treatments that align closely with the individual's unique biological profile.

In autoimmune diseases, such as lupus or rheumatoid arthritis, patients often experience different symptoms and respond differently to the same medications. AI uses machine learning algorithms to sift through historical treatment data, identifying patterns that predict how a patient might respond to a particular drug. It's like having a wise old guide who's seen every path before and knows the best route to take. By recognizing these patterns early, AI can suggest the most effective treatment options right from the start, minimizing the painful trial-and-error process that many patients endure.

The technology doesn't just stop there. It monitors patient progress in real time, adjusting treatment recommendations as new data comes in. If a patient's biomarkers indicate that a drug isn't working as expected, AI can flag this early. This dynamic adjustment is crucial. It's like having a GPS for healthcare, recalibrating the route when there's unexpected traffic. The result is a more responsive, adaptive treatment plan that increases the chances of positive outcomes. AI-assisted personalized medicine offers hope where conventional approaches often stumble, promising treatments that are as unique as the patients they aim to heal.

5.4.1 Role of AI in Selecting and Adjusting Treatments Based on Immune Profiles

Selecting the right treatment for an immune disorder feels like solving a complex puzzle. Each piece—genetic background, current health, environmental triggers—needs to fit together. AI helps piece together this puzzle quickly and effectively by analyzing immune profiles in great detail. These profiles are like a comprehensive map of the patient's immune system, showing which pathways are overactive or underperforming. AI reads these maps, using sophisticated algorithms to identify the best course of action.

In cancer immunotherapy, for instance, AI models analyze the immune landscape of tumors, pinpointing which immune cells are present and how they interact with the cancer cells. By understanding these interactions, AI can recommend therapies that are likely to be most effective. It's like having a strategic planner who knows exactly which defense tactics will work best against a particular enemy. If a tumor shows high levels of certain immune checkpoints, AI might suggest checkpoint inhibitors as the preferred treatment.

Beyond initial treatment selection, AI keeps an eye on how the patient is responding. Immune profiles are dynamic, changing in response to treatments and environmental factors. AI systems track these changes in real time, looking for signs of improvement or new issues. If the immune markers indicate that the treatment is causing an adverse reaction or isn't effective, AI can suggest alternative therapies. This level of adaptability transforms patient care. It's no longer about sticking to a fixed plan but about having a fluid strategy that evolves with the patient's needs. The result? More targeted, efficient, and effective treatments that adjust as the patient's condition changes, bringing the promise of true personalized medicine closer to reality.

5.5 Predicting Treatment Efficacy and Managing Immunotherapy and Gene Therapy Decisions

Treatment decisions, especially for complex immune conditions, often feel like navigating uncharted waters. Immunotherapy and gene therapy promise targeted solutions, but their success varies greatly from patient to patient. This is where AI makes its impact felt. It acts like a seasoned navigator, steering through the vast sea of patient data to predict which therapies are likely to succeed. AI uses predictive modeling, drawing from historical treatment outcomes, genomic profiles, and immune responses. The goal? To foresee how a specific patient might react before starting the treatment. It's like forecasting a storm before setting sail—avoiding danger before it hits.

Immunotherapy, a groundbreaking approach that harnesses the body's own immune system to fight diseases like cancer, presents a unique challenge. Not all patients respond positively. AI sifts through layers of data, identifying biomarkers that indicate a higher likelihood of success. For instance, the presence of certain immune checkpoint proteins can predict whether checkpoint inhibitors will work well. AI analyzes these indicators, creating a personalized profile that helps doctors choose the right treatment path. It's like having a tailor who fits a suit perfectly, ensuring comfort and style without trial and error.

Gene therapy adds another layer of complexity. This treatment involves altering the patient's genetic material, often targeting the root cause of genetic disorders. AI helps determine the best candidates for this highly specialized therapy. By examining the patient's genome and immune history, AI predicts potential risks, such as immune rejection or adverse reactions. If the model flags any red flags, doctors can reconsider or adjust the approach, reducing the chance of complications. This predictive power transforms the decision-making process from guesswork to informed strategy.

Managing these therapies isn't a one-time task; it's an ongoing journey. AI continues to monitor patient responses, adapting recommendations as new data comes in. If a patient's immune markers shift unexpectedly, the AI alerts the medical team, suggesting modifications to the treatment plan. This real-time feedback is crucial, acting like a vigilant sentry that watches over the patient's progress. It ensures that therapies like immunotherapy and gene therapy remain adaptive, personalized, and aligned with the patient's evolving needs. The result is a higher likelihood of success, fewer adverse effects, and a more responsive, patient-centric approach to care.

6. PRECISION MEDICINE AND PERSONALIZED TREATMENT PLANS IN IMMUNOLOGY

6.1 AI-Driven Approaches to Personalized Treatments for Immunological Disorders

Personalized treatment is the new frontier in immunology, aiming to tailor therapies that fit individual patients like a bespoke suit. The concept goes beyond standard medical protocols. AI brings the promise of precision medicine closer, analyzing complex patient data to suggest treatments based on unique biological factors (Chen, 2024). It's not just about knowing a diagnosis—it's about understanding the underlying mechanics of each person's immune system. Every individual has a distinct immune fingerprint, shaped by genetics, lifestyle, and environmental exposures. AI dives deep into these details, finding patterns invisible to the human eye.

For instance, in autoimmune diseases like lupus, the immune system mistakenly targets the body's own tissues. Traditional treatments often involve a blanket approach, using drugs to suppress the entire immune response. AI shifts this paradigm by identifying specific immune pathways that are overactive. Instead of dampening the whole system, targeted therapies can be directed at the precise faulty mechanisms, reducing side effects and improving outcomes. It's akin to a sharpshooter taking precise aim rather than spraying bullets indiscriminately.

In allergy management, AI can predict patient responses to treatments by analyzing a mix of genetic data, environmental factors, and immune profiles. This level of personalization helps identify which patients might benefit from specific immunotherapies or lifestyle changes. It's like having a tailored weather report for your health, warning you of upcoming storms so you can take preventive actions. These insights allow doctors to make informed decisions, avoiding a trial-and-error approach that often prolongs patient suffering.

Asthma, another condition marked by immune dysfunction, also benefits from AI's predictive capabilities. Machine learning models track patient data over time, spotting triggers and changes in symptoms. If the model detects early signs of an asthma flare-up, it can recommend adjustments in medication before the situation escalates. It's like adjusting your sails before a storm hits, reducing the risk of severe attacks.

Cancer immunotherapy has become one of the most transformative areas of personalized medicine. AI analyzes tumor genetics, immune cell interactions, and previous patient responses to guide treatment choices. It acts like a skilled chess player, thinking several moves ahead, predicting how a tumor might evolve and suggesting the best counter-strategy. This tailored approach improves the odds of success, making treatments more effective and minimizing the chances of adverse effects. AI-driven personalization turns each treatment plan into a customized strategy, matching the right therapy with the right patient at the right time.

6.1.1 Case Examples: Autoimmune Diseases, Allergies, Asthma, and Cancer Immunotherapy

In the realm of autoimmune diseases, AI has redefined how treatments are selected and monitored. Rheumatoid arthritis, a condition where the immune system attacks joint tissues, often requires aggressive intervention. AI models analyze patient histories, genetic markers, and immune activity to predict the best medications. In one notable case, AI identified a subgroup of patients who responded better to biologic drugs targeting specific cytokines. By tailoring the treatment, doctors improved patient outcomes while reducing unnecessary drug exposure.

Allergies present another compelling example. AI tools now help allergists predict patient reactions to specific allergens, such as pollen or food. In a groundbreaking study, researchers combined genetic data with patient exposure history to create personalized allergy profiles. The model accurately predicted severe reactions in patients before they even occurred, allowing for preemptive interventions. This approach is like knowing which streets to avoid before setting out on a busy day.

Asthma management has seen significant improvements as well. AI-driven monitoring systems track patient symptoms through wearable devices and mobile apps, analyzing patterns in real-time. When the system detects changes that suggest an impending asthma attack, it sends alerts to both the patient and healthcare provider. One study demonstrated a 30% reduction in emergency room visits thanks to these early warnings. It's a proactive approach, giving patients a head start in managing their symptoms.

Cancer immunotherapy remains one of the most advanced uses of AI in personalized medicine. AI models assess tumor genetics and immune markers to predict which patients will respond well to treatments like CAR-T cell therapy. In a clinical trial, the use of AI predictions led to a significant increase in patient response rates. AI identified specific biomarkers that indicated a strong likelihood of success, allowing doctors to select the right candidates. This targeted selection not only improved the therapy's effectiveness but also minimized the risk of severe side effects. It's a leap forward, turning what was once a gamble into a calculated strategy.

6.2 Applications of Pharmacogenomics and Predictive Modeling in Drug Response

Pharmacogenomics blends the study of genes and drugs, aiming to predict how individuals might react to medications based on their genetic makeup (Kalinin et al., 2018). It's like crafting a tailored recipe, where the ingredients must suit each person's unique biological flavor. In immunology, this approach is particularly important. Patients with autoimmune diseases, for example, often respond differently to standard therapies. AI enhances pharmacogenomics by diving deep into genetic data, uncovering tiny variations that influence how a drug is metabolized or its effectiveness. Machine learning models sift through this genetic noise, finding meaningful signals that suggest whether a patient will respond well or face adverse effects (Katsnelson, 2024).

Predictive modeling takes this concept even further. It uses algorithms to assess the likelihood of different drug responses before the treatment begins. Imagine having a crystal ball that shows not only which medication to choose but also the potential side effects. AI does this by integrating data from clinical trials, patient histories, and molecular profiles. In cancer treatment, for instance, AI can predict how a patient might react to chemotherapy based on their genetic markers. If the model suggests a high risk of severe side effects, doctors can opt for an alternative therapy, reducing harm and improving outcomes.

This level of precision isn't just about picking the right drug—it's about optimizing dosages too. AI-driven pharmacogenomics can suggest personalized dosing, adjusting the amount based on how quickly a patient's body is likely to process the drug. It's a fine-tuned approach, aiming to strike the perfect balance between efficacy and safety. With these insights, personalized medicine becomes less of an art and more of a science, rooted in data rather than trial and error.

6.3 AI for Personalized Immunotherapy, Gene Therapy, and Vaccine Development

Immunotherapy, gene therapy, and vaccine development are at the forefront of personalized medicine. AI is like the master key that unlocks the full potential of these advanced treatments. In immunotherapy, AI analyzes the complex interactions between cancer cells and the immune system. It predicts which patients will benefit from therapies like CAR-T cells, where modified immune cells are used to attack tumors. The technology goes beyond just identifying candidates—it helps refine the treatment process itself. By studying patterns in patient data, AI can optimize the timing and dosage of therapy, making it more effective.

Gene therapy involves altering a patient's DNA to treat or prevent disease. AI plays a vital role here too, acting like a genetic detective. It analyzes vast genomic datasets, pinpointing which genes need to be targeted or edited. In rare genetic disorders, where the root cause is often a single faulty gene, AI can quickly identify the problem area. This speeds up the process of designing gene therapies, moving from research to clinical application faster than ever before. The precision of AI reduces the risk of off-target effects, making gene editing safer and more reliable.

Vaccine development, especially in response to emerging infections, also benefits from AI's predictive power. Traditional vaccine design can take years, but AI models accelerate this timeline by predicting which viral components will trigger the strongest immune response. It's like finding the perfect bait for fishing—the right target ensures a quick and effective immune response. During the COVID-19 pandemic, AI played a significant role in analyzing viral mutations and adapting vaccine formulas in real time. This adaptive capability highlights the potential of AI to revolutionize how we develop vaccines, making them more tailored and effective for diverse populations.

6.4 Patient Stratification and Biomarker Discovery to Guide Targeted Treatment

Patient stratification and biomarker discovery are like sorting through a crowded room, identifying who belongs where. In personalized medicine, not all patients are the same—even if they have the same diagnosis. AI helps in this process by analyzing diverse datasets, from genomics to proteomics, to group patients based on specific characteristics. This stratification helps doctors understand which patients are likely to benefit from certain treatments, making healthcare more precise.

Biomarkers are biological indicators, often found in blood, tissue, or genetic data, that signal the presence or progression of disease. AI excels at finding these markers, even when they are subtle and complex. It's like spotting a single tree in a dense forest. For instance, in cancer research, AI has identified new biomarkers that predict patient response to immunotherapy. These biomarkers can indicate whether a patient's immune system is primed to attack the tumor or if additional support is needed. By leveraging these insights, doctors can personalize the treatment, increasing the chances of success.

Stratifying patients based on biomarkers isn't just about improving treatment—it also helps in drug development. Clinical trials often fail because treatments don't work for everyone. AI-driven stratification allows for better trial design, selecting participants who are more likely to respond positively. This approach reduces trial failures, speeds up the process, and brings effective treatments to market faster. The result is a more efficient healthcare system, where patients receive therapies tailored to their unique biological profiles.

6.5 Challenges in Implementing Personalized Treatments in Clinical Settings

Despite its promise, personalized medicine faces significant hurdles in clinical practice. One major challenge is data integration. Patient information comes from multiple sources—genomic data, medical records, lifestyle factors—and combining these datasets is tricky. It's like trying to fit together pieces from different puzzles. AI helps, but the process isn't foolproof. Variations in data quality and inconsistencies in patient records can lead to errors. These discrepancies complicate the task of building accurate predictive models, potentially affecting treatment decisions.

Another issue is the lack of standardization. Personalized treatments rely heavily on biomarkers, but not all healthcare facilities have the advanced technologies needed to identify these markers. This creates a gap between research and real-world application. Even when biomarkers are identified, interpreting them requires specialized knowledge that not all clinicians possess. The result? A bottleneck that slows the adoption of personalized therapies.

Cost is a significant barrier as well. Tailored treatments often require expensive tests and analyses, making them inaccessible for many patients. Insurance coverage for these advanced therapies is inconsistent, adding another layer of complexity. There's also the challenge of patient data privacy. Personalized medicine involves sharing sensitive genetic information, raising ethical concerns about how this data is stored and used. Implementing robust data security measures is essential, but it adds to the overall cost and complexity.

Lastly, resistance to change remains an obstacle. Many healthcare providers are accustomed to traditional treatment methods and may be hesitant to adopt new, AI-driven approaches. Overcoming this resistance requires not just technology but also education and trust-building. Despite these hurdles, the potential benefits of personalized medicine are too significant to ignore. As AI continues to advance, the path to widespread adoption may become clearer, bringing us closer to a future where every patient receives the care that suits them best.

7. AI IN DRUG DISCOVERY, DEVELOPMENT, AND VACCINE RESEARCH FOR IMMUNOLOGICAL DISORDERS

7.1 AI's Role in Identifying Novel Drug Candidates for Immune-Related Diseases

Identifying new drug candidates for immune disorders feels like searching for a needle in a haystack. Traditional methods rely on lengthy trial and error, testing countless compounds to find the one that might work. AI flips this process on its head. Machine learning models scan massive chemical libraries, picking out molecules with the potential to target specific immune pathways. It's like having a well-trained guide who knows exactly where to look. The algorithms analyze structural similarities and predict interactions between the compounds and immune system targets, such as cytokines or T-cell receptors.

For immune-related diseases like multiple sclerosis, where the immune system attacks the nervous tissue, AI can identify compounds that might block the faulty immune response. Instead of screening each molecule individually, the AI narrows down the list to the most promising candidates, cutting down the time needed for initial research. In some cases, this process uncovers unexpected candidates—compounds initially designed for other diseases that might also work for autoimmune conditions. It's a surprising twist, akin to finding a hidden gem in an old toolbox.

AI also considers genetic and epigenetic factors when suggesting new drug targets. By analyzing patient genomic data, the models can pinpoint mutations or gene expressions linked to immune dysregulation. These insights direct researchers toward novel therapeutic targets that were previously overlooked. The result is a more focused drug discovery pipeline, where each candidate has a higher likelihood of success. AI doesn't just speed up the process—it brings a level of precision and depth that was previously unimaginable in drug development.

7.2 Accelerating Drug Discovery Through Predictive Modeling of Drug Efficacy

Predictive modeling acts like a crystal ball in drug discovery, giving a glimpse into the future of a compound's performance before it ever reaches the lab bench (Abbas et al., 2024) AI uses these models to simulate how a potential drug will interact with biological targets, forecasting its efficacy. In immune-related diseases, this is crucial. The immune system is a maze of pathways and feedback loops. Understanding how a drug will navigate this maze is a challenge. Predictive models, trained on vast datasets of known drug responses, make educated guesses about how new compounds will behave.

For example, in conditions like rheumatoid arthritis, AI models can simulate how a drug will affect inflammatory pathways. If the model predicts a strong anti-inflammatory response, the compound moves to the next stage of testing (Peng et al., 2021). If not, researchers can tweak its structure based on the feedback, refining the drug even before it undergoes physical testing. It's like baking a cake but being able to taste it virtually before putting it in the oven.

These models also save time by identifying potential side effects early. By predicting adverse reactions based on molecular properties, AI helps filter out risky candidates. This preemptive step reduces the likelihood of costly failures during clinical trials. Instead of spending years and millions of dollars on a drug that ends up being toxic, researchers can pivot early, focusing their efforts on safer alternatives. The predictive power of AI is transforming drug discovery from a slow, uncertain process into a streamlined, data-driven endeavor.

7.3 Applications in Clinical Trial Design, Patient Selection, and Monitoring

Clinical trials are the bridge between lab research and real-world treatments, yet they're often plagued by inefficiencies. AI steps in to reshape this process, making it faster and more targeted. One of the key areas where AI shines is in patient selection. The right patients make or break a trial. AI analyzes medical histories, genetic profiles, and even lifestyle data to identify participants who are most likely to respond well to the experimental drug. It's like curating a guest list for an exclusive event, ensuring only those who fit the criteria are invited.

In designing the trial itself, AI helps determine the optimal dosage, timing, and endpoints. By analyzing data from previous studies, the system suggests parameters that maximize the chances of success. For example, in trials for new cancer immunotherapies, AI can predict which biomarkers should be tracked to gauge the treatment's effectiveness. This level of precision reduces uncertainty, guiding researchers toward more meaningful results.

During the trial, AI continuously monitors patient data. It's not just about collecting numbers—it's about interpreting them in real time. If a participant's biomarkers start showing unexpected changes, the system flags it. This early warning allows for quick adjustments, either in the treatment plan or in patient care. The dynamic nature of AI-driven monitoring keeps the trial on track, minimizing risks and improving safety. It's a proactive approach, turning clinical trials into adaptive, responsive experiments rather than rigid tests.

7.4 Case Studies of AI in Developing Immunotherapies and Vaccines

Real-world examples showcase the transformative impact of AI in immunotherapy and vaccine development. One striking case comes from the development of a new cancer immunotherapy. Researchers used AI to analyze patient tumor data, identifying specific immune cells involved in attacking the cancer. The AI model suggested a combination of checkpoint inhibitors that had a high likelihood of success based on the tumor's genetic makeup. In clinical trials, this personalized approach led to a significant increase in response rates, demonstrating the power of AI in guiding immunotherapy decisions.

Another compelling example is the rapid development of COVID-19 vaccines. During the early stages of the pandemic, AI models analyzed viral genetic sequences, predicting which components would elicit the strongest immune response (Floresta et al., 2022). These predictions guided the selection of spike protein targets, speeding up vaccine design. AI also played a role in tracking virus mutations, helping researchers adapt vaccine formulas as new variants emerged. This adaptive strategy would have been nearly impossible with traditional methods alone.

In autoimmune disease research, AI-driven drug discovery led to the identification of a novel therapy for lupus (Fleming, 2018). By integrating patient genetic data with immune response profiles, the AI model pinpointed a new drug target—an inflammatory pathway previously overlooked. The resulting therapy showed promising results in early trials, offering hope for patients with limited treatment options. These case studies highlight AI's role not just as a tool but as a collaborative partner in cutting-edge medical research.

7.5 AI Models for Simulating Immune Responses and Predicting Therapeutic Outcomes

Simulating immune responses is like playing a high-stakes game of chess—each move can trigger a cascade of reactions. AI models take on this challenge, using vast amounts of data to create virtual simulations of how the immune system might respond to a treatment. These models incorporate variables like genetic makeup, immune cell interactions, and even environmental factors, painting a comprehensive picture of the body's defense mechanisms.

In vaccine research, AI simulations predict how different formulations might perform in diverse populations. It's not a one-size-fits-all scenario. A vaccine that works well in one group might be less effective in another due to genetic differences or variations in immune history. By running these virtual trials, AI helps researchers fine-tune the vaccine before it reaches human testing. It's like conducting a dress rehearsal to ensure everything runs smoothly on opening night.

For autoimmune diseases, simulating immune responses helps in understanding the root causes of immune attacks. AI models map out the entire sequence of events—from the initial trigger, like a viral infection, to the subsequent misfiring of immune cells. This deep understanding allows for more targeted therapies, designed to interrupt the process at key points. Predicting therapeutic outcomes isn't about making guesses—it's about using data to make informed, strategic decisions. AI provides a window into the future of treatment effects, helping doctors and researchers choose the best path forward.

8. ETHICAL AND REGULATORY CONSIDERATIONS IN AI-DRIVEN IMMUNOLOGY

8.1 Data Privacy Concerns in Managing High-Dimensional Patient Data

Handling patient data feels like walking a tightrope—one misstep, and the consequences are severe. In AI-driven immunology, the datasets are enormous, often containing sensitive information from genomics, proteomics, and clinical records. Each entry offers a glimpse into a person's biological identity. When merged, these data points create a comprehensive profile, making privacy a significant concern. Protecting this information is like guarding a treasure chest filled with the most personal details of a patient's health. Any breach could expose genetic vulnerabilities or undisclosed medical conditions, putting individuals at risk of discrimination.

AI systems require access to this vast array of data for accurate predictions and analyses. Yet, sharing such high-dimensional information poses challenges. Anonymization helps, but it isn't foolproof. Complex algorithms might still trace data back to an individual, especially when combined with other datasets. This risk calls for robust encryption methods, secure storage solutions, and strict access controls. Patients need assurance that their data is safe. Trust is the cornerstone here. If people fear their genetic information could be misused or leaked, the entire promise of personalized medicine could crumble. Balancing the need for comprehensive data with stringent privacy safeguards is crucial for the future of AI in immunology.

8.2 Ethical Challenges in Using AI for Clinical Decision-Making in Immunology

AI in clinical decision-making feels like adding a new player to the team—a smart, tireless assistant. But it comes with its own set of ethical dilemmas. Physicians rely on their experience and intuition, shaped by years of practice, while AI offers data-driven insights. Integrating these two approaches can lead to conflicts. What happens if the AI suggests a treatment that contradicts the doctor's judgment? The tension between human expertise and machine recommendations creates an ethical gray area.

In immunology, decisions often impact patients with chronic and severe conditions. Mistakes are costly, and trust is delicate. Relying solely on AI may seem tempting due to its analytical prowess, yet doing so risks undermining the doctor-patient relationship. Ethical use of AI means recognizing its limitations, acknowledging that algorithms can miss nuances only a human can perceive. It's about finding a balance where AI aids decision-making without becoming the sole authority. Ensuring the patient's voice remains central is key. Involving them in discussions about AI-generated recommendations fosters transparency and respects their autonomy, making them active participants in their own care.

8.3 Addressing Biases and Fairness in AI Models to Ensure Equitable Outcomes

Bias in AI models is like a hidden trap—one that can skew results and deepen disparities in healthcare. When training data lacks diversity, the models tend to reflect and reinforce existing biases. In immunology, this can be particularly harmful. Immune responses vary across different populations, influenced by genetics, environment, and lifestyle. If an AI model is built on data that mostly represents one group, it might fail to make accurate predictions for others. It's like designing a one-size-fits-all garment that ends up fitting only a small portion of the population.

Addressing this issue requires deliberate action. Diverse datasets are the first step, ensuring that the AI learns from a broad spectrum of patients. Beyond that, fairness metrics must be integrated into the model evaluation process. These metrics act like quality checks, highlighting when the AI's predictions disproportionately favor or disadvantage certain groups. Regular audits and updates are necessary, too, as models can drift over time, inadvertently amplifying biases. Creating equitable AI isn't just a technical challenge—it's an ethical imperative. The goal is to develop tools that serve all patients fairly, regardless of their background, ensuring that everyone benefits from advances in personalized medicine.

8.4 Regulatory Requirements for AI-Based CDSS and Precision Medicine Applications

Navigating the regulatory landscape for AI in healthcare feels like charting a new course through uncharted waters. Clinical Decision Support Systems (CDSS) powered by AI, along with precision medicine applications, must meet stringent standards to gain approval (Taherdoost & Ghofrani, 2024). Regulatory bodies like the FDA in the United States or the EMA in Europe demand rigorous validation. These systems aren't just tools—they influence life-and-death decisions. Ensuring they work as intended is non-negotiable. The validation process involves extensive testing, including clinical trials that prove the AI's accuracy and reliability.

Meeting these requirements often means striking a balance between innovation and caution. Developers must provide clear documentation, detailing how the AI model was trained, what data was used, and how decisions are made. It's like writing a detailed blueprint for a complex machine—every part must be accounted for. Regulatory frameworks also require ongoing monitoring after the AI is deployed, ensuring it continues to perform well in real-world settings. This post-market surveillance acts as a safety net, catching issues that might only appear outside controlled environments. Rigorous regulation isn't a barrier—it's a safeguard, ensuring that these powerful tools enhance patient care without compromising safety.

8.5 The Importance of Transparency, Explainability, and Trust in AI Models for Clinical Use

Trust is the bedrock of clinical practice, and AI must earn it. For doctors to rely on AI recommendations, they need to understand how the model reached its conclusions. Explainability is key here. It's like having a transparent window into the AI's decision-making process. Instead of presenting a black box result, the model should provide clear reasons for its suggestions—whether it's highlighting a specific biomarker or noting patterns in patient data. This transparency helps clinicians feel confident integrating AI insights into their care plans.

Patients, too, deserve to know how AI is influencing their treatment. When an AI-driven system recommends a particular therapy, it should be able to explain why. This isn't just about building trust—it's about respecting patient autonomy. People have the right to understand the tools shaping their healthcare. Explainable AI acts like a bridge, connecting advanced technology with human understanding. By making its inner workings visible, the model becomes less of a mysterious gadget and more of a trusted partner. Trust, once established, forms a strong foundation for the widespread adoption of AI in clinical practice.

8.6 Role of Interdisciplinary Collaboration in Setting Ethical Standards

Creating ethical AI for immunology requires a team effort—no single discipline can do it alone. It's like constructing a bridge, with each expert providing a vital piece of the structure. Computer scientists bring the technical expertise, designing algorithms that process complex biological data. Clinicians contribute their practical experience, highlighting the nuances of patient care that data alone can't capture. Ethicists ensure that the development process aligns with principles of fairness, transparency, and respect for patient autonomy.

Regulators play a crucial role too, providing the framework that guides the ethical use of AI. Together, this interdisciplinary team tackles the big questions: How do we ensure that AI decisions are unbiased? How do we protect patient data while allowing for meaningful analysis? It's a continuous dialogue, not a one-time discussion. The landscape of AI in healthcare evolves rapidly, and so must the ethical guidelines that govern it.

Collaboration also fosters innovation. By pooling knowledge from different fields, the team can anticipate challenges and create solutions that a single discipline might overlook. It's a holistic approach, one that recognizes the complexity of healthcare and the diversity of patient needs. Setting ethical standards isn't about limiting progress—it's about guiding it in a way that benefits everyone, ensuring AI becomes a tool that enhances care without compromising values.

8.7 Patient and Clinician Perspectives on AI in Immunology

8.7.1 Patient Perspectives

Patients express significant concerns regarding data privacy, consent, and the unauthorized access to their health information when artificial intelligence (AI) systems are employed in healthcare. A study by Blease et al. (2023) highlighted that many patients are often unaware of how their data is utilized in AI applications, leading to apprehensions about potential misuse.

Furthermore, the notion of AI making autonomous decisions without human oversight contributes to patient anxiety. Longoni et al. (2022) found that patients are more comfortable with AI applications that operate under human supervision, as this alleviates fears of machines making independent medical decisions.

Trust in automated recommendations remains a critical issue. Patients often question the transparency of AI systems, fearing that opaque algorithms might lead to errors in diagnosis or treatment. A study by Jauk et al. (2023) revealed that patients prefer AI systems whose decision-making processes are transparent and understandable.

Clear communication and explainability of AI-driven decisions are paramount for patient acceptance. Patients expect healthcare providers to elucidate how AI contributes to their care, which enhances trust and compliance. Research by Blease et al. (2023) emphasizes the necessity for clinicians to effectively communicate the role of AI in treatment plans.

Patients also express a desire for personalized care, fearing that AI might promote a one-size-fits-all approach. They value individualized treatment plans and are concerned that AI could overlook personal nuances. Longoni et al. (2022) noted that patients are apprehensive about AI potentially depersonalizing healthcare services.

Balancing the perceived benefits and risks of AI in healthcare is crucial. While patients acknowledge advantages such as faster diagnoses and reduced hospital visits, they remain wary of potential drawbacks, including loss of control over personal health information and data misuse. Jauk et al. (2023) reported that patients weigh these benefits against the risks when considering AI integration into their care.

8.7.2 Clinician Perspectives

Clinicians emphasize the importance of usability in AI tools, focusing on interface design, workflow integration, and time efficiency. A study by Oh et al. (2022) highlighted that user-friendly interfaces and seamless integration into existing workflows are critical for clinician adoption of AI technologies.

There is a prevailing view among clinicians that AI should serve as a supportive tool rather than a replacement for clinical judgment. They perceive AI as an adjunct to enhance decision-making, not as a substitute for their expertise. Oh et al. (2022) found that clinicians are cautious about AI encroaching upon their professional roles.

Concerns about the reliability of AI systems persist, particularly regarding the potential for false positives and negatives in AI predictions. Clinicians are wary of over-reliance on AI, which could lead to diagnostic errors. A study by Wysocki et al. (2022) emphasized the need for rigorous validation of AI tools to ensure their reliability in clinical settings.

Responsibility and liability issues arise when AI provides incorrect advice. Clinicians question who is accountable for errors stemming from AI recommendations. Weiner et al. (2024) discussed the ethical challenges and evolving strategies in integrating AI into clinical practice, highlighting concerns about accountability.

Training needs are evident, as clinicians seek to enhance their comfort level with using AI tools in everyday practice. They recognize the necessity for education and training to effectively incorporate AI into patient care. Harris and Wong (2020) underscored the role of education in integrating AI into clinical practice, noting that adequate training is essential for successful adoption.

Clinicians exhibit openness to AI when systems provide transparent reasoning and real-time feedback. They are more likely to trust and adopt AI tools that offer clear explanations for their recommendations. Wysocki et al. (2022) found that explainability enhances clinicians' trust in AI-driven clinical decision-making.

8.7.3 Aligning Perspectives for Better Adoption

Co-designing AI systems by involving both patients and clinicians in development processes is crucial for better adoption. This collaborative approach ensures that AI tools meet the needs and expectations of end-users. Nguyen and Brown (2023) demonstrated that co-designing AI tools with clinicians enhances usability in healthcare settings.

Implementing continuous feedback loops between users and developers is vital for refining AI systems. Regular input from patients and clinicians allows for iterative improvements, leading to more effective and trusted AI applications. Wysocki et al. (2022) highlighted the importance of assessing the communication gap between AI models and healthcare professionals to enhance trust in AI-driven clinical decision-making (Fan et al., 2020).

Building mutual trust requires transparency, education, and inclusion in AI governance. Educating users about AI functionalities and involving them in governance fosters trust and acceptance. Weiner et al. (2024) emphasized that addressing ethical challenges and involving stakeholders in AI integration strategies are essential for responsible AI implementation in healthcare.

9. CHALLENGES AND LIMITATIONS OF AI IN IMMUNOLOGY

9.1 Technical Limitations in Data Processing, Model Training, and Algorithmic Bias

AI in immunology faces several technical barriers. The first challenge is handling vast amounts of high-dimensional data from sources like genomics, transcriptomics, and proteomics. These datasets are enormous, often containing millions of variables, making it hard to process efficiently. Even with advanced computational resources, training models on such complex data requires significant time and energy, often stretching the limits of current technology. In addition, many AI models are susceptible to algorithmic bias. This bias creeps in during the training phase, when the model learns from datasets that do not fully represent the diversity of the population. For instance, if an AI model is trained predominantly on data from one ethnic group, it might fail to make accurate predictions for individuals from other groups. Such biases can lead to skewed results, reducing the reliability of AI applications in immunology, particularly when dealing with diverse patient groups.

9.2 Issues with Data Quality, Labeling, and Generalization Across Populations

High-quality data is the backbone of reliable AI models. In immunology, obtaining clean, well-annotated data is a persistent issue. Often, datasets are noisy, incomplete, or incorrectly labeled, leading to errors during model training. For example, mislabeled cell types in single-cell RNA sequencing data can significantly affect the accuracy of downstream analyses. Beyond labeling, generalization poses another challenge. AI models trained on specific datasets may struggle to perform well when applied to new data from different populations or environments. For instance, a model trained on data from a European cohort may not generalize well to patients in Asia due to genetic and environmental differences. This lack of generalizability can hinder the application of AI in global healthcare, limiting its effectiveness across diverse patient groups.

9.3 Limitations in Current AI Models for Accurately Predicting Immune Responses

Current AI models, while impressive, often fall short in predicting complex immune responses accurately. The immune system is highly dynamic, involving numerous interacting components, such as cells, proteins, and signaling pathways. AI models struggle to capture this complexity because they typically rely on static datasets that may not reflect the evolving nature of immune responses. For instance, predicting how a patient's immune system will react to a novel pathogen or vaccine is challenging, as it requires understanding intricate cellular interactions that are not fully captured in existing data. Moreover, most AI models are black boxes, offering limited interpretability. Clinicians are often hesitant to trust predictions when they cannot understand the underlying decision-making process, further limiting the adoption of AI in clinical immunology.

9.4 Challenges in Translating Research Models to Clinical Applications

Transitioning AI models from research settings to clinical environments is a significant hurdle. In research, AI models are often developed and validated on carefully curated datasets. However, real-world clinical data is messier, with inconsistencies, missing values, and varying formats. Models trained on clean research data may falter when exposed to the unpredictable nature of clinical datasets (Yu et al., 2019). Additionally, integrating AI models into existing healthcare workflows requires robust infrastructure, regulatory approvals, and clinician training. Many healthcare facilities lack the necessary resources and expertise to implement AI solutions effectively. Furthermore, the regulatory landscape for AI in healthcare is still evolving (Yu et al., 2018). Models must meet stringent standards for safety, efficacy, and privacy, which can delay their deployment in clinical settings.

9.5 Balancing AI-Driven Insights with Clinician Expertise and Judgment

One of the core challenges in using AI in immunology is striking the right balance between AI-generated insights and clinician expertise. AI can process vast datasets and identify patterns that may not be apparent to human experts. Yet, the context and experience of clinicians remain crucial. For instance, an AI model might suggest a specific treatment plan based on data patterns, but a clinician might reject it due to unique patient factors or contextual knowledge not captured in the data. Over-reliance on AI can lead to a loss of human oversight, while disregarding AI insights can mean missing valuable data-driven recommendations. Thus, fostering a collaborative approach where AI tools augment rather than replace human expertise is essential for successful integration in immunology.

10. FUTURE DIRECTIONS AND EMERGING TRENDS IN AI FOR IMMUNOLOGY

10.1 Emerging AI Technologies and Their Potential Impact on Immunological Research

AI technologies are evolving at lightning speed, transforming the landscape of immunology. New advancements in machine learning and deep learning are enhancing our ability to understand complex immune systems. These technologies operate like powerful lenses, bringing clarity to intricate immune processes. Machine learning excels at detecting patterns in large datasets, uncovering relationships that were previously hidden. Deep learning goes even deeper, mimicking the neural networks of the brain to analyze multi-layered data, such as genomics and single-cell RNA sequencing (Esteva et al., 2019). This kind of analysis offers insights into how specific genes influence immune responses, leading to better-targeted therapies.

Federated learning introduces a new way to handle sensitive patient data without compromising privacy. It allows multiple healthcare institutions to collaborate on AI models without sharing raw data. Imagine a team of researchers working together on a puzzle, but each only sees their own piece. The full picture comes together without anyone having to reveal their individual piece. This method strengthens data privacy while still enabling robust AI training. These emerging technologies are not just incremental steps forward—they are revolutionary, reshaping how we approach immunological research and paving the way for breakthroughs that were once beyond reach.

10.2 Prospects of Integrating AI with Real-World Clinical Practices for Sustainable Healthcare

Bringing AI into real-world clinical settings feels like bridging two worlds—one of cutting-edge technology and one of hands-on patient care. AI has immense potential to streamline workflows, enhance diagnostics, and offer personalized treatment plans. Imagine a scenario where an AI system assists doctors during consultations, instantly analyzing patient data, lab results, and medical histories to provide tailored recommendations. It's like having a knowledgeable assistant that never tires, always ready to offer insights.

Sustainable healthcare requires efficient use of resources, and AI can help achieve this. By predicting disease outbreaks or patient surges, AI systems can optimize staffing, supply chains, and treatment protocols. Hospitals in densely populated areas or regions with limited medical infrastructure can benefit greatly from these predictive capabilities. AI doesn't just assist in treatment—it also aids in prevention, identifying patients at risk of chronic diseases and suggesting early interventions. This proactive approach can reduce hospital admissions, lower healthcare costs, and lead to better outcomes overall. The integration of AI into clinical practice isn't a distant dream; it's already taking shape, promising a more efficient, responsive, and patient-centered healthcare system.

10.3 Potential for AI to Uncover Novel Therapeutic Targets and Biomarkers

Discovering new therapeutic targets and biomarkers often feels like searching for a needle in a haystack. The immune system is vast and complex, with countless interactions happening at any given moment. AI changes the game by analyzing data from multiple sources—genomics, proteomics, and clinical studies—to find patterns that hint at new targets. These insights are like uncovering hidden clues that lead researchers down new paths of exploration.

For instance, in autoimmune diseases, AI has identified unexpected molecular pathways that play a critical role in triggering immune attacks. By highlighting these pathways, AI points researchers toward new drug targets, offering hope for therapies that address the root cause of disease rather than just the symptoms. In cancer immunology, AI models have discovered novel biomarkers that predict which patients are likely to respond well to specific treatments. These biomarkers act like signposts, guiding doctors in selecting the most effective therapies for each patient. The potential here is enormous. AI isn't just speeding up the research process—it's expanding the horizon, making discoveries that might have been overlooked without its analytical power.

10.4 Expansion of AI-Assisted Immunology Applications to Underserved and Remote Populations

AI holds the promise of bringing advanced healthcare to regions that have historically been left behind. Rural areas and underserved communities often struggle with limited access to specialists, making it hard to diagnose and manage complex immune conditions. AI-assisted tools, accessible via smartphones or low-cost devices, can bridge this gap. Imagine a rural clinic equipped with an AI diagnostic system that scans patient data for early signs of autoimmune disease. The technology analyzes symptoms, compares them against vast databases, and offers a preliminary diagnosis, guiding local healthcare providers.

Telemedicine, powered by AI, can also extend the reach of immunology experts. Patients in remote areas can upload their data, including lab results and genetic information, to cloud-based AI systems. The AI offers analysis, which is then reviewed by a specialist who provides guidance remotely. It's like bringing the expertise of a top-tier medical center to the patient's doorstep. This expansion of AI applications democratizes access to quality healthcare, ensuring that even those in the most isolated areas benefit from the latest advances in immunology.

10.5 Prospects for Advancing Precision Medicine with Improved Data Integration and Real-Time Analytics

Precision medicine thrives on detailed, integrated data. AI takes this concept to the next level by seamlessly merging diverse data streams—genomics, electronic health records, lifestyle factors—into a unified analysis (Primorac et al., 2020). This integration is like assembling a mosaic, where each tile represents a piece of the patient's health story. AI doesn't just see individual pieces; it visualizes the entire picture, offering insights that can drive personalized treatment plans.

Real-time analytics bring an added dimension. Instead of analyzing static datasets, AI systems process incoming data continuously, adjusting predictions and recommendations as new information becomes available. This dynamic approach is especially useful in managing conditions like asthma or severe allergies, where symptoms can change rapidly. If a patient's immune markers start to spike, the AI system can alert the healthcare provider immediately, suggesting timely interventions. The prospect of real-time, integrated analysis transforms precision medicine from a reactive approach to a proactive one, where treatments adapt to the patient's current needs rather than relying solely on past data.

10.6 Vision for AI in Building More Resilient, Adaptable Healthcare Systems in Immunology

The future of healthcare, especially in immunology, demands systems that can adapt quickly to new challenges. AI offers a vision of a resilient, responsive healthcare model that can withstand sudden changes, like pandemics or unexpected outbreaks of immune-related diseases. AI systems can analyze global health data in real time, identifying emerging threats before they become widespread crises. It's like having a vigilant sentinel, constantly scanning the horizon for potential dangers.

In day-to-day operations, AI enhances the flexibility of healthcare delivery. By optimizing resource allocation, predicting patient surges, and automating routine tasks, AI frees up medical staff to focus on more critical aspects of care. This adaptability is crucial in immunology, where patient responses can be unpredictable. Whether it's adjusting treatment protocols based on the latest research or scaling up care during an epidemic, AI-powered systems provide the backbone for a healthcare model that can evolve in real time. It's not just about handling today's challenges—it's about preparing for tomorrow's unknowns, building a healthcare system that can pivot and thrive no matter what comes its way.

11. CONCLUSION

11.1 Summary of AI's Transformative Role in Immunology

AI has rewritten the playbook in immunology. It's like introducing a new, highly skilled player into a well-worn game, shaking up old strategies and offering a fresh perspective. Traditional methods struggled to capture the intricate details of the immune system, often relying on generalized approaches. AI has changed this by diving deep into data—analyzing genomics, proteomics, and clinical records all at once. Machine learning and deep learning models identify patterns that human eyes might miss. This shift has turned reactive healthcare into a proactive, predictive practice. Diseases are spotted earlier, treatments tailored more precisely, and patient care optimized on an unprecedented scale. AI's role isn't merely supportive; it's transformative, reshaping how we diagnose, treat, and understand immune-related diseases. This new era of immunology promises more personalized, efficient, and effective solutions, fundamentally altering the landscape of medical science.

11.2 Key Insights into the Potential of AI to Improve Decision Support, Diagnostics, and Patient Outcomes

AI has emerged as a vital tool in decision support systems, acting like a digital advisor with a wealth of experience. In clinical settings, AI provides real-time recommendations by analyzing patient data against vast databases of medical histories and research findings. This capability helps doctors make informed choices quickly, especially in complex cases like autoimmune disorders or cancer immunotherapy. Diagnostics have also improved dramatically. AI-driven models process complex biological data, pinpointing subtle markers that indicate early stages of disease. It's like having a highly trained sniffer dog that detects hidden dangers long before they become visible. By catching diseases early, AI-driven diagnostics pave the way for timely interventions, which directly enhance patient outcomes. Personalized medicine benefits as well, with AI suggesting tailored treatments based on individual immune profiles. The result? Higher success rates, fewer adverse effects, and a more patient-centered approach. These advancements demonstrate AI's vast potential to enhance every stage of patient care, from diagnosis to treatment planning (Rezaei et al., 2023).

11.3 Reflections on Ethical, Regulatory, and Collaborative Considerations for Future Advancements

AI's integration into immunology isn't without its challenges. The journey feels like navigating a winding road, where ethical and regulatory hurdles pop up unexpectedly. Privacy concerns loom large as AI systems require access to sensitive patient data, including genetic information. Ensuring that this data is handled with care is crucial. Ethical dilemmas also arise when AI-generated recommendations differ from a physician's judgment. Striking a balance between trusting the algorithm and valuing human expertise is a delicate task. Regulatory bodies play a key role here, setting standards that ensure

AI models are safe, transparent, and reliable. Yet, creating these regulations isn't straightforward. The technology evolves faster than the rules can keep up, demanding ongoing adjustments.

Collaboration is the linchpin for future success. Bringing together computer scientists, clinicians, ethicists, and regulators forms a robust foundation for responsible innovation. This interdisciplinary approach encourages a holistic view, where each perspective contributes to the ethical use of AI in healthcare. It's a collective effort, aimed at harnessing AI's full potential while safeguarding patient rights and well-being. The path forward isn't simple, but it's promising. With careful planning and a collaborative spirit, AI can continue to revolutionize immunology, setting a new standard for patient care and medical research.

REFERENCES

Abbas, M. K. G., Rassam, A., Karamshahi, F., Abunora, R., & Abouseada, M. (2024). The role of AI in drug discovery. *ChemBioChem*, *25*(14), e202300816. Advance online publication. DOI: 10.1002/cbic.202300816 PMID: 38735845

Ahuja, A. S. (2019). The impact of artificial intelligence in medicine on the future role of the physician. *PeerJ*, *7*, e7702. DOI: 10.7717/peerj.7702 PMID: 31592346

Aliper, A., Plis, S., Artemov, A., Ulloa, A., Mamoshina, P., & Zhavoronkov, A. (2016). Deep learning applications for predicting pharmacological properties of drugs and drug repurposing using transcriptomic data. *Molecular Pharmaceutics*, *13*(7), 2524–2530. DOI: 10.1021/acs.molpharmaceut.6b00248 PMID: 27200455

Alsharif, F. (2024). Artificial intelligence in oncology: Applications, challenges and future frontiers. *International Journal of Pharmaceutical Investigation*, *14*(3), 647–656. DOI: 10.5530/ijpi.14.3.76

Banks, G. (1986). Artificial intelligence in medical diagnosis: The INTERNIST/CADUCEUS approach. *Critical Reviews in Medical Informatics*, *1*(1), 23–54. PMID: 3331578

Beam, A. L., & Kohane, I. S. (2018). Big data and machine learning in health care. *Journal of the American Medical Association*, *319*(13), 1317–1318. DOI: 10.1001/jama.2017.18391 PMID: 29532063

Blease, C., Kaptchuk, T. J., Bernstein, M. H., & Mandl, K. D. (2023). Artificial intelligence and informed consent: A scoping review. *BMJ Health & Care Informatics*, *30*(1), e100647. DOI: 10.1136/bmjhci-2023-100647

Chen, R., & Snyder, M. (2013). Promise of personalized omics to precision medicine. *Wiley Interdisciplinary Reviews. Systems Biology and Medicine*, *5*(1), 73–82. DOI: 10.1002/wsbm.1198 PMID: 23184638

Chen, X. (2024). Analyses and concerns in precision medicine: A statistical perspective. arXiv preprint arXiv:2401.06899. https://doi.org//arXiv.2401.06899DOI: 10.48550

Ching, T., Himmelstein, D. S., Beaulieu-Jones, B. K., Kalinin, A. A., Do, B. T., Way, G. P., & Greene, C. S. (2018). Opportunities and obstacles for deep learning in biology and medicine. Journal of the Royal Society Interface, 15(2017), 0387. DOI: 10.1098/rsif.2017.0387

Deo, R. C. (2015). Machine learning in medicine. *Circulation*, *132*(20), 1920–1930. DOI: 10.1161/CIRCULATIONAHA.115.001593 PMID: 26572668

Ekins, S., Puhl, A. C., Zorn, K. M., Lane, T. R., Russo, D. P., Klein, J. J., & Siqueira-Neto, J. L. (2019). Exploring deep learning applications for predicting pharmacological properties of drugs. *Journal of Chemical Information and Modeling*, *59*(8), 3347–3356. DOI: 10.1021/acs.jcim.9b00348

Esteva, A., Chou, K., Yeung, S., Naik, N., Madani, A., Mottaghi, A., Liu, Y., Topol, E., Dean, J., & Socher, R. (2021). Deep learning-enabled medical computer vision. npj. *Digital Medicine*, *4*(1), 5. DOI: 10.1038/s41746-020-00376-2 PMID: 33420381

Esteva, A., Robicquet, A., Ramsundar, B., Kuleshov, V., DePristo, M., Chou, K., Cui, C., Corrado, G., Thrun, S., & Dean, J. (2019). A guide to deep learning in healthcare. *Nature Medicine*, *25*(1), 24–29. DOI: 10.1038/s41591-018-0316-z PMID: 30617335

Fan, W., Liu, J., Zhu, S., & Pardalos, P. M. (2020). Investigating the impacting factors for healthcare professionals to adopt artificial intelligence-based medical diagnosis support systems (AIMDSS). *Annals of Operations Research*, *294*(1), 567–592. DOI: 10.1007/s10479-018-2818-y

Fatima, G., Allami, R. H., & Yousif, M. G. (2023). Integrative AI-driven strategies for advancing precision medicine in infectious diseases and beyond: A novel multidisciplinary approach. arXiv preprint arXiv:2307.15228. https://doi.org//arXiv.2307.15228DOI: 10.48550

Fleming, N. (2018). How artificial intelligence is changing drug discovery. *Nature*, *557*(7706), S55–S57. DOI: 10.1038/d41586-018-05267-x PMID: 29849160

Floresta, G., Zagni, C., Gentile, D., Patamia, V., & Rescifina, A. (2022). Artificial intelligence technologies for COVID-19 de novo drug design. *International Journal of Molecular Sciences*, *23*(6), 3261. DOI: 10.3390/ijms23063261 PMID: 35328682

Ghassemi, M., Naumann, T., Schulam, P., Beam, A. L., Chen, I. Y., & Ranganath, R. (2020). A review of challenges and opportunities in machine learning for health. *AMIA Joint Summits on Translational Science Proceedings AMIA Summit on Translational Science*, *2020*, 191–200. PMID: 32477638

Ghebrehiwet, I., Zaki, N., Damseh, R., & Mohamad, M. S. (2024). Revolutionizing personalized medicine with generative AI: A systematic review. *Artificial Intelligence Review*, *57*(5), 128. Advance online publication. DOI: 10.1007/s10462-024-10768-5

Gómez-González, E. (2020). *Artificial intelligence in medicine and healthcare: Applications, availability, and societal impact. EUR 30197 EN*. Publications Office of the European Union., DOI: 10.2760/047666

Harris, P., & Wong, J. (2020). The role of education in integrating AI into clinical practice. *Medical Education*, *54*(11), 993–1001. DOI: 10.1111/medu.14210 PMID: 32350873

Jiang, F., Jiang, Y., Zhi, H., Dong, Y., Li, H., Ma, S., Wang, Y., Dong, Q., Shen, H., & Wang, Y. (2017). Artificial intelligence in healthcare: Past, present, and future. *Stroke and Vascular Neurology*, *2*(2), 59–67. DOI: 10.1136/svn-2017-000101 PMID: 29507784

Kalinin, A. A., Higgins, G. A., Reamaroon, N., Soroushmehr, S., Allyn-Feuer, A., Dinov, I. D., & Athey, B. D. (2018). Deep learning in pharmacogenomics: From gene regulation to patient stratification. *Pharmacogenomics*, *19*(7), 629–650.

Katsnelson, A. (2024). A drug to call one's own. Scientific American. https://www.scientificamerican.com/article/a-drug-to-call-ones-own/

Kourou, K., Exarchos, T. P., Exarchos, K. P., Karamouzis, M. V., & Fotiadis, D. I. (2015). Machine learning applications in cancer prognosis and prediction. *Computational and Structural Biotechnology Journal*, *13*, 8–17. DOI: 10.1016/j.csbj.2014.11.005 PMID: 25750696

Krittanawong, C., Johnson, K. W., Rosenson, R. S., Wang, Z., Aydar, M., Baber, U., Min, J. K., Tang, W. H. W., Halperin, J. L., & Narayan, S. M. (2019). Deep learning for cardiovascular medicine: A practical primer. *European Heart Journal, 40*(25), 2058–2073. DOI: 10.1093/eurheartj/ehz056 PMID: 30815669

Longoni, C., Bonezzi, A., & Morewedge, C. K. (2019). Resistance to medical artificial intelligence. *The Journal of Consumer Research, 46*(4), 629–650. DOI: 10.1093/jcr/ucz013

Moy, S., Irannejad, M., Manning, S. J., Farahani, M., Ahmed, Y., Gao, E., & Klinger, C. (2024). Patient perspectives on the use of artificial intelligence in health care: A scoping review. *Journal of Patient-Centered Research and Reviews, 11*(1), 51.

Nguyen, T., & Brown, M. (2023). Co-designing AI tools with clinicians: Enhancing usability in healthcare settings. *International Journal of Medical Informatics, 165*, 104112. DOI: 10.1016/j.ijmedinf.2022.104112

Obermeyer, Z., & Emanuel, E. J. (2016). Predicting the future: Big data, machine learning, and clinical medicine. *The New England Journal of Medicine, 375*(13), 1216–1219. DOI: 10.1056/NEJMp1606181 PMID: 27682033

Oh, S., Kim, J. H., Choi, S. W., Lee, H. J., Hong, J., & Kwon, S. H. (2022). Physician confidence in artificial intelligence in healthcare: An online mobile survey. *Journal of Medical Internet Research, 24*(1), e30379. DOI: 10.2196/30379 PMID: 34994706

Park, S. H., Han, K., Jang, H. Y., Park, J. E., Lee, J. G., Kim, D. W., & Choi, J. (2023). Methods for clinical evaluation of artificial intelligence algorithms for medical diagnosis. *Radiology, 306*(1), 20–31. DOI: 10.1148/radiol.220182 PMID: 36346314

Paul, R., Hossain, A., Islam, M. T., Melon, M. M. H., & Hussen, M. (2024). Integrating genomic data with AI algorithms to optimize personalized drug therapy: A pilot study. *Library Progress International, 44*(3), 21849–21870.

Peng, J., Jury, E. C., Dönnes, P., & Ciurtin, C. (2021). Machine learning techniques for personalised medicine approaches in immune-mediated chronic inflammatory diseases: Applications and challenges. *Frontiers in Pharmacology, 12*, 720694. Advance online publication. DOI: 10.3389/fphar.2021.720694 PMID: 34658859

Pinto-Coelho, L. (2023). How artificial intelligence is shaping medical imaging technology: A survey of innovations and applications. *Bioengineering (Basel, Switzerland), 10*(12), 1435. DOI: 10.3390/bioengineering10121435 PMID: 38136026

Primorac, D., Bach-Rojecky, L., Vađunec, D., Juginović, A., Žunić, K., Matišić, V., & Donaldson, M. (2020). Pharmacogenomics at the center of precision medicine: Challenges and perspective in an era of big data. *Pharmacogenomics, 21*(2), 141–156. DOI: 10.2217/pgs-2019-0134 PMID: 31950879

Rajkomar, A., Dean, J., & Kohane, I. (2019). Machine learning in medicine. *The New England Journal of Medicine, 380*(14), 1347–1358. DOI: 10.1056/NEJMra1814259 PMID: 30943338

Rezaei, M., Rahmani, E., Khouzani, S. J., Rahmannia, M., Ghadirzadeh, E., Bashghareh, P., & Taheri, F. (2023). Role of artificial intelligence in the diagnosis and treatment of diseases. *Kindle, 3*(1), 1–160.

Shah, P., Kendall, F., & Khozin, S. (2019). Artificial intelligence in clinical development: Translational perspectives. npj. *Digital Medicine*, *2*(1), 69. DOI: 10.1038/s41746-019-0148-3 PMID: 31372505

Snyder, M., & Chen, R. (2013). Promise of personalized omics to precision medicine. *Wiley Interdisciplinary Reviews. Systems Biology and Medicine*, *5*(1), 73–82. DOI: 10.1002/wsbm.1198 PMID: 23184638

Taherdoost, H., & Ghofrani, A. (2024). *AI and the evolution of personalized medicine in pharmacogenomics*. Intelligent Pharmacy.

Topol, E. J. (2019). High-performance medicine: The convergence of human and artificial intelligence. *Nature Medicine*, *25*(1), 44–56. DOI: 10.1038/s41591-018-0300-7 PMID: 30617339

Warner, E., Lee, J., Hsu, W., Syeda-Mahmood, T., Kahn, C. E.Jr, Gevaert, O., & Rao, A. (2024). Multimodal machine learning in image-based and clinical biomedicine: Survey and prospects. *International Journal of Computer Vision*, *132*(9), 1–17. DOI: 10.1007/s11263-024-02032-8 PMID: 39211895

Weiner, S., Lynch, C., & Halamka, J. (2024). Integrating artificial intelligence into clinical practice: Evolving strategies and ethical challenges. arXiv preprint arXiv:2412.03576. https://arxiv.org/abs/2412.03576

Wysocki, K., McBride, J., & Ventresca, M. (2022). Assessing the communication gap between AI models and healthcare professionals. arXiv preprint arXiv:2204.05030. https://arxiv.org/abs/2204.05030

Yang, X., Huang, K., Yang, D., Zhao, W., & Zhou, X. (2024). Biomedical big data technologies, applications, and challenges for precision medicine: A review. *Global Challenges (Hoboken, NJ)*, *8*(1), 2300163. DOI: 10.1002/gch2.202300163 PMID: 38223896

Yu, K. H., Beam, A. L., & Kohane, I. S. (2018). Artificial intelligence in healthcare. *Nature Biomedical Engineering*, *2*(10), 719–731. DOI: 10.1038/s41551-018-0305-z PMID: 31015651

Yu, Y., Li, M., Liu, L., & Wang, J. (2019). Clinical big data and deep learning: Applications, challenges, and future outlooks. *Big Data Mining and Analytics*, *2*(4), 288–305. DOI: 10.26599/BDMA.2019.9020007

Zahid, A., Syeda-Mahmood, T., & Gevaert, O. (2024). Machine learning-enabled diagnostics in personalized medicine: Challenges and opportunities. *Biomedical AI Journal*, *5*(3), 112–138.

Zhang, Y., Xu, J., & Lee, D. (2023). Generative AI models in clinical prediction and personalized treatments. *Medical AI Insights*, *7*(2), 55–75.

Zou, J., Huss, M., Abid, A., Mohammadi, P., Torkamani, A., & Telenti, A. (2019). A primer on deep learning in genomics. *Nature Genetics*, *51*(1), 12–18. DOI: 10.1038/s41588-018-0295-5 PMID: 30478442

KEY TERMS AND DEFINITIONS

Algorithmic Bias: The tendency of an AI algorithm to produce systematic errors due to biases present in the training data. In immunology, addressing algorithmic bias is crucial to ensure fair and equitable healthcare recommendations.

Artificial Intelligence (AI): A branch of computer science that aims to create systems capable of performing tasks that typically require human intelligence, such as pattern recognition, decision-making, and predictive analytics. In immunology, AI is used to analyze complex datasets to identify disease mechanisms and develop personalized treatments.

Autoimmune Diseases: Conditions where the immune system mistakenly attacks the body's own tissues. AI can help identify early signs of autoimmune diseases and assist in developing targeted treatments.

Bias in AI Models: The presence of systematic errors in AI predictions due to biased training data. Addressing bias is crucial for ensuring that AI models provide equitable healthcare recommendations across diverse patient populations.

Big Data Analytics: The process of examining large and diverse datasets to uncover patterns, correlations, and insights. In the context of immunology, big data analytics helps manage high-dimensional omics data and extract valuable clinical insights.

Bioinformatics: A multidisciplinary field that combines biology, computer science, and statistics to analyze and interpret biological data. In immunology, bioinformatics tools are crucial for analyzing omics datasets and identifying immune-related biomarkers.

Biomarkers: Biological indicators, often measured in blood or tissue samples, that provide information about a disease state or response to treatment. In immunology, biomarkers help identify specific immune responses and guide personalized therapy.

Cancer Immunotherapy: A treatment method that uses the immune system to fight cancer. AI is used to analyze tumor-immune interactions and predict which patients are most likely to benefit from immunotherapy.

Clinical Data Integration: The process of combining patient data from various sources, such as electronic health records (EHRs), laboratory tests, and imaging results, to create a unified dataset for analysis. AI facilitates efficient integration, aiding in comprehensive clinical assessments.

Clinical Decision Support Systems (CDSS): AI-driven tools designed to assist healthcare professionals in making informed clinical decisions. In immunology, CDSS can analyze patient data in real time to suggest diagnostic and therapeutic options, improving patient outcomes.

Computational Biology: The use of data analysis, mathematical modeling, and computational simulations to understand biological systems. It plays a pivotal role in interpreting complex immune responses using AI-driven techniques.

Computational Drug Design: The application of computational techniques to design new therapeutic drugs. AI aids in modeling molecular interactions and predicting drug efficacy, accelerating the drug discovery process.

Cytometry: A technique used to measure the physical and chemical characteristics of cells. AI enhances the analysis of cytometry data, aiding in the identification of immune cell types and their functional states.

Data Privacy: The protection of sensitive patient data, including genetic and clinical information. In AI applications for immunology, data privacy is a major concern due to the sensitive nature of the datasets used.

Deep Learning: An advanced subset of ML that uses neural networks with multiple layers (deep networks) to model complex patterns in data. Deep learning is particularly effective in analyzing high-dimensional omics data, such as genomics and proteomics, for insights into immune system behavior.

Deep Reinforcement Learning: A type of AI where algorithms learn optimal actions through trial and error, guided by feedback. In immunology, it's used to develop adaptive treatment strategies based on evolving patient data.

Disease Biomarkers: Specific molecules, genes, or characteristics used to detect the presence or progression of a disease. AI algorithms can identify novel biomarkers for diagnosing immune-related disorders.

Electronic Health Records (EHRs): Digital versions of patients' medical histories maintained by healthcare providers. AI analyzes EHR data to predict patient outcomes, optimize treatments, and enhance clinical decision-making.

Epigenomics: The study of the complete set of epigenetic modifications on the genetic material of a cell. Epigenomic data, when analyzed with AI, help uncover how gene expression is regulated in immune cells.

Explainability: The degree to which an AI model's decision-making process can be understood by humans. Explainability is critical in clinical settings, as it helps healthcare providers trust and effectively use AI recommendations.

Explainable AI (XAI): AI models designed to provide clear and interpretable explanations for their predictions. In clinical settings, XAI helps healthcare providers understand the reasoning behind AI-driven recommendations, enhancing trust and adoption.

Federated Data Learning: A decentralized approach to machine learning where data remains at its source while models are trained collaboratively across multiple locations. This method is beneficial in immunology for training models on sensitive patient data without compromising privacy.

Federated Learning: An AI technique that allows multiple institutions to train machine learning models collaboratively without sharing raw data. This method is particularly useful for protecting patient privacy while leveraging large, diverse datasets.

Gene Editing: Techniques such as CRISPR/Cas9 that allow for precise modifications of the DNA sequence. AI guides gene editing by identifying target sites and predicting potential off-target effects.

Gene Therapy: A medical approach that involves modifying a patient's genes to treat or prevent disease. AI aids in the identification of target genes and the design of effective gene therapies.

Generative AI: A type of AI that can generate new data instances based on learned patterns from existing data. In drug discovery and immunotherapy, generative AI is used to design novel molecules and predict immune responses.

Genomics: The study of the complete set of DNA (genome) in an organism. Genomics data in immunology help identify genetic variations linked to immune system disorders and potential therapeutic targets.

High-Dimensional Data: Complex datasets with a large number of variables or features. In immunology, high-dimensional data from omics studies require AI techniques for effective analysis and interpretation.

High-Performance Computing (HPC): The use of supercomputers and parallel processing to analyze large datasets quickly. HPC is vital in processing high-throughput omics data and running complex simulations in immunological research.

High-Throughput Sequencing: A rapid DNA sequencing technology that generates large volumes of genetic data. AI algorithms are used to process and analyze high-throughput sequencing data for insights into immune system function.

Immune Profiling: The process of analyzing the components and activity of the immune system. AI-driven immune profiling helps identify specific patterns associated with diseases and tailor personalized therapies.

Immunology: The branch of biomedical science focused on the study of the immune system, its components, and its role in protecting the body from pathogens. Immunology research often leverages AI to understand immune responses and identify therapeutic targets.

Machine Learning (ML): A subset of AI that involves training algorithms on data to learn patterns and make predictions. ML is commonly used in immunology for analyzing patient data, predicting disease outcomes, and suggesting personalized treatment plans.

Multi-Modal AI: An AI approach that combines data from multiple sources (e.g., imaging, genomics, clinical data) for comprehensive analysis. This is particularly useful in immunology for integrating diverse datasets to improve diagnosis and treatment strategies.

Multi-Omics Integration: The process of combining multiple omics datasets (e.g., genomics, transcriptomics, proteomics) to provide a comprehensive view of biological processes. AI models are used to integrate these datasets for enhanced insights into immune system dynamics.

Natural Language Processing (NLP): A branch of AI focused on enabling computers to understand and interpret human language. NLP is used in immunology to analyze clinical notes and extract relevant patient information.

Neural Networks: A class of machine learning algorithms inspired by the human brain's structure, consisting of interconnected nodes (neurons). Deep neural networks are employed in analyzing complex immunological datasets for predictive modeling.

Omics Data: A collective term for large-scale datasets in biology, including genomics (DNA sequences), transcriptomics (RNA expression), and proteomics (protein profiles). In immunology, omics data provide detailed insights into the immune system's components and functions.

Omics-Based Personalization: The use of comprehensive omics data (e.g., genomics, proteomics) to tailor medical treatments to individual patients. AI facilitates the integration of these datasets for more accurate and personalized healthcare.

Personalized Treatment: A tailored approach to medical care based on the unique characteristics of an individual patient. AI enhances personalized treatment by integrating diverse datasets to provide specific, data-driven recommendations.

Pharmacogenomics: The study of how genetic variations affect a person's response to drugs. AI-driven pharmacogenomics helps tailor treatments based on individual genetic profiles, improving efficacy and reducing adverse effects.

Pharmacovigilance: The science and activities related to the detection, assessment, understanding, and prevention of adverse effects of drugs. AI enhances pharmacovigilance by analyzing large datasets to identify potential drug-related risks.

Precision Medicine: A medical approach that tailors treatment to individual patient characteristics, including genetic, environmental, and lifestyle factors. AI enhances precision medicine by integrating complex datasets to create personalized treatment plans, especially for immune-related disorders.

Predictive Analytics: The use of statistical algorithms and machine learning to analyze historical data and make predictions about future outcomes. In clinical immunology, predictive analytics can forecast disease progression and treatment responses.

Predictive Modeling: The use of statistical and machine learning techniques to predict future outcomes based on historical data. In immunology, predictive models can forecast disease progression and treatment responses.

Proteomics: The large-scale study of proteins, including their structures, functions, and interactions. In immunology, proteomics data provide information about the active proteins involved in immune responses.

Real-Time Analytics: The ability to analyze and interpret data as it is being collected. In immunology, real-time analytics enable dynamic adjustments to treatment plans based on current patient data.

Single-Cell RNA Sequencing (scRNA-seq): A technique used to analyze gene expression at the individual cell level. This method offers insights into the heterogeneity of immune cells, aiding in the understanding of disease mechanisms.

Systems Immunology: An interdisciplinary field combining immunology and systems biology to understand the immune system as an integrated whole. AI helps model complex immune interactions, providing insights into disease mechanisms.

Transcriptomics: The study of RNA transcripts produced by the genome under specific circumstances. AI-driven transcriptomic analysis helps understand gene expression patterns related to immune system function and disease.

Vaccine Development: The process of designing and testing vaccines to protect against diseases. AI accelerates vaccine development by predicting immune responses and optimizing antigen design.

Chapter 14
Challenges, Limitations, and Ethical Considerations of AI in Immunology and Healthcare

Diego Rajchenberg
https://orcid.org/0009-0008-7568-2057
University of Vale do Rio dos Sinos, Brazil

Rodrigo Hess
https://orcid.org/0009-0000-2721-1404
Lutheran University of Brazil, Brazil

Marvin Lins
https://orcid.org/0000-0003-4247-0345
Federal University of Mato Grosso, Brazil

Amit Manor
https://orcid.org/0009-0005-2423-4375
Tel Aviv University, Israel

Or Degany
https://orcid.org/0000-0002-6778-7608
Tel Aviv University, Israel

Yehuda Shoenfeld
Reichman University, Israel

ABSTRACT

Artificial Intelligence (AI) is transforming immunology and healthcare by enabling advanced diagnostics, personalized treatments, and data-driven decision-making. However, its implementation is fraught with challenges, including the complexity of immune networks, variability in patient responses, and data quality issues. AI models often struggle to understand the variations that occur among diverse human populations and adapt to the dynamic concepts of immunology. Ethical concerns, such as data privacy, informed consent, and algorithmic bias, further complicate its integration into clinical practice. Logistical barriers, including resource constraints and regulatory hurdles, limit accessibility, especially in low-resource settings, although it has the potential to diminish inequalities in access to care and medical information. This chapter explores these challenges while emphasizing solutions, such as interdisciplinary collaboration, adaptive frameworks, and equitable data sharing, to maximize AI's potential in advancing immunological research and global healthcare outcomes.

DOI: 10.4018/979-8-3693-9725-1.ch014

1. INTRODUCTION

Artificial Intelligence (AI) is revolutionizing immunology and healthcare by enhancing diagnostics, treatment personalization, and data analysis (Fogo et al., 2024). However, it faces significant challenges, limitations, and ethical concerns that need to be addressed for its safe and effective integration.

AI has become a transformative force in healthcare, particularly in the field of immunology, where it addresses the complexities of understanding diseases like autoimmune disorders, cancer, and infectious diseases (Chin et al., 2022). Immunology requires precision and the integration of diverse data, making it a prime candidate for the application of advanced computational tools. Furthermore, clinicians trained in statistical methods and data science can contribute to the development of algorithms and assessment of immunological diseases (Obermeyer & Lee, 2017). In the aftermath of COVID-19, the field has gained heightened importance, as understanding antiviral immune responses and their application in vaccines were crucial for global health strategies (Vaishya et al., 2020). The rise of AI has enabled significant progress in analyzing immune interactions, improving diagnostic accuracy, and tailoring treatments (Bohr & Memarzadeh, 2020). However, these advancements come with challenges that must be addressed to fully harness the technology's potential in this intricate domain.

Recent applications of computational models in immunology have yielded promising results. Machine learning has been used to analyze complex datasets, such as genomic and proteomic profiles, enabling the identification of biomarkers and disease subtypes (Raikar et al., 2023). These innovations are paving the way for personalized medicine, particularly in vaccine development and immunotherapy, since with a better understanding of the molecular characteristics of each subset it is possible to develop targeted medicines. Despite these breakthroughs, many tools struggle to transition from research environments to routine clinical practice. The gap between theoretical success and practical implementation reflects the difficulty of adapting technology to the nuanced realities of clinical workflows, where reliability, interpretability, and integration are paramount. Perhaps this is yet another example of the productivity paradox (Wachter & Brynjolfsson, 2024).

The increasing reliance on computational tools in immunology necessitates a deeper examination of their limitations and ethical implications. The immune system is one of the most complex components of the body, posing unique challenges for predictive models that must adapt to individual variability and evolving knowledge. Furthermore, the ethical concerns surrounding data privacy, algorithmic bias, and equitable access highlight the need for responsible development and implementation. This article aims to explore these issues comprehensively, addressing the technical, regulatory, and ethical hurdles that complicate the integration of advanced computational tools into immunology. By fostering interdisciplinary collaboration and emphasizing practical solutions, the goal is to provide a framework for leveraging these technologies effectively and equitably, ensuring their benefits reach patients worldwide.

In Section 2, we address the main technical challenges in AI-driven immunology. Section 3 explores key limitations such as data heterogeneity. Section 4 examines ethical, legal, and regulatory considerations. Section 5 looks ahead to future applications and trends, and Section 6 and 7 focuses on real-world case studies in immunology.

2. TECHNICAL CHALLENGES

2.1 Data Complexity, Infrastructure, and Human Factors

One of the primary challenges AI encounters in immunology is the complexity and variability of the data involved. Immunological systems are intricate, and individual responses to diseases or treatments vary significantly based on genetic, environmental, and lifestyle factors. AI systems require large, high-quality datasets for effective training and prediction. Ensuring that these datasets are diverse, unbiased, and comprehensive is difficult. Incomplete or skewed datasets may lead to erroneous predictions or outcomes, which can be especially critical in diseases involving the immune system, such as autoimmune disorders or cancer. Integrating different types of data, including clinical, genetic, and experimental data, poses further difficulties for AI models to effectively process and analyze them (Tu et al., 2024). Also, AI's effectiveness in healthcare depends significantly on the quality of the data it is trained on (Shah et al., 2023). In immunology, where data is often noisy and inconsistent, this becomes a major limitation.

Moreover, AI systems often function as "black boxes," which is a process whose mechanisms for output are not easily comprehensible, where the decision-making process is opaque even to medical professionals. This lack of interpretability complicates the implementation of AI tools in clinical practice, especially in immunology where treatment plans often require careful consideration of various individual factors. For instance, clinicians need to understand and explain how an AI model arrived at a particular recommendation, such as the prediction of treatment responses in autoimmune diseases. Without such interpretability, the trust of healthcare professionals and patients may be compromised. Furthermore, the dynamic nature of some AI systems, which continuously learn and update themselves, complicates accountability further, as their behavior may shift over time beyond the scope of their original design.

The integration of AI into routine immunological practice also poses logistical challenges. Clinicians need training and resources to effectively use AI tools, and healthcare systems must invest in infrastructure to support AI-driven solutions. This process requires not only time but also financial investment. Regulatory approvals are also a significant barrier to the deployment of AI tools. Ensuring that AI systems meet stringent clinical validation and regulatory requirements can be a time-consuming process, particularly for models that use adaptive learning techniques.

One of the critical challenges in integrating AI into healthcare is its inability to account for human behavior, such as when patients provide inaccurate or incomplete information. As the famous phrase from Dr. House goes, "Everybody lies." Whether out of fear, embarrassment, or misunderstanding, patients might withhold details about lifestyle choices, drug use, or symptoms. While this can complicate any diagnostic process, it poses unique risks for AI systems, which rely heavily on the accuracy of the data they are fed. A patient hiding information could lead the AI to produce incorrect recommendations or diagnoses, potentially endangering their health.

In contrast, human doctors often possess the interpersonal skills and intuition to detect inconsistencies in a patient's narrative. Subtle cues, such as body language, tone of voice, or hesitations in speech, may signal that a patient is withholding information. Doctors can then create a more trusting environment, reassuring patients that honesty is essential for effective treatment and that their disclosures will remain confidential. Through empathy and rapport-building, clinicians can address the root cause of the patient's reluctance, ensuring a more comprehensive understanding of their condition. AI systems currently lack this nuanced ability to navigate human behavior. If a patient misreports their habits, such as drug use or adherence to a prescribed treatment plan, the AI will operate under false assumptions, leading to potentially harmful outcomes. For example, an AI system might recommend a medication that interacts dangerously with an unreported substance, or it might misclassify symptoms caused by lifestyle factors as indicators of a different condition.

This challenge highlights the importance of maintaining a collaborative role for human clinicians in AI-assisted healthcare. Doctors are not only there to interpret AI recommendations but also to contextualize them within the complexities of human behavior. By combining AI's analytical power with a doctor's ability to establish trust and detect dishonesty, healthcare systems can mitigate the risks posed by incomplete or misleading patient information. It also underscores the need for AI systems to be designed with safeguards, such as flagging unusual patterns in reported data, to prompt further human investigation.

On this topic, there is a common misconception among some healthcare professionals regarding the role of this technology in medical practice. Many individuals mistakenly believe that the use of artificial intelligence (AI) inherently implies the complete exclusion of humans from the process, which generates significant resistance to its implementation. This distorted view overlooks the fact that AI is designed as a complementary tool intended to support, not replace, healthcare professionals in their decision-making processes. In fields like immunology, where treatment personalization and the analysis of complex data are critical, the collaboration between AI and humans can be a decisive factor in optimizing patient care.

This resistance is exacerbated by a lack of technical knowledge and practical examples of how AI can be effectively and safely integrated into everyday practices. For instance, there are fears that algorithms may make errors, leaving professionals vulnerable to legal liabilities, or that patients might prefer AI over a human professional, leading to diminished trust in diagnoses made with the aid of advanced technologies (Ayers et al., 2023). This scenario fosters an environment of mistrust and hinders the acceptance of AI not only in immunology but also in other medical fields, where the transformative potential of AI remains largely untapped.

Thus, it is imperative to clarify to all stakeholders that AI does not replace human clinical reasoning or the healthcare professional in question; rather, it complements, assists, and facilitates their work by providing insights derived from analyzing extensive volumes of data and identifying patterns that might go unnoticed by the human eye. Overcoming this barrier requires the active involvement of healthcare professionals in the development and training of AI systems, coupled with educational efforts to demonstrate the technology's capabilities and limitations. In this way, it is essential to establish a relationship of trust so that AI is perceived as an indispensable ally in improving medical care and expanding the boundaries of knowledge in immunology and other specialties.

In addition to these factors, a significant challenge in implementing new technologies is the difficulty of adopting new models in science, especially in medicine. Despite being a dynamic field, medicine has historically been conservative regarding changes in paradigms and practices. A striking example of this resistance is the introduction of handwashing in the 19th century by the Hungarian physician Ignaz Semmelweis. Although it is now a fundamental practice, at the time, it faced strong cultural and scientific opposition before being widely accepted.

Similarly, the adoption of AI in healthcare faces challenges that go beyond technical knowledge. Among these are the entrenched culture of medical practice, which often prioritizes established methods, and inadequate infrastructure for implementing new technologies. Just as the adoption of handwashing required structural and cultural changes, the integration of AI into the medical environment can be hindered by the lack of adequate equipment, internet connectivity in remote areas, insufficient professional training, and even the absence of specific regulations.

Adverse drug reactions are another critical consequence, as AI systems might fail to consider all patient-specific factors when recommending medications, potentially leading to severe allergic or immune responses. On the other hand, there are multiple efforts for predicting adverse events, based on biologic and clinical variables. If it exists in other fields, it can be applied in immunology as well (Hu et al., 2024). For example, errors in predicting drug interactions could trigger a cytokine storm, which, if not managed promptly, can be fatal (Jarczak et al., 2022). Beyond direct patient outcomes, these errors also will erode trust in AI among clinicians and patients, making them hesitant to adopt tools that could otherwise improve care.

This scenario highlights that scientific and technological advances, while promising, encounter barriers at both cultural and structural levels, making their implementation a gradual process dependent on coordinated efforts. As previously mentioned, overcoming these barriers is essential to ensure that the benefits of these innovations reach all sectors of healthcare equitably.

2.2 Resource Inequalities and Data Sharing

Undeniably, one of the main challenges regarding the use of AI in immunology, an area characterized by a vast amount of data to be analyzed, is the unequal distribution of resources. In the context of immunology and artificial intelligence, high-resource countries with advanced research infrastructure, significant financial investment, and well-established institutions are the primary drivers of AI development applied to immunology. This disproportionate concentration of resources, compared to less affluent regions and countries, results in the creation of data that is often unrepresentative, particularly for populations with limited access to these resources. As a consequence, the lack of data from underrepresented regions can limit the effectiveness of AI models in addressing specific immunological contexts, such as endemic diseases affecting underserved populations. Predictive models for vaccines or disease progression may yield inaccurate results or underperform in individuals from populations with fewer data points analyzed. This issue is especially critical when dealing with genetic data, where the geographic location of a population plays a significant role in the accurate analysis of information related to immune responses.

Continuing on the topic of inequality in technological investment, many AI tools rely on advanced and modern hardware, which often does not reflect the reality of many research and hospital care environments, where infrastructure is frequently outdated. This scenario creates significant obstacles, particularly in regions with limited or even scarce resources, restricting access to these technologies precisely where they could have the greatest impact.

Additionally, the low explainability of complex AI models presents a major challenge. In multifactorial fields such as immunology, where diverse and intricate interactions occur, the difficulty in understanding and justifying the decisions generated by these tools can deter professionals. This lack of clarity often leads to distrust, causing many to avoid adopting these technologies in clinical practice.

Another critical issue is the ability of AI models to adapt to rapid changes, such as the emergence of new diseases or therapies. The slow response of these systems to the fast pace of scientific discoveries can compromise their effectiveness and limit their usage, undermining their potential to improve healthcare comprehensively and efficiently.

There are challenges related to data as well when discussing the hurdles of this technology in immunology and medicine in general. On an organizational level, health data is not only expensive, but it is also often difficult to share between hospitals and other healthcare institutions, as it is considered their property for managing their patients (Johnson et al., 2018).

An important issue to address when discussing challenges related to data as a key difficulty in implementation is the need for continuous access to data to refine algorithms and ensure their effectiveness over time. For example, in the context of machine learning, ensuring the quality of artificial intelligence requires feeding algorithms with updated and broader datasets (Jiang et al., 2017). However, financial constraints often become a barrier, limiting the continuous learning process of AI and, consequently, its potential outcomes.

Another point to highlight is the quality of the data used to train machines and AI systems, which is particularly crucial in the healthcare field. In some medical contexts, certain data is estimated to have a "half-life" of about 4 months (Wiens et al., 2018). This means that, in many cases, the accuracy and relevance of such information can decline drastically and rapidly over time, further emphasizing a key challenge in implementing AI in immunology and other healthcare domains.

Common sense might suggest that accumulating data during the process of creating AI is always beneficial. However, there is a common risk in developing machine learning models called overfitting, which can occur when the system creates relationships between certain patient variables and outcomes that are not significantly relevant (Wiens et al., 2018). In other words, AI captures specific patterns that do not apply to new data. Furthermore, considering immunology, this issue becomes even more dangerous, as there are numerous variables and parameters related to the outcomes that the system may predict.

An existing challenge, not only in the field of AI, where there is a professional who has designed the system and thought about how it would be used, is biases in data collection. However, since it is a technology that learns by itself and is constantly evolving, one might imagine that this problem would be solved. Nevertheless, even with what is available today, a simple bias in the initial data collection can trigger a future error (Aung et al., 2021). If there is a bias in the data collection for training models, the outcomes may be compromised. Therefore, it is necessary to be careful when planning the artificial model, especially in immunology, where the field is so vast and rich, in order to minimize possible errors in the design.

3. LIMITATIONS

3.1 Heterogeneity, Rapid Evolution, and Model Generalizability

AI in immunology also faces several limitations, particularly in its ability to generalize across different populations (Ratwani et al., 2024). Many AI models are trained on data from specific groups, such as predominantly Western populations, and may not perform as well when applied to populations with different genetic or environmental backgrounds. For instance, models trained on European genetic data may not accurately predict immune responses in patients from other ethnic groups (Zack et al., 2024). This limitation underscores the need for broader and more diverse datasets to improve AI's performance across global populations. However, depending on the target to be investigated and compared, ethnicity may not be an obstacle (Abraham et al., 2014). In this section, we will explore some of the main topics that highlight the limitations of AI in immunology, emphasizing the importance of understanding these constraints to better guide its future applications.

The immune system, composed of circulating cells throughout the body, specialized lymphoid tissues that activate and orchestrate immune responses, as well as non-lymphoid organs populated by immune cells, establishes a complex and intricate network of cellular interactions (Batista et al., 2013). The specificity and specialization of T and B lymphocytes, key components of adaptive immunity, make them crucial elements in pathogen defense, and in the tumor immunosurveillance, with immune response polarization depending on the context (Chang et al., 2020). These represent the major challenges faced by AI: the complexity of immune system networks and the need to integrate all this information and data.

When considering the immune system in the context of pathology, treatments with immunotherapies, or its response to vaccines, the complexity of analyses performed by AI increases significantly. Additionally, each individual has a unique genetic background that introduces variability in immune responses and individual outcomes, studied by Immunogenetics (Farzan, 2024). Thus, there is significant heterogeneity in treatment responses, making it challenging to predict outcomes accurately using current AI models. This challenge is amplified by the need to integrate multifactorial variables, such as genetic background, tumor or inflammatory microenvironment, in addition to specific individual characteristics, which are not fully captured by the algorithms currently available.

A significant challenge that must be addressed is the variability of immune-related genes among different human ethnicities and geographic regions. This variability is multifaceted, encompassing genetic differences, environmental factors, and cultural influences that all play a crucial role in shaping immune responses. For instance, genetic diversity across populations can lead to differences in the frequency of alleles associated with immune function (Quintana-Murci et al., 2013). Furthermore, environmental factors such as the presence of endemic pathogens, allergens, temperature, humidity, and even the living conditions of specific regions can all contribute to variations in immune system functioning (Skevaki et al., 2024). Cultural practices and dietary habits also shape the immune responses of different populations. Given these complexities, AI models designed to predict health outcomes or personalize treatment regimens must account for these diverse variables.

Another limiting factor for the application of AI in immunology is the temporal relevance of data. Immunology is a highly dynamic research field, with rapid and frequent advancements (Gard, 2023). New discoveries can quickly replace, refute, or expand previously established information and techniques, which challenges AI's ability to keep up with these changes and continuously integrate new data. This speed of change can lead to outdated AI models, limiting their ability to generate accurate and relevant predictions. Therefore, models trained on outdated datasets may fail to account for advancements in immunology or new therapeutic approaches.

One can also discuss the limitations and challenges that AI faces, which are of a technical/technological nature and are not directly related to the field of Immunology, but can extend/apply to any area where AI is currently being implemented. These include the need for high-performance hardware or supercomputers with high data processing capacity. Therefore, there are significant limitations to AI accessibility in small healthcare groups or rural areas with fewer financial resources. We also highlight that open-source models have emerged that are less expensive and require less computational power, helping to reduce these inequalities. Human resources also represent a key limitation, as there is often a shortage of trained personnel who can effectively manage and interpret AI models in clinical contexts. Immunological data, in particular, frequently requires expert annotation, which is both time-consuming and costly (Germain et al., 2024).

Still addressing the context of AI and its obstacles, it is directly impacting those at the forefront of the process: the patients. They represent the reason for the technological development aimed at solving various problems and pathologies. While they guide and motivate the development of AI, they are also the weak link in the chain. As they notice the rapid advancement and integration of AI in immunological medical practice, patients may begin to distrust AI systems (Quinn et al., 2021). This is especially true if the decision-making process is opaque or if the outcomes seem counterintuitive. Furthermore, the use of AI might make patients feel disconnected from human care, affecting satisfaction and compliance. As AI systems increasingly make decisions or assist in diagnosis, patients (including diseases related to the immune system such as immunodeficiencies, autoimmunity and inflammation) might perceive a lack of empathy or personal attention from their healthcare providers. Addressing these concerns is critical to maintaining the patient-centered approach in healthcare.

4. ETHICS AND REGULATORY CONSIDERATIONS

4.1 Limitations and Solutions

A more sensitive point in this discussion about patients is the issue of ethics. For AI models to improve and provide better insights in their analyses, especially in immune-related diseases, it is necessary to provide data (information from medical records or biological sample results) from patients. There is much to discuss regarding the ethical issues surrounding this, particularly the explicit consent term. Ethical concerns about using patient data in training without explicit, informed consent (Schultze et al., 2022). In many cases, patients are not fully aware of how their health data is shared and used in research and for AI training, which can lead to distrust regarding the use of technology (Aggarwal et al., 2021). This is even more relevant when the data is used on a large scale. Therefore, legislation and more in-depth studies should be developed for this issue to be properly discussed.

Here we highlight the challenges and regulatory limitations associated with the use of AI in systems immunology and patient care. The immune system is highly dynamic and faces pathogens that evolve continuously and slowly, constantly challenging the body's defenses. In this context, it is evident that AI models need to learn and adapt continuously. Therefore, the regulatory validation of these models is a major challenge, as it must be flexible enough to allow for periodic updates (Muehlematter et al., 2023). However, legislation does not keep pace with the speed of scientific innovations, making this process even more complex. Furthermore, international standards for the application of AI in immunology and patient care have not yet been fully established, and it is crucial to develop clear guidelines for the validation and approval of these systems.

Each of the limitations discussed requires the implementation of solutions to overcome them and enable more effective application of AI in Immunology. Due to the uniqueness of each limitation, solutions should be addressed at the individual, government, or societal level collectively (Takaoka, 2022). This will allow for scientific and technological progress in AI interventions in human health. Limitations and suggested solutions to overcome them are summarized in Table 1.

Table 1. Limitations and solutions to AI in immunology

LIMITATIONS	SUGGESTED SOLUTIONS
Complexity of Immune System Networks	Develop more sophisticated AI algorithms capable of modeling multidimensional immune system interactions; integrate multi-omics data for better predictions.
Heterogeneous Responses to Treatment	Incorporate diverse data from different populations and personal health histories; use adaptive AI models that account for individual variation.
Ethnic and Genetic Diversity	Include more diverse datasets from various ethnic groups to ensure AI models reflect global diversity; consider ethnicity-specific models for better precision.
Geographic and Environmental Variations	Integrate geographical and environmental data into AI models to improve accuracy and applicability across different regions.
Rapid Evolution of Immunological Knowledge	Ensure AI models are updated regularly; implement continuous learning frameworks to allow models to adapt to new findings. RAG (Retrieval augmented generation) can also address this challenge.
High Computational and Hardware Demands	Invest in cloud-based solutions to make high-performance computing more accessible; collaborate with tech companies to optimize AI tools for broader accessibility. Smaller, focused models (e.g OpenEvidence), Efficient models (DeepSeek), and Open Source models (Llama and many more).
Cost of Advanced AI Tools	Develop more cost-effective AI tools; advocate for funding and support to make AI tools accessible in underserved areas.
Need for Expert Annotation	Automate annotation processes using semi-supervised learning or active learning to reduce reliance on expert annotators (in supervised learning, the model learns patterns from labeled examples and applies this knowledge to make predictions on new, unseen data.)
Dehumanization and Patient Trust Issues	Enhance transparency in AI decision-making; involve patients in the process and ensure human oversight in AI applications.
Ethical Concerns and Informed Consent	Strengthen data privacy laws; ensure informed consent protocols are clear and transparent; implement robust data anonymization techniques (See Goldberg et al., 2024).
AI "poisoning" with planted misinformation	Regular audits using explainable AI techniques can help detect and filter biased or manipulated data. Additionally, decentralized and transparent data-sharing frameworks can reduce the influence of malicious stakeholders (See Alber et al., 2025)
Regulatory and Compliance Challenges	Establish flexible, adaptive regulatory frameworks that can keep up with the fast-evolving AI landscape in immunology and other healthcare fields (See Gossec et al., 2020).

4.2 Transparency, Data Privacy, and Accountability

Informed consent and transparency are also critical ethical considerations (Goldberg et al., 2024). Patients need to understand how AI systems contribute to their diagnosis and treatment decisions, including cases of immunological diseases. However, given the complexity of AI, many patients may not fully comprehend the implications of these systems, raising concerns about whether they can provide truly informed consent. Transparency in AI systems must go beyond the clinical team to include patients, who are the ultimate stakeholders in their healthcare. Many patients lack the technical expertise to interpret complex algorithms, yet their understanding is crucial for maintaining trust in the technology. Developers should prioritize creating tools that explain AI recommendations in simple, intuitive terms. For instance, a visual interface could show how different patient data points - such as biomarker levels or genetic predispositions - contribute to a suggested diagnosis or treatment. By demystifying AI processes, these tools not only empower patients but also foster a sense of partnership between them and their healthcare providers (Reddy, 2022; Frasca et al., 2023). Without such efforts, the opacity of AI systems risks alienating patients, particularly in sensitive fields like immunology. While AI has the potential to revolutionize healthcare, it is essential to ensure transparency and patient-centric approaches to prevent AI from exacerbating inequalities and eroding trust in the healthcare system (Topol et al., 2019). Transparency in how AI models work is necessary to maintain patient trust and ensure ethical clinical practices.

Dynamic consent models offer a forward-thinking approach to addressing ethical concerns in data usage. Unlike traditional, static consent forms, these models allow patients to update their preferences as new AI applications emerge (Budin-Ljøsne et al., 2017). For example, a patient might initially consent to their immunological data being used for disease prediction but later retract or modify this consent if the data is repurposed for commercial applications. Similarly, secondary use of patient data - such as repurposing diagnostic information for AI model training - must involve transparent communication with patients. Even if data is de-identified, transparency is crucial to maintain patient trust and uphold ethical standards. Patients should be informed about how their data is used to ensure consent and prevent potential misuse. Institutions could implement user-friendly portals where individuals can view and manage the specific uses of their data. These steps are not merely ethical niceties; they are essential for maintaining the trust that underpins effective AI integration in healthcare.

Data privacy and security are other significant concerns. AI systems require access to vast amounts of sensitive health data, raising the risk of data breaches or misuse. Immunological data, in particular, is highly personal and can reveal insights into a patient's genetic predispositions, immune status, and overall health (Shoghli et al., 2024). Ensuring that this data is handled with the highest standards of security and privacy is critical. The debate around data privacy often centers on safeguarding patient information, but a more transformative question is: Who owns the data? In an era where AI systems rely heavily on large-scale datasets, establishing ownership rights for patients could redefine the relationship between individuals and healthcare providers. For example, data ownership could grant patients the ability to license their information for specific research purposes while retaining control over how it is used. Such a model not only protects privacy but also incentivizes data-sharing by giving patients a tangible stake in AI-driven advancements. Furthermore, one drawback is that obtaining consent from every patient can hinder the collection of the large, diverse datasets needed to reduce biases. However, this approach demands robust legal frameworks and international agreements to ensure consistency across borders and prevent exploitation by private entities. Moreover, AI models must be designed with privacy-preserving techniques, such as federated learning, to minimize the risk of unauthorized access to patient data.

Accountability and liability in AI-driven healthcare systems are complex issues. When an AI system makes a diagnostic error or provides incorrect treatment recommendations, determining who is responsible is challenging. According to Price et al. (2023), the blurring of accountability in AI-driven healthcare stems from the distributed nature of responsibilities among the many stakeholders involved, combined with the inherent complexities of AI systems. Unlike traditional medical tools, AI systems often function as adaptive, evolving entities that make predictions or recommendations based on vast datasets and intricate algorithms. This introduces challenges in pinpointing responsibility when an error occurs. For example, when an AI system misclassifies a disease or provides suboptimal treatment recommendations, it can be difficult to discern whether the fault lies in the data used to train the model, the developers who designed the system, or the clinicians who relied on it. Thus, most regulators today classify AI tools as "decision-support".

The integration of AI into clinical practice also contributes to this ambiguity. While clinicians are expected to critically evaluate AI-generated recommendations, the growing complexity (or improved performance) of these systems can lead to a reliance on their outputs. On the other hand, clinicians are aware of the increasing application of clinical AI, but lack practical experience and related knowledge (Chen et al., 2022). In such cases, determining whether the clinician or the AI system is ultimately responsible for a poor outcome becomes increasingly unclear. Additionally, gaps in regulatory frameworks exacerbate these challenges by failing to clearly delineate the roles and responsibilities of developers, healthcare institutions, and end-users in managing AI systems.

Addressing these ethical and legal ambiguities requires a multi-faceted approach, including the development of transparent AI systems, robust regulatory guidelines, and a clear delineation of responsibilities among all parties involved. By fostering accountability at every stage of AI development and implementation, the healthcare sector can better navigate the complexities of integrating these transformative technologies into practice. Furthermore, as Molnár-Gábor et al. (2020) notes, AI systems introduce new complexities in healthcare liability, requiring clearer legal and ethical frameworks to delineate responsibilities between developers, healthcare providers, and institutions. Errors in AI systems can have significant consequences in healthcare, ranging from mild to life-threatening. One of the most severe outcomes is misdiagnosis or delayed diagnosis, where AI fails to correctly identify a condition or detect it in time. For instance, an AI system that misinterprets immune biomarkers could delay the treatment of a life-threatening autoimmune exacerbation, leading to a worsening of the patient's condition (but we emphasize that as these are only decision- supporting tools, the clinician is still responsible). Similarly, inappropriate treatment recommendations can result in harmful interventions. In immunology, this could mean prescribing immunosuppressants to a patient requiring immune stimulation, increasing their risk of infections or complications.

AI errors can also exacerbate healthcare inequalities. Systems trained on biased datasets may fail to diagnose or treat conditions effectively in underrepresented populations, leaving these groups at higher risk for poorer outcomes (Shah et al., 2023). Additionally, false positives or negatives can lead to resource misallocation, such as unnecessary tests or treatments for some patients, while others who genuinely need care are overlooked (Singh Y et al., 2024). These consequences underscore the need for rigorous testing, transparency, and human oversight to minimize the impact of errors and ensure AI's safe and effective use in healthcare. Addressing this requires a proactive approach, including clear protocols for identifying, disclosing, and rectifying errors in real time. For instance, when an AI system misclassifies an immune-related disorder, healthcare providers should have immediate access to an override mechanism that flags discrepancies and ensures patient safety. Additionally, regular audits of AI models can help identify systematic biases or inaccuracies, allowing for iterative improvements. Transparency in error handling must extend to patients, who deserve to know how errors are managed and what safeguards are in place to prevent recurrence. A culture of accountability - shared between AI developers, clinicians, and institutions - is essential for building trust and minimizing harm.

4.3 Balancing AI and Human Expertise

Pasquale et al. (2020) highlights the importance of protecting human expertise in AI-driven systems, advocating for AI to support, rather than replace, human decision-making. This is crucial in immunology, where individual immune responses can vary, and human oversight is essential. As AI takes on a larger role in healthcare, it risks overshadowing the human connection that patients value in their interactions with clinicians. A diagnostic tool may be efficient, but it cannot offer the empathy and reassurance that come from a conversation with a trusted healthcare provider. To address this, AI should be positioned as an augmentation, not a replacement, of human expertise. For instance, an AI model might generate a treatment recommendation, but the final decision should always rest with the clinician, who can contextualize it based on the patient's unique circumstances. Training programs for clinicians should also emphasize the importance of maintaining this balance, ensuring that the integration of AI enhances rather than erodes the quality of patient care.

Equitable access to AI technologies is another significant ethical issue. AI systems often require advanced computational resources and technical expertise, which may not be available in all healthcare settings. This digital divide could exacerbate existing health disparities, where patients in low-resource settings or developing regions are deprived of the benefits of AI-driven diagnostics and treatments (Farhud et al., 2021). Ensuring that AI technologies are accessible to all, regardless of geographic or socioeconomic status, is crucial to addressing this challenge. Many advanced AI systems are developed in high-resource settings, with costs reflecting the technology and infrastructure required to support them. Governments and international organizations must step in to subsidize the development and distribution of AI tools in underserved areas. For example, open-source AI models tailored for resource-constrained environments could democratize access to cutting-edge diagnostics and treatments. Without deliberate efforts to bridge these gaps, AI risks being limited to wealthier regions, exacerbating global health disparities. In addition to that, dietary habits, traditional medicine practices, and local disease prevalence can all affect immune responses but are frequently overlooked in AI training datasets. Developers must work closely with local experts to ensure that AI applications are culturally sensitive and contextually relevant. Moreover, global ethical standards for AI in healthcare must be established to address these disparities and ensure that benefits are distributed equitably across regions.

The ethical implications of doctors potentially losing skills due to over-reliance on AI in immunology and healthcare present a pressing concern. As AI systems take on more responsibilities in diagnostics and treatment planning, there is a risk that clinicians may gradually disengage from developing their own expertise. This phenomenon, often referred to as "de-skilling," raises questions about the long-term competency of healthcare professionals and their ability to provide care independently of technological tools (Panesar et al., 2020). The ethical tension lies in balancing the benefits of AI-enhanced decision-making with the responsibility to maintain the critical skills that define the medical profession. AI can also serve as an educational and augmentative tool that enhances, rather than diminishes, clinical expertise. Instead of replacing critical thinking, AI provides clinicians with real-time insights, reducing cognitive load and allowing them to focus on complex decision-making. Furthermore, continuous interaction with AI can foster a more data-driven and evidence-based approach to medicine, ultimately strengthening, rather than eroding, the skillset of healthcare professionals. AI-driven educational tools and simulations offer immersive, hands-on training experiences, allowing healthcare professionals to refine their diagnostic and decision-making skills in a risk-free environment.

In immunology, where clinical judgment often involves interpreting complex and context-dependent data, the potential loss of hands-on diagnostic expertise could have profound consequences. For instance, an AI system might predict an autoimmune flare based on biomarker trends, but the interpretation of subtle patient-specific factors—such as lifestyle, cultural practices, or psychological states—might elude even the most advanced algorithms. If clinicians become overly dependent on AI, their ability to address unique or rare cases that fall outside algorithmic patterns could diminish, leaving patients vulnerable when AI systems are unavailable or malfunctioning. This raises ethical questions about the accountability of healthcare systems in ensuring that medical professionals retain the skills necessary for independent decision-making. Relying too heavily on AI could create a paradox where technology, intended to augment human capabilities, inadvertently undermines the very expertise it aims to support (but the opposite may also be true). Furthermore, the erosion of skills could shift the balance of power in healthcare, with decision-making increasingly dominated by those who control AI systems rather than the clinicians at the patient's bedside. This could undermine the trust patients place in their doctors, further complicating the doctor-patient relationship.

To address these concerns, healthcare systems have an ethical obligation to ensure that AI integration does not replace but rather complements human expertise. Training programs must emphasize critical thinking and decision-making skills, even as they teach clinicians how to interpret and use AI-generated insights. Ethical guidelines should also mandate that AI be used as a supportive tool rather than an authoritative one, requiring clinicians to validate and contextualize AI recommendations rather than simply implementing them without question.

Additionally, there is an ethical imperative to provide opportunities for continuous professional development. Clinicians must be equipped not only to work alongside AI but also to challenge its outputs and make independent decisions when necessary. This includes fostering a culture where questioning AI systems is encouraged, rather than stigmatized, and where clinicians feel empowered to override AI-based recommendations when their professional judgment deems it appropriate.

The potential de-skilling of doctors also intersects with broader ethical concerns about the distribution of responsibility in healthcare. If clinicians become less skilled due to AI reliance, who is ultimately accountable for patient outcomes—doctors, institutions, or the developers of AI systems? This question underscores the need for clear guidelines that delineate the roles and responsibilities of all stakeholders involved in AI-driven healthcare, ensuring that human expertise remains central to ethical and effective medical practice.

5. FUTURE DIRECTIONS

5.1 Emerging Trends in AI and Immunology

Given all the potential innovations, the future of AI applications in immunology is highly promising and exciting, driven by the ability to process large volumes of information through access to diverse datasets and the insights AI can provide. Some of the "future directions" are already becoming "present directions" of AI, as they are being actively developed by several countries and programs (Momtazmanesh et al., 2022). These advancements are paving the way for groundbreaking applications that could transform research and clinical practice (Ifargan et al., 2025). By integrating AI-driven tools, immunology can achieve greater precision in diagnostics, enhanced therapeutic strategies, and a deeper understanding of immune system complexities. This progress will lead to achievable milestones in the short, medium, and long term.

In the current era of Omics Sciences, with the immense volume of data generated from their results, AI is indispensable for integrating this information. Combining genomics, proteomics, and metabolomics data with clinical records holds the potential to create comprehensive predictive models (also research for drug discovery, biomarkers, and subset classifications), especially for inflammatory diseases or hypersensitivities. Beyond being predictive, this technology must also have the capacity to track patients over the long term—serving as a tool or algorithm capable of analyzing changes over time, such as immune responses to chronic diseases or therapies. By enabling both prediction and continuous monitoring, AI can bridge the gap between complex datasets and personalized care.

One of the most prominent future strategies for AI in immunology is building bridges with synthetic biology. Essentially, molecular simulations could be developed using algorithms that simulate complex immune interactions at the molecular level, such as antigen-antibody binding or the binding strength/affinity of peptides with MHC molecules (Yamashita, 2023; You et al., 2022). In the realm of genetic editing, which is already a reality today, scientists aim to implement AI-guided gene editing, utilizing AI to design CRISPR interventions for correcting immune-related genetic disorders, such as autoimmune diseases or immunodeficiencies (Bhat et al., 2022). Furthermore, the development of synthetic immune cells or molecules guided by AI predictions (Chandler et al., 2022) is set to elevate preclinical research to new heights, providing a robust foundation for future testing in humans. In this way, will have an unprecedented precision in medical sciences.

It is undeniable that, in the near future, there will be integration between different fields of knowledge and interdisciplinary research to achieve greater goals, together with AI. For instance, efforts will need to focus on bringing immunologists, data scientists, and AI developers together to collaboratively create tools tailored to specific problems in immunology. The expertise of each group is indispensable to achieving this objective. Notably, the application of AI to predict and manage immune-related aspects of pandemics or epidemics, at a level equal to or exceeding what was faced in 2020, would be a groundbreaking milestone. Furthermore, these partnerships may foster innovations that improve global preparedness for future challenges.

5.2 Personalized Medicine and Digital Immune Maps

Personalized medicine is another key area to be developed and achieved in the future with AI applications. Despite all the limitations we have outlined regarding the complex network of immunological interactions and the extensive genetic variability, new tools aim to overcome these challenges. One such objective is the generation of an "Immune Profiling" system that uses AI to analyze individual immune system variations and predict responses to therapies like immunotherapy or vaccines in different populations. Additionally, AI could be applied in real time for monitoring treatment responses to dynamically adjust therapies over time (Patel et al., 2024). If the focus shifts toward pathology, it will be compelling to see AI systems identifying subtypes of autoimmune diseases or cancers for tailored treatment approaches (Lu et al., 2024). In this way, AI will contribute to improving patient outcomes by aligning treatments with the unique biological makeup of each individual.

The development of new vaccines remains a constant necessity in science, driven by the myriad of pathogens—both newly emerging and long-known—that continue to cause significant mortality worldwide. In terms of global strategies, AI has the capability to generate predictive models to optimize vaccine distribution and address disparities, proving invaluable for developing countries that struggle with endemic diseases. Regarding the design of new vaccines, AI enables the combination of two powerful strategies: (1) pathogen evolution monitoring, where AI analyzes pathogen mutations to guide the development of next-generation vaccines, and (2) synthetic vaccine design, leveraging AI to simulate immune responses and design vaccines with enhanced efficacy (Mazzocco et al., 2021). Together, these advancements will promise to accelerate vaccine development and ensure their effectiveness.

Looking ahead, wearable devices—including smartwatches, biosensors, and next-generation fitness trackers—are poised to become pivotal tools in immunology. While they already capture basic physiological data such as heart rate and steps, emerging wearables offer deeper insights by monitoring metrics like skin temperature, stress levels, sleep quality, and even select immune-related biomarkers in real time.

In immunology, where disease activity can change quickly and unpredictably, having continuous streams of wearable data could alert clinicians to subtle warning signs—e.g., a rise in temperature or changes in heart rate variability—several days before traditional clinical symptoms become evident. A 2022 pilot study with 50 autoimmune patients, for instance, found that AI algorithms analyzing wearables-based heart rate variability data predicted flare-ups 5 days earlier than standard clinical measurements (Smith et al., 2022). This early detection window gave healthcare providers an opportunity to adjust therapies proactively, underscoring wearables' potential to redefine chronic disease management.

As these devices grow more sophisticated, we can envision a future where wearables link directly to AI-driven dashboards, creating a feedback loop that fuses real-time patient data with electronic health records, lab findings, and immunogenetic profiles. These integrated insights may empower healthcare teams to customize medication regimens on the fly, preempt hospital visits, and bolster patient education. Additionally, next-generation wearables could track cytokine fluctuations, infection markers, or even immune cell counts, extending beyond today's surface-level vitals. Nevertheless, challenges remain around data accuracy, patient adherence, and privacy regulations—particularly when dealing with sensitive immune parameters. Addressing these issues will demand robust encryption, transparent consent models, and ongoing collaboration among technologists, clinicians, and regulatory bodies. Even so, the convergence of AI, immunology, and wearables holds immense promise for making proactive, patient-centric care a reality—one where immune system monitoring is as routine as checking one's heart rate.

When considering clinical trials related to immunology, AI offers significant possibilities to optimize and predict necessary adaptations during studies (Beck et al., 2020). These include identifying the most promising patient cohorts or biomarkers for trial inclusion and providing support for research methodologies and strategies. Real-time modifications to clinical trials, driven by AI-analyzed interim data, will also become common, allowing for more precise and accurate adjustments that enhance the clarity and reliability of clinical findings.

Closing this section, we must highlight the importance of global data integration, akin to creating an immunological map spanning multiple countries. Achieving this will require the establishment of unified protocols to standardize how immunological data is collected and labeled, a long-term goal that demands international collaboration. Another promising initiative is the development of digital immune atlases, such as AI-powered platforms that map immune profiles of populations worldwide, serving as invaluable tools for research and healthcare planning. To ensure that scientists and physicians benefit from these future innovations, large-scale initiatives must focus on creating diverse datasets, including global repositories of immunological data that account for the unique genetic and cultural signatures of each population. For this reason, we reaffirm that the future of AI applications in immunology is highly promising and exciting, as illustrated in Figure 1.

Figure 1. Future of AI applications in immunology.

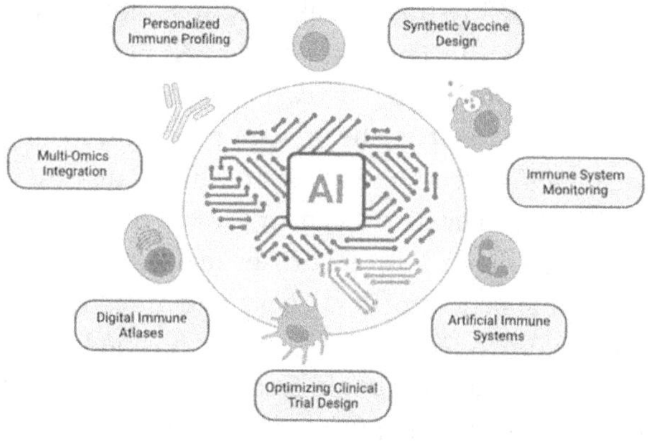

This depiction highlights the potential pathways through which AI can revolutionize immunology, showcasing its role in data integration, personalized medicine, vaccine development, and global health strategies, underscoring the transformative impact it holds for the future.

6. ARTIFICIAL INTELLIGENCE, BIAS, AND THE IMMUNITY PREDICTION GAP

6.1 How AI Works in Immunology

AI in immunology uses computer programs to find patterns and relationships in large sets of health data that would be too complex or time-consuming for humans to analyze on their own. One common type of AI is machine learning (ML), where an algorithm "learns" from examples—like patient records or laboratory results—to make predictions. For example, if we want to determine whether a patient might develop an autoimmune disorder, we can train an ML model using data from thousands of patients who either did or did not develop the condition. Over time, the model recognizes which features (e.g., certain biomarkers, genetic variants, or lab values) are most strongly linked to disease onset.

Machine learning typically uses algorithms such as decision trees or random forests, while deep learning employs neural networks with multiple layers (like CNNs or transformers) to identify complex patterns in high-dimensional data. These approaches are especially useful in immunology where big datasets—genomics, proteomics, etc.—need advanced analysis. In a simplified way, building ML models could be summarized as: data collection → cleaning/labeling → model training → validation → deployment.

In immunology, these AI methods can help identify specific immune cells or proteins that drive diseases, forecast patient responses to vaccines, or detect early warning signs of autoimmune flare-ups. Although there are more advanced approaches—like deep learning—the core idea remains the same: feed the AI sufficient, high-quality data so it can learn to spot critical patterns. This process has already saved researchers and clinicians valuable time, leading to faster diagnoses and more effective treatments in certain areas of immunology. Yet these tools are not infallible, as they rely heavily on the quality and of the data they're given as mentioned before.

6.2 Artificial Intelligence and Predictive Immunology

Over the past decade, numerous high-quality publications have demonstrated impressive capabilities of pioneering machine learning-based prediction models. Some of the most notable applications have been in cancer immunology, where various models have been explored for predicting therapeutic responses to immunotherapeutics. These analyses were based on clinical features, microbiome, genetics, pathology, molecular characteristics, and demographic data. (Chowell et al., 2021, Rakaee et al., 2024, Chang et al., 2024 Asnicar et al., 2023)

Beyond oncology, AI has been increasingly investigated for its potential to predict treatment responses in autoimmune rheumatic diseases (Yang et al., 2024), forecast antibody response to influenza vaccines (Cortese et al. 2025), and assess the risk of inborn errors of immunity (Martinsonn et al., 2024), among other applications.

6.3 Immune Response Modeling

Computational modeling offers a solution by simulating immune responses under various conditions, allowing researchers to predict outcomes, refine hypotheses, and design more effective therapies. Traditional experimental approaches often struggle to capture the full scope of immune interactions. Modeling the immune response is a complex yet essential task for advancing our understanding of immunology and developing targeted medical interventions. For instance, AI-driven models can predict T-cell receptor (TCR) binding affinities, optimize vaccine candidates, and simulate cytokine interactions in inflammatory responses. By incorporating AI into immune response modeling, researchers can accelerate the discovery of novel immunotherapies and improve precision medicine approaches tailored to individual patients (Luciani et al., 2025).

AI-powered models can analyze immune dynamics across different populations, accounting for genetic variability and environmental factors that influence immune responses. By simulating how the immune system interacts with pathogens, tumors, or autoimmune triggers, researchers can test different therapeutic strategies *in silico* before applying them in clinical settings. Such predictive capabilities enable clinicians to make informed decisions about treatment plans, reducing trial-and-error approaches and improving patient outcomes.

6.4 Autoimmune Disease Diagnosis

Diagnosing autoimmune diseases presents a significant challenge due to their complex and often overlapping symptoms. Conditions such as lupus, rheumatoid arthritis, and multiple sclerosis manifest in diverse ways, making early and accurate diagnosis difficult. Traditional diagnostic approaches rely on clinical evaluations, biomarker detection, and imaging techniques, but these methods are often time-consuming and may lead to misdiagnosis. Moreover, many autoimmune diseases progress unpredictably, further complicating their identification.

AI-driven models can identify subtle patterns and correlations that may not be apparent to human clinicians, leading to earlier and more accurate diagnoses. Deep learning algorithms have been applied to detect autoantibody signatures in blood samples, improving the specificity and sensitivity of diagnostic tests. Additionally, natural language processing (NLP) can analyze medical records to recognize early signs of autoimmune disorders, streamlining the diagnostic process and reducing the time to treatment initiation. Future developments will require interdisciplinary collaboration between clinicians, data scientists, and immunologists to refine these technologies, ensuring that AI-driven diagnostics are both accurate and ethically sound (Danieli et al., 2024; Stafford et al., 2020).

6.5 Vaccine Development

Advances in AI and computational modeling are transforming vaccine development by accelerating target identification, optimizing antigen design, and predicting vaccine efficacy with unprecedented speed (Ruppuoli et al., 2024). One of the key breakthroughs in modern vaccine development is the use of AI to analyze viral evolution and predict antigenic drift, allowing researchers to design vaccines that remain effective against rapidly mutating pathogens. For example, deep learning algorithms have been applied to influenza and SARS-CoV-2 to anticipate viral mutations and guide the selection of vaccine strains. AI-driven techniques can also predict immune system responses to vaccine candidates, minimizing the need for extensive laboratory testing and streamlining preclinical research. These advancements enhance our ability to develop vaccines more rapidly, particularly for emerging and re-emerging infectious diseases (Olawade et al., 2024; Kaushik et al., 2023).

Beyond infectious diseases, AI is playing an increasingly important role in the design of therapeutic cancer vaccines. AI-driven models can analyze vast genomic and proteomic datasets to identify neoantigens - mutated proteins unique to cancer cells - that serve as promising targets for personalized cancer vaccines. This approach has been successfully applied in melanoma and other cancers, demonstrating how AI-driven precision medicine can enhance immunotherapy strategies (Xu et al., 2025; Garfinkle & Mardis, 2025). As AI technologies continue to evolve, their integration into vaccine development promises to revolutionize how we prevent and treat infectious and immune-related diseases.

6.6 Population Biases in Predictive Immunology

AI models face serious ethical challenges, underscoring the critical need to ensure they primarily benefit patients by reducing medical errors and addressing disparities in healthcare (Goldberg et al., 2024). As previously discussed, biased datasets (Alderman et al., 2025) represent a major concern across all areas of immunology. For instance, immune responses to vaccination can vary across different ethnic groups (Haralambieva et al., 2014).

A relevant example comes from recent studies on pan–allele peptide-HLA binding predictors, which are designed to predict peptides binding to a given HLA alleles. These models have potential applications in vaccine development, individualized immunotherapy, and beyond.

One recent study found that NetMHCpan4.1 and MHCFlurry2.0 models performed poorly in lower-income populations, which are underrepresented in the training dataset. (Conev et al., 2023). In contrast, Atkins et al. evaluated NetMHCpan-4.1 and 4.0, on a subset of non-European HLA alleles absent from its training data. Despite the model training dataset being heavily skewed toward European Caucasian individuals, they did not observe significant differences in prediction accuracy for the specific non-European alleles tested. This surprising consistency in model performance is noteworthy, as AI models trained on narrow datasets are typically prone to “overfitting”, where the model performs well on its training data but struggles with new, unseen inputs.

The authors suggested that the diversity of sequenced alleles in the training data, along with the broad coverage of genetic sequence space, may have enabled the model to generalize effectively to alleles it had not encountered before. The model's high accuracy on no-European alleles may stem from the model's ability to capture patterns associated with key amino acid residues that influence peptide binding; however, since NetMHCpan is closed-source, its inner workings remain opaque, giving it a 'black box' nature.

6.7 Trust, Bias, and Explainability in AI for Immunology

We should keep in mind that AI models, as revolutionary as they are, represent the latest evolution in a long history of probabilistic models that have been incorporated into medical research and clinical decision-making to support value-based judgment. They face many of the same challenges that medical experts have for decades (Yu et al., 2024). Just as earlier models require careful interpretation, AI systems also demand expert interpretation and careful value judgment. Therefore, researchers and clinicians play a critical role in ensuring that AI implementation in medicine aligns with clinical reasoning and ethical principles.

Recognizing biases of AI models for immune response predictions can be challenging, particularly due to publication biases. Studies that reveal significant biases or null findings are less likely to be accepted for publication, and when such studies are published, they often fail to explore or acknowledge these biases in their limitations. Additionally, there remains a paucity of studies that explore the prevalence of bias among predictive models in immunology.

It is essential to always consider study size, study population, training methods, and statistical methods.

A continuous discussion has been taking place on "Annals of Rheumatic Diseases" in 2019, raising concerns regarding an AI-driven approach to defining subgroups of patients with idiopathic inflammatory myopathy (Pinal-Fernandez et al., 2019). Without delving into the technical aspects of this statistical debate, it underscored the importance of augmented intelligence: the integration of with expert judgment (Mahler et al., 2019).

Moreover, the challenges detailed above highlight the importance of explainable AI models in enhancing trust among patients and clinicians. Recently, Keyl et al., 2025, reported an explainable AI model that predicted treatment outcomes for more than 15,000 patients across various solid cancers, based on multimodal real-world data. The model identified prognostic interactions between markers and, most importantly, demonstrated the ability to quantify the "risk contribution" of each clinical variable to the predicted treatment outcome. Using layer-wise relevance propagation, the model works backward from its prediction, assigning a "relevance score" to each neuron in the network, based on its contribution to the output.

Another interesting example is the development of an explainable AI system to differentiate inflammatory conditions, such as infections, autoimmune diseases, and graft-versus-host diseases. Hoffman et al., 2024, have analyzed the peripheral blood of 118 patients with inflammatory conditions, using complete blood count, CRP analysis, and flow cytometry. The cohorts were designated for training and cross-validation cohorts. Reported accuracy was 81%, with the explainable system allows physicians to understand which clinically relevant parameters contributed to the diagnostic process and identify potential gaps. However, it is important to note the small cohort and the absence of external validation.

The challenges of data collection, including restrictions on data sharing, limit the scope of immunological research. The rarity of some immunological diseases further constrains ambitious studies to small datasets, necessitating data amplification for model training. Additionally, the absence of external validation in some cases, increases the risk of overfitting (Danieli et al., 2022).

To address these limitations, researchers have proposed using decentralized technologies such as blockchain and Swarm Learning in immunology research. Blockchain is a secure system originally developed for cryptocurrencies like "Bitcoin", where information is stored across multiple computers instead of a central server, making data more secured and transparent. Swarm Learning, on the other hand, allows each medical center to function as an independent node within the collaborative network. In this approach, centers train their AI models locally on their own patient data, and then only share the resulting model updates—not the raw patient data—with the network. This ensures that patient privacy is maintained while still benefiting from the collective learning process. Additionally, using standardized datasets helps ensure that information from different centers is compatible and can be effectively integrated (Schultze et al., 2022).

Finally, in the era of AI and amid justified concerns regarding its potential harms, it is important to acknowledge that humans are no less biased. AI tools have the potential to enhance patient care globally and advance health equity - not by achieving superhuman abilities, but more simply by outperforming the average physician.

Moreover, AI models, particularly large language models (LLMs), can aid in bias detection and contribute to the development of structured datasets, further supporting health equity (Pierson et al., 2024).

6.8 Regulatory Hurdles

Regulatory oversight of AI-driven immunological tools, including vaccine development, has intensified as agencies strive to keep pace with rapid innovation. In the United States, the Food and Drug Administration (FDA) uses a risk-based classification system to evaluate software that can influence patient outcomes—known as Software as a Medical Device (SaMD). Per the FDA SaMD Guidelines (2022), developers must demonstrate analytical validity (does the AI model do what it claims?), clinical validity (does it apply correctly in real-world conditions?), and user needs (is it designed with clinicians and patients in mind?). Importantly, if an AI tool continuously retrains on new patient data, it may require ongoing or "real-time" submissions to maintain compliance (FDA, 2022). Elsewhere, the Centers for Biologics Evaluation and Research (CBER) has begun reviewing machine learning–enhanced assays that predict vaccine potency or characterize immune responses, demanding clear documentation of data sources and model performance thresholds (CBER, 2023).

In the European Union, the proposed EU AI Act (European Commission, 2023) categorizes AI systems used in healthcare—particularly for diagnostic or therapeutic purposes—as high-risk. Under this Act, developers must provide detailed risk management strategies, transparency documentation, and evidence of human oversight. Failure to comply may result in substantial penalties, with fines that can reach up to 6% of a company's global annual turnover for serious breaches. Meanwhile, GDPR regulations (European Parliament & Council, 2016) impose strict rules around data processing and consent, requiring de-identification or pseudonymization of patient information used in AI training. These regulations differ from HIPAA in the United States, which focuses on protected health information (PHI) but lacks a single, unified framework for AI's adaptive algorithms. Finally, liability rules also vary: in some European jurisdictions, if an AI tool is viewed merely as "decision support," the clinician might shoulder most of the responsibility for errors, whereas in the U.S., software developers or device manufacturers can face lawsuits if an algorithm's flaw leads to patient harm (Price et al., 2023). Navigating these region-specific guidelines requires robust compliance strategies, transparent reporting, and often direct consultations with regulatory bodies, but doing so can expedite the path from AI innovation to patient-ready solutions.

Below is a quick comparison of the main regulatory frameworks and guidelines relevant to AI in healthcare, each with its own unique approach."

- FDA SaMD: Risk-based classification, re-approval for adaptive AI, etc.
- EU AI Act: High-risk classification, strict fines, mandated human oversight.
- GDPR: Right to be forgotten, explicit consent, heavy data processing rules.
- HIPAA: Focus on PHI protection, less about adaptive AI.

7. WHEN DR. AI SUGGESTS THE WRONG DIAGNOSIS

7.1 Misdiagnoses Caused by Incomplete Patient-Reported Data in AI Systems

Artificial intelligence is transforming immunology by improving diagnostics, predicting disease progression, and personalizing treatments. Machine learning models have demonstrated significant advancements in identifying undiagnosed conditions and optimizing treatment decisions. However, the reliability of AI-driven models is heavily dependent on the quality and completeness of the data they process. Given the crucial role of such data in medical decision-making, ensuring its accuracy is particularly important when applied by large language models. These models, originally trained on diverse datasets, must now adapt to analyzing and interpreting information at the level of an individual patient.

7.2 The Problem of Incomplete Patient-Reported Data

Machine learning algorithms leverage vast amounts of data from electronic health records (EHRs), enabling comprehensive analysis that would be impractical for human review (Rajkomar, 2018). However, these algorithms are inherently limited to the available data, including patient-reported information, which may be missing in a nonrandom manner. This can lead to biases and inaccurate predictions, particularly in immunological disorders where subtle clinical differences significantly impact diagnosis. Inaccurate or missing patient-reported information can cause AI models to misdiagnose conditions, resulting in delayed or inappropriate treatment decisions.

Vulnerable populations, such as those with low socioeconomic status, psychosocial challenges, or immigrant backgrounds (Arpey, 2017; Ng, 2017, Ramoni, 2001), are particularly at risk of being overlooked. These individuals often receive care across multiple institutions and undergo fewer diagnostic tests and treatments, leading to fragmented records that fail to meet algorithmic thresholds for diagnosis or intervention. Missing demographic variables, such as race, ethnicity, and language, exacerbate these issues, particularly when algorithms trained in one institution are applied elsewhere, leading to flawed predictions and inequitable healthcare outcomes due to "overfitting" to the training data. While machine learning techniques exist to account for missing data, they are inconsistently applied. Expanding data integration across institutions and ensuring diverse representation in datasets and clinical trials could mitigate these biases, though challenges persist in capturing information for individuals who remain outside traditional healthcare systems (Gianfrancesco et al., 2018).

7.3 Limitations of Large Language Models: Misdiagnoses and Biases

Although AI models offer great potential, they are not infallible. The use of LLMs does not inherently improve physicians' diagnostic reasoning beyond traditional resources (Goh et al., 2024). General-purpose LLMs lack rigorous medical validation, making them susceptible to producing inaccurate or misleading outputs that may appear authoritative, potentially contributing to clinical misjudgments.

Only recently, a study conducted in July 2023 on ChatGPT-3.5's diagnostic accuracy in pediatric cases found an 83% error rate, with only 56.7% of incorrect diagnoses belonging to the same organ system as the correct diagnosis (e.g., psoriasis misdiagnosed as seborrheic dermatitis) (Barile, 2024). AI systems are evolving rapidly, yet another evaluation of GPT-4 revealed biases in modeling the demographic diversity of medical conditions. The model consistently generated stereotyped clinical vignettes, disproportionately associating certain diagnoses with specific races, ethnicities, and genders, raising concerns about bias in AI-driven medical applications. For example, GPT-4 exhibited bias in differential diagnoses, altering rankings by gender (21%) and race (32%). It recommended fewer imaging tests for Black patients (-9%) and showed biases in pain perception and substance use assessments. Notably, many of the clinical vignettes used in the study were immunology-related, including cases of rheumatoid arthritis, systemic sclerosis, HIV, sarcoidosis, and more, highlighting the significance of this issue in clinical immunology (Zack et al., 2024). A broader study assessing multiple LLMs (Llama 2, Open Assistant (OASST), WizardLM) and medical-domain-aligned models (Clinical Camel, Meditron) found that they performed significantly worse than clinicians across all four chosen diseases and failed to mimic a physician's decision-making process (Hager et al., 2024).

However, with the rapid advancements in LLM reasoning and medical capabilities, newer models such as ChatGPT-o3 (optimized for reasoning) and OpenEvidence (trained on medical literature) have yet to be evaluated in high-quality, peer-reviewed studies.

7.4 The Human-in-the-Loop: Cognitive Shortcuts and Automation Bias

A significant challenge in recognizing AI-related misdiagnoses stems from the human tendency to adopt cognitive shortcuts, leading to an overestimation of AI model capabilities and an overreliance on automation systems. This phenomenon, known as automation bias, can cause clinicians to accept AI-generated recommendations without sufficient scrutiny. However, a careful review of AI-generated outputs is essential to maintaining accurate and comprehensive documentation.

A "human-in-the-loop" approach is necessary, wherein physician oversight plays a critical role in mitigating the risk of errors and ensuring diagnostic reliability (Ohde et al., 2025). Without such oversight, AI models can reinforce existing biases and contribute to erroneous clinical decisions, ultimately compromising patient safety.

7.5 Examples of AI-Related Misdiagnoses

AI-driven misdiagnoses are not limited to LLM-based models; they have been observed across various medical specialties.

In neurology, AI systems frequently misclassify Parkinsonian tremor as essential tremor (Landi et al., 2020). In cardiology, AI struggles to distinguish between sepsis-induced cardiomyopathy and acute myocardial infarction (AMI) in patients with sepsis due to substantial overlap in clinical presentation and biomarker profiles. This ambiguity may lead to inappropriate treatment strategies, potentially worsening patient outcomes (Fang et al., 2024).

7.6 Successful Applications of Diagnostic AI in Immunology

Despite these challenges, artificial intelligence and machine learning models specifically trained on clinical data derived from electronic health records (EHRs), have shown promising results in immunology, particularly in disease detection and predicting treatment responses.

In the field of early diagnosis using EHRs, Johnson et al. developed PheNet, a machine learning model designed to analyze EHRs and rank individuals based on their likelihood of having common variable immunodeficiency (CVID). CVID is often diagnosed 5 to 15 years after symptom onset, but PheNet, which relies exclusively on phenotypic characteristics, has demonstrated greater accuracy than existing risk scores in predicting CVID, enabling earlier intervention (Johnson et al., 2024). Forrest et al. developed a machine learning model to identify patients needing rheumatological evaluation for systemic autoimmune rheumatic diseases (SARDs). The model, trained on longitudinal EHRs from 161,584 individuals, outperformed clinical standards by detecting autoantibody carriers up to five years before conventional assessments (Forrest et al., 2024).

Yang et al. developed nine machine learning models for predicting proliferative lupus nephritis (PLN), with seven demonstrating excellent accuracy in testing cohort. These models confirmed the efficacy of known biomarkers and identified new predictive indicators, such as serum chloride, neutrophil percentage, and serum cystatin C, which could improve patient management. However, the authors warned that since the model was trained on a single-center Chinese cohort, it is crucial to refine it with multicenter data from various populations (Yang et al., 2024).

AI holds immense promise for transforming immunology and other medical fields by enhancing diagnostics, improving disease risk stratification, and optimizing treatment decisions. However, its effectiveness is limited by incomplete patient-reported data, biases in training datasets, and automation bias in clinical settings. To mitigate these risks, AI-driven models must be developed and implemented with rigorous medical validation, physician oversight, and robust data integration. As AI continues to evolve, balancing its benefits with necessary safeguards will be critical to ensuring its safe and effective use in healthcare.

8. CONCLUSION

Building on these observations, the future of AI in immunology lies in fostering collaboration between technologists, immunologists, ethicists, and policymakers. Addressing challenges such as de-skilling among clinicians, biases in AI models, and disparities in access to AI technologies requires concerted efforts across multiple domains. Ensuring that AI systems are designed with inclusivity, adaptability, and patient-centered care at their core is essential to bridging the gap between technological advancements and real-world healthcare needs.

Moreover, the dynamic nature of immunology necessitates that AI models are not only continuously updated but also subjected to rigorous oversight. Ethical frameworks must evolve in parallel, focusing on transparency, patient autonomy, and equitable benefits distribution. By embedding these principles into the development and deployment of AI systems, the healthcare community can mitigate risks while maximizing the transformative potential of AI.

Ultimately, AI's integration into immunology should not replace human expertise but rather amplify it, creating a synergy where technology and clinicians together provide more accurate, efficient, and empathetic care. By addressing the technical, ethical, and practical barriers comprehensively, AI can become a cornerstone of modern immunology, driving breakthroughs that benefit patients and global health alike. The path forward requires balance - leveraging AI's capabilities while preserving the irreplaceable human elements of medical practice.

The future of AI in immunology holds exciting potential, as advancements in AI technologies continue to accelerate. With the growing complexity of immunological diseases and the increasing availability of large-scale data, AI could play a pivotal role in revolutionizing the way we understand and treat immune-related disorders. Future applications may include the development of personalized immunotherapies by integrating genomic, proteomic, and clinical data to identify individualized treatment strategies. The potential to transform diagnostic, therapeutic, and preventative strategies in immunology promises a future where AI enhances the speed and accuracy of medical advances and the accessibility of tailored treatments.

REFERENCES

Abraham, G., Tye-Din, J. A., Bhalala, O. G., Kowalczyk, A., Zobel, J., & Inouye, M. (2014, February 13). Accurate and robust genomic prediction of celiac disease using statistical learning. *PLOS Genetics, 10*(2), e1004137. DOI: 10.1371/journal.pgen.1004137 PMID: 24550740

Aggarwal, R., Farag, S., Martin, G., Ashrafian, H., & Darzi, A. (2021, August 26). Patient Perceptions on Data Sharing and Applying Artificial Intelligence to Health Care Data: Cross-sectional Survey. *Journal of Medical Internet Research, 23*(8), e26162. DOI: 10.2196/26162 PMID: 34236994

Alber, D. A., Yang, Z., Alyakin, A., Yang, E., Rai, S., Valliani, A. A., Zhang, J., Rosenbaum, G. R., Amend-Thomas, A. K., Kurland, D. B., Kremer, C. M., Eremiev, A., Negash, B., Wiggan, D. D., Nakatsuka, M. A., Sangwon, K. L., Neifert, S. N., Khan, H. A., Save, A. V., & Oermann, E. K. (2025, January 8). Medical large language models are vulnerable to data-poisoning attacks. *Nature Medicine, 31*(2), 618–626. Advance online publication. DOI: 10.1038/s41591-024-03445-1 PMID: 39779928

Alderman, J. E., Palmer, J., Laws, E., McCradden, M. D., Ordish, J., Ghassemi, M., Pfohl, S. R., Rostamzadeh, N., Cole-Lewis, H., Glocker, B., Calvert, M., Pollard, T. J., Gill, J., Gath, J., Adebajo, A., Beng, J., Leung, C. H., Kuku, S., Farmer, L. A., & Liu, X. (2025, January). Tackling algorithmic bias and promoting transparency in health datasets: The STANDING Together consensus recommendations. *The Lancet. Digital Health, 7*(1), e64–e88. DOI: 10.1016/S2589-7500(24)00224-3 PMID: 39701919

Arpey, N. C., Gaglioti, A. H., & Rosenbaum, M. E. (2017, July). How Socioeconomic Status Affects Patient Perceptions of Health Care: A Qualitative Study. *Journal of Primary Care & Community Health, 8*(3), 169–175. DOI: 10.1177/2150131917697439 PMID: 28606031

Asnicar, F., Thomas, A. M., Passerini, A., Waldron, L., & Segata, N. (2024, April). Machine learning for microbiologists. *Nature Reviews. Microbiology, 22*(4), 191–205. DOI: 10.1038/s41579-023-00984-1 PMID: 37968359

Atkins, T. K., Solanki, A., Vasmatzis, G., Cornette, J., & Riedel, M. (2024, January 16). Evaluating NetMHCpan performance on non-European HLA alleles not present in training data. *Frontiers in Immunology, 14*, 1288105. DOI: 10.3389/fimmu.2023.1288105 PMID: 38292493

Aung, Y. Y. M., Wong, D. C. S., & Ting, D. S. W. (2021, September 10). The promise of artificial intelligence: A review of the opportunities and challenges of artificial intelligence in healthcare. *British Medical Bulletin, 139*(1), 4–15. DOI: 10.1093/bmb/ldab016 PMID: 34405854

Ayers, J. W., Poliak, A., Dredze, M., Leas, E. C., Zhu, Z., Kelley, J. B., Faix, D. J., Goodman, A. M., Longhurst, C. A., Hogarth, M., & Smith, D. M. (2023, June 1). Comparing Physician and Artificial Intelligence Chatbot Responses to Patient Questions Posted to a Public Social Media Forum. *JAMA Internal Medicine, 183*(6), 589–596. DOI: 10.1001/jamainternmed.2023.1838 PMID: 37115527

Barile, J., Margolis, A., Cason, G., Kim, R., Kalash, S., Tchaconas, A., & Milanaik, R. (2024, March 1). Diagnostic Accuracy of a Large Language Model in Pediatric Case Studies. *JAMA Pediatrics, 178*(3), 313–315. DOI: 10.1001/jamapediatrics.2023.5750 PMID: 38165685

Batista, F. D., & Dustin, M. L. (2013, January). Cell:cell interactions in the immune system. *Immunological Reviews*, *251*(1), 7–12. DOI: 10.1111/imr.12025 PMID: 23278736

Beck, J. T., Rammage, M., Jackson, G. P., Preininger, A. M., Dankwa-Mullan, I., Roebuck, M. C., Torres, A., Holtzen, H., Coverdill, S. E., Williamson, M. P., Chau, Q., Rhee, K., & Vinegra, M. (2020, January). Artificial Intelligence Tool for Optimizing Eligibility Screening for Clinical Trials in a Large Community Cancer Center. *JCO Clinical Cancer Informatics*, *4*(4), 50–59. DOI: 10.1200/CCI.19.00079 PMID: 31977254

Bhat, A. A., Nisar, S., Mukherjee, S., Saha, N., Yarravarapu, N., Lone, S. N., Masoodi, T., Chauhan, R., Maacha, S., Bagga, P., Dhawan, P., Akil, A. A., El-Rifai, W., Uddin, S., Reddy, R., Singh, M., Macha, M. A., & Haris, M. (2022, November 18). Integration of CRISPR/Cas9 with artificial intelligence for improved cancer therapeutics. *Journal of Translational Medicine*, *20*(1), 534. DOI: 10.1186/s12967-022-03765-1 PMID: 36401282

Bohr, A., & Memarzadeh, K. (2020). The rise of artificial intelligence in healthcare applications. In *Artificial Intelligence in healthcare* (pp. 25–60). Academic Press.

Budin-Ljøsne, I., Teare, H. J., Kaye, J., Beck, S., Bentzen, H. B., Caenazzo, L., Collett, C., D'Abramo, F., Felzmann, H., Finlay, T., Javaid, M. K., Jones, E., Katić, V., Simpson, A., & Mascalzoni, D. (2017, January 25). Dynamic Consent: A potential solution to some of the challenges of modern biomedical research. *BMC Medical Ethics*, *18*(1), 4. DOI: 10.1186/s12910-016-0162-9 PMID: 28122615

Chandler, M., Jain, S., Halman, J., Hong, E., Dobrovolskaia, M. A., Zakharov, A. V., & Afonin, K. A. (2022, November). Artificial Immune Cell, AI-cell, a New Tool to Predict Interferon Production by Peripheral Blood Monocytes in Response to Nucleic Acid Nanoparticles. *Small*, *18*(46), e2204941. DOI: 10.1002/smll.202204941 PMID: 36216772

Chang, R. B., & Beatty, G. L. (2020, July). The interplay between innate and adaptive immunity in cancer shapes the productivity of cancer immunosurveillance. *Journal of Leukocyte Biology*, *108*(1), 363–376. DOI: 10.1002/JLB.3MIR0320-475R PMID: 32272502

Chang, T. G., Cao, Y., Sfreddo, H. J., Dhruba, S. R., Lee, S. H., Valero, C., Yoo, S. K., Chowell, D., Morris, L. G. T., & Ruppin, E. (2024, August). LORIS robustly predicts patient outcomes with immune checkpoint blockade therapy using common clinical, pathologic and genomic features. *Nature Cancer*, *5*(8), 1158–1175. DOI: 10.1038/s43018-024-00772-7 PMID: 38831056

Chen, M., Zhang, B., Cai, Z., Seery, S., Gonzalez, M. J., Ali, N. M., Ren, R., Qiao, Y., Xue, P., & Jiang, Y. (2022, August 31). Acceptance of clinical artificial intelligence among physicians and medical students: A systematic review with cross-sectional survey. *Frontiers in Medicine*, *9*, 990604. DOI: 10.3389/fmed.2022.990604 PMID: 36117979

Chin, A., & Rider, N. L. (2022). Artificial Intelligence in Clinical Immunology. In Lidströmer, N., & Ashrafian, H. (Eds.), *Artificial Intelligence in Medicine*. Springer., DOI: 10.1007/978-3-030-64573-1_83

Chowell, D., Yoo, S. K., Valero, C., Pastore, A., Krishna, C., Lee, M., Hoen, D., Shi, H., Kelly, D. W., Patel, N., Makarov, V., Ma, X., Vuong, L., Sabio, E. Y., Weiss, K., Kuo, F., Lenz, T. L., Samstein, R. M., Riaz, N., & Chan, T. A. (2022, April). Improved prediction of immune checkpoint blockade efficacy across multiple cancer types. *Nature Biotechnology*, *40*(4), 499–506. DOI: 10.1038/s41587-021-01070-8 PMID: 34725502

Conev, A., Fasoulis, R., Hall-Swan, S., Ferreira, R., & Kavraki, L. E. (2023, December 2). HLAEquity: Examining biases in pan-allele peptide-HLA binding predictors. *iScience*, *27*(1), 108613. DOI: 10.1016/j.isci.2023.108613 PMID: 38188519

Cortese, M., Hagan, T., Rouphael, N., Wu, S. Y., Xie, X., Kazmin, D., Wimmers, F., Gupta, S., van der Most, R., Coccia, M., Aranuchalam, P. S., Nakaya, H. I., Wang, Y., Coyle, E., Horiuchi, S., Wu, H., Bower, M., Mehta, A., Gunthel, C., & Pulendran, B. (2025, January). System vaccinology analysis of predictors and mechanisms of antibody response durability to multiple vaccines in humans. *Nature Immunology*, *26*(1), 116–130. DOI: 10.1038/s41590-024-02036-z PMID: 39747435

Danieli, M. G., Brunetto, S., Gammeri, L., Palmeri, D., Claudi, I., Shoenfeld, Y., & Gangemi, S. (2024, February). Machine learning application in autoimmune diseases: State of art and future prospectives. *Autoimmunity Reviews*, *23*(2), 103496. DOI: 10.1016/j.autrev.2023.103496 PMID: 38081493

Danieli, M. G., Tonacci, A., Paladini, A., Longhi, E., Moroncini, G., Allegra, A., Sansone, F., & Gangemi, S. (2022, June). A machine learning analysis to predict the response to intravenous and subcutaneous immunoglobulin in inflammatory myopathies. A proposal for a future multi-omics approach in autoimmune diseases. *Autoimmunity Reviews*, *21*(6), 103105. DOI: 10.1016/j.autrev.2022.103105 PMID: 35452850

Fang, S., Jin, H., Zhang, J., Wang, Y., Nan, W., Feng, Y., Su, W., & Jiang, X. (2024, December 24). Machine learning for predicting acute myocardial infarction in patients with sepsis. *Scientific Reports*, *14*(1), 30629. DOI: 10.1038/s41598-024-80575-z PMID: 39719483

Farhud, D. D., & Zokaei, S. (2021, November). Ethical Issues of Artificial Intelligence in Medicine and Healthcare. *Iranian Journal of Public Health*, *50*(11), i–v. DOI: 10.18502/ijph.v50i11.7600 PMID: 35223619

Farzan, R. (2024, January 31). Artificial intelligence in Immuno-genetics. *Bioinformation*, *20*(1), 29–35. DOI: 10.6026/973206300200029 PMID: 38352901

Fogo, A. B., Kronbichler, A., & Bajema, I. M. A. (2024, February 13). I's Threat to the Medical Profession. *Journal of the American Medical Association*, *331*(6), 471–472. DOI: 10.1001/jama.2024.0018 PMID: 38241042

Forrest, I. S., Petrazzini, B. O., Duffy, Á., Park, J. K., O'Neal, A. J., Jordan, D. M., Rocheleau, G., Nadkarni, G. N., Cho, J. H., Blazer, A. D., & Do, R. (2023, April 25). A machine learning model identifies patients in need of autoimmune disease testing using electronic health records. *Nature Communications*, *14*(1), 2385. DOI: 10.1038/s41467-023-37996-7 PMID: 37169741

Frasca, M., La Torre, D., Pravettoni, G., & Cutica, I. (2024). Explainable and interpretable artificial intelligence in medicine: A systematic bibliometric review. *Discover Artificial Intelligence*, *4*(1), 15. DOI: 10.1007/s44163-024-00114-7

Garfinkle, E. A., & Mardis, E. R. (2025). Cancer Immunogenomics Approaches and Applications to Cancer Vaccines. *Cancer Journal (Sudbury, Mass.)*, *31*(2), e0762.

Garg, A. D. (2023, August). The dynamic interface of genetics and immunity: Toward future horizons in health & disease. *Genes and Immunity*, *24*(4), 155–158. DOI: 10.1038/s41435-023-00213-y PMID: 37464025

Germain, R. N., Van Allen, E. M., Trynka, G., Tsang, J. S., Grün, D., Kiemen, A. L., Shi, Y., Pugh Bernard, A., & Nolan, G. P. (2024, June 11). AI and immunology. *Immunity*, *57*(6), 1177–1181. DOI: 10.1016/j.immuni.2024.05.016 PMID: 38865960

Gianfrancesco, M. A., Tamang, S., Yazdany, J., & Schmajuk, G. (2018, November 1). Potential Biases in Machine Learning Algorithms Using Electronic Health Record Data. *JAMA Internal Medicine*, *178*(11), 1544–1547. DOI: 10.1001/jamainternmed.2018.3763 PMID: 30128552

Goh, E., Gallo, R., Hom, J., Strong, E., Weng, Y., Kerman, H., Cool, J. A., Kanjee, Z., Parsons, A. S., Ahuja, N., Horvitz, E., Yang, D., Milstein, A., Olson, A. P. J., Rodman, A., & Chen, J. H. (2024, October 1). Large Language Model Influence on Diagnostic Reasoning: A Randomized Clinical Trial. *JAMA Network Open*, *7*(10), e2440969. DOI: 10.1001/jamanetworkopen.2024.40969 PMID: 39466245

Goldberg, C. B., Adams, L., Blumenthal, D., Brennan, P. F., Brown, N., Butte, A. J., Cheatham, M., deBronkart, D., Dixon, J., Drazen, J., Evans, B. J., Hoffman, S. M., Holmes, C., Lee, P., Manrai, A. K., Omenn, G. S., Perlin, J. B., Ramoni, R., Sapiro, G., & Kohane, I. S. (2024, March). RAISE Consortium. To do no harm - and the most good - with AI in health care. *Nature Medicine*, *30*(3), 623–627. DOI: 10.1038/s41591-024-02853-7 PMID: 38388841

Goldberg, C. B., Adams, L., Blumenthal, D., Brennan, P. F., Brown, N., Butte, A. J., Cheatham, M., deBronkart, D., Dixon, J., Drazen, J., Evans, B. J., Hoffman, S. M., Holmes, C., Lee, P., Manrai, A. K., Omenn, G. S., Perlin, J. B., Ramoni, R., Sapiro, G., & Kohane, I. S. (2024, March). RAISE Consortium. To do no harm - and the most good - with AI in health care. *Nature Medicine*, *30*(3), 623–627. DOI: 10.1038/s41591-024-02853-7 PMID: 38388841

Gossec, L., Kedra, J., Servy, H., Pandit, A., Stones, S., Berenbaum, F., Finckh, A., Baraliakos, X., Stamm, T. A., Gomez-Cabrero, D., Pristipino, C., Choquet, R., Burmester, G. R., & Radstake, T. R. D. J. (2020, January). EULAR points to consider for the use of big data in rheumatic and musculoskeletal diseases. *Annals of the Rheumatic Diseases*, *79*(1), 69–76. DOI: 10.1136/annrheumdis-2019-215694 PMID: 31229952

Hager, P., Jungmann, F., Holland, R., Bhagat, K., Hubrecht, I., Knauer, M., Vielhauer, J., Makowski, M., Braren, R., Kaissis, G., & Rueckert, D. (2024, September). Evaluation and mitigation of the limitations of large language models in clinical decision-making. *Nature Medicine*, *30*(9), 2613–2622. DOI: 10.1038/s41591-024-03097-1 PMID: 38965432

Haralambieva, I. H., Salk, H. M., Lambert, N. D., Ovsyannikova, I. G., Kennedy, R. B., Warner, N. D., Pankratz, V. S., & Poland, G. A. (2014, April 7). Associations between race, sex and immune response variations to rubella vaccination in two independent cohorts. *Vaccine*, *32*(17), 1946–1953. DOI: 10.1016/j.vaccine.2014.01.090 PMID: 24530932

Hoffmann, J., Rheude, A., Neubauer, A., Brendel, C., & Thrun, M. C. (2024, March 6). Development of an explainable AI system using routine clinical parameters for rapid differentiation of inflammatory conditions. *Frontiers in Immunology*, *15*, 1364954. DOI: 10.3389/fimmu.2024.1364954 PMID: 38510238

Hu, Q., Chen, Y., Zou, D., He, Z., & Xu, T. (2024, November 13). Predicting adverse drug event using machine learning based on electronic health records: A systematic review and meta-analysis. *Frontiers in Pharmacology*, *15*, 1497397. DOI: 10.3389/fphar.2024.1497397 PMID: 39605909

Ifargan, T., Hafner, L., Kern, M., Alcalay, O., & Kishony, R. (2025). Autonomous LLM-driven research from data to human-verifiable research papers. *NEJM AI*, *2*(1). Advance online publication. DOI: 10.1056/AIoa2400555

Jarczak, D., & Nierhaus, A. (2022, October 3). Cytokine Storm-Definition, Causes, and Implications. *International Journal of Molecular Sciences*, *23*(19), 11740. DOI: 10.3390/ijms231911740 PMID: 36233040

Jiang, F., Jiang, Y., Zhi, H., Dong, Y., Li, H., Ma, S., Wang, Y., Dong, Q., Shen, H., & Wang, Y. (2017). Artificial intelligence in healthcare: Past, present and future. *Stroke and Vascular Neurology*, *2*(4), e000101. DOI: 10.1136/svn-2017-000101 PMID: 29507784

Johnson, K. W., Torres Soto, J., Glicksberg, B. S., Shameer, K., Miotto, R., Ali, M., Ashley, E., & Dudley, J. T. (2018, June 12). Artificial Intelligence in Cardiology. *Journal of the American College of Cardiology*, *71*(23), 2668–2679. DOI: 10.1016/j.jacc.2018.03.521 PMID: 29880128

Johnson, R., Stephens, A. V., Mester, R., Knyazev, S., Kohn, L. A., Freund, M. K., Bondhus, L., Hill, B. L., Schwarz, T., Zaitlen, N., Arboleda, V. A. A., Bastarache, L., Pasaniuc, B., & Butte, M. J. (2024, May). Electronic health record signatures identify undiagnosed patients with common variable immunodeficiency disease. *Science Translational Medicine*, *16*(745), eade4510. Advance online publication. DOI: 10.1126/scitranslmed.ade4510 PMID: 38691621

Kaushik, R., Kant, R., & Christodoulides, M. (2023). Artificial intelligence in accelerating vaccine development - current and future perspectives. *Front. Bacteriol.*, *2*, 1258159. DOI: 10.3389/fbrio.2023.1258159

Keyl, J., Keyl, P., Montavon, G., Hosch, R., Brehmer, A., Mochmann, L., Jurmeister, P., Dernbach, G., Kim, M., Koitka, S., Bauer, S., Bechrakis, N., Forsting, M., Führer-Sakel, D., Glas, M., Grünwald, V., Hadaschik, B., Haubold, J., Herrmann, K., & Kleesiek, J. (2025, January 30). Decoding pan-cancer treatment outcomes using multimodal real-world data and explainable artificial intelligence. *Nature Cancer*, *6*(2), 307–322. Advance online publication. DOI: 10.1038/s43018-024-00891-1 PMID: 39885364

Landi, I., Glicksberg, B. S., Lee, H. C., Cherng, S., Landi, G., Danieletto, M., Dudley, J. T., Furlanello, C., & Miotto, R. (2020, July 17). Deep representation learning of electronic health records to unlock patient stratification at scale. *NPJ Digital Medicine*, *3*(1), 96. DOI: 10.1038/s41746-020-0301-z PMID: 32699826

Lu, M. Y., Chen, B., Williamson, D. F. K., Chen, R. J., Zhao, M., Chow, A. K., Ikemura, K., Kim, A., Pouli, D., Patel, A., Soliman, A., Chen, C., Ding, T., Wang, J. J., Gerber, G., Liang, I., Le, L. P., Parwani, A. V., Weishaupt, L. L., & Mahmood, F. (2024, October). A multimodal generative AI copilot for human pathology. *Nature*, *634*(8033), 466–473. DOI: 10.1038/s41586-024-07618-3 PMID: 38866050

Luciani, F., Safavi, A., Guruprasad, P., Chen, L., & Ruella, M. (2025, March 28). Advancing CAR T-cell Therapies with Artificial Intelligence: Opportunities and Challenges. *Blood Cancer Discovery*, •••, OF1–OF4. Advance online publication. DOI: 10.1158/2643-3230.BCD-23-0240 PMID: 40152695

Luxton, D. D. (2014, September). Recommendations for the ethical use and design of artificial intelligent care providers. *Artificial Intelligence in Medicine*, *62*(1), 1–10. DOI: 10.1016/j.artmed.2014.06.004 PMID: 25059820

Mahler, M., Rossin, B., & Kubassova, O. (2020, December). Augmented versus artificial intelligence for stratification of patients with myositis. *Annals of the Rheumatic Diseases*, *79*(12), e162. DOI: 10.1136/annrheumdis-2019-216000 PMID: 31362996

Martinson, A. K., Chin, A. T., Butte, M. J., & Rider, N. L. (2024, October). Artificial Intelligence and Machine Learning for Inborn Errors of Immunity: Current State and Future Promise. *The Journal of Allergy and Clinical Immunology. In Practice*, *12*(10), 2695–2704. DOI: 10.1016/j.jaip.2024.08.012 PMID: 39127104

Mazzocco, G., Niemiec, I., Myronov, A., Skoczylas, P., Kaczmarczyk, J., Sanecka-Duin, A., Gruba, K., Król, P., Drwal, M., Szczepanik, M., Pyrc, K., & St pniak, P. (2021, March 25). AI Aided Design of Epitope-Based Vaccine for the Induction of Cellular Immune Responses Against SARS-CoV-2. *Frontiers in Genetics*, *12*, 602196. DOI: 10.3389/fgene.2021.602196 PMID: 33841493

Meszaros, J., Minari, J., & Huys, I. (2022, October 4). The future regulation of artificial intelligence systems in healthcare services and medical research in the European Union. *Frontiers in Genetics*, *13*, 927721. DOI: 10.3389/fgene.2022.927721 PMID: 36267404

Molnár-Gábor, F. (2019). Artificial intelligence in healthcare: doctors, patients and liabilities. In *Regulating artificial intelligence* (pp. 337–360). Springer International Publishing.

Momtazmanesh, S., Nowroozi, A., & Rezaei, N. (2022, October). Artificial Intelligence in Rheumatoid Arthritis: Current Status and Future Perspectives: A State-of-the-Art Review. *Rheumatology and Therapy*, *9*(5), 1249–1304. DOI: 10.1007/s40744-022-00475-4 PMID: 35849321

Muehlematter, U. J., Bluethgen, C., & Vokinger, K. N. (2023, September). FDA-cleared artificial intelligence and machine learning-based medical devices and their 510(k) predicate networks. *The Lancet. Digital Health*, *5*(9), e618–e626. DOI: 10.1016/S2589-7500(23)00126-7 PMID: 37625896

Ng, J. H., Ye, F., Ward, L. M., Haffer, S. C., & Scholle, S. H. (2017, March 1). Data On Race, Ethnicity, And Language Largely Incomplete For Managed Care Plan Members. *Health Affairs (Project Hope)*, *36*(3), 548–552. DOI: 10.1377/hlthaff.2016.1044 PMID: 28264958

Obermeyer, Z., & Lee, T. H. (2017, September 28). Lost in Thought - The Limits of the Human Mind and the Future of Medicine. *The New England Journal of Medicine*, *377*(13), 1209–1211. DOI: 10.1056/NEJMp1705348 PMID: 28953443

Ohde, J. W., Rost, L. M., & Overgaard, J. D. (2025, January 13). The burden of reviewing LLM-generated content. *NEJM AI*, *2*(2). Advance online publication. DOI: 10.1056/AIp2400979

Olawade, D. B., Teke, J., Fapohunda, O., Weerasinghe, K., Usman, S. O., Ige, A. O., & Clement David-Olawade, A. (2024, September). Leveraging artificial intelligence in vaccine development: A narrative review. *Journal of Microbiological Methods*, *224*, 106998. DOI: 10.1016/j.mimet.2024.106998 PMID: 39019262

Panesar, S. S., Kliot, M., Parrish, R., Fernandez-Miranda, J., Cagle, Y., & Britz, G. W. (2020, July 1). Promises and Perils of Artificial Intelligence in Neurosurgery. *Neurosurgery*, *87*(1), 33–44. DOI: 10.1093/neuros/nyz471 PMID: 31748800

Pasquale, F. (2020). *New Laws of Robotics: Defending Human Expertise in the Age of AI*. The Belknap Press of Harvard University Press.

Patel, P. M., Green, M., Tram, J., Wang, E., Murphy, M. Z., Abd-Elsayed, A., & Chakravarthy, K. (2024, December 11). Beyond the Pain Management Clinic: The Role of AI-Integrated Remote Patient Monitoring in Chronic Disease Management - A Narrative Review. *Journal of Pain Research*, *17*, 4223–4237. DOI: 10.2147/JPR.S494238 PMID: 39679431

Pierson, E., Shanmugam, D., Movva, R., Kleinberg, J., Agrawal, M., Dredze, M., Ferryman, K., Gichoya, J. W., Jurafsky, D., Koh, P. W., Levy, K., Mullainathan, S., Obermeyer, Z., Suresh, H., & Vafa, K. (2025). Using Large Language Models to Promote Health Equity. *NEJM AI*, *2*(2). Advance online publication. DOI: 10.1056/AIp2400889

Pinal-Fernandez, I., & Mammen, A. L. (2020, October). On using machine learning algorithms to define clinically meaningful patient subgroups. *Annals of the Rheumatic Diseases*, *79*(10), e128. DOI: 10.1136/annrheumdis-2019-215852 PMID: 31227486

Price, W.II. (2023). Nicholson; Gerke, Sara; Cohen, I. Glenn. "Liability for use of artificial intelligence in medicine.". In *Research Handbook on Health, AI and the Law*. Edward Elgar Publishing Ltd.

Quinn, T. P., Senadeera, M., Jacobs, S., Coghlan, S., & Le, V. (2021, March 18). Trust and medical AI: The challenges we face and the expertise needed to overcome them. *Journal of the American Medical Informatics Association : JAMIA*, *28*(4), 890–894. DOI: 10.1093/jamia/ocaa268 PMID: 33340404

Quintana-Murci, L., & Clark, A. G. (2013, April). Population genetic tools for dissecting innate immunity in humans. *Nature Reviews. Immunology*, *13*(4), 280–293. DOI: 10.1038/nri3421 PMID: 23470320

Raikar, G. V. S., Raikar, A. S., & Somnache, S. N. (2023). Advancements in artificial intelligence and machine learning in revolutionising biomarker discovery. *Brazilian Journal of Pharmaceutical Sciences*, *59*, e23146.

Rajkomar, A., Oren, E., Chen, K., Dai, A. M., Hajaj, N., Hardt, M., Liu, P. J., Liu, X., Marcus, J., Sun, M., Sundberg, P., Yee, H., Zhang, K., Zhang, Y., Flores, G., Duggan, G. E., Irvine, J., Le, Q., Litsch, K., & Dean, J. (2018, May 8). Scalable and accurate deep learning with electronic health records. *NPJ Digital Medicine*, *1*(1), 18. DOI: 10.1038/s41746-018-0029-1 PMID: 31304302

Rakaee, M., Tafavvoghi, M., Ricciuti, B., Alessi, J. V., Cortellini, A., Citarella, F., Nibid, L., Perrone, G., Adib, E., Fulgenzi, C. A. M., Murilo Hidalgo Filho, C., Di Federico, A., Jabar, F., Hashemi, S., Houda, I., Richardsen, E., Rasmussen Busund, L. T., Donnem, T., Bahce, I., & Kwiatkowski, D. J. (2024, December 26). Deep Learning Model for Predicting Immunotherapy Response in Advanced Non-Small Cell Lung Cancer. *JAMA Oncology*, ●●●. Advance online publication. DOI: 10.1001/jamaoncol.2024.5356 PMID: 39724105

Ramoni, M., & Sebastiani, P. (2001, November). Robust learning with missing data. *Machine Learning*, *45*(2), 147–170. DOI: 10.1023/A:1010968702992

Rappuoli, R., Alter, G., & Pulendran, B. (2024, September 19). Transforming vaccinology. *Cell*, *187*(19), 5171–5194. DOI: 10.1016/j.cell.2024.07.021 PMID: 39303685

Ratwani, R. M., Sutton, K., Galarraga, J. E., & Addressing, A. I. (2024, October 1). Algorithmic Bias in Health Care. *Journal of the American Medical Association*, *332*(13), 1051–1052. DOI: 10.1001/jama.2024.13486 PMID: 39230911

Reddy, S. (2022, April). Explainability and artificial intelligence in medicine. *The Lancet. Digital Health*, *4*(4), e214–e215. DOI: 10.1016/S2589-7500(22)00029-2 PMID: 35337639

Schultze, J. L., Büttner, M., & Becker, M. (2022, July). Swarm immunology: Harnessing blockchain technology and artificial intelligence in human immunology. *Nature Reviews. Immunology*, *22*(7), 401–403. DOI: 10.1038/s41577-022-00740-1 PMID: 35624333

Schultze, J. L., Büttner, M., & Becker, M. (2022, July). Swarm immunology: Harnessing blockchain technology and artificial intelligence in human immunology. *Nature Reviews. Immunology*, *22*(7), 401–403. DOI: 10.1038/s41577-022-00740-1 PMID: 35624333

Shah, N. H., Entwistle, D., & Pfeffer, M. A. (2023, September 5). Creation and Adoption of Large Language Models in Medicine. *Journal of the American Medical Association*, *330*(9), 866–869. DOI: 10.1001/jama.2023.14217 PMID: 37548965

Shah, N. H., Entwistle, D., & Pfeffer, M. A. (2023, September 5). Creation and Adoption of Large Language Models in Medicine. *Journal of the American Medical Association*, *330*(9), 866–869. DOI: 10.1001/jama.2023.14217 PMID: 37548965

Shoghli, A., Darvish, M., & Sadeghian, Y. (2024). Balancing Innovation and Privacy: Ethical Challenges in AI-Driven Healthcare. *Journal of Research in Medical Sciences : the Official Journal of Isfahan University of Medical Sciences*, *4*(1), 1–11. DOI: 10.22034/jrms.2024.494112.1034

Singh, Y., Patel, H., Vera-Garcia, D. V., Hathaway, Q. A., Sarkar, D., & Quaia, E. (2024, November 7). Beyond the hype: Navigating bias in AI-driven cancer detection. *Oncotarget*, *15*(1), 764–766. DOI: 10.18632/oncotarget.28665 PMID: 39513852

Skevaki, C., Nadeau, K. C., Rothenberg, M. E., Alahmad, B., Mmbaga, B. T., Masenga, G. G., Sampath, V., Christiani, D. C., Haahtela, T., & Renz, H. (2024, May). Impact of climate change on immune responses and barrier defense. *The Journal of Allergy and Clinical Immunology*, *153*(5), 1194–1205. DOI: 10.1016/j.jaci.2024.01.016 PMID: 38309598

Stafford, I. S., Kellermann, M., Mossotto, E., Beattie, R. M., MacArthur, B. D., & Ennis, S. (2020, March 9). A systematic review of the applications of artificial intelligence and machine learning in autoimmune diseases. *NPJ Digital Medicine*, *3*(1), 30. DOI: 10.1038/s41746-020-0229-3 PMID: 32195365

Takaoka, K. (2022, April 5). AI Implementation Science for Social Issues: Pitfalls and Tips. *Journal of Epidemiology*, *32*(4), 155–162. DOI: 10.2188/jea.JE20210278 PMID: 35095090

Topol, E. (2019). *Deep Medicine: How Artificial Intelligence Can Make Healthcare Human Again*. Basic Books.

Tu, T., Azizi, S., Driess, D., Schaekermann, M., Amin, M., Chang, B. S. P. C., Carroll, A., Lau, C., Tanno, M. B. A. R., Ktena, I., Palepu, A., Mustafa, B., Chowdhery, A., Liu, Y., Kornblith, S., Fleet, D., Mansfield, P., Prakash, S., Wong, R., & Natarajan, V. (2024). Towards Generalist Biomedical AI. *NEJM AI*, *1*(3). Advance online publication. DOI: 10.1056/AIoa2300138

Vaishya, R., Javaid, M., Khan, I. H., & Haleem, A. (2020, July-August). Artificial Intelligence (AI) applications for COVID-19 pandemic. *Diabetes & Metabolic Syndrome*, *14*(4), 337–339. DOI: 10.1016/j.dsx.2020.04.012 PMID: 32305024

Wachter, R. M., & Brynjolfsson, E. (2024, January 2). Will Generative Artificial Intelligence Deliver on Its Promise in Health Care? *Journal of the American Medical Association*, *331*(1), 65–69. DOI: 10.1001/jama.2023.25054 PMID: 38032660

Wiens, J., & Shenoy, E. S. (2018, January 6). Machine Learning for Healthcare: On the Verge of a Major Shift in Healthcare Epidemiology. *Clinical Infectious Diseases*, *66*(1), 149–153. DOI: 10.1093/cid/cix731 PMID: 29020316

Xu, Q. H., Yin, X. Y., Chen, Z. Q., Huang, E. K., Yao, X., Li, X., & Liu, P. N. (2025, March 25). Construction of In Situ Personalized Cancer Vaccines by Bioorthogonal Catalytic Microneedles for Augmented Melanoma Immunotherapy. *Small*, *e2500015*, 2500015. Advance online publication. DOI: 10.1002/smll.202500015 PMID: 40130650

Yamashita, T. (2023). Molecular Dynamics Simulation for Investigating Antigen-Antibody Interaction. *Methods in Molecular Biology (Clifton, N.J.)*, *2552*, 101–107. DOI: 10.1007/978-1-0716-2609-2_4 PMID: 36346587

Yang, P., Liu, Z., Lu, F., Sha, Y., Li, P., Zheng, Q., Wang, K., Zhou, X., Zeng, X., & Wu, Y. (2024, June 11). Machine learning models predicts risk of proliferative lupus nephritis. *Frontiers in Immunology*, *15*, 1413569. DOI: 10.3389/fimmu.2024.1413569 PMID: 38919623

Yang, Y., Liu, Y., Chen, Y., Luo, D., Xu, K., & Zhang, L. (2024, October 22). Artificial intelligence for predicting treatment responses in autoimmune rheumatic diseases: Advancements, challenges, and future perspectives. *Frontiers in Immunology*, *15*, 1477130. DOI: 10.3389/fimmu.2024.1477130 PMID: 39502698

You, R., Qu, W., Mamitsuka, H., & Zhu, S. (2022, June 24). DeepMHCII: A novel binding core-aware deep interaction model for accurate MHC-II peptide binding affinity prediction. *Bioinformatics (Oxford, England)*, *38*(Suppl 1), i220–i228. DOI: 10.1093/bioinformatics/btac225 PMID: 35758790

Yu, K. H., Healey, E., Leong, T. Y., Kohane, I. S., & Manrai, A. K. (2024, May 30). Medical Artificial Intelligence and Human Values. *The New England Journal of Medicine*, *390*(20), 1895–1904. DOI: 10.1056/NEJMra2214183 PMID: 38810186

Zack, T., Lehman, E., Suzgun, M., Rodriguez, J. A., Celi, L. A., Gichoya, J., Jurafsky, D., Szolovits, P., Bates, D. W., Abdulnour, R. E., Butte, A. J., & Alsentzer, E. (2024, January). Assessing the potential of GPT-4 to perpetuate racial and gender biases in health care: A model evaluation study. *The Lancet. Digital Health*, *6*(1), e12–e22. DOI: 10.1016/S2589-7500(23)00225-X PMID: 38123252

Compilation of References

"Healthily: Medically Verified Health Information You Need for Self-Care." n.d. Healthily. Accessed January 20, 2025. https://www.livehealthily.com/

1. Witkowski, K., Okhai, R., & Neely, S. R. (2024). Public perceptions of artificial intelligence in healthcare: Ethical concerns and opportunities for patient-centered care. *BMC Medical Ethics*, *25*(1), 1–11. DOI: 10.1186/s12910-024-01066-4 PMID: 38909180

63. Trugenberger, C. A., Wälti, C., Peregrim, D., Sharp, M. E., & Bureeva, S. (2013). Discovery of novel biomarkers and phenotypes by semantic technologies. *BMC Bioinformatics*, *14*(1), 1–17. DOI: 10.1186/1471-2105-14-51 PMID: 23402646

8. Yamamoto, T. N., Kishton, R. J., & Restifo, N. P. (2019). Developing neoantigen-targeted T cell–based treatments for solid tumors. *Nature Medicine*, *25*(10), 1488–1499. DOI: 10.1038/s41591-019-0596-y PMID: 31591590

Abbas, M. K. G., Rassam, A., Karamshahi, F., Abunora, R., & Abouseada, M. (2024). The role of AI in drug discovery. *ChemBioChem*, *25*(14), e202300816. Advance online publication. DOI: 10.1002/cbic.202300816 PMID: 38735845

Abdallah, S., Sharifa, M., Almadhoun, M. K. I. K., Khawar, M. M.Sr, Shaikh, U., Balabel, K. M., Saleh, I., Manzoor, A., Mandal, A. K., & Ekomwereren, O. (2023). The impact of artificial intelligence on optimizing diagnosis and treatment plans for rare genetic disorders. *Cureus*, *15*(10). Advance online publication. DOI: 10.7759/cureus.46860 PMID: 37954711

Abdelmageed, M. I., Abdelmoneim, A. H., Mustafa, M. I., Elfadol, N. M., Murshed, N. S., Shantier, S. W., & Makhawi, A. M. (2020). Design of a multiepitope-based peptide vaccine against the E protein of human COVID-19: An immunoinformatics approach. *BioMed Research International*, *2683286*(1), 2683286. Advance online publication. DOI: 10.1155/2020/2683286 PMID: 32461973

Abelin, J. G., Keskin, D. B., Sarkizova, S., Hartigan, C. R., Zhang, W., Sidney, J., Stevens, J., Lane, W., Zhang, G. L., Eisenhaure, T. M., Clauser, K. R., Hacohen, N., Rooney, M. S., Carr, S. A., & Wu, C. J. (2017). Mass spectrometry profiling of HLA-associated peptidomes in mono-allelic cells enables more accurate Epitope prediction. *Immunity*, *46*(2), 315–326. DOI: 10.1016/j.immuni.2017.02.007 PMID: 28228285

Abiodun, O. I., Jantan, A., Omolara, A. E., Dada, K. V., Mohamed, N. A., & Arshad, H. (2018). State-of-the-art in artificial neural network applications: A survey. *Heliyon*, *4*(11), e00938. DOI: 10.1016/j.heliyon.2018.e00938 PMID: 30519653

Abou Ghayda, R.. (2024). Artificial intelligence in andrology: From semen analysis to image diagnostics. *The World Journal of Men's Health*, *42*(1), 39. DOI: 10.5534/wjmh.230050 PMID: 37382282

Abraham, G., Tye-Din, J. A., Bhalala, O. G., Kowalczyk, A., Zobel, J., & Inouye, M. (2014, February 13). Accurate and robust genomic prediction of celiac disease using statistical learning. *PLOS Genetics*, *10*(2), e1004137. DOI: 10.1371/journal.pgen.1004137 PMID: 24550740

Achilles, S. L., Creinin, M. D., Stoner, K. A., Chen, B. A., Meyn, L., & Hillier, S. L. (2014). Changes in genital tract immune cell populations after initiation of intrauterine contraception. *American journal of obstetrics and gynecology, 211*(5), 489. e481-489. e489.

Ada. "Health Powered by Ada." Accessed January 20, 2025. https://ada.com/

Adamichou, C., Genitsaridi, I., Nikolopoulos, D., Nikoloudaki, M., Repa, A., Bortoluzzi, A., Fanouriakis, A., Sidiropoulos, P., Boumpas, D. T., & Bertsias, G. K. (2021). Lupus or Not? SLE Risk Probability Index (SLERPI): A Simple, Clinician-Friendly Machine Learning-Based Model to Assist the Diagnosis of Systemic Lupus Erythematosus. *Annals of the Rheumatic Diseases*, *80*(6), 758–766. DOI: 10.1136/annrheumdis-2020-219069 PMID: 33568388

Aderibigbe, A. O.Adebayo Olusegun AderibigbePeter Efosa OhenhenNwabueze Kelvin NwaobiaJoachim Osheyor GidiagbaEmmanuel Chigozie Ani. (2023). Artificial intelligence in developing countries: Bridging the gap between potential and implementation. *Computer Science & IT Research Journal*, *4*(3), 185–199. DOI: 10.51594/csitrj.v4i3.629

Adytia, G. J., Sutanto, H., Pratiwi, L., & Fetarayani, D. (2025). Advances in Synthetic Immunology for Targeted Treatment of Systemic Autoimmune Diseases: Opportunities, Challenges, and Future Directions. *Immuno*, *5*(1), 6. DOI: 10.3390/immuno5010006

Agache, I., Canelo-Aybar, C., Annesi-Maesano, I., Cecchi, L., Rigau, D., Rodríguez-Tanta, L. Y., Nieto-Gutierrez, W., Song, Y., Cantero-Fortiz, Y., Roqué, M., Vasquez, J. C., Sola, I., Biagioni, B., Chung, F., D'Amato, G., Damialis, A., del Giacco, S., Vecillas, L., Dominguez-Ortega, J., & Akdis, C. A. (2024). The Impact of Outdoor Pollution and Extreme Temperatures on Asthma-Related Outcomes: A Systematic Review for the EAACI Guidelines on Environmental Science for Allergic Diseases and Asthma. *Allergy*, *79*(7), 1725–1760. DOI: 10.1111/all.16041 PMID: 38311978

Aggarwal, R., Farag, S., Martin, G., Ashrafian, H., & Darzi, A. (2021, August 26). Patient Perceptions on Data Sharing and Applying Artificial Intelligence to Health Care Data: Cross-sectional Survey. *Journal of Medical Internet Research*, *23*(8), e26162. DOI: 10.2196/26162 PMID: 34236994

Aghamiri, S. S., Amin, R., & Helikar, T. (2022). Recent applications of quantitative systems pharmacology and machine learning models across diseases. *Journal of Pharmacokinetics and Pharmacodynamics*, *49*(1), 19–37. DOI: 10.1007/s10928-021-09790-9 PMID: 34671863

Aguirre, J., Schwarz, M., Garzorz, N., Omar, M., Buehler, A., Eyerich, K., & Ntziachristos, V. (2017). Precision Assessment of Label-Free Psoriasis Biomarkers with Ultra-Broadband Optoacoustic Mesoscopy. *Nature Biomedical Engineering*, *1*(5), 1–8. DOI: 10.1038/s41551-017-0068

Agu, P. C., & Obulose, C. N. (2024). Piquing artificial intelligence towards drug discovery: Tools, techniques, and applications. *Drug Development Research, 85*(2), e22159. DOI: 10.1002/ddr.22159 PMID: 38375772

Ahanin, E., Sade, A. B., & Tat, H. H. (2022). Applications of artificial intelligence and voice assistant in healthcare. *International Journal of Academic Research in Business & Social Sciences, 12*(12), 2545–2554. DOI: 10.6007/IJARBSS/v12-i12/16048

Ahmed, A., & Adil, K. (2023). *Transforming Healthcare Systems with Artificial Intelligence: Revolutionizing Efficiency*. Quality, and Patient Care.

Ahmed, Z., Mohamed, K., Zeeshan, S., & Dong, X. (2020). Artificial intelligence with multi-functional machine learning platform development for better healthcare and precision medicine. *Database : The Journal of Biological Databases and Curation, 2020*, baaa010. DOI: 10.1093/database/baaa010 PMID: 32185396

Ahn, B., Moon, D., Kim, H.-S., Lee, C., Cho, N. H., Choi, H.-K., Kim, D., Lee, J.-Y., Nam, E. J., Won, D., An, H. J., Kwon, S. Y., Shin, S.-J., Jung, H. R., Kwon, D., Park, H., Kim, M., Cha, Y. J., Park, H., & Park, E. (2024). Histopathologic image-based deep learning classifier for predicting platinum-based treatment responses in high-grade serous ovarian cancer. *Nature Communications, 15*(1), 4253. DOI: 10.1038/s41467-024-48667-6 PMID: 38762636

Ahuja, A. S. (2019). The impact of artificial intelligence in medicine on the future role of the physician. *PeerJ, 7*, e7702. DOI: 10.7717/peerj.7702 PMID: 31592346

Aijaz, , S. FKhan, , S. JAzim, , FShakeel, , C. SHassan, , U. (2022). Deep learning application for effective classification of different types of psoriasis. *Journal of Healthcare Engineering,* (1), 7541583.

Aileni, M., Rohela, G. K., Jogam, P., Soujanya, S., & Zhang, B. (2022). Biotechnological perspectives to combat the COVID-19 pandemic: Precise diagnostics and inevitable vaccine paradigms. *Cells, 11*(7), 1182. DOI: 10.3390/cells11071182 PMID: 35406746

Akgun, S., & Greenhow, C. (2022). Artificial intelligence in education: Addressing ethical challenges in K-12 settings. *AI and Ethics, 2*(3), 431–440. DOI: 10.1007/s43681-021-00096-7 PMID: 34790956

Al Kuwaiti, A., Nazer, K., Al-Reedy, A., Al-Shehri, S., Al-Muhanna, A., Subbarayalu, A. V., Al Muhanna, D., & Al-Muhanna, F. A. (2023). A review of the role of artificial intelligence in healthcare. *Journal of Personalized Medicine, 13*(6), 951. DOI: 10.3390/jpm13060951 PMID: 37373940

Alag, A. (2019). Machine Learning Approach Yields Epigenetic Biomarkers of Food Allergy: A Novel 13-Gene Signature to Diagnose Clinical Reactivity. *PLoS One, 14*(6), e0218253. DOI: 10.1371/journal.pone.0218253 PMID: 31216310

Alahmari, N., Alswedani, S., Alzahrani, A., Katib, I., Albeshri, A., & Mehmood, R. (2022). Musawah: A data-driven ai approach and tool to co-create healthcare services with a case study on cancer disease in Saudi Arabia. *Sustainability (Basel), 14*(6), 3313. DOI: 10.3390/su14063313

Alami, H., Rivard, L., Lehoux, P., Hoffman, S. J., Cadeddu, S. B. M., Savoldelli, M., Samri, M. A., Ag Ahmed, M. A., Fleet, R., & Fortin, J.-P. (2020). Artificial intelligence in health care: Laying the Foundation for Responsible, sustainable, and inclusive innovation in low-and middle-income countries. *Globalization and Health*, *16*(1), 1–6. DOI: 10.1186/s12992-020-00584-1 PMID: 32580741

Alasasfeh, H. O., Alomari, T., & Ibbini, M. S. (2021, March). Deep Learning Approach for COVID-19 Detection Based on X-Ray Images. In 2021 18th International Multi-Conference on Systems, Signals & Devices (SSD) (pp. 1-6). IEEE.

Alawam, A. S., & Alwethaynani, M. S. (2024). Construction of an aerolysin-based multi-epitope vaccine against Aeromonas hydrophila: An in-silico machine learning and artificial intelligence-supported approach. *Frontiers in Immunology*, *15*, 1369890. DOI: 10.3389/fimmu.2024.1369890 PMID: 38495891

Alber, D. A., Yang, Z., Alyakin, A., Yang, E., Rai, S., Valliani, A. A., Zhang, J., Rosenbaum, G. R., Amend-Thomas, A. K., Kurland, D. B., Kremer, C. M., Eremiev, A., Negash, B., Wiggan, D. D., Nakatsuka, M. A., Sangwon, K. L., Neifert, S. N., Khan, H. A., Save, A. V., & Oermann, E. K. (2025, January 8). Medical large language models are vulnerable to data-poisoning attacks. *Nature Medicine*, *31*(2), 618–626. Advance online publication. DOI: 10.1038/s41591-024-03445-1 PMID: 39779928

Aldea, M., Andre, F., Marabelle, A., Dogan, S., Barlesi, F., & Soria, J.-C. (2021). Overcoming resistance to tumor-targeted and immune-targeted therapies. *Cancer Discovery*, *11*(4), 874–899. DOI: 10.1158/2159-8290.CD-20-1638 PMID: 33811122

Alderman, J. E., Palmer, J., Laws, E., McCradden, M. D., Ordish, J., Ghassemi, M., Pfohl, S. R., Rostamzadeh, N., Cole-Lewis, H., Glocker, B., Calvert, M., Pollard, T. J., Gill, J., Gath, J., Adebajo, A., Beng, J., Leung, C. H., Kuku, S., Farmer, L. A., & Liu, X. (2025, January). Tackling algorithmic bias and promoting transparency in health datasets: The STANDING Together consensus recommendations. *The Lancet. Digital Health*, *7*(1), e64–e88. DOI: 10.1016/S2589-7500(24)00224-3 PMID: 39701919

Aldousari, E., & Kithinji, D. (2024). Artificial intelligence and health information: A bibliometric analysis of three decades of research. *Health Informatics Journal*, *30*(3), 14604582241283969. DOI: 10.1177/14604582241283969 PMID: 39262107

Algohary, A., Shiradkar, R., Pahwa, S., Purysko, A., Verma, S., Moses, D., Shnier, R., Haynes, A.-M., Delprado, W., Thompson, J., Tirumani, S., Mahran, A., Rastinehad, A. R., Ponsky, L., Stricker, P. D., & Madabhushi, A. (2020). Combination of peri-tumoral and intra-tumoral radiomic features on bi-parametric MRI accurately stratifies prostate cancer risk: A multi-site study. *Cancers (Basel)*, *12*(7), 2200. DOI: 10.3390/cancers12082200 PMID: 32781640

Al-Haija, Q. A., & Adebanjo, A. (2020, September). Breast cancer diagnosis in histopathological images using ResNet-50 convolutional neural network. In *2020 IEEE International IOT, Electronics and Mechatronics Conference (IEMTRONICS)* (pp. 1-7). IEEE.DOI: DOI: 10.1109/IEMTRONICS51293.2020.9216455

Alhasan, M., & Hasaneen, M. (2021). Digital imaging, technologies and artificial intelligence applications during COVID-19 pandemic. *Computerized Medical Imaging and Graphics*, *91*, 101933. DOI: 10.1016/j.compmedimag.2021.101933 PMID: 34082281

Alhejaily, A.-M. G. (2024). Artificial intelligence in healthcare. *Biomedical Reports*, *22*(1), 11. DOI: 10.3892/br.2024.1889 PMID: 39583770

Ali, H. R., Jackson, H. W., Zanotelli, V. R. T., Danenberg, E., Fischer, J. R., Bardwell, H., Provenzano, E., Ali, H. R., Al Sa'd, M., Alon, S., Aparicio, S., Battistoni, G., Balasubramanian, S., Becker, R., Bodenmiller, B., Boyden, E. S., Bressan, D., Bruna, A., Marcel, B., & Bodenmiller, B. (2020). Imaging mass cytometry and multiplatform genomics define the phenogenomic landscape of breast cancer. *Nature Cancer*, *1*(2), 163–175. DOI: 10.1038/s43018-020-0026-6 PMID: 35122013

Ali, K. A., Mohin, S., Mondal, P., Goswami, S., Ghosh, S., & Choudhuri, S. (2024). Influence of artificial intelligence in modern pharmaceutical formulation and drug development. *Future Journal of Pharmaceutical Sciences*, *10*(1), 53. DOI: 10.1186/s43094-024-00625-1

Alipanahi, B., Delong, A., Weirauch, M. T., & Frey, B. J. (2015). Predicting the sequence specificities of DNA- and RNA-binding proteins by deep learning. *Nature Biotechnology*, *33*(8), 831–838. DOI: 10.1038/nbt.3300 PMID: 26213851

Aliper, A., Plis, S., Artemov, A., Ulloa, A., Mamoshina, P., & Zhavoronkov, A. (2016). Deep Learning Applications for Predicting Pharmacological Properties of Drugs and Drug Repurposing Using Transcriptomic Data. *Molecular Pharmaceutics*, *13*(7), 2524–2530. DOI: 10.1021/acs.molpharmaceut.6b00248 PMID: 27200455

Ali, S., Akhlaq, F., Imran, A. S., Kastrati, Z., Daudpota, S. M., & Moosa, M. (2023). The enlightening role of explainable artificial intelligence in medical & healthcare domains: A systematic literature review. *Computers in Biology and Medicine*, *166*, 107555. DOI: 10.1016/j.compbiomed.2023.107555 PMID: 37806061

Alizadeh, A. A., Aranda, V., Bardelli, A., Blanpain, C., Bock, C., Borowski, C., Caldas, C., Califano, A., Doherty, M., Elsner, M., Esteller, M., Fitzgerald, R., Korbel, J. O., Lichter, P., Mason, C. E., Navin, N., Pe'er, D., Polyak, K., Roberts, C. W. M., & Zucman-Rossi, J. (2015). Toward understanding and exploiting tumor heterogeneity. *Nature Medicine*, *21*(8), 846–853. DOI: 10.1038/nm.3915 PMID: 26248267

Aljabali, A. A. A., Obeid, M. A., Gammoh, O., El-Tanani, M., Mishra, V., Mishra, Y., Kapre, S., Srivatsa Palakurthi, S., Hassan, S. S., Nawn, D., Lundstrom, K., Hromić-Jahjefendić, A., Serrano-Aroca, Á., Redwan, E. M., Uversky, V. N., & Tambuwala, M. M. (2024). Nanomaterial-Driven Precision Immunomodulation: A New Paradigm in Therapeutic Interventions. *Cancers (Basel)*, *16*(11), 2030. DOI: 10.3390/cancers16112030 PMID: 38893150

Aljabali, A. A., Obeid, M. A., Bashatwah, R. M., Serrano-Aroca, Á., Mishra, V., Mishra, Y., El-Tanani, M., Hromić-Jahjefendić, A., Kapoor, D. N., Goyal, R., Naikoo, G. A., & Tambuwala, M. M. (2023). Nanomaterials and Their Impact on the Immune System. *International Journal of Molecular Sciences*, *24*(3), 2008. DOI: 10.3390/ijms24032008 PMID: 36768330

Al-Karawi, D., Al-Zaidi, S., Helael, K. A., Obeidat, N., Mouhsen, A. M., Ajam, T., Alshalabi, B. A., Salman, M., & Ahmed, M. H. (2024). A Review of Artificial Intelligence in Breast Imaging. *Tomography : a Journal for Imaging Research*, *10*(5), 705–726. DOI: 10.3390/tomography10050055 PMID: 38787015

Ally, A., Balasundaram, M., Carlsen, R., Chuah, E., Clarke, A., Dhalla, N., Holt, R. A., Jones, S. J. M., Lee, D., Ma, Y., Marra, M. A., Mayo, M., Moore, R. A., Mungall, A. J., Schein, J. E., Sipahimalani, P., Tam, A., Thiessen, N., Cheung, D., & Laird, P. W.Cancer Genome Atlas Research Network. (2017). Comprehensive and integrative genomic characterization of hepatocellular carcinoma. *Cell, 169*(7), 1327–1341.e1323. DOI: 10.1016/j.cell.2017.05.046 PMID: 28622513

Almeida, J., & Costa, F. (2021). Image-Based Diagnosis of Oral Lichen Planus Using Machine Learning. *International Journal of Oral Science.*

Almeida, P. M., Rivest, F., Juppet, Q., Kowal, J., Pelz, B., Cassano, M., Eroglu, D., & Dupouy, D. (2022). Abstract 1716: Mapping the cellular architecture of the tumor microenvironment by integrating hyperplex immunofluorescence and automated image analysis. *Cancer Research, 82*(12, Supplement), 1716. DOI: 10.1158/1538-7445.AM2022-1716

Almuhanna, H., Alenezi, M., Abualhasan, M., Alajmi, S., Alfadhli, R., & Karar, A. S. (2024). AI Asthma Guard: Predictive Wearable Technology for Asthma Management in Vulnerable Populations. *Applied System Innovation, 7*(5), 78. DOI: 10.3390/asi7050078

Alnasser, B. (2023). A Review of Literature on the Economic Implications of Implementing Artificial Intelligence in Healthcare. *E-Health Telecommunication Systems and Networks, 12*(3), 35–48. DOI: 10.4236/etsn.2023.123003

Alowais, S. A., Alghamdi, S. S., Alsuhebany, N., Alqahtani, T., Alshaya, A. I., Almohareb, S. N., Aldairem, A., Alrashed, M., Bin Saleh, K., Badreldin, H. A., Al Yami, M. S., Al Harbi, S., & Albekairy, A. M. (2023). Revolutionizing healthcare: The role of artificial intelligence in clinical practice. *BMC Medical Education, 23*(1), 689. DOI: 10.1186/s12909-023-04698-z PMID: 37740191

Alsharif, F. (2024). Artificial intelligence in oncology: Applications, challenges and future frontiers. *International Journal of Pharmaceutical Investigation, 14*(3), 647–656. DOI: 10.5530/ijpi.14.3.76

Alshehri, S., Alahmari, K. A., & Alasiry, A. (2024). A Comprehensive Evaluation of AI-Assisted Diagnostic Tools in ENT Medicine: Insights and Perspectives from Healthcare Professionals. *Journal of Personalized Medicine, 14*(4), 354. DOI: 10.3390/jpm14040354 PMID: 38672981

Alter, O., Newman, E., Ponnapalli, S. P., & Tsai, J. W. (2024). AI/ML-Derived Mechanistically Interpretable Whole-Genome Biomarkers of Patient Survival in Pre-Treatment Primary Neuroblastoma Tumors and Whole Blood. *Journal of Clinical Oncology, 42*(16, suppl), 10043–10043. DOI: 10.1200/JCO.2024.42.16_suppl.10043

Aluthge Don, Y., *Regulatory Perspectives of AI as Medical Device: a scoping review.* 2024.

Amir, E.-D., Davis, K. L., Tadmor, M. D., Simonds, E. F., Levine, J. H., Bendall, S. C., Shenfeld, D. K., Krishnaswamy, S., Nolan, G. P., & Pe'er, D. (2013). viSNE enables visualization of high dimensional single-cell data and reveals phenotypic heterogeneity of leukemia. *Nature Biotechnology, 31*(6), 545–552. DOI: 10.1038/nbt.2594 PMID: 23685480

Anagnostou, V., Landon, B. V., Medina, J. E., Forde, P., & Velculescu, V. E. (2022). Translating the evolving molecular landscape of tumors to biomarkers of response for cancer immunotherapy. *Science Translational Medicine*, *14*(670), eabo3958. Advance online publication. DOI: 10.1126/scitranslmed.abo3958 PMID: 36350985

Anaya, J., Sidhom, J.-W., Mahmood, F., & Baras, A. S. (2024). Multiple-instance learning of somatic mutations for the classification of tumor type and the prediction of microsatellite status. *Nature Biomedical Engineering*, *8*(1), 57–67. DOI: 10.1038/s41551-023-01120-3 PMID: 37919367

Anderson, J., & Mooney, C. (2021). AI in medical diagnostics: Applications and challenges. *Journal of Artificial Intelligence in Healthcare*, *12*(3), 45–67.

Anderson, K., Kline, C., Tuck, T., & Collins, M. (2020). Challenges in translating stem cell therapy to clinical applications. *Journal of Cellular Therapy*, *25*(3), 389–398.

André, T., Shiu, K.-K., Kim, T. W., Jensen, B. V., Jensen, L. H., Punt, C., Smith, D., Garcia-Carbonero, R., Benavides, M., Gibbs, P., de la Fouchardiere, C., Rivera, F., Elez, E., Bendell, J., Le, D. T., Yoshino, T., Van Cutsem, E., Yang, P., Farooqui, M. Z. H., & Diaz, L. A.Jr. (2020). Pembrolizumab in microsatellite-instability-high advanced colorectal cancer. *The New England Journal of Medicine*, *383*(23), 2207–2218. DOI: 10.1056/NEJMoa2017699 PMID: 33264544

Anklam, E., Bahl, M. I., Ball, R., Beger, R. D., Cohen, J., Fitzpatrick, S., Girard, P., Halamoda-Kenzaoui, B., Hinton, D., Hirose, A., Hoeveler, A., Honma, M., Hugas, M., Ishida, S., Kass, G. E. N., Kojima, H., Krefting, I., Liachenko, S., Liu, Y., & Slikker, W.Jr. (2022). Emerging technologies and their impact on regulatory science. *Experimental Biology and Medicine*, *247*(1), 1–75. DOI: 10.1177/15353702211052280 PMID: 34783606

Ankley, G. T., & Edwards, S. W. (2018). The Adverse Outcome Pathway: A Multifaceted Framework Supporting 21st Century Toxicology. *Current Opinion in Toxicology*, *9*, 1–7. DOI: 10.1016/j.cotox.2018.03.004 PMID: 29682628

Antonelli, G., Rizkala, T., Iacopini, F., & Hassan, C. (2023). Current and future implications of artificial intelligence in colonoscopy. *Annals of Gastroenterology*, *36*(2), 114. DOI: 10.20524/aog.2023.0781 PMID: 36864946

Anyanwu, E. C.. (2024). Artificial intelligence in healthcare: A review of ethical dilemmas and practical applications. *International Medical Science Research Journal*, *4*(2), 126–140. DOI: 10.51594/imsrj.v4i2.755

Aquino, Y. S. J., Carter, S. M., Houssami, N., Braunack-Mayer, A., Win, K. T., Degeling, C., Wang, L., & Rogers, W. A. (2023). Practical, epistemic and normative implications of algorithmic bias in healthcare artificial intelligence: A qualitative study of multidisciplinary expert perspectives. *Journal of Medical Ethics*, jme-2022-108850. DOI: 10.1136/jme-2022-108850 PMID: 36823101

Aquino, Y. S. J., Rogers, W. A., Braunack-Mayer, A., Frazer, H., Win, K. T., Houssami, N., Degeling, C., Semsarian, C., & Carter, S. M. (2023). Utopia versus dystopia: Professional perspectives on the impact of healthcare artificial intelligence on clinical roles and skills. *International Journal of Medical Informatics*, *169*, 104903. DOI: 10.1016/j.ijmedinf.2022.104903 PMID: 36343512

Ara, A., & Mifa, A. F. (2024). Integrating artificial intelligence and big data in mobile health: A systematic review of innovations and challenges in healthcare systems. Global Mainstream Journal of Business, Economics, Development & Project Management, 3(01), 01-16.

Ardila, D., Kiraly, A. P., Bharadwaj, S., Choi, B., Reicher, J. J., Peng, L., Tse, D., Etemadi, M., Ye, W., Corrado, G., Naidich, D. P., & Shetty, S. (2019). End-to-end lung cancer screening with three-dimensional deep learning on low-dose chest computed tomography. *Nature Medicine*, *25*(6), 954–961. DOI: 10.1038/s41591-019-0447-x PMID: 31110349

Argelaguet, R., Velten, B., Arnol, D., Dietrich, S., Zenz, T., Marioni, J. C., Buettner, F., Huber, W., & Stegle, O. (2018). Multi-omics factor analysis—A framework for unsupervised integration of multi-omics datasets. *Molecular Systems Biology*, *14*(6), e8124. DOI: 10.15252/msb.20178124 PMID: 29925568

Arigbabu, A. T., Olaniyi, O. O., Adigwe, C. S., Adebiyi, O. O., & Ajayi, S. A. (2024). Data governance in AI-enabled healthcare systems: A case of the project nightingale. *Asian Journal of Research in Computer Science*, *17*(5), 85–107. DOI: 10.9734/ajrcos/2024/v17i5441

Armin, M. (2018). The potential of stem cell therapy in regenerative medicine: A review. *Stem Cell Journal*, *8*(2), 95–105.

Arnar, D. O., Oddsson, S. J., Gunnarsdottir, T., Gudlaugsdottir, G. J., Gudmundsson, E. F., Ketilsdóttir, A., Halldorsdottir, H., Hrafnkelsdottir, T. J., Hallsson, H., Amundadottir, M. L., & Thorgeirsson, T. (2022). Improving outpatient care for heart failure through digital innovation: A feasibility study. *Pilot and Feasibility Studies*, *8*(1), 242. DOI: 10.1186/s40814-022-01206-w PMID: 36451212

Arpey, N. C., Gaglioti, A. H., & Rosenbaum, M. E. (2017, July). How Socioeconomic Status Affects Patient Perceptions of Health Care: A Qualitative Study. *Journal of Primary Care & Community Health*, *8*(3), 169–175. DOI: 10.1177/2150131917697439 PMID: 28606031

Artsi, Y., & Vera Sorin, B. S. (2024). Advancing Clinical Practice: The Potential of Multimodal Technology in Modern Medicine. *Journal of Clinical Medicine*, *13*(20), 6246. DOI: 10.3390/jcm13206246 PMID: 39458196

Ashwini, T., Narayan, R., Shenoy, P. A., & Nayak, U. Y. (2022). Computational modeling for the design and development of nano based drug delivery systems. *Journal of Molecular Liquids*, *368*, 120596.

Asiniwasis, R., Merati, N., Roesler, J., Simpson, E. L., Aubry, R., McMullen, E., Fraess, L., Choi, U. Y., Hinther, K., Chu, D. K., & Jack, C. (2024). The Social and Home Environment: Impacts of Determinants of Health on Atopic Dermatitis, Pathways Toward Solutions, and Unique Considerations for Rural and Remote North American Indigenous Populations. *The Journal of Allergy and Clinical Immunology. In Practice*, *12*(2), 290–299. DOI: 10.1016/j.jaip.2023.11.034 PMID: 38013155

Aslam, R., Herrles, L., Aoun, R., Pioskowik, A., & Pietrzyk, A. (2024). Link between Gut Microbiota Dysbiosis and Childhood Asthma: Insights from a Systematic Review. *The Journal of Allergy and Clinical Immunology. Global*, *3*(3), 100289. DOI: 10.1016/j.jacig.2024.100289 PMID: 39105129

Asnicar, F., Thomas, A. M., Passerini, A., Waldron, L., & Segata, N. (2024, April). Machine learning for microbiologists. *Nature Reviews. Microbiology*, *22*(4), 191–205. DOI: 10.1038/s41579-023-00984-1 PMID: 37968359

Atkins, T. K., Solanki, A., Vasmatzis, G., Cornette, J., & Riedel, M. (2024, January 16). Evaluating NetMHCpan performance on non-European HLA alleles not present in training data. *Frontiers in Immunology*, *14*, 1288105. DOI: 10.3389/fimmu.2023.1288105 PMID: 38292493

Attia, Z. I., Noseworthy, P. A., Lopez-Jimenez, F., Asirvatham, S. J., Deshmukh, A. J., Gersh, B. J., Carter, R. E., Yao, X., Rabinstein, A. A., Erickson, B. J., Kapa, S., & Friedman, P. A. (2019). An artificial intelligence-enabled ECG algorithm for the identification of patients with atrial fibrillation during sinus rhythm: A retrospective analysis of outcome prediction. *Lancet*, *394*(10201), 861–867. DOI: 10.1016/S0140-6736(19)31721-0 PMID: 31378392

Atzeni, F., Talotta, R., Masala, I. F., Bongiovanni, S., Boccassini, L., & Sarzi-Puttini, P. (2017). Biomarkers in rheumatoid arthritis. *The Israel Medical Association Journal*, *19*(8), 512–516. PMID: 28825772

Aung, Y. Y. M., Wong, D. C. S., & Ting, D. S. W. (2021, September 10). The promise of artificial intelligence: A review of the opportunities and challenges of artificial intelligence in healthcare. *British Medical Bulletin*, *139*(1), 4–15. DOI: 10.1093/bmb/ldab016 PMID: 34405854

Avorn, J. (2015). The $2.6 billion pill—Methodologic and policy considerations. *The New England Journal of Medicine*, *372*(20), 1877–1879. DOI: 10.1056/NEJMp1500848 PMID: 25970049

Awuah, W. A., Aderinto, N., Poornaselvan, J., Tan, J. K., Shah, M. H., Ashinze, P., Pujari, A. G., Bharadwaj, H. R., Abdul-Rahman, T., & Atallah, O. (2024). Empowering health care consumers & understanding patients' perspectives on AI integration in oncology and surgery: A perspective. *Health Science Reports*, *7*(7), e2268. DOI: 10.1002/hsr2.2268 PMID: 39050906

Ayers, J. W., Poliak, A., Dredze, M., Leas, E. C., Zhu, Z., Kelley, J. B., Faix, D. J., Goodman, A. M., Longhurst, C. A., Hogarth, M., & Smith, D. M. (2023, June 1). Comparing Physician and Artificial Intelligence Chatbot Responses to Patient Questions Posted to a Public Social Media Forum. *JAMA Internal Medicine*, *183*(6), 589–596. DOI: 10.1001/jamainternmed.2023.1838 PMID: 37115527

Babarinde, A. O.. (2023). Review of AI applications in Healthcare: Comparative insights from the USA and Africa. *International Medical Science Research Journal*, *3*(3), 92–107. DOI: 10.51594/imsrj.v3i3.641

Bäckel, C., & Capponi, A. (2023). Enhancing cell therapy research through AI-based genetic engineering. *Biotechnology Advances*, *15*(1), 233–250.

Badawy, M. (2023). *Integrating Artificial Intelligence and Big Data into Smart Healthcare Systems: A Comprehensive Review of Current Practices and Future Directions*. Artificial Intelligence Evolution.

Baek, M., DiMaio, F., Anishchenko, I., Dauparas, J., Ovchinnikov, S., Lee, G. R., … Baker, D. (2021). Accurate prediction of protein structures and interactions using a three-track neural network. *Science (New York, N.Y.)*, *373*(6557), 871–876. doi:. abj8754DOI: 10.1126/science

Bae, S., Choi, H., Lee, J., Kang, M., Ahn, S., Lee, Y., & Nam, J. (2024). Rational Design of Lipid Nanoparticles for Enhanced mRNA Vaccine Delivery via Machine Learning. *Small*, •••, 2405618. PMID: 39264000

Bae, W. D., Alkobaisi, S., Horak, M., Park, C.-S., Kim, S., & Davidson, J. (2022). Predicting Health Risks of Adult Asthmatics Susceptible to Indoor Air Quality Using Improved Logistic and Quantile Regression Models. *Life (Chicago, Ill.)*, *12*(10), 1631. DOI: 10.3390/life12101631 PMID: 36295066

Bagger, F. O., Borgwardt, L., Jespersen, A. S., Hansen, A. R., Bertelsen, B., Kodama, M., & Nielsen, F. C. (2024). Whole genome sequencing in clinical practice. *BMC Medical Genomics*, *17*(1), 39. DOI: 10.1186/s12920-024-01795-w PMID: 38287327

Bakare, S. S., Adeniyi, A. O., Akpuokwe, C. U., & Eneh, N. E.Seun Solomon BakareAdekunle Oyeyemi AdeniyiChidiogo Uzoamaka AkpuokweNkechi Emmanuella Eneh. (2024). Data Privacy Laws and Compliance: A Comparative Review Of The Eu GDPR And USA Regulations. *Computer Science & IT Research Journal*, *5*(3), 528–543. DOI: 10.51594/csitrj.v5i3.859

Bakker, D. S., Nierkens, S., Knol, E. F., Giovannone, B., Delemarre, E. M., van der Schaft, J., van Wijk, F., de Bruin-Weller, M. S., Drylewicz, J., & Thijs, J. L. (2021). Confirmation of Multiple Endotypes in Atopic Dermatitis Based on Serum Biomarkers. *The Journal of Allergy and Clinical Immunology*, *147*(1), 189–198. DOI: 10.1016/j.jaci.2020.04.062 PMID: 32526312

Balakrishna, S., & Solanki, V. K. (2024). A Comprehensive Review on AI-Driven Healthcare Transformation. *Ingeniería Solidaria*, *20*(2), 1–30. DOI: 10.16925/2357-6014.2024.02.07

Banegas-Luna, A. J., Cerón-Carrasco, J. P., & Pérez-Sánchez, H. (2018). A review of ligand-based virtual screening web tools and screening algorithms in large molecular databases in the age of big data. *Future Medicinal Chemistry*, *10*(22), 2641–2658. DOI: 10.4155/fmc-2018-0076 PMID: 30499744

Banerjee, S., & Patel, R. (2022). Machine learning for early disease detection: A systematic review. *Medical AI Review*, *15*(4), 89–105.

Banka, R., Das, P., Das, S., & Ghosh, J. (2025). Tailored nutrition and diet plan using AI and machine learning for precision wellness. In *Harnessing AI and machine learning for precision wellness*. IGI Global., DOI: 10.4018/979-8-3693-9521-9.ch007

Banks, G. (1986). Artificial intelligence in medical diagnosis: The INTERNIST/CADUCEUS approach. *Critical Reviews in Medical Informatics*, *1*(1), 23–54. PMID: 3331578

Bardhan, I., Oh, J. H., Zheng, Z., & Kirksey, K. (2015). Predictive analytics for readmission of patients with congestive heart failure. *Information Systems Research*, *26*(1), 19–39. DOI: 10.1287/isre.2014.0553

Barile, J., Margolis, A., Cason, G., Kim, R., Kalash, S., Tchaconas, A., & Milanaik, R. (2024, March 1). Diagnostic Accuracy of a Large Language Model in Pediatric Case Studies. *JAMA Pediatrics*, *178*(3), 313–315. DOI: 10.1001/jamapediatrics.2023.5750 PMID: 38165685

Barja-Martinez, S., Aragüés-Peñalba, M., Munné-Collado, Í., Lloret-Gallego, P., Bullich-Massagué, E., & Villafafila-Robles, R. (2021). Artificial intelligence techniques for enabling Big Data services in distribution networks: A review. *Renewable & Sustainable Energy Reviews*, *150*, 111459. DOI: 10.1016/j.rser.2021.111459

Baronzio, G., Parmar, G., & Baronzio, M. (2015). Overview of Methods for Overcoming Hindrance to Drug Delivery to Tumors, with Special Attention to Tumor Interstitial Fluid. *Frontiers in Oncology*, *5*, 165. DOI: 10.3389/fonc.2015.00165 PMID: 26258072

Barragán-Montero, A., Javaid, U., Valdés, G., Nguyen, D., Desbordes, P., Macq, B., Willems, S., Vandewinckele, L., Holmström, M., Löfman, F., Michiels, S., Souris, K., Sterpin, E., & Lee, J. A. (2021). Artificial intelligence and machine learning for medical imaging: A technology review. *Physica Medica*, *83*, 242–256. DOI: 10.1016/j.ejmp.2021.04.016 PMID: 33979715

Barriga, A., Rutle, A., & Heldal, R. (2020). Improving Model Repair through Experience Sharing. *Journal of Object Technology*, *19*(2), 13–1.

Barturen, G., Babaei, S., Català-Moll, F., Martínez-Bueno, M., Makowska, Z., Martorell-Marugán, J., Carmona-Sáez, P., Toro-Domínguez, D., Carnero-Montoro, E., Teruel, M., Kerick, M., Acosta-Herrera, M., Le Lann, L., Jamin, C., Rodríguez-Ubreva, J., García-Gómez, A., Kageyama, J., Buttgereit, A., Hayat, S., & Alarcón-Riquelme, M. E. (2021). Integrative Analysis Reveals a Molecular Stratification of Systemic Autoimmune Diseases. *Arthritis & Rheumatology (Hoboken, N.J.)*, *73*(6), 1073–1085. DOI: 10.1002/art.41610 PMID: 33497037

Basile, A. O., Yahi, A., & Tatonetti, N. P. (2019). Artificial Intelligence for Drug Toxicity and Safety. *Trends in Pharmacological Sciences*, *40*(9), 624–635. DOI: 10.1016/j.tips.2019.07.005 PMID: 31383376

Bassel, A., Abdulkareem, A. B., Alyasseri, Z. A. A., Sani, N. S., & Mohammed, H. J. (2022). Automatic malignant and benign skin cancer classification using a hybrid deep learning approach. *Diagnostics (Basel)*, *12*(10), 2472. DOI: 10.3390/diagnostics12102472 PMID: 36292161

Batista, F. D., & Dustin, M. L. (2013, January). Cell:cell interactions in the immune system. *Immunological Reviews*, *251*(1), 7–12. DOI: 10.1111/imr.12025 PMID: 23278736

Batra, A. M., & Reche, A. (2023). A new era of dental care: Harnessing artificial intelligence for better diagnosis and treatment. *Cureus*, *15*(11). PMID: 38143639

Baxi, V., Edwards, R., Montalto, M., & Saha, S. (2022). Digital pathology and artificial intelligence in translational medicine and clinical practice. *Modern Pathology*, *35*(1), 23–32. DOI: 10.1038/s41379-021-00919-2 PMID: 34611303

Beam, A. L., & Kohane, I. S. (2018). Big data and machine learning in health care. *Journal of the American Medical Association*, *319*(13), 1317–1318. DOI: 10.1001/jama.2017.18391 PMID: 29532063

Beaudart, C., Zaaria, M., Pasleau, F., Reginster, J. Y., & Bruyère, O. (2017). Health outcomes of sarcopenia: A systematic review and meta-analysis. *PLoS One*, *12*(1), e0169548. DOI: 10.1371/journal.pone.0169548 PMID: 28095426

Beaulieu, A., & Leonelli, S. (2021). Data and society: A critical introduction.

Becker, S., Miron-Shatz, T., Schumacher, N., Krocza, J., Diamantidis, C., & Albrecht, U. V. (2014). mHealth 2.0: Experiences, possibilities, and perspectives. *JMIR mHealth and uHealth*, *2*(2), e3328. DOI: 10.2196/mhealth.3328 PMID: 25099752

Beck, J. T., Rammage, M., Jackson, G. P., Preininger, A. M., Dankwa-Mullan, I., Roebuck, M. C., Torres, A., Holtzen, H., Coverdill, S. E., Williamson, M. P., Chau, Q., Rhee, K., & Vinegra, M. (2020, January). Artificial Intelligence Tool for Optimizing Eligibility Screening for Clinical Trials in a Large Community Cancer Center. *JCO Clinical Cancer Informatics*, *4*(4), 50–59. DOI: 10.1200/CCI.19.00079 PMID: 31977254

Belciug, S. (2020). *Artificial intelligence in cancer: diagnostic to tailored treatment*. Academic Press.

Bellanti, J. A. (2024). IgE and Non-IgE Food Allergy: A Review of Immunological Mechanisms. *Journal of Food Allergy*, *6*(1), 37–46. DOI: 10.2500/jfa.2024.6.240003 PMID: 39257598

Bellinghausen, I., Khatri, R., & Saloga, J. (2022). Current Strategies to Modulate Regulatory T Cell Activity in Allergic Inflammation. *Frontiers in Immunology*, *13*(May), 912529. Advance online publication. DOI: 10.3389/fimmu.2022.912529 PMID: 35720406

Beneke, F., & Mackenrodt, M. O. (2019). Artificial intelligence and collusion. *IIC Int. Rev.IIC; International Review of Industrial Property and Copyright Law*, *50*(1), 109–134. DOI: 10.1007/s40319-018-00773-x

Bengio, Y., Goodfellow, I., & Courville, A. (2017). *Deep learning* (Vol. 1). MIT press.

Benjamens, S., Dhunnoo, P., & Mesko, B. (2020). The state of artificial intelligence-based FDA-approved medical devices and algorithms: An online database. *NPJ Digital Medicine*, *3*(1), 118. DOI: 10.1038/s41746-020-00324-0 PMID: 32984550

Benkirane, H., Pradat, Y., Michiels, S., & Cournède, P.-H. (2023). CustOmics: A Versatile Deep-Learning Based Strategy for Multi-Omics Integration. *PLoS Computational Biology*, *19*(3), e1010921. DOI: 10.1371/journal.pcbi.1010921 PMID: 36877736

Berbís, M. A., Godino, F. P., Del Val, J. R., Mata, L. A., & Luna, A. (2023). Clinical impact of artificial intelligence-based solutions on imaging of the pancreas and liver. *World Journal of Gastroenterology*, *29*(9), 1427–1445. DOI: 10.3748/wjg.v29.i9.1427 PMID: 36998424

Bezbaruah, R., Chavda, V. P., Nongrang, L., Alom, S., Deka, K., Kalita, T., Ali, F., Bhattacharjee, B., & Vora, L. (2022). Nanoparticle-Based Delivery Systems for Vaccines. *Vaccines*, *10*(11), 1946. DOI: 10.3390/vaccines10111946 PMID: 36423041

Bhange, M., & Telange, D. (2025a). Convergence of nanotechnology and artificial intelligence in the fight against liver cancer: A comprehensive review. *Discover. Oncology*, *16*(1), 77. DOI: 10.1007/s12672-025-01821-y PMID: 39841330

Bhat, A. A., Nisar, S., Mukherjee, S., Saha, N., Yarravarapu, N., Lone, S. N., Masoodi, T., Chauhan, R., Maacha, S., Bagga, P., Dhawan, P., Akil, A. A., El-Rifai, W., Uddin, S., Reddy, R., Singh, M., Macha, M. A., & Haris, M. (2022, November 18). Integration of CRISPR/Cas9 with artificial intelligence for improved cancer therapeutics. *Journal of Translational Medicine*, *20*(1), 534. DOI: 10.1186/s12967-022-03765-1 PMID: 36401282

Bhattacharya, S., Dunn, P., Thomas, C. G., Smith, B., Schaefer, H., Chen, J., & Butte, A. J. (2018). ImmPort, toward repurposing of open access immunological assay data for translational and clinical research. *Scientific Data*, *5*(1), 180015. DOI: 10.1038/sdata.2018.15 PMID: 29485622

Bhol, N. K., Bhanjadeo, M. M., Singh, A. K., Dash, U. C., Ojha, R. R., Majhi, S., Duttaroy, A. K., & Jena, A. B. (2024). The interplay between cytokines, inflammation, and antioxidants: Mechanistic insights and therapeutic potentials of various antioxidants and anti-cytokine compounds. *Biomedicine and Pharmacotherapy*, *178*, 117177. DOI: 10.1016/j.biopha.2024.117177 PMID: 39053423

Bianchini, S., Müller, M., & Pelletier, P. (2022). Artificial intelligence in science: An emerging general method of invention. *Research Policy*, *51*(10), 104604. DOI: 10.1016/j.respol.2022.104604

Bielecki, A., & Bielecki, A. (2019). Foundations of artificial neural networks. In Kacprzyk, J. (Ed.), *Models of Neurons and Perceptrons: Selected Problems and Challenges* (pp. 15–28). Springer International Publishing. DOI: 10.1007/978-3-319-90140-4_3

Bilsen, J. H. M. (2019). A Network-Based Approach for Identifying Suitable Biomarkers for Oral Immunotherapy of Food Allergy. *BMC Bioinformatics*, *20*(1), 206. DOI: 10.1186/s12859-019-2802-9 PMID: 31014233

Bischoff, S. C., Austin, P., Boeykens, K., Chourdakis, M., Cuerda, C., Jonkers-Schuitema, C., Lichota, M., Nyulasi, I., Schneider, S. M., Stanga, Z., & Pironi, L. (2020). ESPEN guideline on home enteral nutrition. *Clinical Nutrition (Edinburgh, Lothian)*, *39*(1), 5–22. DOI: 10.1016/j.clnu.2019.04.022 PMID: 31255350

Biswas, I., & Singh, R. (2024). "Application Of AI And Blockchain In Healthcare Industry"–A Review. *Journal of Advanced Zoology*, *45*(2). Advance online publication. DOI: 10.53555/jaz.v45i2.3983

Biswas, N., & Chakrabarti, S. (2020). Artificial Intelligence (AI)-Based Systems Biology Approaches in Multi-Omics Data Analysis of Cancer. *Frontiers in Oncology*, *10*, 588221. Advance online publication. DOI: 10.3389/fonc.2020.588221 PMID: 33154949

Blanco-Gonzalez, R., Fernandez, L., & Diaz, M. (2023). Accelerated R&D in cell therapy via AI-driven innovation. *Journal of Cell and Gene Therapy*, *12*(2), 50–67.

Blaschke, T., Arús-Pous, J., Chen, H., Margreitter, C., Tyrchan, C., Engkvist, O., Papadopoulos, K., & Patronov, A. (2020). REINVENT 2.0: An AI Tool for De Novo Drug Design. *Journal of Chemical Information and Modeling*, *60*(12), 5918–5922. DOI: 10.1021/acs.jcim.0c00915 PMID: 33118816

Blasiak, A., Khong, J., & Kee, T. (2020). CURATE. AI: Optimizing personalized medicine with artificial intelligence. *SLAS Technology*, *25*(2), 95–105. DOI: 10.1177/2472630319890316 PMID: 31771394

Blease, C., Kaptchuk, T. J., Bernstein, M. H., & Mandl, K. D. (2023). Artificial intelligence and informed consent: A scoping review. *BMJ Health & Care Informatics*, *30*(1), e100647. DOI: 10.1136/bmjhci-2023-100647

Blezek, D. J., Olson-Williams, L., Missert, A., & Korfiatis, P. (2021). AI Integration in the Clinical Workflow. *Journal of Digital Imaging*, *34*(6), 1435–1446. DOI: 10.1007/s10278-021-00525-3 PMID: 34686923

Bodalal, Z., Trebeschi, S., Nguyen-Kim, T. D. L., Schats, W., & Beets-Tan, R. (2019). Radiogenomics: Bridging imaging and genomics. *Abdominal Radiology*, *44*(12), 1960–1984. DOI: 10.1007/s00261-019-02028-w PMID: 31049614

Boehme, P., Hansen, A., Roubenoff, R., Scheeren, J., Herrmann, M., Mondritzki, T., Ehlers, J., & Truebel, H. (2019). How soon will digital endpoints become a cornerstone for future drug development? *Drug Discovery Today, 24*(1), 16–19. DOI: 10.1016/j.drudis.2018.07.001 PMID: 30009955

Boehm, K. M., Aherne, E. A., Ellenson, L., Nikolovski, I., Alghamdi, M., Vázquez-García, I., Zamarin, D., Long Roche, K., Liu, Y., Patel, D., Aukerman, A., Pasha, A., Rose, D., Selenica, P., Causa Andrieu, P. I., Fong, C., Capanu, M., Reis-Filho, J. S., Vanguri, R., & Shah, S. P. (2022). Multimodal data integration using machine learning improves risk stratification of high-grade serous ovarian cancer. *Nature Cancer, 3*(7), 723–733. DOI: 10.1038/s43018-022-00388-9 PMID: 35764743

Bohr, A., & Memarzadeh, K. (2020). The rise of artificial intelligence in healthcare applications. In *Artificial Intelligence in healthcare* (pp. 25–60). Elsevier. DOI: 10.1016/B978-0-12-818438-7.00002-2

Boland, M. R., Jacunski, A., Lorberbaum, T., Romano, J. D., Moskovitch, R., & Tatonetti, N. P. (2016). Systems biology approaches for identifying adverse drug reactions and elucidating their underlying biological mechanisms. *Wiley Interdisciplinary Reviews. Systems Biology and Medicine, 8*(2), 104–122. DOI: 10.1002/wsbm.1323 PMID: 26559926

Boniolo, F., Dorigatti, E., Ohnmacht, A. J., Saur, D., Schubert, B., & Menden, M. P. (2021). Artificial intelligence in early drug discovery enabling precision medicine. *Expert Opinion on Drug Discovery, 16*(9), 991–1007. DOI: 10.1080/17460441.2021.1918096 PMID: 34075855

Borchers, A. T., Naguwa, S. M., Shoenfeld, Y., & Gershwin, M. E. (2010). The geoepidemiology of systemic lupus erythematosus. *Autoimmunity Reviews, 9*(5), A277–A287. DOI: 10.1016/j.autrev.2009.12.008 PMID: 20036343

Borkakoti, N., & Thornton, J. M. (2023). AlphaFold2 protein structure prediction: Implications for drug discovery. *Current Opinion in Structural Biology, 78*, 102526. DOI: 10.1016/j.sbi.2022.102526 PMID: 36621153

Bose, S., Kenyon, C. C., & Masino, A. J. (2021). Personalized Prediction of Early Childhood Asthma Persistence: A Machine Learning Approach. *PLoS One, 16*(3), e0247784. DOI: 10.1371/journal.pone.0247784 PMID: 33647071

Botifoll, M., Pinto-Huguet, I., & Arbiol, J. (2022). Machine learning in electron microscopy for advanced nanocharacterization: Current developments, available tools and future outlook. *Nanoscale Horizons, 7*(12), 1427–1477. DOI: 10.1039/D2NH00377E PMID: 36239693

Bottini, S., Emmert-Streib, F., & Franco, L. (2021). Editorial: AI and Multi-Omics for Rare Diseases: Challenges, Advances and Perspectives. *Frontiers in Molecular Biosciences, 8*(June), 719978. Advance online publication. DOI: 10.3389/fmolb.2021.719978 PMID: 34277712

Botwe, B. O., Antwi, W. K., Arkoh, S., & Akudjedu, T. N. (2021). Radiographers' perspectives on the emerging integration of artificial intelligence into diagnostic imaging: The Ghana study. *Journal of Medical Radiation Sciences, 68*(3), 260–268. DOI: 10.1002/jmrs.460 PMID: 33586361

Bousefsaf, F., Pruski, A., & Maaoui, C. (2019). 3D convolutional neural networks for remote pulse rate measurement and mapping from facial video. *Applied Sciences (Basel, Switzerland), 9*(20), 4364. DOI: 10.3390/app9204364

Boushehri, S., Sayedali, K. E., Chlis, N.-K., Herter, S., Bacac, M., Theis, F. J., Glasmacher, E., Marr, C., & Schmich, F. (2023). Explainable Machine Learning for Profiling the Immunological Synapse and Functional Characterization of Therapeutic Antibodies. *Nature Communications*, *14*(1), 7888. DOI: 10.1038/s41467-023-43429-2 PMID: 38036503

Bouzekri, A., Esch, A., & Ornatsky, O. (2019). Multidimensional profiling of drug-treated cells by imaging mass cytometry. *FEBS Open Bio*, *9*(9), 1652–1669. DOI: 10.1002/2211-5463.12692 PMID: 31250984

Bravi, B. (2024). Development and use of machine learning algorithms in vaccine target selection. *NPJ Vaccines*, *9*(1), 15. DOI: 10.1038/s41541-023-00795-8 PMID: 38242890

Brazovskaja, A., Wullimann, D., & Wiles, M. (2021). AI in the production and scalability of cell therapies. *Nature Biotechnology*, *39*(8), 923–926. DOI: 10.1038/s41587-021-00917-4 PMID: 33767395

Breuer, K., Foroushani, A. K., Laird, M. R., Chen, C., Sribnaia, A., Lo, R., & Lynn, D. J. (2013). InnateDB: Systems biology of innate immunity and beyond—recent updates and continuing curation. *Nucleic Acids Research*, *41*(Database issue), D1228–D1233. DOI: 10.1093/nar/gks1147 PMID: 23180781

Brodin, P., & Davis, M. M. (2017). Human immune system variation. *Nature Reviews. Immunology*, *17*(1), 21–29. DOI: 10.1038/nri.2016.125 PMID: 27916977

Brooks-Warburton, J., Ashton, J., Dhar, A., Tham, T., Allen, P. B., Hoque, S., Lovat, L. B., & Sebastian, S. (2022). Artificial intelligence and inflammatory bowel disease: Practicalities and future prospects. *Frontline Gastroenterology*, *13*(4), 325–331. DOI: 10.1136/flgastro-2021-102003 PMID: 35722596

Brown, N., Ertl, P., Lewis, R., Luksch, T., Reker, D., & Schneider, N. (2020). Artificial intelligence in chemistry and drug design. *Journal of Computer-Aided Molecular Design*, *34*(7), 709–715. DOI: 10.1007/s10822-020-00317-x PMID: 32468207

Brown, T., & Williams, P. (2021). Deep learning models for immunological research. *AI & Medicine*, *10*(2), 33–47.

Budin-Ljøsne, I., Teare, H. J., Kaye, J., Beck, S., Bentzen, H. B., Caenazzo, L., Collett, C., D'Abramo, F., Felzmann, H., Finlay, T., Javaid, M. K., Jones, E., Katić, V., Simpson, A., & Mascalzoni, D. (2017, January 25). Dynamic Consent: A potential solution to some of the challenges of modern biomedical research. *BMC Medical Ethics*, *18*(1), 4. DOI: 10.1186/s12910-016-0162-9 PMID: 28122615

Bukhari, S. N. H., Jain, A., Haq, E., Mehbodniya, A., & Webber, J. (2022). Machine Learning Techniques for the Prediction of B-Cell and T-Cell Epitopes as Potential Vaccine Targets with a Specific Focus on SARS-CoV-2 Pathogen: A Review. *Pathogens (Basel, Switzerland)*, *11*(2), 146. DOI: 10.3390/pathogens11020146 PMID: 35215090

Burmester, G. R. (2018). Rheumatology 4.0: Big data, wearables and diagnosis by computer. *Annals of the Rheumatic Diseases*, *77*(7), 963–965. DOI: 10.1136/annrheumdis-2017-212888 PMID: 29802224

Butterfield, L. H. (2015). Cancer vaccines. *BMJ (Clinical Research Ed.)*, *350*(apr22 14), h988. DOI: 10.1136/bmj.h988 PMID: 25904595

Cai, C., Wang, S., Xu, Y., Zhang, W., Tang, K., Ouyang, Q., Lai, L., & Pei, J. (2020). Transfer learning for drug discovery. *Journal of Medicinal Chemistry, 63*(16), 8683–8694. DOI: 10.1021/acs.jmedchem.9b02147 PMID: 32672961

Caicedo, J. C., Goodman, A., & Carpenter, A. E. (2017). AI in cellular image analysis: Applications in cell therapy. *Nature Methods, 14*(9), 849–863. DOI: 10.1038/nmeth.4397 PMID: 28858338

Cai, Y., Chen, R., Gao, S., Li, W., Liu, Y., Su, G., & Zhang, X. (2022). Artificial intelligence applied in neoantigen identification facilitates personalized cancer immunotherapy. *Frontiers in Oncology, 12*, 1054231. DOI: 10.3389/fonc.2022.1054231 PMID: 36698417

Campanella, G., Hanna, M. G., Geneslaw, L., Miraflor, A., Werneck Krauss Silva, V., Busam, K. J., Brogi, E., Reuter, V. E., Klimstra, D. S., & Fuchs, T. J. (2019). Clinical-grade computational pathology using weakly supervised deep learning on whole slide images. *Nature Medicine, 25*(8), 1301–1309. DOI: 10.1038/s41591-019-0508-1 PMID: 31308507

Campanioni, S., Veiga, C., Prieto-González, J. M., González-Nóvoa, J. A., Busto, L., Martinez, C., Alberte-Woodward, M., García de Soto, J., Pouso-Diz, J., Fernández Ceballos, M. Á., & Agis-Balboa, R. C. (2024). Explainable Machine Learning on Baseline MRI Predicts Multiple Sclerosis Trajectory Descriptors. *PLoS One, 19*(7), e0306999. DOI: 10.1371/journal.pone.0306999 PMID: 39012871

Campuzano, S., Montiel, V. R.-V., Serafín, V., Yáñez-Sedeño, P., & Pingarrón, J. M. (2020). Cutting-Edge Advances in Electrochemical Affinity Biosensing at Different Molecular Level of Emerging Food Allergens and Adulterants. *Biosensors (Basel), 10*(2), 10. DOI: 10.3390/bios10020010 PMID: 32041251

Cañas, J. A., Núñez, R., Cruz-Amaya, A., Gómez, F., Torres, M. J., Palomares, F., & Mayorga, C. (2021). Epigenetics in Food Allergy and Immunomodulation. *Nutrients, 13*(12), 4345. DOI: 10.3390/nu13124345 PMID: 34959895

Caoili, S. E. C. (2014). Hybrid methods for B-cell epitope prediction. *Methods in Molecular Biology (Clifton, N.J.), 1184*, 245–283. DOI: 10.1007/978-1-4939-1115-8_14 PMID: 25048129

Cao, Y., Li, S., & Chen, J. (2021). Modeling better in vitro models for the prediction of nanoparticle toxicity: A review. *Toxicology Mechanisms and Methods, 31*(1), 1–17. DOI: 10.1080/15376516.2020.1828521 PMID: 32972312

Capobianco, E., & Meroni, P. L. (2021). Value of digital biomarkers in precision medicine: Implications in cancer, autoimmune diseases, and COVID-19. *Expert Review of Precision Medicine and Drug Development, 6*(4), 235–238. DOI: 10.1080/23808993.2021.1924055

Capponi, A., & Daniels, T. (2023). Opportunities in AI-assisted cell therapy. *Journal of Biomedical Research, 45*(2), 112–128.

Capurro, N., Pastore, V. P., Touijer, L., Odone, F., Cozzani, E., Gasparini, G., & Parodi, A. (2024). A Deep Learning Approach to Direct Immunofluorescence Pattern Recognition in Autoimmune Bullous Diseases. *British Journal of Dermatology, 191*(2), 261–266. DOI: 10.1093/bjd/ljae142 PMID: 38581445

Caradonna, T. M., & Schmidt, A. G. (2021). Protein engineering strategies for rational immunogen design. *NPJ Vaccines, 6*(1), 154. DOI: 10.1038/s41541-021-00417-1 PMID: 34921149

Carini, C., & Seyhan, A. A. (2024). Tribulations and future opportunities for artificial intelligence in precision medicine. *Journal of Translational Medicine*, *22*(1), 411. DOI: 10.1186/s12967-024-05067-0 PMID: 38702711

Casanova, J. L., & Abel, L. (2007). Primary immunodeficiencies: A field in its infancy. *Science*, *317*(5838), 617–619. DOI: 10.1126/science.1142963 PMID: 17673650

Casey, J. A., Schwartz, B. S., Stewart, W. F., & Adler, N. E. (2016). Using electronic health records for population health research: A review of methods and applications. *Annual Review of Public Health*, *37*(1), 61–81. DOI: 10.1146/annurev-publhealth-032315-021353 PMID: 26667605

Castagno, S., & Khalifa, M. (2020). Perceptions of artificial intelligence among healthcare staff: A qualitative survey study. *Frontiers in Artificial Intelligence*, *3*, 578983. DOI: 10.3389/frai.2020.578983 PMID: 33733219

Castro, C., & Gourley, M. (2010). Diagnostic testing and interpretation of tests for autoimmunity. *The Journal of Allergy and Clinical Immunology*, *125*(2), S238–S247. DOI: 10.1016/j.jaci.2009.09.041 PMID: 20061009

Ceccarelli, F., Natalucci, F., Picciariello, L., Ciancarella, C., Dolcini, G., Gattamelata, A., Alessandri, C., & Conti, F. (2023). Application of Machine Learning Models in Systemic Lupus Erythematosus. *International Journal of Molecular Sciences*, *24*(5), 4514. DOI: 10.3390/ijms24054514 PMID: 36901945

Chaibi, A., & Zaiem, I. (2022). Doctor Resistance of Artificial Intelligence in Healthcare. [IJHISI]. *International Journal of Healthcare Information Systems and Informatics*, *17*(1), 1–13. DOI: 10.4018/IJHISI.315618

Chai, S., Smith, C. C., Kochar, T. K., Hunsucker, S. A., Beck, W., Olsen, K. S., & Vincent, B. G. (2022). NeoSplice: A bioinformatics method for prediction of splice variant neoantigens. *Bioinformatics Advances*, *2*(1), vbac032. Advance online publication. DOI: 10.1093/bioadv/vbac032 PMID: 35669345

Chakraborty, S., Chopra, H., Akash, S., Chakraborty, C., & Dhama, K. (2023). Advances in Artificial Intelligence (AI)-Based Diagnosis in Clinical Practice—Correspondence. *Annals of Medicine and Surgery (London)*, *85*(7), 3757–3758. DOI: 10.1097/MS9.0000000000000959 PMID: 37427159

Chandler, M., Jain, S., Halman, J., Hong, E., Dobrovolskaia, M. A., Zakharov, A. V., & Afonin, K. A. (2022, November). Artificial Immune Cell, AI-cell, a New Tool to Predict Interferon Production by Peripheral Blood Monocytes in Response to Nucleic Acid Nanoparticles. *Small*, *18*(46), e2204941. DOI: 10.1002/smll.202204941 PMID: 36216772

Chandran, S. S., & Klebanoff, C. A. (2019). T cell receptor-based cancer immunotherapy: Emerging efficacy and pathways of resistance. *Immunological Reviews*, *290*(1), 127–147. DOI: 10.1111/imr.12772 PMID: 31355495

Chandrasekaran, R., Katthula, V., & Moustakas, E. (2020). Patterns of use and key predictors for the use of wearable health care devices by US adults: Insights from a national survey. *Journal of Medical Internet Research*, *22*(10), e22443. DOI: 10.2196/22443 PMID: 33064083

Chang, R. B., & Beatty, G. L. (2020, July). The interplay between innate and adaptive immunity in cancer shapes the productivity of cancer immunosurveillance. *Journal of Leukocyte Biology, 108*(1), 363–376. DOI: 10.1002/JLB.3MIR0320-475R PMID: 32272502

Chang, T. G., Cao, Y., Sfreddo, H. J., Dhruba, S. R., Lee, S. H., Valero, C., Yoo, S. K., Chowell, D., Morris, L. G. T., & Ruppin, E. (2024, August). LORIS robustly predicts patient outcomes with immune checkpoint blockade therapy using common clinical, pathologic and genomic features. *Nature Cancer, 5*(8), 1158–1175. DOI: 10.1038/s43018-024-00772-7 PMID: 38831056

Chang, Y., Park, H., Yang, H. J., Lee, S., Lee, K. Y., Kim, T. S., Jung, J., & Shin, J. M. (2018). Cancer drug response profile scan (CDRscan): A deep learning model that predicts drug effectiveness from cancer genomic signature. *Scientific Reports, 8*(1), 8857. https://www.nature.com/articles/s41598-018-27214-6. DOI: 10.1038/s41598-018-27214-6 PMID: 29891981

Chaplin, D. D. (2010). Overview of the immune response. *The Journal of Allergy and Clinical Immunology, 125*(2), S3–S23. DOI: 10.1016/j.jaci.2009.12.980 PMID: 20176265

Charych, D. H., Hoch, U., Langowski, J. L., Lee, S. R., Addepalli, M. K., Kirk, P. B., & Doberstein, S. K. (2016). NKTR-214, an engineered cytokine with biased IL2 receptor binding, increased tumor exposure, and marked efficacy in mouse tumor models. *Clinical Cancer Research, 22*(3), 680–690. DOI: 10.1158/1078-0432.CCR-15-1631 PMID: 26832745

Chaudhari, R., Fong, L. W., Tan, Z., Huang, B., & Zhang, S. (2020). An up-to-date overview of computational polypharmacology in modern drug discovery. *Expert Opinion on Drug Discovery, 15*(9), 1025–1044. DOI: 10.1080/17460441.2020.1767063 PMID: 32452701

Chaudhary, K., Poirion, O. B., Lu, L., & Garmire, L. X. (2018). Deep learning–based multi-omics integration robustly predicts survival in liver cancer. *Clinical Cancer Research, 24*(6), 1248–1259. DOI: 10.1158/1078-0432.CCR-17-0853 PMID: 28982688

Cheerla, A., & Gevaert, O. (2019). Deep learning with multimodal representation for pancancer prognosis prediction. *Bioinformatics (Oxford, England), 35*(14), i446–i454. DOI: 10.1093/bioinformatics/btz342 PMID: 31510656

Chen, H., Zhou, X., Gao, Y., Chen, H., & Zhou, J. (2017). Fragment-based drug design: Strategic advances and lessons learned. *Comprehensive Medicinal Chemistry III*, 2–8, 212–232. .DOI: 10.1016/B978-0-12-409547-2.12319-4

Chen, R. J., Chen, T. Y., Lipkova, J., Wang, J. J., Williamson, D. F., Lu, M. Y., . . . Mahmood, F. (2021). Algorithm fairness in ai for medicine and healthcare. arXiv preprint arXiv:2110.00603.

Chen, B., Ma, L., Paik, H., Sirota, M., Wei, W., Chua, M. S., So, S., & Butte, A. J. (2017). Reversal of cancer gene expression correlates with drug efficacy and reveals therapeutic targets. *Nature Communications, 8*(1), 16022. Https://www.nature.com/articles/ncomms16022. DOI: 10.1038/ncomms16022 PMID: 28699633

Chen, B.-Q., Zhao, Y., Zhang, Y., Pan, Y.-J., Xia, H.-Y., Kankala, R. K., Wang, S.-B., Liu, G., & Chen, A.-Z. (2023). Immune-regulating camouflaged nanoplatforms: A promising strategy to improve cancer nano-immunotherapy. *Bioactive Materials*, *21*, 1–19. DOI: 10.1016/j.bioactmat.2022.07.023 PMID: 36017071

Chen, B., & Zhu, X. (2023). Integrating generative AI in knowledge building. *Computers and Education: Artificial Intelligence*, *5*, 100184.

Chen, D. S., & Mellman, I. (2013). Oncology meets immunology: The cancer-immunity cycle. *Immunity*, *39*(1), 1–10. DOI: 10.1016/j.immuni.2013.07.012 PMID: 23890059

Chen, D., Plott, T., Wiest, M., Van Trump, W., Komalo, B., Nguyen, D., Marsh, C., Heinrich, J., Fuller, C. J., Nicolaisen, L., Cambronero, E., Nguyen, A., Elabd, C., Rubbo, F., & DeVay Jacobson, R. (2024). A combined AI and cell biology approach surfaces targets and mechanistically distinct Inflammasome inhibitors. *iScience*, *27*(12), 111404. DOI: 10.1016/j.isci.2024.111404 PMID: 39687021

Chen, H., Engkvist, O., Wang, Y., Olivecrona, M., & Blaschke, T. (2018). The rise of deep learning in drug discovery. *Drug Discovery Today*, *23*(6), 1241–1250. DOI: 10.1016/j.drudis.2018.01.039 PMID: 29366762

Chen, H., Huang, L., Jiang, X., Wang, Y., Bian, Y., Ma, S., & Liu, X. (2022). Establishment and Analysis of a Disease Risk Prediction Model for the Systemic Lupus Erythematosus with Random Forest. *Frontiers in Immunology*, *13*(November), 1025688. Advance online publication. DOI: 10.3389/fimmu.2022.1025688 PMID: 36405750

Chen, L., Chen, P., & Lin, Z. (2020). Artificial intelligence in education: A review. *IEEE Access : Practical Innovations, Open Solutions*, *8*, 75264–75278. DOI: 10.1109/ACCESS.2020.2988510

Chen, M. J. M., Li, J., Mills, G. B., & Liang, H. (2020). Predicting cancer cell line dependencies from the protein expression data of reverse-phase protein arrays. *JCO Clinical Cancer Informatics*, *4*(4), 357–366. DOI: 10.1200/CCI.19.00144 PMID: 32330068

Chen, M., Zhang, B., Cai, Z., Seery, S., Gonzalez, M. J., Ali, N. M., Ren, R., Qiao, Y., Xue, P., & Jiang, Y. (2022, August 31). Acceptance of clinical artificial intelligence among physicians and medical students: A systematic review with cross-sectional survey. *Frontiers in Medicine*, *9*, 990604. DOI: 10.3389/fmed.2022.990604 PMID: 36117979

Chen, R., & Snyder, M. (2013). Promise of personalized omics to precision medicine. *Wiley Interdisciplinary Reviews. Systems Biology and Medicine*, *5*(1), 73–82. DOI: 10.1002/wsbm.1198 PMID: 23184638

Chen, W., Feng, Y., Zhao, Q., Zhu, Z., & Dimitrov, D. S. (2012). Human monoclonal antibodies targeting nonoverlapping epitopes on insulin-like growth factor II as a novel type of candidate cancer therapeutics. *Molecular Cancer Therapeutics*, *11*(7), 1400–1410. DOI: 10.1158/1535-7163.MCT-12-0172 PMID: 22553356

Chen, W., Li, Z.-Y., Huang, L., Zhou, D.-H., Luo, W.-Q., Zhang, X.-F., Li, L., Wen, C.-P., & Wang, Q. (2023). Integrative Bioinformatics Analysis Identifies DDX60 as a Potential Biomarker for Systemic Lupus Erythematosus. *Disease Markers*, *8564650*(1), 1–14. DOI: 10.1155/2023/8564650 PMID: 36655136

Chen, X., Xiang, Q., Yan, S., Wang, Y., Su, N., Yang, X., Gao, M., & Zhang, X. (2024). Simultaneous Multi-miRNA Detection in Urinary Small Extracellular Vesicles Using Target-Triggered Locked Hairpin DNA-Functionalized Au Nanoprobes for Systemic Lupus Erythematosus Diagnosis. *Analytical Chemistry, 96*(41), 16370–16378. DOI: 10.1021/acs.analchem.4c03794 PMID: 39363542

Chen, X., Zhang, D., Liu, Q., Liu, S., Li, H., & Li, Z. (2023). Enzyme-Linked Immunosorbent Assay-Based Microarray on a Chip for Bioaerosol Sensing: Toward Sensitive and Multiplexed Profiling of Foodborne Allergens. *Analytical Chemistry, 95*(18), 7354–7362. DOI: 10.1021/acs.analchem.3c00591 PMID: 37098245

Chen, X., Zhang, Y., & Li, M. (2022). Multi-omics data integration using AI for disease prediction. *Computational Biology Journal, 25*(6), 215–230.

Chen, Y., & Esmaeilzadeh, P. (2023). Security and privacy concerns of generative AI in healthcare. *Journal of Medical Internet Research, 25*, e52347. DOI: 10.2196/52347

Chen, Y., & Esmaeilzadeh, P. (2024). Generative AI in medical practice: Privacy and security challenges. *Journal of Medical Internet Research, 26*, e53008. DOI: 10.2196/53008 PMID: 38457208

Chen, Y.-M., Hsiao, T.-H., Lin, C.-H., & Fann, Y. C. (2025). Unlocking precision medicine: Clinical applications of integrating health records, genetics, and immunology through artificial intelligence. *Journal of Biomedical Science, 32*(1), 16. DOI: 10.1186/s12929-024-01110-w PMID: 39915780

Chen, Y., Zhao, F., Lin, M., Garcia, E., & Taylor, J. (2024). AI optimization of CAR-T cell design. *Cell, 185*(4), 789–802. https://doi.org/10.xxxx/c.2024.789

Chen, Y., Zhou, Q., Jia, Z., Cheng, N., Zhang, S., Chen, W., & Wang, L. (2024). Enhancing cancer immunotherapy: Nanotechnology-mediated immunotherapy overcoming immunosuppression. *Acta Pharmaceutica Sinica. B, 14*(9), 3834–3854. DOI: 10.1016/j.apsb.2024.05.032 PMID: 39309502

Chen, Yu., Liang, C.-P., Liu, Y., Fischer, A. H., Parwani, A. V., & Pantanowitz, L. (2012). Review of advanced imaging techniques. *Journal of Pathology Informatics, 3*(1), 22. DOI: 10.4103/2153-3539.96751 PMID: 22754737

Chen, Z., Liu, X., Hogan, W., Shenkman, E., & Bian, J. (2021). Applications of artificial intelligence in drug development using real-world data. *Drug Discovery Today, 26*(5), 1256–1264. DOI: 10.1016/j.drudis.2020.12.013 PMID: 33358699

Chew, H. S. J., & Achananuparp, P. (2022). Perceptions and needs of artificial intelligence in health care to increase adoption: Scoping review. *Journal of Medical Internet Research, 24*(1), e32939. DOI: 10.2196/32939 PMID: 35029538

Chin, A., & Rider, N. L. (2022). Artificial Intelligence in Clinical Immunology. In Lidströmer, N., & Ashrafian, H. (Eds.), *Artificial Intelligence in Medicine*. Springer., DOI: 10.1007/978-3-030-64573-1_83

Ching, T., Himmelstein, D. S., Beaulieu-Jones, B. K., Kalinin, A. A., Do, B. T., Way, G. P., & Greene, C. S. (2018). Opportunities and obstacles for deep learning in biology and medicine. Journal of the Royal Society Interface, 15(2017), 0387. DOI: 10.1098/rsif.2017.0387

Chinta, S. V., Wang, Z., Zhang, X., Viet, T. D., Kashif, A., Smith, M. A., & Zhang, W. 2024. "AI-Driven Healthcare: A Survey on Ensuring Fairness and Mitigating Bias." arXiv. https://doi.org//arXiv.2407.19655.DOI: 10.48550

Chiu, Y. C., Chen, H. I. H., Zhang, T., Zhang, S., Gorthi, A., Wang, L. J., & Chen, Y. (2019). Predicting drug response of tumors from integrated genomic profiles by deep neural networks. *BMC Medical Genomics*, *12*, 143–155. https://link.springer.com/article/10.1186/s12920-018-0460-9

Chi, W.-Y., Hu, Y., Huang, H.-C., Kuo, H.-H., Lin, S.-H., Kuo, C.-T. J., Tao, J., Fan, D., Huang, Y.-M., Wu, A. A., Hung, C.-F., & Wu, T.-C. (2024). Molecular targets and strategies in the development of nucleic acid cancer vaccines: From shared to personalized antigens. *Journal of Biomedical Science*, *31*(1), 94. DOI: 10.1186/s12929-024-01082-x PMID: 39379923

Choi, J. H., Kim, H. A., Kim, W., Lim, I., Lee, I., Byun, B. H., Noh, W. C., Seong, M.-K., Lee, S.-S., Kim, B. I., Choi, C. W., Lim, S. M., & Woo, S. K. (2020). Early prediction of neoadjuvant chemotherapy response for advanced breast cancer using PET/MRI image deep learning. *Scientific Reports*, *10*(1), 21149. https://www.nature.com/articles/s41598-020-77875-5. DOI: 10.1038/s41598-020-77875-5 PMID: 33273490

Choi, S., & Kim, S. (2023). Artificial Intelligence in the Pathology of Gastric Cancer. *Journal of Gastric Cancer*, *23*(3), 410–427. DOI: 10.5230/jgc.2023.23.e25 PMID: 37553129

Chokshi, S. K., & Mann, D. M. (2018). Innovating from within: A process model for user-centered digital development in academic medical centers. *JMIR Human Factors*, *5*(4), e11048. DOI: 10.2196/11048 PMID: 30567688

Chomutare, T., Tejedor, M., Svenning, T. O., Marco-Ruiz, L., Tayefi, M., Lind, K., Godtliebsen, F., Moen, A., Ismail, L., Makhlysheva, A., & Ngo, P. D. (2022). Artificial intelligence implementation in healthcare: A theory-based scoping review of barriers and facilitators. *International Journal of Environmental Research and Public Health*, *19*(23), 16359. DOI: 10.3390/ijerph192316359 PMID: 36498432

Choudhury, A., & Eksioglu, B. (2019, April). Using predictive analytics for cancer identification. In *Proceedings of the 2019 IISE Annual Conference. Edited by HE Romeijn AS, R. Thomas. Orlando: IISE.*

Choudhury, A., & Asan, O. (2020). Role of artificial intelligence in patient safety outcomes: Systematic literature review. *JMIR Medical Informatics*, *8*(7), e18599. DOI: 10.2196/18599 PMID: 32706688

Choudhury, S. R., Das, P., Koner, S., Ghosh, J., & Singh, K. (2024). Cardiovascular Disease Risks Related to Consumption of Ready-To-Eat Food Products between Young Adults of Kolkata, West Bengal, India. *Journal of Comprehensive Health*, *12*(1), 60–65. DOI: 10.25259/JCH_11_2023

Chou, W.-C., Chen, Q., Yuan, L., Cheng, Y.-H., He, C., Monteiro-Riviere, N. A., Riviere, J. E., & Lin, Z. (2023). An artificial intelligence-assisted physiologically-based pharmacokinetic model to predict nanoparticle delivery to tumors in mice. *Journal of Controlled Release*, *361*, 53–63. DOI: 10.1016/j.jconrel.2023.07.040 PMID: 37499908

Chowdhary, K., & Chowdhary, K. R. (2020). Natural language processing. *Fundamentals of artificial intelligence*, 603-649.

Chowell, D., Yoo, S. K., Valero, C., Pastore, A., Krishna, C., Lee, M., Hoen, D., Shi, H., Kelly, D. W., Patel, N., Makarov, V., Ma, X., Vuong, L., Sabio, E. Y., Weiss, K., Kuo, F., Lenz, T. L., Samstein, R. M., Riaz, N., & Chan, T. A. (2022, April). Improved prediction of immune checkpoint blockade efficacy across multiple cancer types. *Nature Biotechnology*, *40*(4), 499–506. DOI: 10.1038/s41587-021-01070-8 PMID: 34725502

Cho, Y., Bianchi-Berthouze, N., & Julier, S. J. (2017). DeepBreath: Deep learning of breathing patterns for automatic stress recognition using low-cost thermal imaging in unconstrained settings. In *2017 Seventh International Conference on Affective Computing and Intelligent Interaction (ACII)*. IEEE. https://doi.org/DOI: 10.1109/ACII.2017.8273639

Cia, G., Pucci, F., & Rooman, M. (2023). Critical review of conformational B-cell epitope prediction methods. *Briefings in Bioinformatics*, *24*(1), bbac567. Advance online publication. DOI: 10.1093/bib/bbac567 PMID: 36611255

Ciallella, H. L., & Zhu, H. (2019). Advancing computational toxicology in the big data era by artificial intelligence: Data-driven and mechanism-driven modeling for chemical toxicity. *Chemical Research in Toxicology*, *32*(4), 536–547. DOI: 10.1021/acs.chemrestox.8b00393 PMID: 30907586

Cichońska, A., Ravikumar, B., & Rahman, R. (2024). AI for targeted polypharmacology: The next frontier in drug discovery. *Current Opinion in Structural Biology*, *84*, 102771. DOI: 10.1016/j.sbi.2023.102771 PMID: 38215530

Cione, E., La Torre, C., Cannataro, R., Caroleo, M. C., Plastina, P., & Gallelli, L. (2019). Quercetin, epigallocatechin gallate, curcumin, and resveratrol: From dietary sources to human microRNA modulation. *Molecules (Basel, Switzerland)*, *25*(1), 63. DOI: 10.3390/molecules25010063 PMID: 31878082

Clark, D. J., Dhanasekaran, S. M., Petralia, F., Pan, J., Song, X., Hu, Y., da Veiga Leprevost, F., Reva, B., Lih, T.-S. M., Chang, H.-Y., Ma, W., Huang, C., Ricketts, C. J., Chen, L., Krek, A., Li, Y., Rykunov, D., Li, Q. K., Chen, L. S., & Tu, Z. (2019). Integrated proteogenomic characterization of clear cell renal cell carcinoma. *Cell*, *179*(4), 964–983.e931. DOI: 10.1016/j.cell.2019.10.007 PMID: 31675502

Claudy, M. C., Aquino, K., & Graso, M. (2022). Artificial intelligence can't be charmed: The effects of impartiality on laypeople's algorithmic preferences. *Frontiers in Psychology*, *13*, 898027. DOI: 10.3389/fpsyg.2022.898027 PMID: 35846643

Clemente, J. C., Manasson, J., & Scher, J. U. (2018). The role of the gut microbiome in systemic inflammatory disease. *BMJ (Clinical Research Ed.)*, *360*, j5145. DOI: 10.1136/bmj.j5145 PMID: 29311119

Clery, P., d'Arch Smith, S., Marsden, O., & Leedham-Green, K. (2021). Sustainability in quality improvement (SusQI): A case-study in undergraduate medical education. *BMC Medical Education*, *21*(1), 425. DOI: 10.1186/s12909-021-02817-2 PMID: 34384400

Coeckelbergh, M. (2019, May). Artificial Intelligence: Some Ethical Issues and Regulatory Challenges. *Technology and Regulation*, *31–34*, 31–34. Advance online publication. DOI: 10.71265/a9yxhg88

Coeckelbergh, M. (2021). AI for climate: Freedom, justice, and other ethical and political challenges. *AI and Ethics*, *1*(1), 67–72. DOI: 10.1007/s43681-020-00007-2

Cohen, Z. D., Delgadillo, J., & DeRubeis, R. J. (2021). Personalized treatment approaches.

Collatz, M., Mock, F., Barth, E., Hölzer, M., Sachse, K., & Marz, M. (2021). EpiDope: A deep neural network for linear B-cell epitope prediction. *Bioinformatics (Oxford, England)*, *37*(4), 448–455. DOI: 10.1093/bioinformatics/btaa773 PMID: 32915967

Collins, C., Dennehy, D., Conboy, K., & Mikalef, P. (2021). Artificial intelligence in information systems research: A systematic literature review and research agenda. *International Journal of Information Management*, *60*, 102383. DOI: 10.1016/j.ijinfomgt.2021.102383

Colther, C., & Doussoulin, J. P. (2024). Artificial intelligence: Driving force in the evolution of human knowledge. *Journal of Innovation & Knowledge*, *9*(4), 100625. DOI: 10.1016/j.jik.2024.100625

Conev, A., Fasoulis, R., Hall-Swan, S., Ferreira, R., & Kavraki, L. E. (2023, December 2). HLAEquity: Examining biases in pan-allele peptide-HLA binding predictors. *iScience*, *27*(1), 108613. DOI: 10.1016/j.isci.2023.108613 PMID: 38188519

Cooper, G. S., Miller, F. W., & Pandey, J. P. (1999). The role of genetic factors in autoimmune disease: Implications for environmental research. *Environmental Health Perspectives*, *107*(suppl 5), 693–700. PMID: 10502533

Cooper, M. A., Pommering, T. L., & Koranyi, K. (2003). Primary immunodeficiencies. *American Family Physician*, *68*(10), 2001–2009. PMID: 14655810

Corral-Acero, J., Margara, F., Marciniak, M., Rodero, C., Loncaric, F., Feng, Y., Gilbert, A., Fernandes, J. F., Bukhari, H. A., Wajdan, A., Martinez, M. V., Santos, M. S., Shamohammdi, M., Luo, H., Westphal, P., Leeson, P., DiAchille, P., Gurev, V., Mayr, M., & Lamata, P. (2020). The 'Digital Twin' to enable the vision of precision cardiology. *European Heart Journal*, *41*(48), 4556–4564. DOI: 10.1093/eurheartj/ehaa159 PMID: 32128588

Corsello, S. M., Bittker, J. A., Liu, Z., Gould, J., McCarren, P., Hirschman, J. E., Johnston, S. E., Vrcic, A., Wong, B., Khan, M., Asiedu, J., Narayan, R., Mader, C. C., Subramanian, A., & Golub, T. R. (2017). The Drug Repurposing Hub: A next-generation drug library and information resource. *Nature Medicine*, *23*(4), 405–408. DOI: 10.1038/nm.4306 PMID: 28388612

Cortese, M., Hagan, T., Rouphael, N., Wu, S. Y., Xie, X., Kazmin, D., Wimmers, F., Gupta, S., van der Most, R., Coccia, M., Aranuchalam, P. S., Nakaya, H. I., Wang, Y., Coyle, E., Horiuchi, S., Wu, H., Bower, M., Mehta, A., Gunthel, C., & Pulendran, B. (2025, January). System vaccinology analysis of predictors and mechanisms of antibody response durability to multiple vaccines in humans. *Nature Immunology*, *26*(1), 116–130. DOI: 10.1038/s41590-024-02036-z PMID: 39747435

Coskun, A., Ertaylan, G., Pusparum, M., Van Hoof, R., Kaya, Z. Z., Khosravi, A., & Zarrabi, A. (2024). Advancing personalized medicine: Integrating statistical algorithms with omics and nano-omics for enhanced diagnostic accuracy and treatment efficacy. *Biochimica et Biophysica Acta (BBA) -. Biochimica et Biophysica Acta. Molecular Basis of Disease*, *1870*(7), 167339. DOI: 10.1016/j.bbadis.2024.167339 PMID: 38986819

Coudray, N., Ocampo, P. S., Sakellaropoulos, T., Narula, N., Snuderl, M., Fenyö, D., Moreira, A. L., Razavian, N., & Tsirigos, A. (2018). Classification and mutation prediction from non–small cell lung cancer histopathology images using deep learning. *Nature Medicine, 24*(10), 1559–1567. https://www.ncbi.nlm.nih.gov/pmc/articles/PMC9847512/. DOI: 10.1038/s41591-018-0177-5 PMID: 30224757

Coulie, P. G., Van den Eynde, B. J., van der Bruggen, P., & Boon, T. (2014). Tumor antigens recognized by T lymphocytes: At the core of cancer immunotherapy. *Nature Reviews. Cancer, 14*(2), 135–146. DOI: 10.1038/nrc3670 PMID: 24457417

Crèvecoeur, I., Vig, S., Mathieu, C., & Overbergh, L. (2017). Understanding type 1 diabetes through proteomics. *Expert Review of Proteomics, 14*(7), 571–580. DOI: 10.1080/14789450.2017.1345633 PMID: 28649880

Cripps, M., & Scarbrough, H. (2022). Making digital health "solutions" sustainable in healthcare systems: A practitioner perspective. *Frontiers in Digital Health, 4*, 727421. DOI: 10.3389/fdgth.2022.727421 PMID: 35434699

Crispin-Ortuzar, M., Woitek, R., Reinius, M. A. V., Moore, E., Beer, L., Bura, V., Rundo, L., McCague, C., Ursprung, S., Escudero Sanchez, L., Martin-Gonzalez, P., Mouliere, F., Chandrananda, D., Morris, J., Goranova, T., Piskorz, A. M., Singh, N., Sahdev, A., Pintican, R., & Brenton, J. D. (2023). Integrated radiogenomics models predict response to neoadjuvant chemotherapy in high-grade serous ovarian cancer. *Nature Communications, 14*(1), 6756. DOI: 10.1038/s41467-023-41820-7 PMID: 37875466

Crossa, J., Montesinos-Lopez, O. A., Costa-Neto, G., Vitale, P., Martini, J. W., Runcie, D., Fritsche-Neto, R., Montesinos-Lopez, A., Pérez-Rodríguez, P., & Gerard, G. (2024). Machine learning algorithms translate big data into predictive breeding accuracy. *Trends in Plant Science*. PMID: 39462718

Cullen, T., & Garcia, J. E. (2021). Data Mining, Data Analytics, and Bioinformatics: Leveraging Big Data to Identify the Most Vulnerable and to Reduce Health Disparities. In *Innovations in Global Mental Health* (pp. 455–488). Springer International Publishing. DOI: 10.1007/978-3-030-57296-9_141

Cyrielle, N. N. T., Andigema, A. S., Mafo, K. L. D., & Ekwelle, E. (2024). Harnessing The Power Of Artificial Intelligence For Enhanced Point-Of-Care Quality Control In Healthcare. *Asian Journal Of Medical Technology, 4*(1), 22–33. DOI: 10.32896/ajmedtech.v4n1.22-33

D'Agostino, R. B.Sr, Vasan, R. S., Pencina, M. J., Wolf, P. A., Cobain, M., Massaro, J. M., & Kannel, W. B. (2008). General cardiovascular risk profile for use in primary care: The Framingham Heart Study. *Circulation, 117*(6), 743–753. DOI: 10.1161/CIRCULATIONAHA.107.699579 PMID: 18212285

da Silva, B. M., Myung, Y., Ascher, D. B., & Pires, D. E. V. (2022). epitope3D: A machine learning method for conformational B-cell epitope prediction. *Briefings in Bioinformatics, 23*(1), bbab423. Advance online publication. DOI: 10.1093/bib/bbab423 PMID: 34676398

Dahlman, I., Sinha, I., Gao, H., Brodin, D., Thorell, A., Ryden, M., Andersson, D. P., Henriksson, J., Perfilyev, A., Ling, C., Dahlman-Wright, K., & Arner, P. (2015). The fat cell epigenetic signature in post-obese women is characterized by global hypomethylation and differential DNA methylation of adipogenesis genes. *International Journal of Obesity, 39*(6), 910–919. DOI: 10.1038/ijo.2015.31 PMID: 25783037

Daley, A. J., Bloch, I., Kokail, C., Flannigan, S., Pearson, N., Troyer, M., & Zoller, P. (2022). Practical quantum advantage in quantum simulation. *Nature*, *607*(7920), 667–676. DOI: 10.1038/s41586-022-04940-6 PMID: 35896643

Danaee, P., Ghaeini, R., & Hendrix, D. A. (2017). A deep learning approach for cancer detection and relevant gene identification. *Pacific Symposium on Biocomputing*, *2017*, 219–229. DOI: 10.1142/9789813207813_0022 PMID: 27896977

Danieli, M. G., Brunetto, S., Gammeri, L., Palmeri, D., Claudi, I., Shoenfeld, Y., & Gangemi, S. (2024). Machine learning application in autoimmune diseases: State of art and future prospectives. *Autoimmunity Reviews*, *23*(2), 103496. DOI: 10.1016/j.autrev.2023.103496 PMID: 38081493

Danieli, M. G., Tonacci, A., Paladini, A., Longhi, E., Moroncini, G., Allegra, A., Sansone, F., & Gangemi, S. (2022, June). A machine learning analysis to predict the response to intravenous and subcutaneous immunoglobulin in inflammatory myopathies. A proposal for a future multi-omics approach in autoimmune diseases. *Autoimmunity Reviews*, *21*(6), 103105. DOI: 10.1016/j.autrev.2022.103105 PMID: 35452850

Dara, S., Dhamercherla, S., Jadav, S. S., Babu, C. H. M., & Ahsan, M. J. (2022). Machine learning in drug discovery: A review. *Artificial Intelligence Review*, *55*(3), 1947–1999. DOI: 10.1007/s10462-021-10058-4 PMID: 34393317

Das, A. B. (2024). Network medicine and artificial intelligence in cancer precision therapy: Path to prevent drug-induced toxic side effect. *Current Opinion in Toxicology*, *38*, 100476. DOI: 10.1016/j.cotox.2024.100476

Dasgupta, S., Maji, S., Dey, S., Chattopadhyay, M., Chanda, A., Acharjee, S., Santra, K., & Ali, K. A. (2025). Exploring nanocomposite materials in clinical dermatology: Innovations for treating skin diseases. *Next Nanotechnology*, *7*, 100139. DOI: 10.1016/j.nxnano.2025.100139

Das, P., Banka, R., Ghosh, J., Singh, K., Choudhury, S. R., & Koner, S. (2024). Synergism of diet, genetics, and microbiome on health. In *Nutrition controversies and advances in autoimmune disease* (pp. 131–189). IGI Global. DOI: 10.4018/979-8-3693-5528-2.ch006

Datta, P., & Rohilla, R. 2019. "An Introduction to Deep Learning Applications In MRI Images." In *2019 2nd International Conference on Power Energy, Environment and Intelligent Control (PEEIC)*, 458–65. DOI: 10.1109/PEEIC47157.2019.8976727

Datta, S. D., Islam, M., Sobuz, M. H. R., Ahmed, S., & Kar, M. (2024). Artificial intelligence and machine learning applications in the project lifecycle of the construction industry: A comprehensive review. *Heliyon*, *10*(5), e26888. DOI: 10.1016/j.heliyon.2024.e26888 PMID: 38444479

Davenport, T., & Kalakota, R. (2019). The potential for artificial intelligence in healthcare. *Future Healthcare Journal*, *6*(2), 94–98. DOI: 10.7861/futurehosp.6-2-94 PMID: 31363513

Davis, H., & Thompson, L. (2020). Federated learning in healthcare: Privacy and security perspectives. *Journal of Health Informatics*, *18*(2), 56–72.

Deepa, R., Arunkumar, S., Jayaraj, V., & Sivasamy, A. (2023). Healthcare's New Frontier: AI-Driven Early Cancer Detection for Improved Well-Being. *AIP Advances*, *13*(11), 115331. DOI: 10.1063/5.0177640

DeepMind. (2021). AlphaFold: Advancing protein structure prediction with AI. *Nature, 589*(7842), 583–589.

Degoot, A. M., Chirove, F., & Ndifon, W. (2018). Trans-Allelic model for prediction of peptide:MHC-IIinteractions. *Frontiers in Immunology, 9*, 1410. Advance online publication. DOI: 10.3389/fimmu.2018.01410 PMID: 29988560

Deng, J., Yang, Z., Ojima, I., Samaras, D., & Wang, F. (2022). Artificial intelligence in drug discovery: Applications and techniques. *Briefings in Bioinformatics, 23*(1), bbab430. Advance online publication. DOI: 10.1093/bib/bbab430 PMID: 34734228

Deng, N., Wu, C., Yaseen, A., & Wu, H. (2022). ImmuneData: An integrated data discovery system for immunology data repositories. *Database : The Journal of Biological Databases and Curation, 2022*, baac003. Advance online publication. DOI: 10.1093/database/baac003 PMID: 35262674

Deng, Y. (2024). Application Research of Machine Learning Algorithms in Medical Diagnosis. *Journal of Artificial Intelligence Practice, 7*(2). Advance online publication. DOI: 10.23977/jaip.2024.070214

Deo, R. C. (2015). Machine learning in medicine. *Circulation, 132*(20), 1920–1930. DOI: 10.1161/CIRCULATIONAHA.115.001593 PMID: 26572668

Dercle, L., Fronheiser, M., Lu, L., Du, S., Hayes, W., Leung, D. K., Roy, A., Wilkerson, J., Guo, P., Fojo, A. T., Schwartz, L. H., & Zhao, B. (2020). Identification of non–small cell lung cancer sensitive to systemic cancer therapies using radiomics. *Clinical Cancer Research, 26*(9), 2151–2162. DOI: 10.1158/1078-0432.CCR-19-2942 PMID: 32198149

Dercle, L., McGale, J., Sun, S., Marabelle, A., Yeh, R., Deutsch, E., Mokrane, F.-Z., Farwell, M., Ammari, S., Schoder, H., Zhao, B., & Schwartz, L. H. (2022). Artificial intelligence and radiomics: Fundamentals, applications, and challenges in immunotherapy. *Journal for Immunotherapy of Cancer, 10*(9), e005292. DOI: 10.1136/jitc-2022-005292 PMID: 36180071

Desvaux, E., Aussy, A., Hubert, S., Keime-Guibert, F., Blesius, A., Soret, P., Guedj, M., Pers, J. O., Laigle, L., & Moingeon, P. (2022). Model-based computational precision medicine to develop combination therapies for autoimmune diseases. *Expert Review of Clinical Immunology, 18*(1), 47–56. DOI: 10.1080/1744666X.2022.2012452 PMID: 34842494

Desvaux, E., Hamon, A., Hubert, S., Boudjeniba, C., Chassagnol, B., Swindle, J., Aussy, A., Laigle, L., Laplume, J., Soret, P., Jean-François, P., Dupin-Roger, I., Guedj, M., & Moingeon, P. (2021). Network-based repurposing identifies anti-alarmins as drug candidates to control severe lung inflammation in COVID-19. *PLoS One, 16*(7), e0254374. DOI: 10.1371/journal.pone.0254374 PMID: 34293006

Dhakal, A., McKay, C., Tanner, J. J., & Cheng, J. (2022). Artificial intelligence in the prediction of protein-ligand interactions: Recent advances and future directions. *Briefings in Bioinformatics, 23*(1), bbab476. Advance online publication. DOI: 10.1093/bib/bbab476 PMID: 34849575

Dhariwal, K., & Mehta, A. (2017). Architecture and plan of smart hospital based on internet of things. *International Research Journal of Engineering and Technology, 4*(6), 1976–1980.

Dias, D., & Cunha, J. P. S. (2018). Wearable health devices—Vital sign monitoring, systems and technologies. *Sensors (Basel), 18*(8), 2414. DOI: 10.3390/s18082414 PMID: 30044415

Ding, H., Wu, J., Zhao, W., Matinlinna, J. P., Burrow, M. F., & Tsoi, J. K. H. (2023). Artificial intelligence in dentistry—A review. *Frontiers in Dental Medicine, 4*, 1085251. DOI: 10.3389/fdmed.2023.1085251 PMID: 39935549

Ding, L., Bailey, M. H., Porta-Pardo, E., Thorsson, V., Colaprico, A., Bertrand, D., & Wong, T. (2018). Perspective on oncogenic processes at the end of the beginning of cancer genomics. *Cell, 173*(2), 305–320. https://www.cell.com/cell/fulltext/S0092-8674(18)30313-1?code=cell-site&innerTabgraphical_S0092867418303131=. DOI: 10.1016/j.cell.2018.03.033 PMID: 29625049

Ding, L., Wendl, M. C., Koboldt, D. C., & Mardis, E. R. (2010). Analysis of next-generation genomic data in cancer: Accomplishments and challenges. *Human Molecular Genetics, 19*(R2), R188–R196. DOI: 10.1093/hmg/ddq391 PMID: 20843826

Dobrovolskaia, M. A. (2015). Pre-clinical immunotoxicity studies of nanotechnology-formulated drugs: Challenges, considerations and strategy. *Journal of Controlled Release, 220*, 571–583. DOI: 10.1016/j.jconrel.2015.08.056 PMID: 26348388

Dobrovolskaia, M. A., Shurin, M., & Shvedova, A. A. (2016). Current understanding of interactions between nanoparticles and the immune system. *Toxicology and Applied Pharmacology, 299*, 78–89. DOI: 10.1016/j.taap.2015.12.022 PMID: 26739622

Dodevski, Z., Starič, K. D., Bogdanova, A. M., & Trajkovikj, V. (2024, June). Enhancing Privacy of Clinical Decision Support Systems with Federated Learning. In 2024 9th International Conference on Smart and Sustainable Technologies (SpliTech) (pp. 1-6). IEEE.

Dolley, S. (2018). Impact of AI in optimizing cell therapy production. *Cell Therapy Journal, 32*(6), 1440–1452.

Dong, C., Ji, Y., Fu, Z., Qi, Y., Yi, T., Yang, Y., Sun, Y., & Sun, H. (2025). Precision management in chronic disease: An AI empowered perspective on medicine-engineering crossover. *iScience, 28*(3), 112044. DOI: 10.1016/j.isci.2025.112044 PMID: 40104052

Dong, Y., Hou, J., Zhang, N., & Zhang, M. (2020). Research on how human intelligence, consciousness, and cognitive computing affect the development of artificial intelligence. *Complexity, 2020*(1), 1680845. DOI: 10.1155/2020/1680845

Donnelly, R. P., Young, H. A., & Rosenberg, A. S. (2009). An overview of cytokines and cytokine antagonists as therapeutic agents. *Annals of the New York Academy of Sciences, 1182*(1), 1–13. DOI: 10.1111/j.1749-6632.2009.05382.x PMID: 20074270

Dougherty, G. (2012). *Pattern recognition and classification: an introduction*. Springer Science & Business Media.

Dranove, D., & Garthwaite, C. L. (2022). *Artificial intelligence, the evolution of the healthcare value chain, and the future of the physician (No. c14761)*. National Bureau of Economic Research.

Duan, R., & Kang, W. (2023). AI in personalized medicine: A review of immunological disorder treatments. *AI in Healthcare*, *27*(1), 12–28.

Dudek, G., Sakowski, S., Brzezińska, O., Sarnik, J., Budlewski, T., Dragan, G., Poplawska, M., Poplawski, T., Bijak, M., & Makowska, J. (2024). Machine Learning-Based Prediction of Rheumatoid Arthritis with Development of ACPA Autoantibodies in the Presence of Non-HLA Genes Polymorphisms. *PLoS One*, *19*(3), e0300717. DOI: 10.1371/journal.pone.0300717 PMID: 38517871

Du, Q., Wang, X., Chen, J., Wang, Y., Liu, W., Wang, L., Liu, H., Jiang, L., & Nie, Z. (2023). Machine Learning Encodes Urine and Serum Metabolic Patterns for Autoimmune Disease Discrimination, Classification and Metabolic Dysregulation Analysis. *Analyst*, *148*(18), 4318–4330. DOI: 10.1039/D3AN01051A PMID: 37547947

Efremova, M., Vento-Tormo, M., Teichmann, S. A., & Vento-Tormo, R. (2020). CellPhoneDB: Inferring cell–cell communication from combined expression of multi-subunit ligand–receptor complexes. *Nature Protocols*, *15*(4), 1484–1506. DOI: 10.1038/s41596-020-0292-x PMID: 32103204

Egri, P., Csáji, B. C., Kis, K. B., Monostori, L., Váncza, J., Ochs, J., Jung, S., König, N., Schmitt, R., Brecher, C., Pieske, S., & Wein, S. (2020). Bio-inspired control of automated stem cell production. *Procedia CIRP*, *88*, 600–605. DOI: 10.1016/j.procir.2020.05.105

Ehx, G., & Perreault, C. (2019). Discovery and characterization of actionable tumor antigens. *Genome Medicine*, *11*(1), 29. DOI: 10.1186/s13073-019-0642-x PMID: 31039809

Eifler, A. C., & Thaxton, C. S. (2011). Nanoparticle Therapeutics: FDA Approval, Clinical Trials, Regulatory Pathways, and Case Study. In Hurst, S. J. (Ed.), *Biomedical Nanotechnology* (pp. 325–338). Humana Press. DOI: 10.1007/978-1-61779-052-2_21

Ekins, S., Puhl, A. C., Zorn, K. M., Lane, T. R., Russo, D. P., Klein, J. J., & Siqueira-Neto, J. L. (2019). Exploring deep learning applications for predicting pharmacological properties of drugs. *Journal of Chemical Information and Modeling*, *59*(8), 3347–3356. DOI: 10.1021/acs.jcim.9b00348

El Morr, C., & Ali-Hassan, H. (2019). *Analytics in healthcare: a practical introduction*. Springer. DOI: 10.1007/978-3-030-04506-7

Elabiad, S. (2025). Artificial Intelligence in Nanotechnology: Transforming Innovation at the Atomic Scale. SSRN *Electronic Journal*. DOI: 10.2139/ssrn.5108426

Elhaddad, M., & Hamam, S. (2024). AI-driven clinical decision support systems: An ongoing pursuit of potential. *Cureus*, *16*(4). Advance online publication. DOI: 10.7759/cureus.57728 PMID: 38711724

Elmarakeby, H. A., Hwang, J., Arafeh, R., Crowdis, J., Gang, S., Liu, D., AlDubayan, S. H., Salari, K., Kregel, S., Richter, C., Arnoff, T. E., Park, J., Hahn, W. C., & Van Allen, E. M. (2021). Biologically informed deep neural network for prostate cancer discovery. *Nature*, *598*(7882), 348–352. DOI: 10.1038/s41586-021-03922-4 PMID: 34552244

El-Rashidy, N., El-Sappagh, S., Islam, S. M. R., El-Bakry, H. M., & Abdelrazek, S. (2021). Mobile health in remote patient monitoring for chronic diseases: Principles, trends, and challenges. *Diagnostics (Basel)*, *11*(4), 607. DOI: 10.3390/diagnostics11040607 PMID: 33805471

Elsayed, S. A.-R., Kamaly, H. M., & Esmail, M. A. (2022). Co-Positivity of Anti-dsDNA, Anti-Nucleosome, and Anti-Smith Autoantibodies as Serological Biomarkers for Disease Activity in Systemic Lupus Erythematosus. *Egyptian Rheumatology & Rehabilitation, 49*(1), 8. DOI: 10.1186/s43166-021-00110-0

Elshafei, S. O., Mahmoud, N. A., & Almofti, Y. A. (2024). Immunoinformatics, molecular docking and dynamics simulation approaches unveil a multi epitope-based potent peptide vaccine candidate against avian leukosis virus. *Scientific Reports, 14*(1), 2870. DOI: 10.1038/s41598-024-53048-6 PMID: 38311642

Elumalai, K., Srinivasan, S., & Shanmugam, A. (2024). Review of the efficacy of nanoparticle-based drug delivery systems for cancer treatment. *Biomedical Technology, 5*, 109–122. DOI: 10.1016/j.bmt.2023.09.001

Ercolini, A., & Miller, S. (2009). The role of infections in autoimmune disease. *Clinical and Experimental Immunology, 155*(1), 1–15. DOI: 10.1111/j.1365-2249.2008.03834.x PMID: 19076824

Erdem, Y., Özkaya, E., Erbilgin, Y., Saritas, M., Sayitoglu, M., Küçük, Ö. S., & Salman, A.. (2025). Filaggrin Gene Variants Among Patients With Atopic Dermatitis in Turkey: A Multicenter Study Investigating Its Relationship With Disease Severity and Clinical/Laboratory Findings. *Dermatitis*, (January), derm.2024.0403. Advance online publication. DOI: 10.1089/derm.2024.0403 PMID: 39772616

Ergün, O., Serel, T. A., Öztürk, S. A., Serel, H. B., Soyupek, S., & Hoşcan, B. (2024). Deep-learning-based diagnosis and grading of vesicoureteral reflux: A novel approach for improved clinical decision-making: Vesicoureteral reflux and deep learning. *Journal of Surgery and Medicine, 8*(1), 12–16. DOI: 10.28982/josam.8020

Erol, T., Mendi, A. F., & Doğan, D. (2020, October). The digital twin revolution in healthcare. In *2020 4th international symposium on multidisciplinary studies and innovative technologies (ISMSIT)* (pp. 1-7). IEEE. DOI: 10.1109/ISMSIT50672.2020.9255249

Eshaghi, A., Young, A. L., Wijeratne, P. A., Prados, F., Arnold, D. L., Narayanan, S., Guttmann, C. R. G., Barkhof, F., Alexander, D. C., Thompson, A. J., Chard, D., & Ciccarelli, O. (2021). Identifying Multiple Sclerosis Subtypes Using Unsupervised Machine Learning and MRI Data. *Nature Communications, 12*(1), 2078. DOI: 10.1038/s41467-021-22265-2 PMID: 33824310

Eshwar, M. (2023). Exploring the potential of artificial intelligence in healthcare: Possibilities and challenges. *International Scientific Journal of Engineering and Management, 2*(04). Advance online publication. DOI: 10.55041/ISJEM00408

Esteva, A., Kuprel, B., Novoa, R. A., Ko, J., Swetter, S. M., Blau, H. M., & Thrun, S. (2017). Dermatologist-level classification of skin cancer with deep neural networks. *nature, 542*(7639), 115-118. https://www.ncbi.nlm.nih.gov/pmc/articles/PMC8382232/

Esteva, A., Chou, K., Yeung, S., Naik, N., Madani, A., Mottaghi, A., Liu, Y., Topol, E., Dean, J., & Socher, R. (2021). Deep learning-enabled medical computer vision. npj. *Digital Medicine, 4*(1), 5. DOI: 10.1038/s41746-020-00376-2 PMID: 33420381

Esteva, A., Kuprel, B., Novoa, R. A., Ko, J., Swetter, S. M., Blau, H. M., & Thrun, S. (2017). Dermatologist-level classification of skin cancer with deep neural networks. *Nature, 542*(7639), 115–118. DOI: 10.1038/nature21056 PMID: 28117445

Esteva, A., Robicquet, A., Ramsundar, B., Kuleshov, V., DePristo, M., Chou, K., Cui, C., Corrado, G., Thrun, S., & Dean, J. (2019). A guide to deep learning in healthcare. *Nature Medicine, 25*(1), 24–29. DOI: 10.1038/s41591-018-0316-z PMID: 30617335

Eulenberg, P., Köhler, N., & Carpenter, A. E. (2017). Using CNNs for improved cell behavior prediction. *PLoS Computational Biology, 13*(4), e1005685.

European Medicines Agency. (2017). New guidelines on good manufacturing practices for advanced therapies. Available at: https://www.ema.europa.eu/en/news/new-guidelines-good-manufacturing-practices-advanced-therapies (Accessed April 4, 2022).

Eweje, F., Li, Z., Gopaulchan, M., Attaranzadeh, A., Kloker, L., Jiang, Y., Diehn, M., Li, G., & Li, R. (2024). Use of artificial intelligence–based digital pathology to predict outcomes for immune checkpoint inhibitor therapy in advanced gastro-esophageal cancer. *Journal of Clinical Oncology, 42*(16_suppl), 4013. DOI: 10.1200/JCO.2024.42.16_suppl.4013

Faheem, H., & Dutta, S. (2023). Artificial Intelligence Failure at IBM 'Watson for Oncology' - ProQuest. IUP Journal of Knowledge Management. 21(3). Accessed March 4, 2025. https://www.proquest.com/openview/5d55d56634fb060f97ae707091489ec9/1?pq-origsite=gscholar&cbl=54461

Familoni, B.Babajide Tolulope Familoni. (2024). Ethical frameworks for AI in healthcare entrepreneurship: A theoretical examination of challenges and approaches. *International Journal of Frontiers in Biology and Pharmacy Research, 5*(1), 57–65. DOI: 10.53294/ijfbpr.2024.5.1.0032

Fang, S., Jin, H., Zhang, J., Wang, Y., Nan, W., Feng, Y., Su, W., & Jiang, X. (2024, December 24). Machine learning for predicting acute myocardial infarction in patients with sepsis. *Scientific Reports, 14*(1), 30629. DOI: 10.1038/s41598-024-80575-z PMID: 39719483

Fang, W., An, Y., Sugimori, H., Kiuch, S., & Kamishima, T. (2022). Pos1391 Deep Learning-Based Pannus Localization Software in the Hands of Inflammatory Arthritis Using Time-Intensity Curve (Tic) Shape Classification on Dynamic Mri Dataset. *Annals of the Rheumatic Diseases, 81*(Suppl 1), 1036–1036. DOI: 10.1136/annrheumdis-2022-eular.2196

Fan, W., Liu, J., Zhu, S., & Pardalos, P. M. (2020). Investigating the impacting factors for healthcare professionals to adopt artificial intelligence-based medical diagnosis support systems (AIMDSS). *Annals of Operations Research, 294*(1), 567–592. DOI: 10.1007/s10479-018-2818-y

Farhud, D. D., & Zokaei, S. (2021, November). Ethical Issues of Artificial Intelligence in Medicine and Healthcare. *Iranian Journal of Public Health, 50*(11), i–v. DOI: 10.18502/ijph.v50i11.7600 PMID: 35223619

Farias, A. S., Pradella, F., Schmitt, A., Santos, L. M., & Martins-de-Souza, D. (2014). Ten years of proteomics in multiple sclerosis. *Proteomics, 14*(4-5), 467–480. DOI: 10.1002/pmic.201300268 PMID: 24339438

Farzan, R. (2024, January 31). Artificial intelligence in Immuno-genetics. *Bioinformation, 20*(1), 29–35. DOI: 10.6026/973206300200029 PMID: 38352901

Fass, L. (2008). Imaging and cancer: A review. *Molecular Oncology*, *2*(2), 115–152. DOI: 10.1016/j.molonc.2008.04.001 PMID: 19383333

Feng, Y., Wang, Y., Zeng, C., & Mao, H. (2021). Artificial Intelligence and Machine Learning in Chronic Airway Diseases: Focus on Asthma and Chronic Obstructive Pulmonary Disease. *International Journal of Medical Sciences*, *18*(13), 2871–2889. DOI: 10.7150/ijms.58191 PMID: 34220314

Feng, Z., Bethmann, D., Kappler, M., Ballesteros-Merino, C., Eckert, A., Bell, R. B., Cheng, A., Bui, T., Leidner, R., Urba, W. J., Johnson, K., Hoyt, C., Bifulco, C. B., Bukur, J., Wickenhauser, C., Seliger, B., & Fox, B. A. (2017). Multiparametric immune profiling in HPV-oral squamous cell cancer. *JCI Insight*, *2*(14), e93652. Advance online publication. DOI: 10.1172/jci.insight.93652 PMID: 28724788

Fernández-Nebro, A., Marsal, S., Chatham, W., & Rahman, A. (2012). Systemic lupus erythematosus: Genomics, mechanisms, and therapies. *Clinical & Developmental Immunology*, *2012*, 2012. DOI: 10.1155/2012/926931 PMID: 22844327

Ferrara, R., & Matos, I. (2020). Atypical patterns of response and progression in the era of immunotherapy combinations. *Future Oncology (London, England)*, *16*(23), 1707–1713. DOI: 10.2217/fon-2020-0186 PMID: 32687405

Filipp, F. V. (2019). Opportunities for artificial intelligence in advancing precision medicine. *Current Genetic Medicine Reports*, *7*(4), 208–213. DOI: 10.1007/s40142-019-00177-4 PMID: 31871830

Fleming, N. (2018). How artificial intelligence is changing drug discovery. *Nature*, *557*(7706), S55–S57. DOI: 10.1038/d41586-018-05267-x PMID: 29849160

Fleri, W., Paul, S., Dhanda, S. K., Mahajan, S., Xu, X., Peters, B., & Sette, A. (2017). The Immune Epitope Database and Analysis Resource in Epitope discovery and synthetic vaccine design. *Frontiers in Immunology*, *8*, 278. DOI: 10.3389/fimmu.2017.00278 PMID: 28352270

Floresta, G., Zagni, C., Gentile, D., Patamia, V., & Rescifina, A. (2022). Artificial intelligence technologies for COVID-19 de novo drug design. *International Journal of Molecular Sciences*, *23*(6), 3261. DOI: 10.3390/ijms23063261 PMID: 35328682

Fogo, A. B., Kronbichler, A., & Bajema, I. M. A. (2024, February 13). I's Threat to the Medical Profession. *Journal of the American Medical Association*, *331*(6), 471–472. DOI: 10.1001/jama.2024.0018 PMID: 38241042

Folorunso, A.. (2024). A policy framework on AI usage in developing countries and its impact. *Global Journal of Engineering and Technology Advances*, *21*(01), 154–166. DOI: 10.30574/gjeta.2024.21.1.0192

Forrest, I. S., Petrazzini, B. O., Duffy, Á., Park, J. K., O'Neal, A. J., Jordan, D. M., Rocheleau, G., Nadkarni, G. N., Cho, J. H., Blazer, A. D., & Do, R. (2023, April 25). A machine learning model identifies patients in need of autoimmune disease testing using electronic health records. *Nature Communications*, *14*(1), 2385. DOI: 10.1038/s41467-023-37996-7 PMID: 37169741

Fountzilas, E., Pearce, T., Baysal, M. A., Chakraborty, A., & Tsimberidou, A. M. (2025). Convergence of evolving artificial intelligence and machine learning techniques in precision oncology. *npj. Digital Medicine*, *8*(1), 75. PMID: 39890986

Fox, T. A., & Booth, C. (2021). Gene Therapy for Primary Immunodeficiencies. *British Journal of Haematology*, *193*(6), 1044–1059. DOI: 10.1111/bjh.17269 PMID: 33336808

Frasca, M., La Torre, D., Pravettoni, G., & Cutica, I. (2024). Explainable and interpretable artificial intelligence in medicine: A systematic bibliometric review. *Discover Artificial Intelligence*, *4*(1), 15. DOI: 10.1007/s44163-024-00114-7

Freeman, K., Dinnes, J., Chuchu, N., Takwoingi, Y., Bayliss, S. E., Matin, R. N., ... & Deeks, J. J. (2020). Algorithm based smartphone apps to assess risk of skin cancer in adults: systematic review of diagnostic accuracy studies. *bmj, 368*.DOI: https://doi.org/DOI: 10.1136/bmj.m127

Freitag, F., Maucher, M., Riester, Z., & Hudecek, M. (2020). New targets and technologies for CAR-T cells. *Current Opinion in Oncology*, *32*(5), 510–517. DOI: 10.1097/CCO.0000000000000653 PMID: 32657796

Fridman, W. H., Pages, F., Sautes-Fridman, C., & Galon, J. (2012). The immune contexture in human tumours: Impact on clinical outcome. *Nature Reviews. Cancer*, *12*(4), 298–306. DOI: 10.1038/nrc3245 PMID: 22419253

Frishberg, M. (2025). Peering Inside AI's Black Box. *Research Technology Management*, *68*(2), 59–60. DOI: 10.1080/08956308.2025.2448388

Furxhi, I., Faccani, L., Zanoni, I., Brigliadori, A., Vespignani, M., & Costa, A. L. (2024). Design rules applied to silver nanoparticles synthesis: A practical example of machine learning application. *Computational and Structural Biotechnology Journal*, *25*, 20–33. DOI: 10.1016/j.csbj.2024.02.010 PMID: 38444982

Galal, A., Talal, M., & Moustafa, A. (2022). Applications of machine learning in metabolomics: Disease modeling and classification. *Frontiers in Genetics*, *13*, 1017340. DOI: 10.3389/fgene.2022.1017340 PMID: 36506316

Gama, F., Tyskbo, D., Nygren, J., Barlow, J., Reed, J., & Svedberg, P. (2022). Implementation frameworks for artificial intelligence translation into health care practice: Scoping review. *Journal of Medical Internet Research*, *24*(1), e32215. DOI: 10.2196/32215 PMID: 35084349

Gani, R., Isty, M. N., Rimi, R. A., Parsub, W. R., Islam, M. S., Priyanka, M. M., . . . Adnan, M. N. (2024, March). Impact of ai in healthcare services: Analysis using medical synthetic data. In 2024 International Conference on Advances in Computing, Communication, Electrical, and Smart Systems (iCACCESS) (pp. 01-06). IEEE.

Gao, Y., K., Fokoue, A., Luo, H., Iyengar, A., Dey, S., & Zhang, P. (2018). Interpretable drug target prediction using deep neural representation. *IJCAI International Joint Conference on Artificial Intelligence*, 7, 3371– 3377. https://doi.org/DOI: 10.24963/ijcai.2018/468

Gao, P., & Li, S. (2020). Bayesian networks for disease risk prediction. *Statistical AI*, *8*(4), 122–138.

Gao, Y., Zhang, Y., & Liu, X. (2024). Rheumatoid arthritis: Pathogenesis and therapeutic advances. *MedComm*, *5*(3), e509. DOI: 10.1002/mco2.509 PMID: 38469546

Garfinkle, E. A., & Mardis, E. R. (2025). Cancer Immunogenomics Approaches and Applications to Cancer Vaccines. *Cancer Journal (Sudbury, Mass.)*, *31*(2), e0762.

Garg, A. D. (2023, August). The dynamic interface of genetics and immunity: Toward future horizons in health & disease. *Genes and Immunity*, *24*(4), 155–158. DOI: 10.1038/s41435-023-00213-y PMID: 37464025

Gaudelet, T., Day, B., Jamasb, A. R., Soman, J., Regep, C., Liu, G., Hayter, J. B. R., Vickers, R., Roberts, C., Tang, J., Roblin, D., Blundell, T. L., Bronstein, M. M., & Taylor-King, J. P. (2021). Utilizing graph machine learning within drug discovery and development. *Briefings in Bioinformatics*, *22*(6), bbab159. Advance online publication. DOI: 10.1093/bib/bbab159 PMID: 34013350

Gawriljuk, V. O., Foil, D. H., Puhl, A. C., Zorn, K. M., Lane, T. R., Riabova, O., Makarov, V., Godoy, A. S., Oliva, G., & Ekins, S. (2021). Development of machine learning models and the discovery of a new antiviral compound against yellow fever virus. *Journal of Chemical Information and Modeling*, *61*(8), 3804–3813. DOI: 10.1021/acs.jcim.1c00460 PMID: 34286575

Gebretsadik, G., & Menon, M. K. C. (2016). Proteomics and its applications in diagnosis of auto immune diseases. *Open Journal of Immunology*, *6*(1), 14–33. DOI: 10.4236/oji.2016.61003

Gerke, S., Minssen, T., & Cohen, G. (2020). Ethical and legal challenges of artificial intelligence-driven healthcare. In *Artificial intelligence in healthcare* (pp. 295–336). Elsevier. DOI: 10.1016/B978-0-12-818438-7.00012-5

Germain, R. N., Van Allen, E. M., Trynka, G., Tsang, J. S., Grün, D., Kiemen, A. L., Shi, Y., Pugh Bernard, A., & Nolan, G. P. (2024, June 11). AI and immunology. *Immunity*, *57*(6), 1177–1181. DOI: 10.1016/j.immuni.2024.05.016 PMID: 38865960

Ghassemi, M., Naumann, T., Schulam, P., Beam, A. L., Chen, I. Y., & Ranganath, R. (2020). A review of challenges and opportunities in machine learning for health. *AMIA Joint Summits on Translational Science Proceedings AMIA Summit on Translational Science*, *2020*, 191–200. PMID: 32477638

Ghebrehiwet, I., Zaki, N., Damseh, R., & Mohamad, M. S. (2024). Revolutionizing personalized medicine with generative AI: A systematic review. *Artificial Intelligence Review*, *57*(5), 128. Advance online publication. DOI: 10.1007/s10462-024-10768-5

Ghodke-Puranik, Y., Olferiev, M., & Crow, M. K. (2024). Systemic Lupus Erythematosus Genetics: Insights into Pathogenesis and Implications for Therapy. *Nature Reviews. Rheumatology*, *20*(10), 635–648. DOI: 10.1038/s41584-024-01152-2 PMID: 39232240

Ghofrani, A., & Taherdoost, H. (2024). Biomedical data analytics for better patient outcomes. *Drug Discovery Today*, •••, 104280. PMID: 39732322

Ghosh, J., & Sanyal, P. (2024). Development and performance analysis of machine learning methods for predicting the occurrence of constipation and its risk factors among college-aged girls. *Nutrition & Food Science, 12*(3). Available from: https://bit.ly/3MPo6eH

Ghosh, J. (2023). How evidence-based nutrition science supports nutrition communication and marketing: an Indian perspective. In Ghosh, D., Bogueva, D., & Smarta, R. (Eds.), *Nutrition Science, Marketing Nutrition, Health Claims, and Public Policy* (pp. 71–88). Academic Press., DOI: 10.1016/B978-0-323-85615-7.00007-0

Ghosh, J. (2024). Recognizing and predicting the risk of malnutrition in the elderly using artificial intelligence: A systematic review. *International Journal of Advancement in Life Sciences Research*, *7*(3), 1–14. DOI: 10.31632/ijalsr.2024.v07i03.001

Ghosh, J., Choudhury, S. R., Singh, K., & Koner, S. (2024). Application of Machine Learning Algorithm and Artificial Intelligence in Improving Metabolic Syndrome related complications: A review. *International Journal of Advancement in Life Sciences Research*, *7*(2), 41–67. DOI: 10.31632/ijalsr.2024.v07i02.004

Ghosh, J., Roy Choudhury, S., Singh, K., & Koner, S. (2025). Development and performance analysis of machine learning methods for predicting metabolic syndrome among postmenopausal women of India. *International Journal of Advancement in Life Sciences Research*, *8*(1), 006. Advance online publication. DOI: 10.31632/ijalsr.2025.v08i01.006

Ghosh, S. (2020). *Computational Immunology: Applications* (1st ed.). CRC Press., DOI: 10.1201/9781351023504

Ghosh, S., & Mukherjee, P. (2021). Role of Deep Learning in Diagnosing Oral Lichen Planus: A Review. *Journal of Dental Research.*

Gianfrancesco, M. A., Tamang, S., Yazdany, J., & Schmajuk, G. (2018, November 1). Potential Biases in Machine Learning Algorithms Using Electronic Health Record Data. *JAMA Internal Medicine*, *178*(11), 1544–1547. DOI: 10.1001/jamainternmed.2018.3763 PMID: 30128552

Giardino, G., Gallo, V., Prencipe, R., Gaudino, G., Romano, R., De Cataldis, M., & Pignata, C. (2016). Unbalanced immune system: Immunodeficiencies and autoimmunity. *Frontiers in Pediatrics*, *4*, 107. DOI: 10.3389/fped.2016.00107 PMID: 27766253

Gibney, G. T., Kudchadkar, R. R., DeConti, R. C., Thebeau, M. S., Czupryn, M. P., Tetteh, L., & Weber, J. S. (2015). Safety, correlative markers, and clinical results of adjuvant nivolumab in combination with vaccine in resected high-risk metastatic melanoma. *Clinical Cancer Research*, *21*(4), 712–720. DOI: 10.1158/1078-0432.CCR-14-2468 PMID: 25524312

Gibson, D., Kovanovic, V., Ifenthaler, D., Dexter, S., & Feng, S. (2023). Learning theories for artificial intelligence promoting learning processes. *British Journal of Educational Technology*, *54*(5), 1125–1146. DOI: 10.1111/bjet.13341

Gil Del Alcazar, C. R., Huh, S. J., Ekram, M. B., Trinh, A., Liu, L. L., Beca, F., Zi, X., Kwak, M., Bergholtz, H., Su, Y., Ding, L., Russnes, H. G., Richardson, A. L., Babski, K., Min Hui Kim, E., McDonnell, C. H.III, Wagner, J., Rowberry, R., Freeman, G. J., & Polyak, K. (2017). Immune escape in breast cancer during in situ to invasive carcinoma transition. *Cancer Discovery*, *7*(10), 1098–1115. DOI: 10.1158/2159-8290.CD-17-0222 PMID: 28652380

Gillet, J. P., Varma, S., & Gottesman, M. M. (2013). The clinical relevance of cancer cell lines. *Journal of the National Cancer Institute*, *105*(7), 452–458. DOI: 10.1093/jnci/djt007 PMID: 23434901

Gillette, M. A., Satpathy, S., Cao, S., Dhanasekaran, S. M., Vasaikar, S. V., Krug, K., Petralia, F., Li, Y., Liang, W.-W., Reva, B., Krek, A., Ji, J., Song, X., Liu, W., Hong, R., Yao, L., Blumenberg, L., Savage, S. R., Wendl, M. C., & Shi, Z. (2020). Proteogenomic characterization reveals therapeutic vulnerabilities in lung adenocarcinoma. *Cell*, *182*(1), 200–225.e235. DOI: 10.1016/j.cell.2020.06.013 PMID: 32649874

Gilligan, K. C. (2022). Protecting consumers and regulating data: The need for comprehensive federal oversight of the direct-to-consumer genetic testing industry. *Drexel L. Rev.*, *14*, 207.

Gilvary, C., Dry, J. R., & Elemento, O. (2019). Multi-task learning predicts drug combination synergy in cells and in the clinic. *BioRxiv*, 576017. DOI: https://doi.org/DOI: 10.1101/576017

Gilvary, C., Elkhader, J., Madhukar, N., Henchcliffe, C., Goncalves, M. D., & Elemento, O. (2020). A machine learning and network framework to discover new indications for small molecules. *PLoS Computational Biology*, *16*(8), e1008098. DOI: 10.1371/journal.pcbi.1008098 PMID: 32764756

Goh, E., Gallo, R., Hom, J., Strong, E., Weng, Y., Kerman, H., Cool, J. A., Kanjee, Z., Parsons, A. S., Ahuja, N., Horvitz, E., Yang, D., Milstein, A., Olson, A. P. J., Rodman, A., & Chen, J. H. (2024, October 1). Large Language Model Influence on Diagnostic Reasoning: A Randomized Clinical Trial. *JAMA Network Open*, *7*(10), e2440969. DOI: 10.1001/jamanetworkopen.2024.40969 PMID: 39466245

Goh, G. K. M., Dunker, A. K., Foster, J. A., & Uversky, V. N. (2020). A novel strategy for the development of vaccines for SARS-CoV-2 (COVID-19) and other viruses using AI and viral shell disorder. *Journal of Proteome Research*, *19*(11), 4355–4363. DOI: 10.1021/acs.jproteome.0c00672 PMID: 33006287

Goktas, P., & Damadoglu, E. (2025). Future of allergy and immunology: Is artificial intelligence the key in the digital era? *Annals of Allergy, Asthma & Immunology*, *134*(4), 396–407.

Goldberg, C. B., Adams, L., Blumenthal, D., Brennan, P. F., Brown, N., Butte, A. J., Cheatham, M., deBronkart, D., Dixon, J., Drazen, J., Evans, B. J., Hoffman, S. M., Holmes, C., Lee, P., Manrai, A. K., Omenn, G. S., Perlin, J. B., Ramoni, R., Sapiro, G., & Kohane, I. S. (2024, March). RAISE Consortium. To do no harm - and the most good - with AI in health care. *Nature Medicine*, *30*(3), 623–627. DOI: 10.1038/s41591-024-02853-7 PMID: 38388841

Goldenberg, M. M. (2012). Multiple sclerosis review. *P&T : a Peer-Reviewed Journal for Formulary Management*, *37*(3), 175. PMID: 22605909

Goligher, E. C., Heath, A., & Harhay, M. O. (2024). Bayesian statistics for clinical research. *Lancet*, *404*(10457), 1067–1076. DOI: 10.1016/S0140-6736(24)01295-9 PMID: 39277290

Gómez-Bombarelli, R., Wei, J. N., Duvenaud, D., Hernández-Lobato, J. M., Sánchez-Lengeling, B., Sheberla, D., Aguilera-Iparraguirre, J., Hirzel, T. D., Adams, R. P., & Aspuru-Guzik, A. (2018). Automatic Chemical Design Using a Data-Driven Continuous Representation of Molecules. *ACS Central Science*, *4*(2), 268–276. DOI: 10.1021/acscentsci.7b00572 PMID: 29532027

Gómez-González, E. (2020). *Artificial intelligence in medicine and healthcare: Applications, availability, and societal impact. EUR 30197 EN*. Publications Office of the European Union., DOI: 10.2760/047666

Gomez, M., Patel, S., & Kamat, S. (2019). Safety challenges in stem cell therapy. *Current Stem Cell Reports*, *5*(2), 125–135.

Gong, F., Wang, Y., & Zhang, Y.. (2024). Artificial Intelligence Diagnosing of Oral Lichen Planus. *Bioengineering (Basel, Switzerland)*. PMID: 39593819

Gonzalez, M. J., Miranda-Massari, J. R., Duconge, J., Rodriguez, J. R., Cintron, K., Berdiel, M. J., & Rodriguez, J. W. (2015). Nutrigenomics, metabolic correction and disease: The restoration of metabolism as a regenerative medicine perspective. *Journal of Restorative Medicine*, *4*(1), 74–82. DOI: 10.14200/jrm.2014.4.0109

González-Moles, M. A., & Ramos-García, P.. (2021). A Machine-Learning Algorithm for the Reliable Identification of Oral Lichen Planus. *Oral Diseases*.

González-Moles, M. A., & Ramos-García, P.. (2023). Hypertension in Oral Lichen Planus: A Systematic Review and Meta-Analysis. *Oral Diseases*. PMID: 37725328

Goodfellow, I. J., Shlens, J., & Szegedy, C. (2018). Explaining and harnessing adversarial examples. *Journal of Machine Learning Research*, *20*(1), 1–15.

Goodman, R. E., Ebisawa, M., Ferreira, F., Sampson, H. A., van Ree, R., Vieths, S., Baumert, J. L., Bohle, B., Lalithambika, S., Wise, J., & Taylor, S. L. (2016). AllergenOnline: A peer-reviewed, curated allergen database to assess novel food proteins for potential cross-reactivity. *Molecular Nutrition & Food Research*, *60*(5), 1183–1198. DOI: 10.1002/mnfr.201500769 PMID: 26887584

Gorki, V., & Medhi, B. (2024). Use of artificial intelligence in vaccine development against pathogens: Challenges and future directions. *Indian Journal of Pharmacology*, *56*(2), 77–79. DOI: 10.4103/ijp.ijp_259_24 PMID: 38687309

Gorriz Sáez, J. M., Álvarez Illán, I., Arco Martín, J. E., Castillo Barnes, D., Formoso, M. A., Gallego Molina, N. J., Jiménez Mesa, C., Martínez Murcia, F. J., Ortiz García, A., & Ramírez Pérez De Inestrosa, J. (2023). Computational approaches to Explainable Artificial Intelligence: Advances in theory, applications and trends.

Goshisht, M. K. (2024). Machine Learning and Deep Learning in Synthetic Biology: Key Architectures, Applications, and Challenges. *ACS Omega*, *9*(9), 9921–9945. DOI: 10.1021/acsomega.3c05913 PMID: 38463314

Gossec, L., Kedra, J., Servy, H., Pandit, A., Stones, S., Berenbaum, F., Finckh, A., Baraliakos, X., Stamm, T. A., Gomez-Cabrero, D., Pristipino, C., Choquet, R., Burmester, G. R., & Radstake, T. R. D. J. (2020, January). EULAR points to consider for the use of big data in rheumatic and musculoskeletal diseases. *Annals of the Rheumatic Diseases*, *79*(1), 69–76. DOI: 10.1136/annrheumdis-2019-215694 PMID: 31229952

Gottlieb, A., Stein, G. Y., Ruppin, E., & Sharan, R. (2011). PREDICT: A method for inferring novel drug indications with application to personalized medicine. *Molecular Systems Biology*, *7*(1), 496. DOI: 10.1038/msb.2011.26 PMID: 21654673

Gou, F., Liu, J., Xiao, C., & Wu, J. (2024). Research on artificial-intelligence-assisted medicine: A survey on medical artificial intelligence. *Diagnostics (Basel)*, *14*(14), 1472. DOI: 10.3390/diagnostics14141472 PMID: 39061610

Grebien, F., Heider, M., & Schanda, J. (2019). Advances in stem cell therapy for hematologic malignancies. *Blood Cancer Journal*, *9*(8), 70.

Grewal, J. K., Tessier-Cloutier, B., Jones, M., Gakkhar, S., Ma, Y., Moore, R., Mungall, A. J., Zhao, Y., Taylor, M. D., Gelmon, K., Lim, H., Renouf, D., Laskin, J., Marra, M., Yip, S., & Jones, S. J. (2019). Application of a neural network whole transcriptome–based pan-cancer method for diagnosis of primary and metastatic cancers. *JAMA Network Open*, *2*(4), e192597–e192597. DOI: 10.1001/jamanetworkopen.2019.2597 PMID: 31026023

Guan, Z., Li, H., Liu, R., Cai, C., Liu, Y., Li, J., Wang, X., Huang, S., Wu, L., Liu, D., Yu, S., Wang, Z., Shu, J., Hou, X., Yang, X., Jia, W., & Sheng, B. (2023). Artificial intelligence in diabetes management: Advancements, opportunities, and challenges. *Cell Reports Medicine*, *4*(10), 101213. DOI: 10.1016/j.xcrm.2023.101213 PMID: 37788667

Guarra, F., & Colombo, G. (2023). Computational methods in immunology and vaccinology: Design and development of antibodies and immunogens. *Journal of Chemical Theory and Computation*, *19*(16), 5315–5333. DOI: 10.1021/acs.jctc.3c00513 PMID: 37527403

Gubin, M. M., Artyomov, M. N., Mardis, E. R., & Schreiber, R. D. (2015). Tumor neoantigens: Building a framework for personalized cancer immunotherapy. *The Journal of Clinical Investigation*, *125*(9), 3413–3421. DOI: 10.1172/JCI80008 PMID: 26258412

Guerra, R. (2024). Enhancing risk management in hospitals: Leveraging artificial intelligence for improved outcomes. *Italian Journal of Medicine*, *18*(2). Advance online publication. DOI: 10.4081/itjm.2024.1721

Guida, G., Bagnasco, D., Carriero, V., Bertolini, F., Fabio, L. M. R., Nicola, S., & Brussino, L.. (2022). Critical Evaluation of Asthma Biomarkers in Clinical Practice. *Frontiers in Medicine*, *9*(October), 969243. Advance online publication. DOI: 10.3389/fmed.2022.969243 PMID: 36300189

Guimarães, P., Batista, A., Zieger, M., Kaatz, M., & Koenig, K. (2020). Artificial Intelligence in Multiphoton Tomography: Atopic Dermatitis Diagnosis. *Scientific Reports*, *10*(1), 7968. DOI: 10.1038/s41598-020-64937-x PMID: 32409755

Gulati, S., Mattsson, A. H., Schussek, S., Zheng, B., DeOliveira, R. B., Shaughnessy, J., & Ram, S. (2023). Preclinical efficacy of a cell division protein candidate gonococcal vaccine identified by artificial intelligence. *mBio*, *14*(6), e0250023. DOI: 10.1128/mbio.02500-23 PMID: 37905891

Gunasekeran, D. V., Tseng, R. M. W. W., Tham, Y.-C., & Wong, T. Y. (2021). Applications of digital health for public health responses to COVID-19: A systematic scoping review of artificial intelligence, telehealth and related technologies. *NPJ Digital Medicine*, *4*(1), 40. DOI: 10.1038/s41746-021-00412-9 PMID: 33637833

Guo, Y., Hao, Z., Zhao, S., Gong, J., & Yang, F. (2020). Artificial intelligence in health care: Bibliometric analysis. *Journal of Medical Internet Research*, *22*(7), e18228. DOI: 10.2196/18228 PMID: 32723713

Gupta, A. K., & Srivastava, M. K. (2024). Framework for AI Adoption in Healthcare Sector: Integrated DELPHI, ISM–MICMAC Approach. *IEEE Transactions on Engineering Management*, *71*, 8116–8131. DOI: 10.1109/TEM.2024.3386580

Gupta, N., & Singh, R. (2022). Explainable AI for clinical decision-making. *AI in Medicine*, *30*(5), 99–112.

Gurovich, Y., Hanani, Y., Bar, O., Nadav, G., Fleischer, N., Gelbman, D., Basel-Salmon, L., Krawitz, P. M., Kamphausen, S. B., Zenker, M., Bird, L. M., & Gripp, K. W. (2019). Identifying facial phenotypes of genetic disorders using deep learning. *Nature Medicine*, *25*(1), 60–64. DOI: 10.1038/s41591-018-0279-0 PMID: 30617323

Güvenç Paltun, B., Kaski, S., & Mamitsuka, H. (2021). Machine learning approaches for drug combination therapies. *Briefings in Bioinformatics*, *22*(6), bbab293. DOI: 10.1093/bib/bbab293 PMID: 34368832

Haas, R., Zelezniak, A., Iacovacci, J., Kamrad, S., Townsend, S., & Ralser, M. (2017). Designing and interpreting 'multi-omic' experiments that may change our understanding of biology. *Current Opinion in Systems Biology*, *6*, 37–45. DOI: 10.1016/j.coisb.2017.08.009 PMID: 32923746

Hager, P., Jungmann, F., Holland, R., Bhagat, K., Hubrecht, I., Knauer, M., Vielhauer, J., Makowski, M., Braren, R., Kaissis, G., & Rueckert, D. (2024, September). Evaluation and mitigation of the limitations of large language models in clinical decision-making. *Nature Medicine*, *30*(9), 2613–2622. DOI: 10.1038/s41591-024-03097-1 PMID: 38965432

Haghayegh, F., Norouziazad, A., Haghani, E., Feygin, A. A., Rahimi, R. H., Ghavamabadi, H. A., Sadighbayan, D., Madhoun, F., Papagelis, M., Felfeli, T., & Salahandish, R. (2024). Revolutionary Point-of-Care Wearable Diagnostics for Early Disease Detection and Biomarker Discovery through Intelligent Technologies. *Advancement of Science*, *11*(36), 2400595. DOI: 10.1002/advs.202400595 PMID: 38958517

Hanggi, M., & Moschytz, G. S. (2000). *Cellular Neural Networks: Analysis, Design and Optimization*. Springer Science & Business Media. DOI: 10.1007/978-1-4757-3220-7

Hanna, M. G., Pantanowitz, L., Dash, R., Harrison, J. H., Deebajah, M., Pantanowitz, J., & Rashidi, H. H. (2025). Future of Artificial Intelligence (AI) - Machine Learning (ML) Trends in Pathology and Medicine. *Modern Pathology*, *100705*(January), 100705. DOI: 10.1016/j.modpat.2025.100705 PMID: 39761872

Han, W., Wang, X., Li, L., Wichuk, S., Hutchings, E., Dadashova, R., Paschke, J., & Maksymowych, W. P. (2020). Thu0105 Isotope-Labeling-Lc-Ms-Based Metabolic Profiling Of Multiple Serum Sample Sets For The Discovery Of High-Confidence Rheumatoid Arthritis Biomarkers. *Annals of the Rheumatic Diseases*, *79*(June), 266–267. DOI: 10.1136/annrheumdis-2020-eular.5189

Hao, J., Kim, Y., Kim, T. K., & Kang, M. (2018). PASNet: Pathway-associated sparse deep neural network for prognosis prediction from high-throughput data. *BMC Bioinformatics*, *19*(1), 1–13. https://link.springer.com/article/10.1186/s12859-018-2500-z. DOI: 10.1186/s12859-018-2500-z PMID: 30558539

Haouam, K.-D., & Benmalek, M. (2024). Machine Learning Algorithms for Early Prediction of Multiple Sclerosis Progression: A Comparative Study. *Advances in Artificial Intelligence and Machine Learning*, *04*(01), 2027–2051. DOI: 10.54364/AAIML.2024.41116

Haralambieva, I. H., Salk, H. M., Lambert, N. D., Ovsyannikova, I. G., Kennedy, R. B., Warner, N. D., Pankratz, V. S., & Poland, G. A. (2014, April 7). Associations between race, sex and immune response variations to rubella vaccination in two independent cohorts. *Vaccine*, *32*(17), 1946–1953. DOI: 10.1016/j.vaccine.2014.01.090 PMID: 24530932

Hardy, L. C., Smeekens, J. M., & Kulis, M. D. (2019). Biomarkers in food allergy immunotherapy. *Current Allergy and Asthma Reports*, *19*, 1–9.

Harrison, P. J., Wieslander, H., Sabirsh, A., Karlsson, J., Malmsjö, V., Hellander, A., Wählby, C., & Spjuth, O. (2021). Deep-Learning Models for Lipid Nanoparticle-Based Drug Delivery. *Nanomedicine (London)*, *16*(13), 1097–1110. DOI: 10.2217/nnm-2020-0461 PMID: 33949890

Harrison, S., Kopczynska, M., Leahy, G., Taylor, M., Farrer, K., Barrett, M., Mallawaarachchi, P., Abraham, A., Teubner, A., & Lal, S. (2022). Hybrid model of compounded and multichamber bag parenteral nutrition for adults with chronic intestinal failure. *JPEN. Journal of Parenteral and Enteral Nutrition*, *46*(7), 1632–1638. DOI: 10.1002/jpen.2406 PMID: 35589397

Harris, P., & Wong, J. (2020). The role of education in integrating AI into clinical practice. *Medical Education*, *54*(11), 993–1001. DOI: 10.1111/medu.14210 PMID: 32350873

Hartenfeller, M., & Schneider, G. (2011). Enabling future drug discovery by *de novo* design. *Wiley Interdisciplinary Reviews. Computational Molecular Science*, *1*(5), 742–759. DOI: 10.1002/wcms.49

Hasan, H. E., Jaber, D., Khabour, O. F., & Alzoubi, K. H. (2024). Ethical considerations and concerns in the implementation of AI in pharmacy practice: A cross-sectional study. *BMC Medical Ethics*, *25*(1), 55. DOI: 10.1186/s12910-024-01062-8 PMID: 38750441

Hasan, S. A., & Farri, O. (2019). Clinical Natural Language Processing with Deep Learning. In Consoli, S., Recupero, D. R., & Petković, M. (Eds.), *Data Science for Healthcare: Methodologies and Applications* (pp. 147–171). Springer International Publishing., DOI: 10.1007/978-3-030-05249-2_5

Hasanzadeh, A., Hamblin, M. R., Kiani, J., Noori, H., Hardie, J. M., Karimi, M., & Shafiee, H. (2022). Could artificial intelligence revolutionize the development of nanovectors for gene therapy and mRNA vaccines? *Nano Today*, *47*, 101665. DOI: 10.1016/j.nantod.2022.101665 PMID: 37034382

Hassanien, A. E., & Mononteliza, J. (2020). Autonomous driving path planning based on sarsa-dyna algorithm. *Asia-pacific J Convergent Res Interchange*, *6*(7), 59–70. DOI: 10.47116/apjcri.2020.07.06

Hassan, M., Kushniruk, A., & Borycki, E. (2024). Barriers to and Facilitators of Artificial Intelligence Adoption in Health Care: Scoping Review. *JMIR Human Factors*, *11*(1), e48633. DOI: 10.2196/48633 PMID: 39207831

Hasselgren, C., & Oprea, T. I. (2024). Artificial Intelligence for Drug Discovery: Are We There Yet? *Annual Review of Pharmacology and Toxicology*, *2024*(64), 527–550. DOI: 10.1146/annurev-pharmtox-040323-040828 PMID: 37738505

Havel, J. J., Chowell, D., & Chan, T. A. (2019). The evolving landscape of biomarkers for checkpoint inhibitor immunotherapy. *Nature Reviews. Cancer*, *19*(3), 133–150. DOI: 10.1038/s41568-019-0116-x PMID: 30755690

Heijmans, M., Habets, J., Kuijf, M., Kubben, P., & Herff, C. (2019). Evaluation of Parkinson's disease at home: Predicting tremor from wearable sensors. In *2019 41st Annual International Conference of the IEEE Engineering in Medicine and Biology Society (EMBC)*. IEEE. https://doi.org/DOI: 10.1109/EMBC.2019.8857717

He, J., Baxter, S. L., Xu, J., Xu, J., Zhou, X., & Zhang, K. (2019). The practical implementation of artificial intelligence technologies in medicine. *Nature Medicine*, *25*(1), 30–36. DOI: 10.1038/s41591-018-0307-0 PMID: 30617336

Hemmati, S., Saeidikia, Z., Seradj, H., & Mohagheghzadeh, A. (2024). Immunomodulatory peptides as vaccine adjuvants and antimicrobial agents. *Pharmaceuticals (Basel, Switzerland)*, *17*(2), 201. DOI: 10.3390/ph17020201 PMID: 38399416

Hernandez, J. J., Pryszlak, M., Smith, L., Yanchus, C., Kurji, N., Shahani, V. M., & Molinski, S. V. (2017). Giving Drugs a Second Chance: Overcoming Regulatory and Financial Hurdles in Repurposing Approved Drugs as Cancer Therapeutics. *Frontiers in Oncology*, *7*, 291479. DOI: 10.3389/fonc.2017.00273 PMID: 29184849

Hesse, L., Oude Elberink, J. N. G., Van Oosterhout, A. J. M., & Nawijn, M. C. (2022). Allergen immunotherapy for allergic airway diseases: Use lessons from the past to design a brighter future. *Pharmacology & Therapeutics*, *237*, 108115. DOI: 10.1016/j.pharmthera.2022.108115 PMID: 35063570

Hessel, M., Soyer, H., Espeholt, L., Czarnecki, W., Schmitt, S., & Van Hasselt, H. (2019, July). Multi-task deep reinforcement learning with popart. *Proceedings of the AAAI Conference on Artificial Intelligence*, *33*(01), 3796–3803.

Hessler, G., & Baringhaus, K. H. (2018). Artificial Intelligence in Drug Design. *Molecules (Basel, Switzerland)*, *23*(10), 2520. DOI: 10.3390/molecules23102520 PMID: 30279331

Heydari, S., Masoumi, N., Esmaeeli, E., Ayyoubzadeh, S. M., Ghorbani-Bidkorpeh, F., & Ahmadi, M. (2024). Artificial intelligence in nanotechnology for treatment of diseases. *Journal of Drug Targeting*, *32*(10), 1247–1266. DOI: 10.1080/1061186X.2024.2393417 PMID: 39155708

He, Z., Liu, Z., & Gong, L. (2021). Biomarker Identification and Pathway Analysis of Rheumatoid Arthritis Based on Metabolomics in Combination with Ingenuity Pathway Analysis. *Proteomics*, *21*(11–12), 2100037. DOI: 10.1002/pmic.202100037 PMID: 33969925

Hinshaw, D. C., & Shevde, L. A. (2019). The tumor microenvironment innately modulates cancer progression. *Cancer Research*, *79*(18), 4557–4566. DOI: 10.1158/0008-5472.CAN-18-3962 PMID: 31350295

Ho, D., Quake, S. R., McCabe, E. R., Chng, W. J., Chow, E. K., Ding, X., Gelb, B. D., Ginsburg, G. S., Hassenstab, J., Ho, C.-M., Mobley, W. C., Nolan, G. P., Rosen, S. T., Tan, P., Yen, Y., & Zarrinpar, A. (2020). Enabling technologies for personalized and precision medicine. *Trends in Biotechnology*, *38*(5), 497–518. DOI: 10.1016/j.tibtech.2019.12.021 PMID: 31980301

Hoffmann, J., Rheude, A., Neubauer, A., Brendel, C., & Thrun, M. C. (2024, March 6). Development of an explainable AI system using routine clinical parameters for rapid differentiation of inflammatory conditions. *Frontiers in Immunology*, *15*, 1364954. DOI: 10.3389/fimmu.2024.1364954 PMID: 38510238

Holzinger, A., Carrington, A., & Müller, H. (2017). Implementing explainable AI in cell therapy. *Journal of AI Research in Medicine*, *18*(3), 45–65.

Hoseini, F. (2023). AI Ethics: A Call for Global Standards in Technology Development. *AI and Tech in Behavioral and Social Sciences*, *1*(4), 1–3. DOI: 10.61838/kman.aitech.1.4.1

Hoseini, M. (2023). Patient Experiences with AI in Healthcare Settings. *AI and Tech in Behavioral and Social Sciences, 1*(3), 12–18. DOI: 10.61838/kman.aitech.1.3.3

Hosny, A., Parmar, C., Quackenbush, J., Schwartz, L. H., & Aerts, H. J. W. L. (2018). Artificial intelligence in radiology. *Nature Reviews. Cancer, 18*(8), 500–510. DOI: 10.1038/s41568-018-0016-5 PMID: 29777175

Housley, W. J., Pitt, D., & Hafler, D. A. (2015). Biomarkers in multiple sclerosis. *Clinical Immunology (Orlando, Fla.), 161*(1), 51–58. DOI: 10.1016/j.clim.2015.06.015 PMID: 26143623

Huanbutta, K., Burapapadh, K., Kraisit, P., Sriamornsak, P., Ganokratanaa, T., Suwanpitak, K., & Sangnim, T. (2024). Artificial intelligence-driven pharmaceutical industry: A paradigm shift in drug discovery, formulation development, manufacturing, quality control, and post-market surveillance. *European Journal of Pharmaceutical Sciences, 203*, 106938. DOI: 10.1016/j.ejps.2024.106938 PMID: 39419129

Huang, C., Chen, L., Savage, S. R., Eguez, R. V., Dou, Y., Li, Y., da Veiga Leprevost, F., Jaehnig, E. J., Lei, J. T., Wen, B., Schnaubelt, M., Krug, K., Song, X., Cieślik, M., Chang, H.-Y., Wyczalkowski, M. A., Li, K., Colaprico, A., Li, Q. K., & Zhu, J. (2021). Proteogenomic insights into the biology and treatment of HPV-negative head and neck squamous cell carcinoma. *Cancer Cell, 39*(3), 361–379.e316. DOI: 10.1016/j.ccell.2020.12.007 PMID: 33417831

Huang, J.-D., Wang, J., Ramsey, E., Leavey, G., Chico, T. J. A., & Condell, J. (2022). Applying artificial intelligence to wearable sensor data to diagnose and predict cardiovascular disease: A review. *Sensors (Basel), 22*(20), 8002. DOI: 10.3390/s22208002 PMID: 36298352

Huang, J., Habib, A.-R., Mendis, D., Chong, J., Smith, M., Duvnjak, M., Chiu, C., Singh, N., & Wong, E. (2020). An Artificial Intelligence Algorithm That Differentiates Anterior Ethmoidal Artery Location on Sinus Computed Tomography Scans. *The Journal of Laryngology and Otology, 134*(1), 52–55. DOI: 10.1017/S0022215119002536 PMID: 31865928

Huang, K., Wu, X., Li, Y., Lv, C., Yan, Y., Wu, Z., Zhang, M., Huang, W., Jiang, Z., Hu, K., Li, M., Su, J., Zhu, W., Li, F., Chen, M., Chen, J., Li, Y., Zeng, M., Zhu, J., & Zhao, S. (2023, March 16). Artificial Intelligence-Based Psoriasis Severity Assessment: Real-world Study and Application. *Journal of Medical Internet Research, 25*, e44932. DOI: 10.2196/44932 PMID: 36927843

Huang, M.-H., & Rust, R. T. (2018). Artificial intelligence in service. *Journal of Service Research, 21*(2), 155–172. DOI: 10.1177/1094670517752459

Huang, Q., Zhang, X., & Hu, Z. (2021). Application of artificial intelligence modeling technology based on multi-omics in noninvasive diagnosis of inflammatory bowel disease. *Journal of Inflammation Research, 14*, 1933–1943. DOI: 10.2147/JIR.S306816 PMID: 34017190

Huang, X., Wang, H., She, C., Feng, J., Liu, X., Hu, X., Chen, L., & Tao, Y. (2022). Artificial intelligence promotes the diagnosis and screening of diabetic retinopathy. *Frontiers in Endocrinology, 13*, 946915. DOI: 10.3389/fendo.2022.946915 PMID: 36246896

Huang, Y., Guo, X., Wu, Y., Chen, X., Feng, L., Xie, N., & Shen, G. (2024). Nanotechnology's frontier in combatting infectious and inflammatory diseases: Prevention and treatment. *Signal Transduction and Targeted Therapy, 9*(1), 34. DOI: 10.1038/s41392-024-01745-z PMID: 38378653

Huang, Y., Zhang, Z., & Zhou, Y. (2022). AbAgIntPre: A deep learning method for predicting antibody-antigen interactions based on sequence information. *Frontiers in Immunology, 13*, 1053617. DOI: 10.3389/fimmu.2022.1053617 PMID: 36618397

Hui, X., & Kan, E. C. (2017). Monitoring vital signs over multiplexed radio by near-field coherent sensing. *Nature Electronics, 1*(1), 74–78. DOI: 10.1038/s41928-017-0001-0

Hui, X., & Kan, E. C. (2018). Accurate extraction of heartbeat intervals with near-field coherent sensing. In *2018 IEEE International Conference on Communications (ICC)*. IEEE. https://doi.org/DOI: 10.1109/ICC.2018.8423000

Human Immunome Project. (2020, December 16). Retrieved February 8, 2025, from Human Immunome Project website: https://www.humanimmunomeproject.org/

Hundal, J., Carreno, B. M., Petti, A. A., Linette, G. P., Griffith, O. L., Mardis, E. R., & Griffith, M. (2016). pVAC-Seq: A genome-guided in silico approach to identifying tumor neoantigens. *Genome Medicine, 8*(1), 11. DOI: 10.1186/s13073-016-0264-5 PMID: 26825632

Hu, Q., Chen, Y., Zou, D., He, Z., & Xu, T. (2024, November 13). Predicting adverse drug event using machine learning based on electronic health records: A systematic review and meta-analysis. *Frontiers in Pharmacology, 15*, 1497397. DOI: 10.3389/fphar.2024.1497397 PMID: 39605909

Hurault, G., Roekevisch, E., Schram, M. E., Szegedi, K., Kezic, S., Middelkamp-Hup, M. A., & Tanaka, R. J. (2022). Can serum biomarkers predict the outcome of systemic immunosuppressive therapy in adult atopic dermatitis patients? *Skin Health and Disease, 2*(1), ski2–ski77.

Hurst, J. H., Zhao, C., Hostetler, H. P., Gorveh, M. G., Lang, J. E., & Goldstein, B. A. (2022). Environmental and Clinical Data Utility in Pediatric Asthma Exacerbation Risk Prediction Models. *BMC Medical Informatics and Decision Making, 22*(1), 108. DOI: 10.1186/s12911-022-01847-0 PMID: 35459216

Hurvitz, N., Azmanov, H., Kesler, A., & Ilan, Y. (2021). Establishing a Second-Generation Artificial Intelligence-Based System for Improving Diagnosis, Treatment, and Monitoring of Patients with Rare Diseases. *European Journal of Human Genetics : EJHG, 29*(10), 1485–1490. DOI: 10.1038/s41431-021-00928-4 PMID: 34276056

Hutchison, S., & Pritchard, A. L. (2018). Identifying neoantigens for use in immunotherapy. *Mammalian Genome, 29*(11–12), 714–730. DOI: 10.1007/s00335-018-9771-6 PMID: 30167844

Hwang, D.-K., Hsu, C.-C., Chang, K.-J., Chao, D., Sun, C.-H., Jheng, Y.-C., Yarmishyn, A. A., Wu, J.-C., Tsai, C.-Y., Wang, M.-L., Peng, C.-H., Chien, K.-H., Kao, C.-L., Lin, T.-C., Woung, L.-C., Chen, S.-J., & Chiou, S.-H. (2019). Artificial intelligence-based decision-making for age-related macular degeneration. *Theranostics, 9*(1), 232–245. DOI: 10.7150/thno.28447 PMID: 30662564

Ifargan, T., Hafner, L., Kern, M., Alcalay, O., & Kishony, R. (2025). Autonomous LLM-driven research from data to human-verifiable research papers. *NEJM AI, 2*(1). Advance online publication. DOI: 10.1056/AIoa2400555

Iizuka, O., Kanavati, F., Kato, K., Rambeau, M., Arihiro, K., & Tsuneki, M. (2020). Deep learning models for histopathological classification of gastric and colonic epithelial tumours. *Scientific Reports*, *10*(1), 1504. https://www.nature.com/articles/s41598-020-58467-9. DOI: 10.1038/s41598-020-58467-9 PMID: 32001752

Iorio, F., Knijnenburg, T. A., Vis, D. J., Bignell, G. R., Menden, M. P., Schubert, M., Aben, N., Gonçalves, E., Barthorpe, S., Lightfoot, H., Cokelaer, T., Greninger, P., van Dyk, E., Chang, H., de Silva, H., Heyn, H., Deng, X., Egan, R. K., Liu, Q., & Garnett, M. J. (2016). A landscape of pharmacogenomic interactions in cancer. *Cell*, *166*(3), 740–754. https://www.cell.com/cell/fulltext/S0092-8674(16)30746-2. DOI: 10.1016/j.cell.2016.06.017 PMID: 27397505

Iovino, L., Barriga Rodriguez, A., Rutle, A., & Heldal, R. (2020). Model repair with quality-based reinforcement learning.

Iqbal, F. M., Lam, K., Joshi, M., Khan, S., Ashrafian, H., & Darzi, A. (2021). Clinical Outcomes of Digital Sensor Alerting Systems in Remote Monitoring: A Systematic Review and Meta-Analysis. *NPJ Digital Medicine*, *4*(1), 1–12. DOI: 10.1038/s41746-020-00378-0 PMID: 33420338

Ismail, A. F. M. F., Sam, M. F. M., Bakar, K. A., Ahamat, A., Adam, S., & Qureshi, M. I. (2022). Artificial intelligence in healthcare business ecosystem: a bibliometric study. International journal of online and biomedical engineering, 18(9), 100-114.

Issa, W. B., Shorbagi, A., Al-Sharman, A., Rababa, M., Al-Majeed, K., Radwan, H., Refaat Ahmed, F., Al-Yateem, N., Mottershead, R., Abdelrahim, D. N., Hijazi, H., Khasawneh, W., Ali, I., Abbas, N., & Fakhry, R. (2024). Shaping the future: perspectives on the Integration of Artificial Intelligence in health profession education: a multi-country survey. *BMC Medical Education*, *24*(1), 1166. DOI: 10.1186/s12909-024-06076-9 PMID: 39425151

Izuhara, K., Nunomura, S., Nakahara, T., & Onozuka, D. (n.d.). The Search for Blood Biomarkers Useful in Treating Atopic Dermatitis Patients. *Expert Review of Clinical Pharmacology*, *0*(0), 1–10. DOI: 10.1080/17512433.2024.2438192 PMID: 39631097

Jabarulla, M. Y., & Lee, H.-N. (2021). A blockchain and artificial intelligence-based, patient-centric healthcare system for combating the COVID-19 pandemic: Opportunities and applications. In *Healthcare*. Mdpi.

Jackson, H. W., Fischer, J. R., Zanotelli, V. R. T., Ali, H. R., Mechera, R., Soysal, S. D., Moch, H., Muenst, S., Varga, Z., Weber, W. P., & Bodenmiller, B. (2020). The single-cell pathology landscape of breast cancer. *Nature*, *578*(7796), 615–620. DOI: 10.1038/s41586-019-1876-x PMID: 31959985

Jaffe, C. C. (2012). Imaging and genomics: Is there a synergy? *Radiology*, *264*(3), 329–331. DOI: 10.1148/radiol.12120871 PMID: 22821693

Jamialahmadi, H., Khalili-Tanha, G., Nazari, E., & Rezaei-Tavirani, M. (2024). Artificial intelligence and bioinformatics: A journey from traditional techniques to smart approaches. *Gastroenterology and Hepatology from Bed To Bench*, *17*(3), 241. PMID: 39308539

Jang, H., Lee, A. C., Lee, S., & Kwon, S. (2024). Abstract 3533: Spatially Resolved Laser-Activated Cell Sorting (SLACS) and AI Integration for Enhanced Pathological Analysis and Biomarker Discovery. *Cancer Research, 84*(6, Supplement), 3533. DOI: 10.1158/1538-7445.AM2024-3533

Janjua, T. I., Cao, Y., Kleitz, F., Linden, M., Yu, C., & Popat, A. (2023). Silica nanoparticles: A review of their safety and current strategies to overcome biological barriers. *Advanced Drug Delivery Reviews, 203*, 115115. DOI: 10.1016/j.addr.2023.115115 PMID: 37844843

Jansson, M., Ohtonen, P., Alalääkkölä, T., Heikkinen, J., Mäkiniemi, M., Lahtinen, S., Lahtela, R., Ahonen, M., Jämsä, S., & Liisantti, J. (2022). Artificial intelligence-enhanced care pathway planning and scheduling system: Content validity assessment of required functionalities. *BMC Health Services Research, 22*(1), 1513. DOI: 10.1186/s12913-022-08780-y PMID: 36510176

Jarczak, D., & Nierhaus, A. (2022, October 3). Cytokine Storm-Definition, Causes, and Implications. *International Journal of Molecular Sciences, 23*(19), 11740. DOI: 10.3390/ijms231911740 PMID: 36233040

Jayatunga, M. K. P., Xie, W., Ruder, L., Schulze, U., & Meier, C. (2022). AI in small-molecule drug discovery: A coming wave? *Nature Reviews. Drug Discovery, 21*(3), 175–176. DOI: 10.1038/d41573-022-00025-1 PMID: 35132242

Jeong, D. Y., Park, J., Song, H., Moon, J., Lee, T., Ahn, C., Park, S., Lee, S.-H., Ock, C.-Y., & Lee, H. Y. (2024). Abstract 4170: Artificial Intelligence (AI)-Based Multi-Modal Approach Using H&E and CT Image for Predicting Treatment Response of Immune Checkpoint Inhibitor (ICI) in Non-Small Cell Lung Cancer (NSCLC). *Cancer Research, 84*(6, Supplement), 4170. DOI: 10.1158/1538-7445.AM2024-4170

Jiang, F., Jiang, Y., Zhi, H., Dong, Y., Li, H., Ma, S., Wang, Y., Dong, Q., Shen, H., & Wang, Y. (2017). Artificial intelligence in healthcare: Past, present, and future. *Stroke and Vascular Neurology, 2*(2), 59–67. DOI: 10.1136/svn-2017-000101 PMID: 29507784

Jiang, H., Han, L., & Zhou, Y. (2021). Personalized CAR-T therapy supported by AI-based genetic insights. *Journal of Hematology & Oncology, 14*(1), 47. PMID: 33743795

Jiang, L. Y., Liu, X. C., Nejatian, N. P., Nasir-Moin, M., Wang, D., Abidin, A., Eaton, K., Riina, H. A., Laufer, I., Punjabi, P., Miceli, M., Kim, N. C., Orillac, C., Schnurman, Z., Livia, C., Weiss, H., Kurland, D., Neifert, S., Dastagirzada, Y., & Oermann, E. K. (2023). Health system-scale language models are all-purpose prediction engines. *Nature, 619*(7969), 357–362. DOI: 10.1038/s41586-023-06160-y PMID: 37286606

Jiang, T., Shi, T., Zhang, H., Hu, J., Song, Y., Wei, J., Ren, S., & Zhou, C. (2019). Tumor neoantigens: From basic research to clinical applications. *Journal of Hematology & Oncology, 12*(1), 93. DOI: 10.1186/s13045-019-0787-5 PMID: 31492199

Jiang, X., Zhao, H., Saldanha, O. L., Nebelung, S., Kuhl, C., Amygdalos, I., Lang, S. A., Wu, X., Meng, X., Truhn, D., Kather, J. N., & Ke, J. (2023). An MRI deep learning model predicts outcome in rectal cancer. *Radiology, 307*(2), e222223. DOI: 10.1148/radiol.222223 PMID: 37278629

Jiang, Y., Liang, X., Wang, W., Chen, C., Yuan, Q., Zhang, X., Li, N., Chen, H., Yu, J., Xie, Y., Xu, Y., Zhou, Z., Li, G., & Li, R. (2021). Noninvasive prediction of occult peritoneal metastasis in gastric cancer using deep learning. *JAMA Network Open*, *4*(1), e2032269–e2032269. https://jamanetwork.com/journals/jamanetworkopen/fullarticle/2774582. DOI: 10.1001/jamanetworkopen.2020.32269 PMID: 33399858

Jiao, T., Schnitzer, M. E., Forget, A., & Blais, L. (2022). Identifying Asthma Patients at High Risk of Exacerbation in a Routine Visit: A Machine Learning Model. *Respiratory Medicine*, *198*(July), 106866. DOI: 10.1016/j.rmed.2022.106866 PMID: 35594754

Jimenes-Vargas, K., Pazos, A., Munteanu, C. R., Perez-Castillo, Y., & Tejera, E. (2024). Prediction of compound-target interaction using several artificial intelligence algorithms and comparison with a consensus-based strategy. *Journal of Cheminformatics*, *16*(1), 1–13. DOI: 10.1186/s13321-024-00816-1 PMID: 38449058

Jiménez-Luna, J., Grisoni, F., Weskamp, N., & Schneider, G. (2021). Artificial intelligence in drug discovery: Recent advances and future perspectives. *Expert Opinion on Drug Discovery*, *16*(9), 949–959. DOI: 10.1080/17460441.2021.1909567 PMID: 33779453

Jin, C., Yu, H., Ke, J., Ding, P., Yi, Y., Jiang, X., Duan, X., Tang, J., Chang, D. T., Wu, X., Gao, F., & Li, R. (2021). Predicting treatment response from longitudinal images using multi-task deep learning. *Nature Communications*, *12*(1), 1851. DOI: 10.1038/s41467-021-22188-y PMID: 33767170

Jin, X., Liu, C., Xu, T., Su, L., & Zhang, X. (2020). Artificial intelligence biosensors: Challenges and prospects. *Biosensors & Bioelectronics*, *165*, 112412. DOI: 10.1016/j.bios.2020.112412 PMID: 32729531

Jobin, A., Ienca, M., & Vayena, E. (2019). The global landscape of AI ethics guidelines. *Nature Machine Intelligence*, *1*(9), 389–399. DOI: 10.1038/s42256-019-0088-2

Johnson, D., & Peters, K. (2020). Reinforcement learning for adaptive immunotherapy trials. *AI in Clinical Research*, *6*(1), 45–60.

Johnson, K. B., Wei, W. Q., Weeraratne, D., Frisse, M. E., Misulis, K., Rhee, K., Zhao, J., & Snowdon, J. L. (2021). Precision medicine, AI, and the future of personalized health care. *Clinical and Translational Science*, *14*(1), 86–93. DOI: 10.1111/cts.12884 PMID: 32961010

Johnson, K. W., Torres Soto, J., Glicksberg, B. S., Shameer, K., Miotto, R., Ali, M., Ashley, E., & Dudley, J. T. (2018, June 12). Artificial Intelligence in Cardiology. *Journal of the American College of Cardiology*, *71*(23), 2668–2679. DOI: 10.1016/j.jacc.2018.03.521 PMID: 29880128

Johnson, R., Stephens, A. V., Mester, R., Knyazev, S., Kohn, L. A., Freund, M. K., Bondhus, L., Hill, B. L., Schwarz, T., Zaitlen, N., Arboleda, V. A. A., Bastarache, L., Pasaniuc, B., & Butte, M. J. (2024, May). Electronic health record signatures identify undiagnosed patients with common variable immunodeficiency disease. *Science Translational Medicine*, *16*(745), eade4510. Advance online publication. DOI: 10.1126/scitranslmed.ade4510 PMID: 38691621

Jones, D. R., & Chen, H. M. (2021). Sources of stem cells in regenerative therapy. *Journal of Regenerative Medicine*, *19*(2), 157–164.

Jones, G., Jindal, A., Ghani, U., Kotelnikov, S., Egbert, M., Hashemi, N., & Kozakov, D. (2022). Elucidation of protein function using computational docking and hotspot analysis by ClusPro and FTMap. *Acta Crystallographica. Section D, Structural Biology, 78*(Pt 6), 690–697. DOI: 10.1107/S2059798322002741 PMID: 35647916

Jordan, M. I., & Mitchell, T. M. (2015). Machine learning: Trends, perspectives, and prospects. *Science, 349*(6245), 255–260. DOI: 10.1126/science.aaa8415 PMID: 26185243

Jörg, S., Grohme, D. A., Erzler, M., Binsfeld, M., Haghikia, A., Müller, D. N., Linker, R. A., & Kleinewietfeld, M. (2016). Environmental factors in autoimmune diseases and their role in multiple sclerosis. *Cellular and Molecular Life Sciences : CMLS, 73*(24), 4611–4622. DOI: 10.1007/s00018-016-2311-1 PMID: 27491297

Joshi, N., & Burlina, P. (2021). AI fairness via domain adaptation. arXiv preprint arXiv:2104.01109.

Joshi, M., Archer, S., Morbi, A., Arora, S., Kwasnicki, R., Ashrafian, H., Khan, S., Cooke, G., & Darzi, A. (2021). Short-term wearable sensors for in-hospital medical and surgical patients: Mixed methods analysis of patient perspectives. *JMIR Perioperative Medicine, 4*(1), e18836. DOI: 10.2196/18836 PMID: 33885367

Joyce, J. A., & Pollard, J. W. (2009). Microenvironmental regulation of metastasis. *Nature Reviews. Cancer, 9*(3), 239–252. DOI: 10.1038/nrc2618 PMID: 19279573

Jumper, J., Evans, R., Pritzel, A., Green, T., Figurnov, M., Ronneberger, O., Tunyasuvunakool, K., Bates, R., Žídek, A., Potapenko, A., Bridgland, A., Meyer, C., Kohl, S. A. A., Ballard, A. J., Cowie, A., Romera-Paredes, B., Nikolov, S., Jain, R., Adler, J., & Hassabis, D. (2021). Highly accurate protein structure prediction with AlphaFold. *Nature, 596*(7873), 583–589. DOI: 10.1038/s41586-021-03819-2 PMID: 34265844

Kadurin, A., Nikolenko, S., Khrabrov, K., Aliper, A., & Zhavoronkov, A. (2017). druGAN: An Advanced Generative Adversarial Autoencoder Model for de Novo Generation of New Molecules with Desired Molecular Properties in Silico. *Molecular Pharmaceutics, 14*(9), 3098–3104. DOI: 10.1021/acs.molpharmaceut.7b00346 PMID: 28703000

Kaissis, G. A., Makowski, M. R., Rückert, D., & Braren, R. F. (2020). Secure, privacy-preserving and federated machine learning in medical imaging. *Nature Machine Intelligence, 2*(6), 305–311. DOI: 10.1038/s42256-020-0186-1

Kaladharan, S., Manayath, D., & Gopalakrishnan, R. (2024). Regulatory Challenges in AI/ML-Enabled Medical Devices: A Scoping Review and Conceptual Framework. *Journal of Medical Devices, 18*(040801), 040801. Advance online publication. DOI: 10.1115/1.4066280

Kale, G. A. (2019). Artificial Intelligence in Healthcare-Opportunities and Challenges.

Kalinin, A. A., Higgins, G. A., Reamaroon, N., Soroushmehr, S., Allyn-Feuer, A., Dinov, I. D., & Athey, B. D. (2018). Deep learning in pharmacogenomics: From gene regulation to patient stratification. *Pharmacogenomics, 19*(7), 629–650.

Kalyane, D., Sanap, G., Paul, D., Shenoy, S., Anup, N., Polaka, S., Tambe, V., & Tekade, R. K. (2020). Artificial intelligence in the pharmaceutical sector: current scene and future prospect. In Tekade, R. K. (Ed.), *The Future of Pharmaceutical Product Development and Research* (pp. 73–107). Elsevier. DOI: 10.1016/B978-0-12-814455-8.00003-7

Kamel Boulos, M. N., & Zhang, P. (2021). Digital Twins: From Personalised Medicine to Precision Public Health. *Journal of Personalized Medicine, 11*(8), 745. DOI: 10.3390/jpm11080745 PMID: 34442389

Kamya, P., Ozerov, I. V., Pun, F. W., Tretina, K., Fokina, T., Chen, S., Naumov, V., Long, X., Lin, S., Korzinkin, M., Polykovskiy, D., Aliper, A., Ren, F., & Zhavoronkov, A. (2024). PandaOmics: An AI-Driven Platform for Therapeutic Target and Biomarker Discovery. *Journal of Chemical Information and Modeling, 64*(10), 3961–3969. DOI: 10.1021/acs.jcim.3c01619 PMID: 38404138

Kaplan, A., Cao, H., FitzGerald, J. M., Iannotti, N., Yang, E., Kocks, J. W. H., Kostikas, K., Price, D., Reddel, H. K., Tsiligianni, I., Vogelmeier, C. F., Pfister, P., & Mastoridis, P. (2021). Artificial Intelligence/Machine Learning in Respiratory Medicine and Potential Role in Asthma and COPD Diagnosis. *The Journal of Allergy and Clinical Immunology. In Practice, 9*(6), 2255–2261. DOI: 10.1016/j.jaip.2021.02.014 PMID: 33618053

Kapoor, D. U., Sharma, J. B., Gandhi, S. M., Prajapati, B. G., Thanawuth, K., Limmatvapirat, S., & Sriamornsak, P. (2024). AI-driven design and optimization of nanoparticle-based drug delivery systems. *Science, Engineering and Health Studies*, 24010003.

Kaput, J., & Rodriguez, R. L. (2004). Nutritional genomics: The next frontier in the postgenomic era. *Physiological Genomics, 16*(2), 166–177. DOI: 10.1152/physiolgenomics.00107.2003 PMID: 14726599

Karachaliou, C.-E., & Livaniou, E. (2023). Immunosensors for Autoimmune-Disease-Related Biomarkers: A Literature Review. *Sensors (Basel), 23*(15), 6770. DOI: 10.3390/s23156770 PMID: 37571553

Karahmet Sher, E., Alebić, M., Marković Boras, M., Boškailo, E., Karahmet Farhat, E., Karahmet, A., Pavlović, B., Sher, F., & Lekić, L. (2024). Nanotechnology in medicine revolutionizing drug delivery for cancer and viral infection treatments. *International Journal of Pharmaceutics, 660*, 124345. DOI: 10.1016/j.ijpharm.2024.124345 PMID: 38885775

Karami, P., Gholamin, D., Fathi, F., Afsar, T., & Johari-Ahar, M. (2024). Anti-CCP Biosensors in Rheumatoid Arthritis. *Clinica Chimica Acta, 561*(July), 119767. DOI: 10.1016/j.cca.2024.119767 PMID: 38857671

Kardia. "EKG Anywhere, Anytime". Accessed January 20, 2025. https://www.kardia.com/

Karimi, M., Wu, D., Wang, Z., & Shen, Y. (2019). DeepAffinity: Interpretable deep learning of compound-protein affinity through unified recurrent and convolutional neural networks. *Bioinformatics (Oxford, England), 35*(18), 3329–3338. DOI: 10.1093/bioinformatics/btz111 PMID: 30768156

Karthika, R., Muthusamy, S., & Prabhu, P. R. (2023). InflANNet: A neural network predictor for Influenza A CTL and HTL epitopes to aid robust vaccine design. *Bulletin of the National Research Center, 47*(1), 129. Advance online publication. DOI: 10.1186/s42269-023-01101-1

Kasula, B. Y. (2021). Ethical and regulatory considerations in AI-Driven healthcare solutions. *International Meridian Journal, 3*(3), 1–8.

Katirai, A. (2023). The ethics of advancing artificial intelligence in healthcare: Analyzing ethical considerations for Japan's innovative AI hospital system. *Frontiers in Public Health, 11*, 1142062. DOI: 10.3389/fpubh.2023.1142062 PMID: 37529426

Katsnelson, A. (2024). A drug to call one's own. Scientific American. https://www.scientificamerican.com/article/a-drug-to-call-ones-own/

Kaushik, R., Kant, R., & Christodoulides, M. (2023). Artificial intelligence in accelerating vaccine development - current and future perspectives. *Frontiers in Bacteriology, 2*, 1258159. Advance online publication. DOI: 10.3389/fbrio.2023.1258159

Kaushik, S., & Das, T. (2020). AI in therapeutic cell line development. *Stem Cells Translational Medicine, 9*(2), 123–135.

Kazerooni, A. F., Bagley, S. J., Akbari, H., Saxena, S., Bagheri, S., Guo, J., Chawla, S., Nabavizadeh, A., Mohan, S., & Bakas, S.. (2021). Applications of radiomics and radiogenomics in high-grade gliomas in the era of precision medicine. *Cancers (Basel), 13*(5921), 5921. Advance online publication. DOI: 10.3390/cancers13235921 PMID: 34885031

Kegerreis, B., Catalina, M. D., Bachali, P., Geraci, N. S., Labonte, A. C., Zeng, C., Stearrett, N., Crandall, K. A., Lipsky, P. E., & Grammer, A. C. (2019). Machine Learning Approaches to Predict Lupus Disease Activity from Gene Expression Data. *Scientific Reports, 9*(1), 9617. DOI: 10.1038/s41598-019-45989-0 PMID: 31270349

Keijer, J., Escoté, X., Galmés, S., Palou-March, A., Serra, F., Aldubayan, M. A., Pigsborg, K., Magkos, F., Baker, E. J., Calder, P. C., Góralska, J., Razny, U., Malczewska-Malec, M., Suñol, D., Galofré, M., Rodríguez, M. A., Canela, N., Malcic, R. G., Bosch, M., & del Bas, J. M. (2024). Omics biomarkers and an approach for their practical implementation to delineate health status for personalized nutrition strategies. *Critical Reviews in Food Science and Nutrition, 64*(23), 8279–8307. DOI: 10.1080/10408398.2023.2198605 PMID: 37077157

Kelly, C. J., Karthikesalingam, A., Suleyman, M., Corrado, G., & King, D. (2019). Key Challenges for Delivering Clinical Impact with Artificial Intelligence. *BMC Medicine, 17*(1), 195. DOI: 10.1186/s12916-019-1426-2 PMID: 31665002

Kennedy, R. B., Ovsyannikova, I. G., Palese, P., & Poland, G. A. (2020). Current challenges in vaccinology. *Frontiers in Immunology, 11*, 1181. DOI: 10.3389/fimmu.2020.01181 PMID: 32670279

Keren, L., Bosse, M., Marquez, D., Angoshtari, R., Jain, S., Varma, S., Yang, S.-R., Kurian, A., Van Valen, D., West, R., Bendall, S. C., & Angelo, M. (2018). A structured tumor-immune microenvironment in triple negative breast cancer revealed by multiplexed ion beam imaging. *Cell, 174*(6), 1373–1387.e19. DOI: 10.1016/j.cell.2018.08.039 PMID: 30193111

Keser, G., Bayrakdar, İ. Ş., Pekiner, F. N., Çelik, Ö., & Orhan, K. (2023). A Deep Learning Algorithm for Classification of Oral Lichen Planus Lesions from Photographic Images: A Retrospective Study. *Journal of Stomatology, Oral and Maxillofacial Surgery*, *124*(1), 101264. DOI: 10.1016/j.jormas.2022.08.007 PMID: 35964938

Keyl, J., Keyl, P., Montavon, G., Hosch, R., Brehmer, A., Mochmann, L., Jurmeister, P., Dernbach, G., Kim, M., Koitka, S., Bauer, S., Bechrakis, N., Forsting, M., Führer-Sakel, D., Glas, M., Grünwald, V., Hadaschik, B., Haubold, J., Herrmann, K., & Kleesiek, J. (2025, January 30). Decoding pan-cancer treatment outcomes using multimodal real-world data and explainable artificial intelligence. *Nature Cancer*, *6*(2), 307–322. Advance online publication. DOI: 10.1038/s43018-024-00891-1 PMID: 39885364

Khalid, W. B., Anwar, A., & Waheed, O. T. (2022). Contactless vitals measurement robot. In *2022 8th International Conference on Automation, Robotics and Applications (ICARA)*. IEEE. https://doi.org/ DOI: 10.1109/ICARA55094.2022.9738523

Khalifa, M., & Albadawy, M. (2024). Artificial intelligence for clinical prediction: Exploring key domains and essential functions. *Computer Methods and Programs in Biomedicine Update*, *5*, 100148. DOI: 10.1016/j.cmpbup.2024.100148

Khan, M. S., Umer, H., & Faruqe, F. (2024). Artificial intelligence for low income countries. *Humanities & Social Sciences Communications*, *11*(1), 1–13. DOI: 10.1057/s41599-024-03947-w

Khan, M. T., Islam, M. J., Parihar, A., Islam, R., Jerin, T. J., Dhote, R., & Halim, M. A. (2021). Immunoinformatic and molecular modeling approach to design a universal multi-epitope vaccine for SARS-CoV-2. *Informatics in Medicine Unlocked*, *24*(100578), 100578. DOI: 10.1016/j.imu.2021.100578 PMID: 33898733

Khan, S. R., Al Rijjal, D., Piro, A., & Wheeler, M. B. (2021). Integration of AI and traditional medicine in drug discovery. *Drug Discovery Today*, *26*(4), 982–992. DOI: 10.1016/j.drudis.2021.01.008 PMID: 33476566

Khan, S., Mohan, K., Muzammil, S., Alam, M. A., & Khayyam, K. U. (2024). Current Prospects in Rheumatoid Arthritis: Pathophysiology, Genetics, and Treatments. *Recent Advances in Anti-infective Drug Discovery*, *19*(1), 36–55. DOI: 10.2174/2772434418666230406083149 PMID: 37038682

Khatib, C. M., Klein-Petersen, A. W., Amalie, T. M. R., Egeberg, A., Christensen, M. O., Silverberg, J. I., Thomsen, S. F., Irvine, A. D., & Thyssen, J. P. (2024). Increased Loss-of-Function Filaggrin Gene Mutation Prevalence in Atopic Dermatitis Patients across Northern Latitudes Indicates Genetic Fitness: A Systematic Review and Meta-Analysis. *Experimental Dermatology*, *33*(7), e15130. DOI: 10.1111/exd.15130 PMID: 38989976

Khosravi-Maharlooei, M., Madley, R., Borsotti, C., Ferreira, L. M., Sharp, R. C., Brehm, M. A., Greiner, D. L., Parent, A. V., Anderson, M. S., Sykes, M., & Creusot, R. J. (2022). Modeling human T1D-associated autoimmune processes. *Molecular Metabolism*, *56*, 101417. DOI: 10.1016/j.molmet.2021.101417 PMID: 34902607

Kim, D. N., McNaughton, A. D., & Kumar, N. (2024). Leveraging artificial intelligence to expedite antibody design and enhance antibody-antigen interactions. *Bioengineering (Basel, Switzerland)*, *11*(2), 185. DOI: 10.3390/bioengineering11020185 PMID: 38391671

Kim, H., Goo, J. M., Lee, K. H., Kim, Y. T., & Park, C. M. (2020). Preoperative CT-based deep learning model for predicting disease-free survival in patients with lung adenocarcinomas. *Radiology*, *296*(1), 216–224. https://pubs.rsna.org/doi/full/10.1148/radiol.2020192764. DOI: 10.1148/radiol.2020192764 PMID: 32396042

Kim, S., & Cho, H. (2021). Natural language processing for genomic data analysis. *Bioinformatics and AI*, *11*(2), 210–228.

Kim, S., Kim, H. S., Kim, E., Lee, M. G., Shin, E.-C., Paik, S., & Kim, S. (2018). Neopepsee: Accurate genome-level prediction of neoantigens by harnessing sequence and amino acid immunogenicity information. *Annals of Oncology : Official Journal of the European Society for Medical Oncology*, *29*(4), 1030–1036. DOI: 10.1093/annonc/mdy022 PMID: 29360924

Klangkalya, N., Fleisher, T. A., & Rosenzweig, S. D. (2024). Diagnostic Tests for Primary Immunodeficiency Disorders: Classic and Genetic Testing. *Allergy and Asthma Proceedings*, *45*(5), 355–363. DOI: 10.2500/aap.2024.45.240051 PMID: 39294902

Klein, J., Sprague, D., Lane, M., Hart, M., Petrillo, O., do Valle, I. F., Davis, M., Ferguson, A., Allen, A., Jooss, K., & Dhanik, A. (2024). Abstract 904: AI Platform Provides an EDGE and Enables State-of-the-Art Identification of Peptide-HLAs for the Development of T Cell Inducing Vaccines. *Cancer Research*, *84*(6, Supplement), 904. DOI: 10.1158/1538-7445.AM2024-904

Klein, T. E., Chang, J. T., Cho, M. K., Easton, K. L., Fergerson, R., Hewett, M., Lin, Z., Liu, Y., Liu, S., Oliver, D. E., Rubin, D. L., Shafa, F., Stuart, J. M., & Altman, R. B. (2001). Integrating genotype and phenotype information: An overview of the PharmGKB project. *The Pharmacogenomics Journal*, *1*(3), 167–170. https://www.nature.com/articles/6500035. DOI: 10.1038/sj.tpj.6500035 PMID: 11908751

Klysik, J. (2001). Concept of immunomics: A new frontier in the battle for gene function? *Acta Biotheoretica*, *49*(3), 191–202. DOI: 10.1023/A:1011901410166 PMID: 11558896

Koper-Lenkiewicz, O. M., Sutkowska, K., Wawrusiewicz-Kurylonek, N., Kowalewska, E., & Matowicka-Karna, J. (2022). Proinflammatory Cytokines (IL-1, -6, -8, -15, -17, -18, -23, TNF-α) Single Nucleotide Polymorphisms in Rheumatoid Arthritis—A Literature Review. *International Journal of Molecular Sciences*, *23*(4), 2106. DOI: 10.3390/ijms23042106 PMID: 35216226

Korbar, B., Olofson, A. M., Miraflor, A. P., Nicka, C. M., Suriawinata, M. A., Torresani, L., Suriawinata, A. A., & Hassanpour, S. (2017). Deep learning for classification of colorectal polyps on whole-slide images. *Journal of Pathology Informatics*, *8*(1), 30. https://www.sciencedirect.com/science/article/pii/S2153353922004345. DOI: 10.4103/jpi.jpi_34_17 PMID: 28828201

Korsunskiy, I., Blyuss, O., Gordukova, M., Davydova, N., Zaikin, A., Zinovieva, N., Zimin, S., Molchanov, R., Salpagarova, A., Eremeeva, A., Filipenko, M., Prodeus, A., Korsunskiy, A., Hsu, P., & Munblit, D. (2020). Expanding TREC and KREC Utility in Primary Immunodeficiency Diseases Diagnosis. *Frontiers in Immunology, 11*(March), 320. Advance online publication. DOI: 10.3389/fimmu.2020.00320 PMID: 32194560

Kourou, K., Exarchos, T. P., Exarchos, K. P., Karamouzis, M. V., & Fotiadis, D. I. (2015). Machine learning applications in cancer prognosis and prediction. *Computational and Structural Biotechnology Journal, 13*, 8–17. DOI: 10.1016/j.csbj.2014.11.005 PMID: 25750696

Krassowski, M., Paczkowska, M., Cullion, K., Huang, T., Dzneladze, I., Ouellette, B. F. F., Yamada, J. T., Fradet-Turcotte, A., & Reimand, J. (2018). ActiveDriverDB: Human disease mutations and genome variation in post-translational modification sites of proteins. *Nucleic Acids Research, 46*(D1), D901–D910. DOI: 10.1093/nar/gkx973 PMID: 29126202

Krishnan Ganapathy, M. N. (2021). Artificial intelligence and healthcare regulatory and legal concerns. *Telehealth and Medicine Today, 6*(2).

Krittanawong, C., Johnson, K. W., Rosenson, R. S., Wang, Z., Aydar, M., Baber, U., Min, J. K., Tang, W. H. W., Halperin, J. L., & Narayan, S. M. (2019). Deep learning for cardiovascular medicine: A practical primer. *European Heart Journal, 40*(25), 2058–2073. DOI: 10.1093/eurheartj/ehz056 PMID: 30815669

Kroll, A. V., Jiang, Y., Zhou, J., Holay, M., Fang, R. H., & Zhang, L. (2019). Biomimetic Nanoparticle Vaccines for Cancer Therapy. *Advanced Biosystems, 3*(1), 1800219. DOI: 10.1002/adbi.201800219 PMID: 31728404

Krzyszczyk, P., Acevedo, A., Davidoff, E. J., Timmins, L. M., Marrero-Berrios, I., Patel, M., White, C., Lowe, C., Sherba, J. J., & Hartmanshenn, C. (2018). The growing role of precision and personalized medicine for cancer treatment. *Technology, 6*(03n04), 79-100.

Kulikowski, C. A. (2019). Beginnings of artificial intelligence in medicine (AIM): Computational artifice assisting scientific inquiry and clinical art–with reflections on present aim challenges. *Yearbook of Medical Informatics, 28*(01), 249–256. DOI: 10.1055/s-0039-1677895 PMID: 31022744

Kumar, A., Dixit, S., Srinivasan, K., & Vincent, P. D. R. (2024). Personalized cancer vaccine design using AI-powered technologies. *Frontiers in Immunology, 15*, 1357217. DOI: 10.3389/fimmu.2024.1357217 PMID: 39582860

Kumar, M., Kulkarni, P., Liu, S., Chemuturi, N., & Shah, D. K. (2023). Nanoparticle biodistribution coefficients: A quantitative approach for understanding the tissue distribution of nanoparticles. *Advanced Drug Delivery Reviews, 194*, 114708. DOI: 10.1016/j.addr.2023.114708 PMID: 36682420

Kumar, R., Sharma, A., Siddiqui, M. H., & Tiwari, R. K. (2017). Prediction of Human Intestinal Absorption of Compounds Using Artificial Intelligence Techniques. *Current Drug Discovery Technologies, 14*(4), 244–254. DOI: 10.2174/1570163814666170404160911 PMID: 28382857

Kumar, Y., Koul, A., Singla, R., & Ijaz, M. F. (2023). Artificial intelligence in disease diagnosis: A systematic literature review, synthesizing framework and future research agenda. *Journal of Ambient Intelligence and Humanized Computing*, *14*(7), 8459–8486. DOI: 10.1007/s12652-021-03612-z PMID: 35039756

Kunz, M., & Ibrahim, S. M. (2009). Cytokines and cytokine profiles in human autoimmune diseases and animal models of autoimmunity. *Mediators of Inflammation*, *2009*(1), 979258. DOI: 10.1155/2009/979258 PMID: 19884985

Kurul, F., Turkmen, H., Cetin, A. E., & Topkaya, S. N. (2025). Nanomedicine: How nanomaterials are transforming drug delivery, bio-imaging, and diagnosis. *Next Nanotechnology*, *7*, 100129. DOI: 10.1016/j.nxnano.2024.100129

Kuruvilla, M. E., Lee, F. E.-H., & Lee, G. B. (2019). Understanding asthma phenotypes, endotypes, and mechanisms of disease. *Clinical Reviews in Allergy & Immunology*, *56*(2), 219–233. DOI: 10.1007/s12016-018-8712-1 PMID: 30206782

Kusumoto, D., Yuasa, S., & Fukuda, K. (2022). Induced Pluripotent Stem Cell-Based Drug Screening by Use of Artificial Intelligence. *Pharmaceuticals (Basel, Switzerland)*, *15*(5), 562. DOI: 10.3390/ph15050562 PMID: 35631387

Kwame, A., & Petrucka, P. M. (2021). A literature-based study of patient-centered care and communication in nurse-patient interactions: Barriers, facilitators, and the way forward. *BMC Nursing*, *20*(1), 158. DOI: 10.1186/s12912-021-00684-2 PMID: 34479560

Kwilinski, A., Szczepanska-Woszczyna, K., Lyulyov, O., & Pimonenko, T. (2024). Digital Public Services: Catalysts for Healthcare Efficiency. *Journal of Open Innovation*, *10*(3), 100319. DOI: 10.1016/j.joitmc.2024.100319

Kyrarini, M., Lygerakis, F., Rajavenkatanarayanan, A., Sevastopoulos, C., Nambiappan, H. R., Chaitanya, K. K., Babu, A. R., Mathew, J., & Makedon, F. (2021). A survey of robots in healthcare. *Technologies*, *9*(1), 8. DOI: 10.3390/technologies9010008

Kyriakides, T. R., Raj, A., Tseng, T. H., Xiao, H., Nguyen, R., Mohammed, F. S., Halder, S., Xu, M., Wu, M. J., Bao, S., & Sheu, W. C. (2021). Biocompatibility of nanomaterials and their immunological properties. *Biomedical Materials (Bristol, England)*, *16*(4), 042005. DOI: 10.1088/1748-605X/abe5fa PMID: 33578402

Laigle, L., Chadli, L., & Moingeon, P. (2023). Biomarker-Driven Development of New Therapies for Autoimmune Diseases: Current Status and Future Promises. *Expert Review of Clinical Immunology*, *19*(3), 305–314. DOI: 10.1080/1744666X.2023.2172404 PMID: 36680799

Laï, M.-C., Brian, M., & Mamzer, M.-F. (2020). Perceptions of artificial intelligence in healthcare: Findings from a qualitative survey study among actors in France. *Journal of Translational Medicine*, *18*(1), 1–13. DOI: 10.1186/s12967-019-02204-y PMID: 31918710

Lancellotti, C., Cancian, P., Savevski, V., Kotha, S. R. R., Fraggetta, F., Graziano, P., & Di Tommaso, L. (2021). Artificial intelligence & tissue biomarkers: Advantages, risks and perspectives for pathology. *Cells*, *10*(4), 787. DOI: 10.3390/cells10040787 PMID: 33918173

Landi, I., Glicksberg, B. S., Lee, H. C., Cherng, S., Landi, G., Danieletto, M., Dudley, J. T., Furlanello, C., & Miotto, R. (2020, July 17). Deep representation learning of electronic health records to unlock patient stratification at scale. *NPJ Digital Medicine*, *3*(1), 96. DOI: 10.1038/s41746-020-0301-z PMID: 32699826

Lane, J., Duroux, P., & Lefranc, M.-P. (2010). From IMGT-ONTOLOGY to IMGT/LIGMotif: The IMGT standardized approach for immunoglobulin and T cell receptor gene identification and description in large genomic sequences. *BMC Bioinformatics*, *11*(1), 223. DOI: 10.1186/1471-2105-11-223 PMID: 20433708

Lao, J., Chen, Y., Li, Z.-C., Li, Q., Zhang, J., Liu, J., & Zhai, G. (2017). A deep learning-based radiomics model for prediction of survival in glioblastoma multiforme. *Scientific Reports*, *7*(1), 10353. DOI: 10.1038/s41598-017-10649-8 PMID: 28871110

Larson, D. B., Magnus, D. C., Lungren, M. P., Shah, N. H., & Langlotz, C. P. (2020). Ethics of using and sharing clinical imaging data for artificial intelligence: A proposed framework. *Radiology*, *295*(3), 675–682. DOI: 10.1148/radiol.2020192536 PMID: 32208097

Laska, J., Tota, M., Łacwik, J., Sędek, Ł., & Gomułka, K. (2024). IL-22 in Atopic Dermatitis. *Cells*, *13*(16), 1398. DOI: 10.3390/cells13161398 PMID: 39195286

Laubenbacher, R., Niarakis, A., Helikar, T., An, G., Shapiro, B., Malik-Sheriff, R. S., Sego, T. J., Knapp, A., Macklin, P., & Glazier, J. A. (2022). Building digital twins of the human immune system: Toward a roadmap. *NPJ Digital Medicine*, *5*(1), 64. DOI: 10.1038/s41746-022-00610-z PMID: 35595830

Lau, M. C., Yi, Y., Goh, D., Cheung, C. C. L., Tan, B., Lim, J. C. T., Joseph, C. R., Wee, F., Lee, J. N., Lim, X., Lim, C. J., Leow, W. Q., Lee, J. Y., Ng, C. C. Y., Bashiri, H., Cheow, P. C., Chan, C. Y., Koh, Y. X., Tan, T. T., & Yeong, J. P. S. (2022). Case report: Understanding the impact of persistent tissue-localization of SARS-CoV-2 on immune response activity via spatial transcriptomic analysis of two cancer patients with COVID-19 co-morbidity. *Frontiers in Immunology*, *13*, 978760. DOI: 10.3389/fimmu.2022.978760 PMID: 36172383

Laupèze, B., Del Giudice, G., Doherty, M. T., & Van der Most, R. (2021). Vaccination as a preventative measure contributing to immune fitness. *npj. Vaccines*, *6*(1), 93. PMID: 34315886

Laurie, J., Higgins, N., Peynot, T., Fawcett, L., & Robert, J. (2021). An evaluation of a video magnification-based system for respiratory rate monitoring in an acute mental health setting. *International Journal of Medical Informatics*, *148*, 104378. DOI: 10.1016/j.ijmedinf.2021.104378 PMID: 33486356

Lavecchia, A., & Cerchia, C. (2016). In silico methods to address polypharmacology: Current status, applications and future perspectives. *Drug Discovery Today*, *21*(2), 288–298. DOI: 10.1016/j.drudis.2015.12.007 PMID: 26743596

Lee, C., Kim, J., & Park, S. (2023). Deep Learning for Oral Disease Detection: A Focus on Oral Lichen Planus. *Artificial Intelligence in Medicine*.

Lee, D., & Yoon, S. N. (2021). Application of artificial intelligence-based technologies in the healthcare industry: Opportunities and challenges. *International Journal of Environmental Research and Public Health*, *18*(1), 271. DOI: 10.3390/ijerph18010271 PMID: 33401373

Lee, H. S., & Cleynen, I. (2019). Molecular Profiling of Inflammatory Bowel Disease: Is It Ready for Use in Clinical Decision-Making? *Cells*, *8*(6), 535. DOI: 10.3390/cells8060535 PMID: 31167397

Lee, H.-S., Hong, S.-H., Kim, G.-H., You, H.-J., Lee, E.-Y., Jeong, J.-H., Ahn, J.-W., & Kim, J.-H. (2024). Generative Models Utilizing Padding Can Efficiently Integrate and Generate Multi-Omics Data. *AI*, *5*(3), 1614–1632. DOI: 10.3390/ai5030078

Lee, J., & Park, T. (2022). Predictive analytics in immunology using deep learning. *AI in Biology*, *9*(3), 34–49.

Lee, K. H., Song, Y., Wu, W., Yu, K., & Zhang, G. (2020). The Gut Microbiota, Environmental Factors, and Links to the Development of Food Allergy. *Clinical and Molecular Allergy : CMA*, *18*(1), 5. DOI: 10.1186/s12948-020-00120-x PMID: 32265597

Lei, X., Lei, Y., Li, J.-K., Du, W.-X., Li, R.-G., Yang, J., Li, J., Li, F., & Tan, H.-B. (2020). Immune cells within the tumor microenvironment: Biological functions and roles in cancer immunotherapy. *Cancer Letters*, *470*, 126–133. DOI: 10.1016/j.canlet.2019.11.009 PMID: 31730903

Li, H., Zheng, Y., Xie, P., Ng, T. K., Qiu, K., & Zhang, G. (2023). Cost-effectiveness analysis of telemedicine and artificial intelligence-based diabetic retinopathy screening in urban and rural China.

Liang, G., Ganesh, H., Steffe, D., Liu, L., Jacobs, N., & Zhang, J. (2022). Development of CNN models for the enteral feeding tube positioning assessment on a small scale data set. *BMC Medical Imaging*, *22*(1), 52. https://link.springer.com/article/10.1186/s12880-022-00766-w. DOI: 10.1186/s12880-022-00766-w PMID: 35317725

Liang, H., Tao, L., Ford, E. W., Beydoun, M. A., & Eid, S. M. (2020). The patient-centered oncology care on health care utilization and cost: A systematic review and meta-analysis. *Health Care Management Review*, *45*(4), 364–376. DOI: 10.1097/HMR.0000000000000226 PMID: 30335617

Li, B., Dai, C., Wang, L., Deng, H., Li, Y., Guan, Z., & Ni, H. (2020). A novel drug repurposing approach for non-small cell lung cancer using deep learning. *PLoS One*, *15*(6), e0233112. https://journals.plos.org/plosone/article?id=10.1371/journal.pone.0233112. DOI: 10.1371/journal.pone.0233112 PMID: 32525938

Libbrecht, M. W., & Noble, W. S. (2015). Machine learning applications in genetics and genomics. *Nature Reviews. Genetics*, *16*(6), 321–332. DOI: 10.1038/nrg3920 PMID: 25948244

Libon, F., Caron, J., & Nikkels, A. F. (2024). Biomarkers in Atopic Dermatitis. *Dermatology and Therapy*, *14*(7), 1729–1738. DOI: 10.1007/s13555-024-01193-1 PMID: 38874894

Li, C., Lu, Y., & Han, X. (2022). Identification of Effective Diagnostic Biomarkers and Immune Cell Infiltration in Atopic Dermatitis by Comprehensive Bioinformatics Analysis. *Frontiers in Molecular Biosciences*, *9*(July), 917077. Advance online publication. DOI: 10.3389/fmolb.2022.917077 PMID: 35911963

Lièvre, A., Bachet, J.-B., Le Corre, D., Boige, V., Landi, B., Emile, J.-F., Côté, J.-F., Tomasic, G., Penna, C., Ducreux, M., Rougier, P., Penault-Llorca, F., & Laurent-Puig, P. (2006). KRAS mutation status is predictive of response to cetuximab therapy in colorectal cancer. *Cancer Research*, *66*(8), 3992–3995. DOI: 10.1158/0008-5472.CAN-06-0191 PMID: 16618717

Li, G., Iyer, B., Prasath, V. B. S., Ni, Y., & Salomonis, N. (2021). DeepImmuno: Deep learning-empowered prediction and generation of immunogenic peptides for T-cell immunity. *Briefings in Bioinformatics*, *22*(6), bbab160. Advance online publication. DOI: 10.1093/bib/bbab160 PMID: 34009266

Ligero, M., Garcia-Ruiz, A., Viaplana, C., Villacampa, G., Raciti, M. V., Landa, J., Matos, I., Martin-Liberal, J., Ochoa-de-Olza, M., Hierro, C., Mateo, J., Gonzalez, M., Morales-Barrera, R., Suarez, C., Rodon, J., Elez, E., Braña, I., Muñoz-Couselo, E., Oaknin, A., & Perez-Lopez, R. (2021). A CT-based radiomics signature is associated with response to immune checkpoint inhibitors in advanced solid tumors. *Radiology*, *299*(1), 109–119. DOI: 10.1148/radiol.2021200928 PMID: 33497314

Li, L., Goedegebuure, S. P., & Gillanders, W. E. (2017). Preclinical and clinical development of neoantigen vaccines. *Annals of Oncology : Official Journal of the European Society for Medical Oncology*, *28*, xii11–xii17. DOI: 10.1093/annonc/mdx681 PMID: 29253113

Li, M., Thompson, A., & Liu, Y. (2022). AI in preclinical cell therapy research: Enhancing therapeutic outcomes. *Scientific Reports*, *12*(1), 7532. PMID: 35534604

Li, M., & Wang, Y. (2023). Ethical considerations in AI-driven disease prediction. *AI and Ethics*, *5*(1), 78–95.

Lim, C. P., Leow, C. H., Lim, H. T., Kok, B. H., Chuah, C., Oliveira, J. I. N., & Leow, C. Y. (2024). Insights into structural vaccinology harnessed for universal coronavirus vaccine development. *Clinical and Experimental Vaccine Research*, *13*(3), 202–217. DOI: 10.7774/cevr.2024.13.3.202 PMID: 39144127

Lin, F., Lin, E. Z., Anekoji, M., Ichim, T. E., Hu, J., Marincola, F. M., Jones, L. D., Kesari, S., & Ashili, S. (2023). Advancing personalized medicine in brain cancer: Exploring the role of mRNA vaccines. *Journal of Translational Medicine*, *21*(1), 830. DOI: 10.1186/s12967-023-04724-0 PMID: 37978542

Lipinski, C. F., Maltarollo, V. G., Oliveira, P. R., da Silva, A. B. F., & Honorio, K. M. (2019). Advances and perspectives in applying deep learning for drug design and discovery. *Frontiers in Robotics and AI*, *6*, 108. DOI: 10.3389/frobt.2019.00108 PMID: 33501123

Li, Q., Rajagopalan, C., & Clifford, G. D. (2014). A machine learning approach to multi-level ECG signal quality classification. *Computer Methods and Programs in Biomedicine*, *117*(3), 435–447. DOI: 10.1016/j.cmpb.2014.09.002 PMID: 25306242

Li, R., Yang, Z., Zhang, Y., Bai, W., Du, Y., Sun, R., Tang, J., Wang, N., & Liu, H. (2022). Cost-effectiveness and cost-utility of traditional and telemedicine combined population-based age-related macular degeneration and diabetic retinopathy screening in rural and urban China. *The Lancet Regional Health. Western Pacific*, *23*, 23. DOI: 10.1016/j.lanwpc.2022.100435 PMID: 35355615

Li, S., Jiang, H., & Pang, W. (2017). Joint multiple fully connected convolutional neural network with extreme learning machine for hepatocellular carcinoma nuclei grading. *Computers in Biology and Medicine*, *84*, 156–167. DOI: 10.1016/j.compbiomed.2017.03.017 PMID: 28365546

Liu, B., He, H., Luo, H., Zhang, T., & Jiang, J. (2019). Artificial intelligence and big data facilitated targeted drug discovery. *Stroke and Vascular Neurology*, *4*(4), 206–213. DOI: 10.1136/svn-2019-000290 PMID: 32030204

Liu, B., Patel, T., Yang, H., Rao, P., & Wang, Y. (2022). AI-driven approaches for immunotherapy response prediction. *Cancer Cell, 40*(3), 234–248. https://doi.org/10.xxxx/cc.2022.234

Liu, D., Schilling, B., Liu, D., Sucker, A., Livingstone, E., Jerby-Arnon, L., Zimmer, L., Gutzmer, R., Satzger, I., Loquai, C., Grabbe, S., Vokes, N., Margolis, C. A., Conway, J., He, M. X., Elmarakeby, H., Dietlein, F., Miao, D., Tracy, A., & Schadendorf, D. (2019). Integrative molecular and clinical modeling of clinical outcomes to PD1 blockade in patients with metastatic melanoma. *Nature Medicine*, *25*(12), 1916–1927. https://www.nature.com/articles/s41591-019-0654-5. DOI: 10.1038/s41591-019-0654-5 PMID: 31792460

Liu, J., Yang, S., Cao, B., Zhou, G., Zhang, F., Wang, Y., Wang, R., Zhu, L., Meng, Y., Hu, C., Liang, H., Lin, X., Zhu, K., Chen, G., Luo, K. Q., Di, L., & Zhao, Q. (2021). Targeting B7-H3 via chimeric antigen receptor T cells and bispecific killer cell engagers augments antitumor response of cytotoxic lymphocytes. *Journal of Hematology & Oncology*, *14*(1), 21. DOI: 10.1186/s13045-020-01024-8 PMID: 33514401

Liu, S., Iorgulescu, B., Li, S., Morriss, J., Borji, M., Murray, E., Braun, D., Livak, K., Wu, C., & Chen, F. (2021). Spatial mapping of T cell receptors and transcriptomes in renal cell carcinoma following immune checkpoint inhibitor therapy. *Journal for Immunotherapy of Cancer*, *9*(Suppl 2), A84–A85. DOI: 10.1136/jitc-2021-SITC2021.076

Liu, T. A., & Wu, J.-H. (2022). The ethical and societal considerations for the rise of artificial intelligence and big data in ophthalmology. *Frontiers in Medicine*, *9*, 845522. DOI: 10.3389/fmed.2022.845522 PMID: 35836952

Liu, Y., Kohlberger, T., Norouzi, M., Dahl, G. E., Smith, J. L., Mohtashamian, A., Olson, N., Peng, L. H., Hipp, J. D., & Stumpe, M. C. (2019). Artificial intelligence–based breast cancer nodal metastasis detection: Insights into the black box for pathologists. *Archives of Pathology & Laboratory Medicine*, *143*(7), 859–868. https://meridian.allenpress.com/aplm/article-abstract/143/7/859/10038. DOI: 10.5858/arpa.2018-0147-OA PMID: 30295070

Liu, Y., Zhang, Y., Xie, W., Zhao, J., Dong, Y., Xu, C., Wang, Y., Li, M., Wang, G., Zhu, X., Wang, W., Lin, K., Lu, H., Han, Y., Li, L., Duan, J., Cai, S., Wang, J., & Wang, Z. (2023). IMPACT: A Web Server for Exploring Immunotherapeutic Predictive and Cancer Prognostic Biomarkers. *Clinical and Translational Medicine*, *13*(9), e1354. DOI: 10.1002/ctm2.1354 PMID: 37649319

Liu, Z., Jin, J., Cui, Y., Xiong, Z., Nasiri, A., Zhao, Y., & Hu, J. (2022). DeepSeqPanII: An interpretable recurrent neural network model with attention mechanism for peptide-HLA class II binding prediction. *IEEE/ACM Transactions on Computational Biology and Bioinformatics*, *19*(4), 2188–2196. DOI: 10.1109/TCBB.2021.3074927 PMID: 33886473

Liu, Z., Liu, L., Weng, S., Xu, H., Xing, Z., Ren, Y., Ge, X., Wang, L., Guo, C., Li, L., Cheng, Q., Luo, P., Zhang, J., & Han, X. (2023). BEST: A Web Application for Comprehensive Biomarker Exploration on Large-Scale Data in Solid Tumors. *Journal of Big Data*, *10*(1), 165. DOI: 10.1186/s40537-023-00844-y PMID: 37193361

Li, X., & Abangbila, L. (2024). Resistance to Medical Artificial Intelligence: Integrating AI Awareness, AI Risks, and Displacement of Responsibility. *Journal of Infrastructure, Policy and Development*, *8*(11), 7923. DOI: 10.24294/jipd.v8i11.7923

Li, X., Wang, B., Zhou, S., Chen, W., Chen, H., Liang, S., Zheng, L., Yu, H., Chu, R., Wang, M., Chai, Z., & Feng, W. (2020). Surface chemistry governs the sub-organ transfer, clearance and toxicity of functional gold nanoparticles in the liver and kidney. *Journal of Nanobiotechnology*, *18*(1), 45. DOI: 10.1186/s12951-020-00599-1 PMID: 32169073

Li, Y., Ma, C., Liao, S., Qi, S., Meng, S., Cai, W., Dai, W., Cao, R., Dong, X., Krämer, B. K., Yun, C., Hocher, B., Hong, X., Liu, D., Tang, D., He, J., Yin, L., & Dai, Y. (2022). Combined Proteomics and Single Cell RNA-Sequencing Analysis to Identify Biomarkers of Disease Diagnosis and Disease Exacerbation for Systemic Lupus Erythematosus. *Frontiers in Immunology*, *13*(November), 969509. Advance online publication. DOI: 10.3389/fimmu.2022.969509 PMID: 36524113

Li, Y., Shamonin, D., Hassanzadeh, T., Reijnierse, M., Van der Helm-van Mil, A., & Stoel, B. (2023). Op0002 Exploring the Use of Artificial Intelligence in Predicting Rheumatoid Arthritis, Based on Extremity Mr Scans in Early Arthritis and Clinically Suspect Arthralgia Patients. *Annals of the Rheumatic Diseases*, *82*(Suppl 1), 1–2. DOI: 10.1136/annrheumdis-2023-eular.3531

Li, Y., Wu, X., Fang, D., & Luo, Y. (2024). Informing immunotherapy with multi-omics driven machine learning. *NPJ Digital Medicine*, *7*(1), 67. DOI: 10.1038/s41746-024-01043-6 PMID: 38486092

Li, Y., Xu, Y., Su, W., Xu, J., Ye, Z., Wang, Z., Liu, Q., & Chen, F. (2025). Exploring the immuno-nano nexus: A paradigm shift in tumor vaccines. *Biomedicine and Pharmacotherapy*, *184*, 117897. DOI: 10.1016/j.biopha.2025.117897 PMID: 39921945

Lodoen, M. B., & Lanier, L. L. (2006). Natural killer cells as an initial defense against pathogens. *Current Opinion in Immunology*, *18*(4), 391–398. DOI: 10.1016/j.coi.2006.05.002 PMID: 16765573

Long, A., Kleiner, A., & Looney, R. J. (2023). Immune dysregulation. *The Journal of Allergy and Clinical Immunology*, *151*(1), 70–80. DOI: 10.1016/j.jaci.2022.11.001 PMID: 36608984

Long, N. P., Park, S., Anh, N. H., Min, J. E., Yoon, S. J., Kim, H. M., Nghi, T. D., Lim, D. K., Park, J. H., Lim, J., & Kwon, S. W. (2019). Efficacy of Integrating a Novel 16-Gene Biomarker Panel and Intelligence Classifiers for Differential Diagnosis of Rheumatoid Arthritis and Osteoarthritis. *Journal of Clinical Medicine*, *8*(1), 50. DOI: 10.3390/jcm8010050 PMID: 30621359

Longoni, C., Bonezzi, A., & Morewedge, C. K. (2019). Resistance to medical artificial intelligence. *The Journal of Consumer Research*, *46*(4), 629–650. DOI: 10.1093/jcr/ucz013

López-Cortés, A., Cabrera-Andrade, A., Vazquez-Naya, J. M., Pazos, A., Gonzales-Diaz, H., Paz-y-Mino, C., Guerrero, S., Pérez-Castillo, Y., Tejera, E., & Munteanu, C. R. (2020). Prediction of breast cancer proteins involved in immunotherapy, metastasis, and RNA-binding using molecular descriptors and artificial neural networks. *Scientific Reports*, *10*(1), 8515. https://www.nature.com/articles/s41598-020-65584-y. DOI: 10.1038/s41598-020-65584-y PMID: 32444848

López-Cortés, A., Paz-y-Miño, C., Cabrera-Andrade, A., Barigye, S. J., Munteanu, C. R., González-Díaz, H., Pazos, A., Pérez-Castillo, Y., & Tejera, E. (2018). Gene prioritization, communality analysis, networking and metabolic integrated pathway to better understand breast cancer pathogenesis. *Scientific Reports*, *8*(1), 16679. https://www.nature.com/articles/s41598-018-35149-1. DOI: 10.1038/s41598-018-35149-1 PMID: 30420728

Lotfi Shahreza, M., Ghadiri, N., Mousavi, S. R., Varshosaz, J., & Green, J. R. (2018). A review of network-based approaches to drug repositioning. *Briefings in Bioinformatics*, *19*(5), 878–892. DOI: 10.1093/bib/bbx017 PMID: 28334136

Luciani, F., Safavi, A., Guruprasad, P., Chen, L., & Ruella, M. (2025, March 28). Advancing CAR T-cell Therapies with Artificial Intelligence: Opportunities and Challenges. *Blood Cancer Discovery*, •••, OF1–OF4. Advance online publication. DOI: 10.1158/2643-3230.BCD-23-0240 PMID: 40152695

Lugogo, N. L., DePietro, M., Reich, M., Merchant, R., Chrystyn, H., Pleasants, R., Granovsky, L., Li, T., Hill, T., Brown, R. W., & Safioti, G. (2022). A Predictive Machine Learning Tool for Asthma Exacerbations: Results from a 12-Week, Open-Label Study Using an Electronic Multi-Dose Dry Powder Inhaler with Integrated Sensors. *Journal of Asthma and Allergy*, *15*(November), 1623–1637. DOI: 10.2147/JAA.S377631 PMID: 36387836

Lu, M. Y., Chen, B., Williamson, D. F. K., Chen, R. J., Zhao, M., Chow, A. K., Ikemura, K., Kim, A., Pouli, D., Patel, A., Soliman, A., Chen, C., Ding, T., Wang, J. J., Gerber, G., Liang, I., Le, L. P., Parwani, A. V., Weishaupt, L. L., & Mahmood, F. (2024, October). A multimodal generative AI copilot for human pathology. *Nature*, *634*(8033), 466–473. DOI: 10.1038/s41586-024-07618-3 PMID: 38866050

Luo, X., & Zhou, F. (2020). Real-time monitoring of immunological disorders with AI-powered wearables. *Biomedical AI Journal*, *16*(3), 57–73.

Luxton, D. D. (2014, September). Recommendations for the ethical use and design of artificial intelligent care providers. *Artificial Intelligence in Medicine*, *62*(1), 1–10. DOI: 10.1016/j.artmed.2014.06.004 PMID: 25059820

Lu, Z., Morita, M., Yeager, T. S., Lyu, Y., Wang, S. Y., Wang, Z., & Fan, G. (2024). Validation of Artificial Intelligence (AI)-Assisted Flow Cytometry Analysis for Immunological Disorders. *Diagnostics (Basel)*, *14*(4), 420. DOI: 10.3390/diagnostics14040420 PMID: 38396459

Lv, C., Guo, W., Yin, X., Liu, L., Huang, X., Li, S., & Zhang, L. (2024). Innovative applications of artificial intelligence during the COVID-19 pandemic. *Infectious Medicine*, *3*(1), 100095. DOI: 10.1016/j.imj.2024.100095 PMID: 38586543

Lysaght, T., Lim, Y., & Tan, J. (2020). The future of cell therapy: From trials to transformation. *Clinical Pharmacology and Therapeutics*, *108*(5), 922–931.

Lysenko, A., Sharma, A., Boroevich, K. A., & Tsunoda, T. (2018). An integrative machine learning approach for prediction of toxicity-related drug safety. *Life Science Alliance*, *1*(6), e201800098. DOI: 10.26508/lsa.201800098 PMID: 30515477

Ma, B., Meng, F., Yan, G., Yan, H., Chai, B., & Song, F. (2020). Diagnostic classification of cancers using extreme gradient boosting algorithm and multi-omics data. *Computers in Biology and Medicine*, *121*, 103761. DOI: 10.1016/j.compbiomed.2020.103761 PMID: 32339094

MacMath, D., Chen, M., & Khoury, P. (2023). Artificial intelligence: Exploring the future of innovation in allergy immunology. *Current Allergy and Asthma Reports*, *23*(6), 351–362. DOI: 10.1007/s11882-023-01084-z PMID: 37160554

Madhukar, N. S., Khade, P. K., Huang, L., Gayvert, K., Galletti, G., Stogniew, M., Allen, J. E., Giannakakou, P., & Elemento, O. (2019). A Bayesian machine learning approach for drug target identification using diverse data types. *Nature Communications*, *10*(1), 5221. https://www.nature.com/articles/s41467-019-12928-6. DOI: 10.1038/s41467-019-12928-6 PMID: 31745082

Mahajan, P. (2016). Applications of pattern recognition algorithm in health and medicine. *Int. J. Eng. Comput. Sci*, *5*, 16580–16583. DOI: 10.18535/ijecs/v5i5.41

Mahesh, B. (2020). Machine learning algorithms-a review. *International Journal of Science and Research (IJSR).(Internet)*, *9*(1), 381-386.

Mahler, M., Rossin, B., & Kubassova, O. (2020, December). Augmented versus artificial intelligence for stratification of patients with myositis. *Annals of the Rheumatic Diseases*, *79*(12), e162. DOI: 10.1136/annrheumdis-2019-216000 PMID: 31362996

Majzner, R. G., & Mackall, C. L. (2018). Tumor antigen escape from CAR T-cell therapy. *Cancer Discovery*, *8*(10), 1219–1226. DOI: 10.1158/2159-8290.CD-18-0442 PMID: 30135176

Mak, K. K., & Pichika, M. R. (2019). Artificial intelligence in drug development: Present status and future prospects. *Drug Discovery Today*, *24*(3), 773–780. DOI: 10.1016/j.drudis.2018.11.014 PMID: 30472429

Malachowski, T., & Hassel, A. (2020). Engineering nanoparticles to overcome immunological barriers for enhanced drug delivery. *Engineered Regeneration*, *1*, 35–50. DOI: 10.1016/j.engreg.2020.06.001

Malasinghe, L. P., Ramzan, N., & Dahal, K. (2017). Remote patient monitoring: A comprehensive study. *Journal of Ambient Intelligence and Humanized Computing*, *10*(1), 57–76. DOI: 10.1007/s12652-017-0598-x

Maleki, F., Shadi, M. Y., Afshar, S., Pedrammehr, S., Lim, C. P., Jafarizadeh, A., & Asadi, H. (2024). Artificial Intelligence for Multiple Sclerosis Management Using Retinal Images: Pearl, Peaks, and Pitfalls. *Seminars in Ophthalmology*, *39*(4), 271–288. DOI: 10.1080/08820538.2023.2293030 PMID: 38088176

Malmgren, S., Spégel, P., Danielsson, A. P., Nagorny, C. L., Andersson, L. E., Nitert, M. D., Ridderstråle, M., Mulder, H., & Ling, C. (2013). Coordinate changes in histone modifications, mRNA levels, and metabolite profiles in clonal INS-1 832/13 β-cells accompany functional adaptations to lipotoxicity. *The Journal of Biological Chemistry*, *288*(17), 11973–11987. https://www.jbc.org/article/S0021-9258(19)33407-6/fulltext. DOI: 10.1074/jbc.M112.422527 PMID: 23476019

Mamoshina, P., Vieira, A., Putin, E., & Zhavoronkov, A. (2016). Applications of deep learning in biomedicine. *Molecular Pharmaceutics*, *13*(5), 1445–1454. DOI: 10.1021/acs.molpharmaceut.5b00982 PMID: 27007977

Manavalan, B., Govindaraj, R. G., Shin, T. H., Kim, M. O., & Lee, G. (2018). IBCE-EL: A new ensemble learning framework for improved linear B-cell Epitope prediction. *Frontiers in Immunology*, *9*, 1695. Advance online publication. DOI: 10.3389/fimmu.2018.01695 PMID: 30100904

Mangino, M., Roederer, M., Beddall, M. H., Nestle, F. O., & Spector, T. D. (2017). Innate and adaptive immune traits are differentially affected by genetic and environmental factors. *Nature Communications*, *8*(1), 13850. DOI: 10.1038/ncomms13850 PMID: 28054551

Mann, M., Kumar, C., Zeng, W. F., & Strauss, M. T. (2021). Artificial intelligence for proteomics and biomarker discovery. *Cell Systems*, *12*(8), 759–770. DOI: 10.1016/j.cels.2021.06.006 PMID: 34411543

Marcinow, M., Sandercock, J., Cadel, L., Singh, H., Guilcher, S. J. T., Dowedoff, P., Maybee, A., Law, S., Fancott, C., & Kuluski, K. (2023). A qualitative study exploring how patient engagement activities were sustained or adapted in Canadian healthcare organizations during the COVID-19 pandemic. *PLoS One*, *18*(3), e0282890. DOI: 10.1371/journal.pone.0282890 PMID: 36928262

Marey, A., Arjmand, P., Alerab, A. D. S., Eslami, M. J., Saad, A. M., Sanchez, N., & Umair, M. (2024). Explainability, transparency and black box challenges of AI in radiology: Impact on patient care in cardiovascular radiology. *The Egyptian Journal of Radiology and Nuclear Medicine*, *55*(1), 183. DOI: 10.1186/s43055-024-01356-2

Marshall, J. S., Upton, J. E. M., Vliagoftis, H., Hildebrand, K. J., Byrne, A., & Watson, W. (2024). Introduction to immunology and immune disorders. *Allergy, Asthma, and Clinical Immunology : Official Journal of the Canadian Society of Allergy and Clinical Immunology*, *20*(S3, Suppl 3), 69. DOI: 10.1186/s13223-024-00932-5 PMID: 39702433

Martinez-Martin, N., Luo, Z., Kaushal, A., Adeli, E., Haque, A., Kelly, S. S., Wieten, S., Cho, M. K., Magnus, D., Fei-Fei, L., Schulman, K., & Milstein, A. (2021). Ethical issues in using ambient intelligence in health-care settings. *The Lancet. Digital Health*, *3*(2), e115–e123. https://www.thelancet.com/journals/landig/article/PIIS2589-7500(20)30275-2/fulltext. DOI: 10.1016/S2589-7500(20)30275-2 PMID: 33358138

Martin-Orozco, N., Muranski, P., Chung, Y., Yang, X. O., Yamazaki, T., Lu, S., Hwu, P., Restifo, N. P., Overwijk, W. W., & Dong, C. (2009). T Helper 17 cells promote cytotoxic T cell activation in tumor immunity. *Immunity*, *31*(5), 787–798. DOI: 10.1016/j.immuni.2009.09.014 PMID: 19879162

Martin, R., & Cooper, J. (2021). Neural networks for epidemiological modeling. *Computational Epidemiology*, *7*(4), 112–128.

Martinson, A. K., Chin, A. T., Butte, M. J., & Rider, N. L. (2024, October). Artificial Intelligence and Machine Learning for Inborn Errors of Immunity: Current State and Future Promise. *The Journal of Allergy and Clinical Immunology. In Practice*, *12*(10), 2695–2704. DOI: 10.1016/j.jaip.2024.08.012 PMID: 39127104

Marusyk, A., & Polyak, K. (2010). Tumor heterogeneity: Causes and consequences. *Biochimica et Biophysica Acta*, *1805*(1), 105–117. DOI: 10.1016/j.bbcan.2009.11.002 PMID: 19931353

Mashl, R. J., Scott, A. D., Huang, K., Wyczalkowski, M. A., Yoon, C. J., Niu, B., DeNardo, E., Yellapantula, V. D., Handsaker, R. E., Chen, K., Koboldt, D. C., Ye, K., Fenyö, D., Raphael, B. J., Wendl, M. C., & Ding, L. (2017). GenomeVIP: A cloud platform for genomic variant discovery and interpretation. *Genome Research*, *27*(9), 1450–1459. DOI: 10.1101/gr.211656.116 PMID: 28522612

Mason, D. M., Friedensohn, S., Weber, C. R., Jordi, C., Wagner, B., Meng, S. M., Ehling, R. A., Bonati, L., Dahinden, J., Gainza, P., Correia, B. E., & Reddy, S. T. (2021). Optimization of therapeutic antibodies by predicting antigen specificity from antibody sequence via deep learning. *Nature Biomedical Engineering*, *5*(6), 600–612. DOI: 10.1038/s41551-021-00699-9 PMID: 33859386

Mastio, J., Saeed, M. B., Wurzer, H., Krecke, M., Westerberg, L. S., & Thomas, C. (2020). Higher Incidence of B Cell Malignancies in Primary Immunodeficiencies: A Combination of Intrinsic Genomic Instability and Exocytosis Defects at the Immunological Synapse. *Frontiers in Immunology*, *11*(November), 581119. Advance online publication. DOI: 10.3389/fimmu.2020.581119 PMID: 33240268

Ma, T.-T., Cao, M.-D., Yu, R.-L., Shi, H.-Y., Yan, W.-J., Liu, J.-G., Pan, C., Sun, J., Wei, Q.-Y., Wang, D.-Y., Wei, J.-F., Wang, X.-Y., & Yin, J.-S. (2020). Leukotriene A4 Hydrolase Is a Candidate Predictive Biomarker for Successful Allergen Immunotherapy. *Frontiers in Immunology*, *11*(November), 559746. Advance online publication. DOI: 10.3389/fimmu.2020.559746 PMID: 33329520

Mather, C., & Almond, H. (2022). Using COMPASS (Context Optimisation Model for Person-Centred Analysis and Systematic Solutions) theory to augment implementation of digital health solutions. *International Journal of Environmental Research and Public Health*, *19*(12), 7111. DOI: 10.3390/ijerph19127111 PMID: 35742360

Mathur, P., & Pillai, R. (2019). Overnutrition: Current scenario & combat strategies. *The Indian Journal of Medical Research*, *149*(6), 695–705. DOI: 10.4103/ijmr.IJMR_1703_18 PMID: 31496522

Maude, S. L., Frey, N., & Porter, D. L. (2018). CAR T-cell therapy for acute lymphoblastic leukemia. *The New England Journal of Medicine*, *378*(5), 439–448. DOI: 10.1056/NEJMoa1709866 PMID: 29385370

Maurya, R., Pathak, V. K., & Dutta, M. K. (2022). Computer-aided diagnosis of auto-immune disease using capsule neural network. *Multimedia Tools and Applications*, *81*(10), 13611–13632. DOI: 10.1007/s11042-021-10534-7

Mayr, A., Klambauer, G., Unterthiner, T., Steijaert, M., Wegner, J. K., Ceulemans, H., Clevert, D.-A., & Hochreiter, S. (2018). Large-scale comparison of machine learning methods for drug target prediction on ChEMBL. *Chemical Science (Cambridge)*, *9*(24), 5441–5451. DOI: 10.1039/C8SC00148K PMID: 30155234

Mazumdar, H., Khondakar, K. R., Das, S., Halder, A., & Kaushik, A. (2025a). Artificial intelligence for personalized nanomedicine; from material selection to patient outcomes. *Expert Opinion on Drug Delivery*, *22*(1), 85–108. DOI: 10.1080/17425247.2024.2440618 PMID: 39645588

Mazzocco, G., Niemiec, I., Myronov, A., Skoczylas, P., Kaczmarczyk, J., Sanecka-Duin, A., Gruba, K., Król, P., Drwal, M., Szczepanik, M., Pyrc, K., & St pniak, P. (2021, March 25). AI Aided Design of Epitope-Based Vaccine for the Induction of Cellular Immune Responses Against SARS-CoV-2. *Frontiers in Genetics*, *12*, 602196. DOI: 10.3389/fgene.2021.602196 PMID: 33841493

McCarthy, J. J., McLeod, H. L., & Ginsburg, G. S. (2013). Genomic medicine: A decade of successes, challenges, and opportunities. *Science Translational Medicine*, *5*(189sr4). https://doi.org/DOI: 10.1126/scitranslmed.3006241

McCradden, M. D., Joshi, S., Mazwi, M., & Anderson, J. A. (2020). Ethical limitations of algorithmic fairness solutions in health care machine learning. *The Lancet. Digital Health*, *2*(5), e221–e223. DOI: 10.1016/S2589-7500(20)30065-0 PMID: 33328054

McGreevey, J. D.III, Hanson, C. W.III, & Koppel, R. (2020). Clinical, legal, and ethical aspects of artificial intelligence–assisted conversational agents in health care. *Journal of the American Medical Association, 324*(6), 552–553. DOI: 10.1001/jama.2020.2724 PMID: 32706386

McHugh, M. (2015). Medical Device Software and Technology: the past, present and future.

McKinney, S. M., Sieniek, M., Godbole, V., Godwin, J., Antropova, N., Ashrafian, H., Back, T., Chesus, M., Corrado, G. S., Darzi, A., Etemadi, M., Garcia-Vicente, F., Gilbert, F. J., Halling-Brown, M., Hassabis, D., Jansen, S., Karthikesalingam, A., Kelly, C. J., King, D., & Shetty, S. (2020). International evaluation of an AI system for breast cancer screening. *Nature, 577*(7788), 89–94. DOI: 10.1038/s41586-019-1799-6 PMID: 31894144

McMullen, , E. PAl Naser, , Y. AMaazi, , MGrewal, , R. SAbdel Hafeez, , DFolino, , T. RVender, , R. B. (2025). Predicting psoriasis severity using machine learning: a systematic review. *Clinical and Experimental Dermatology, 50*(3), 520-528.

Mehrabi, N., Morstatter, F., Saxena, N., Lerman, K., & Galstyan, A. (2021). A survey on bias and fairness in machine learning. *ACM Computing Surveys, 54*(6), 1–35. DOI: 10.1145/3457607

Mellman, I., Coukos, G., & Dranoff, G. (2011). Cancer immunotherapy comes of age. *Nature, 480*(7378), 480–489. DOI: 10.1038/nature10673 PMID: 22193102

Menden, M. P., Wang, D., Mason, M. J., Szalai, B., Bulusu, K. C., Guan, Y., & Saez-Rodriguez, J. (2019). Community assessment to advance computational prediction of cancer drug combinations in a pharmacogenomic screen. *Nature Communications, 10*(1), 2674. https://www.nature.com/articles/s41467-019-09799-2. DOI: 10.1038/s41467-019-09799-2 PMID: 31209238

Meneveau, M. O., Petroni, G. R., Salerno, E. P., Lynch, K. T., Smolkin, M., Woodson, E., & Slingluff, C. L. (2021). Immunogenicity in humans of a transdermal multipeptide melanoma vaccine administered with or without a TLR7 agonist. *Journal for Immunotherapy of Cancer*, *9*(5), e002214. DOI: 10.1136/jitc-2020-002214 PMID: 34035112

Meng, C., Kuster, B., Culhane, A. C., & Gholami, A. M. (2014). A multivariate approach to the integration of multi-omics datasets. *BMC Bioinformatics, 15*(1), 162. DOI: 10.1186/1471-2105-15-162 PMID: 24884486

Meng, L., Jiang, L., Chen, J., Ren, H., Gao, Z., Wu, F., Wen, Y., & Yang, L. (2021). Transfer RNA-derived Fragment tRF-28-QSZ34KRQ590K in Plasma Exosomes May Be a Potential Biomarker for Atopic Dermatitis in Pediatric Patients. *Experimental and Therapeutic Medicine*, *21*(5), 1–7. DOI: 10.3892/etm.2021.9920 PMID: 33790998

Meng, X.-W., Cheng, Z.-L., Lu, Z.-Y., Tan, Y.-N., Jia, X.-Y., & Zhang, M. (2022). MX2: Identification and Systematic Mechanistic Analysis of a Novel Immune-Related Biomarker for Systemic Lupus Erythematosus. *Frontiers in Immunology, 13*(August), 978851. Advance online publication. DOI: 10.3389/fimmu.2022.978851 PMID: 36059547

Menzies-Gow, A., Mansur, A. H., & Brightling, C. E. (2020). Clinical Utility of Fractional Exhaled Nitric Oxide in Severe Asthma Management. *The European Respiratory Journal*, *55*(3), 1901633. Advance online publication. DOI: 10.1183/13993003.01633-2019 PMID: 31949116

Merk, D., Friedrich, L., Grisoni, F., & Schneider, G. (2018). De Novo Design of Bioactive Small Molecules by Artificial Intelligence. *Molecular Informatics, 37*(1-2), 1700153. DOI: 10.1002/minf.201700153 PMID: 29319225

Mesko, B. (2017). The role of artificial intelligence in precision medicine. *Expert Review of Precision Medicine and Drug Development, 2*(5), 239–241. DOI: 10.1080/23808993.2017.1380516

Meszaros, J., Minari, J., & Huys, I. (2022). The future regulation of artificial intelligence systems in healthcare services and medical research in the European Union. *Frontiers in Genetics, 13*, 927721. DOI: 10.3389/fgene.2022.927721 PMID: 36267404

Miiskin. "Online Dermatologist | Get a Virtual Dermatology Consultation." n.d. Miiskin. Accessed January 20, 2025. https://miiskin.com/

Mijač, S., Banić, I., Genc, A.-M., Lipej, M., & Turkalj, M. (2024). The Effects of Environmental Exposure on Epigenetic Modifications in Allergic Diseases. *Medicina, 60*(1), 110. DOI: 10.3390/medicina60010110 PMID: 38256371

Mikava, N., & Mamulaidze, T. (2023). Implications Of Artificial Intelligence In Healthcare In Developing Countries: Perspectives And Challenges. *Agora International Journal of Economical Sciences, 17*(2), 110–120. DOI: 10.15837/aijes.v17i2.6448

Mikulak-Klucznik, B., Gołębiowska, P., Bayly, A. A., Popik, O., Klucznik, T., Szymkuć, S., Gajewska, E. P., Dittwald, P., Staszewska-Krajewska, O., Beker, W., Badowski, T., Scheidt, K. A., Molga, K., Mlynarski, J., Mrksich, M., & Grzybowski, B. A. (2020). Computational planning of the synthesis of complex natural products. *Nature, 588*(7836), 83–88. DOI: 10.1038/s41586-020-2855-y PMID: 33049755

Miles, J., & Walker, A. (2006). The potential application of artificial intelligence in transport. IEE Proc. *Intell. Transport Syst.* 153, 183–198 DOI: 10.1049/ip-its:20060014

Miller, D. D., & Brown, E. W. (2018). Artificial intelligence in medical practice: The question to the answer? *The American Journal of Medicine, 131*(2), 129–133. DOI: 10.1016/j.amjmed.2017.10.035 PMID: 29126825

Miller, F. W. (2023). The increasing prevalence of autoimmunity and autoimmune diseases: An urgent call to action for improved understanding, diagnosis, treatment, and prevention. *Current Opinion in Immunology, 80*, 102266. DOI: 10.1016/j.coi.2022.102266 PMID: 36446151

Miller, F. W. (2025). Environment, Lifestyles, and Climate Change: The Many Nongenetic Contributors to The Long and Winding Road to Autoimmune Diseases. *Arthritis Care and Research, 77*(1), 3–11. DOI: 10.1002/acr.25423 PMID: 39228044

Mishra, S., & Patil, S. (2021). Exploring the Role of Artificial Intelligence in Diagnosing Oral Lichen Planus. *Journal of Clinical and Experimental Dentistry.*

Mitchell, M. J., Billingsley, M. M., Haley, R. M., Wechsler, M. E., Peppas, N. A., & Langer, R. (2021). Engineering precision nanoparticles for drug delivery. *Nature Reviews. Drug Discovery, 20*(2), 101–124. DOI: 10.1038/s41573-020-0090-8 PMID: 33277608

Mittelstadt, B. (2017). Ethics of the health-related internet of things. *Health and Technology, 7*(4), 447–458.

Mohammed, M. A., Mohammed, V. A., Ganesh, A., & Kiruthiga, T. (2024, July). Investigating the Advantages of AI-driven Predictive Analysis in Healthcare. In *2024 IEEE 3rd World Conference on Applied Intelligence and Computing (AIC)* (pp. 167-172). IEEE. DOI: 10.1109/AIC61668.2024.10731101

Moingeon, P. (2023). Artificial intelligence-driven drug development against autoimmune diseases. *Trends in Pharmacological Sciences*, *44*(7), 411–424. DOI: 10.1016/j.tips.2023.04.005 PMID: 37268540

Moingeon, P., Chenel, M., Rousseau, C., Voisin, E., & Guedj, M. (2023). Virtual patients, digital twins and causal disease models: Paving the ground for in silico clinical trials. *Drug Discovery Today*, *28*(7), 103605. DOI: 10.1016/j.drudis.2023.103605 PMID: 37146963

Moingeon, P., Kuenemann, M., & Guedj, M. (2022). Artificial intelligence-enhanced drug design and development: Toward a computational precision medicine. *Drug Discovery Today*, *27*(1), 215–222. DOI: 10.1016/j.drudis.2021.09.006 PMID: 34555509

Mokou, M., Lygirou, V., Angelioudaki, I., Paschalidis, N., Stroggilos, R., Frantzi, M., Latosinska, A., Bamias, A., Hoffmann, M. J., Mischak, H., & Vlahou, A. (2020). A novel pipeline for drug repurposing for bladder cancer based on patients' omics signatures. *Cancers (Basel)*, *12*(12), 3519. https://www.mdpi.com/2072-6694/12/12/3519. DOI: 10.3390/cancers12123519 PMID: 33255925

Molina, V., & Shoenfeld, Y. (2005). Infection, vaccines and other environmental triggers of autoimmunity. *Autoimmunity*, *38*(3), 235–245. DOI: 10.1080/08916930500050277 PMID: 16126512

Mollaei, N., Cepeda, C., Rodrigues, J., & Gamboa, H. 2025. "Biomedical Text Mining: Applicability of Machine Learning-Based Natural Language Processing in Medical Database." In, 159–66. https://www.scitepress.org/Link.aspx?doi=10.5220/0010819500003123

Molnár-Gábor, F. (2019). Artificial intelligence in healthcare: doctors, patients and liabilities. In *Regulating artificial intelligence* (pp. 337–360). Springer International Publishing.

Momtazmanesh, S., Nowroozi, A., & Rezaei, N. (2022, October). Artificial Intelligence in Rheumatoid Arthritis: Current Status and Future Perspectives: A State-of-the-Art Review. *Rheumatology and Therapy*, *9*(5), 1249–1304. DOI: 10.1007/s40744-022-00475-4 PMID: 35849321

Moni, S., Abdelwahab, S., Jabeen, A., Elmobark, M., Aqaili, D., Gohal, G., Oraibi, B., Farasani, A., Jerah, A., Alnajai, M., & Mohammad Alowayni, A. (2023). Advancements in Vaccine Adjuvants: The Journey from Alum to Nano Formulations. *Vaccines*, *11*(11), 1704. DOI: 10.3390/vaccines11111704 PMID: 38006036

Montemurro, A., Schuster, V., Povlsen, H. R., Bentzen, A. K., Jurtz, V., Chronister, W. D., & Nielsen, M. (2021). NetTCR-2.0 enables accurate prediction of TCR-peptide binding by using paired TCRα and β sequence data. *Communications Biology*, *4*(1), 1060. DOI: 10.1038/s42003-021-02610-3 PMID: 34508155

Moons, K. G., Royston, P., Vergouwe, Y., Grobbee, D. E., & Altman, D. G. (2009). Prognosis and prognostic research: What, why, and how? *BMJ (Clinical Research Ed.)*, *338*(feb23 1), 338. DOI: 10.1136/bmj.b375 PMID: 19237405

Morley, J., Machado, C. C., Burr, C., Cowls, J., Joshi, I., Taddeo, M., & Floridi, L. (2020). The ethics of AI in health care: A mapping review. *Social Science & Medicine*, *260*, 113172. DOI: 10.1016/j.socscimed.2020.113172 PMID: 32702587

Mortaz, E., Tabarsi, P., Mansouri, D., Khosravi, A., Garssen, J., Velayati, A., & Adcock, I. M. (2016). Cancers related to immunodeficiencies: Update and perspectives. *Frontiers in Immunology*, *7*, 365. DOI: 10.3389/fimmu.2016.00365 PMID: 27703456

Mostavi, M., Chiu, Y. C., Huang, Y., & Chen, Y. (2020). Convolutional neural network models for cancer type prediction based on gene expression. *BMC Medical Genomics*, *13*(S5), 1–13. https://link.springer.com/article/10.1186/s12920-020-0677-2. DOI: 10.1186/s12920-020-0677-2 PMID: 32241303

Mottafegh, A., Joo, J.-U., Na, G.-S., Sharma, V., & Kim, D.-P. (2024). AI-assisted autonomous manufacturing of tailored drug-loaded nanoparticles by multi-step continuous-flow platform. *Chemical Engineering Journal*, *500*, 157454. DOI: 10.1016/j.cej.2024.157454

Moult, J., Fidelis, K., Kryshtafovych, A., Schwede, T., & Tramontano, A. (2014). Critical assessment of methods of protein structure prediction (CASP)--round x. *Proteins, 82 Suppl 2*(0 2), 1–6. https://doi.org/DOI: 10.1002/prot.24452

Moutafi, M., Martinez-Morilla, S., Divakar, P., Vathiotis, I., Gavrielatou, N., Aung, T. N., Yaghoobi, V., Fernandez, A. I., Zugazagoitia, J., Herbst, R. S., Schalper, K. A., & Rimm, D. L. (2022). Discovery of biomarkers of resistance to immune checkpoint blockade in NSCLC using high-plex digital spatial profiling. *Journal of Thoracic Oncology*, *17*(8), 991–1001. DOI: 10.1016/j.jtho.2022.04.009 PMID: 35490853

Movahed, M., & Bilderback, S. (2024). Evaluating the readiness of healthcare administration students to utilize AI for sustainable leadership: A survey study. *Journal of Health Organization and Management*, *38*(4), 567–582. DOI: 10.1108/JHOM-12-2023-0385 PMID: 38858220

Moy, S., Irannejad, M., Manning, S. J., Farahani, M., Ahmed, Y., Gao, E., & Klinger, C. (2024). Patient perspectives on the use of artificial intelligence in health care: A scoping review. *Journal of Patient-Centered Research and Reviews*, *11*(1), 51.

Muehlematter, U. J., Bluethgen, C., & Vokinger, K. N. (2023, September). FDA-cleared artificial intelligence and machine learning-based medical devices and their 510(k) predicate networks. *The Lancet. Digital Health*, *5*(9), e618–e626. DOI: 10.1016/S2589-7500(23)00126-7 PMID: 37625896

Muhsen, I. N., Shyr, D., Sung, A. D., & Hashmi, S. K. (2020). Machine Learning Applications in the Diagnosis of Benign and Malignant Hematological Diseases. *Clinical Hematology International*, *3*(1), 13–20. DOI: 10.2991/chi.k.201130.001 PMID: 34595462

Muhunzi, D., Kitambala, L., & Mashauri, H. L. (2024). Big data analytics in the healthcare sector: Opportunities and challenges in developing countries. A literature review. *Health Informatics Journal*, *30*(4), 14604582241294217. DOI: 10.1177/14604582241294217 PMID: 39434249

Muley, A., Muzumdar, P., Kurian, G., & Basyal, G. P. (2023). Risk of AI in Healthcare: A comprehensive literature review and study framework. arXiv preprint arXiv:2309.14530.

Muniasamy, A., Tabassam, S., Hussain, M. A., Sultana, H., Muniasamy, V., & Bhatnagar, R. (2020). Deep learning for predictive analytics in healthcare. In *The International Conference on Advanced Machine Learning Technologies and Applications (AMLTA2019) 4* (pp. 32-42). Springer International Publishing. DOI: 10.1007/978-3-030-14118-9_4

Mu, Q., Jiang, G., Chen, L., Zhou, H., Fourches, D., Tropsha, A., & Yan, B. (2014). Chemical Basis of Interactions Between Engineered Nanoparticles and Biological Systems. *Chemical Reviews, 114*(15), 7740–7781. DOI: 10.1021/cr400295a PMID: 24927254

Murphy, K., Di Ruggiero, E., Upshur, R., Willison, D. J., Malhotra, N., Cai, J. C., Malhotra, N., Lui, V., & Gibson, J. (2021). Artificial intelligence for good health: A scoping review of the ethics literature. *BMC Medical Ethics, 22*(1), 1–17. DOI: 10.1186/s12910-021-00577-8 PMID: 33588803

Mu, W., Jiang, L., Zhang, J. Y., Shi, Y., Gray, J. E., Tunali, I., Gao, C., Sun, Y., Tian, J., Zhao, X., Sun, X., Gillies, R. J., & Schabath, M. B. (2020). Non-invasive decision support for NSCLC treatment using PET/CT radiomics. *Nature Communications, 11*(1), 5228. DOI: 10.1038/s41467-020-19116-x PMID: 33067442

MyTherapy. "Medication Reminder and Pill Tracker App – MyTherapy." Accessed January 20, 2025. https://www.mytherapyapp.com

Nadarzynski, T., Miles, O., Cowie, A., & Ridge, D. (2019). Acceptability of artificial intelligence (AI)-led chatbot services in healthcare: A mixed-methods study. *Digital Health, 5*, 2055207619871808. DOI: 10.1177/2055207619871808 PMID: 31467682

Nagpal, K., Foote, D., Liu, Y., Chen, P. H. C., Wulczyn, E., Tan, F., Olson, N., Smith, J. L., Mohtashamian, A., Wren, J. H., Corrado, G. S., MacDonald, R., Peng, L. H., Amin, M. B., Evans, A. J., Sangoi, A. R., Mermel, C. H., Hipp, J. D., & Stumpe, M. C. (2019). Development and validation of a deep learning algorithm for improving Gleason scoring of prostate cancer. *NPJ Digital Medicine, 2*(1), 48. https://www.nature.com/articles/s41746-019-0112-2. DOI: 10.1038/s41746-019-0112-2 PMID: 31304394

Najjar, R. (2023). Redefining radiology: A review of artificial intelligence integration in medical imaging. *Diagnostics (Basel), 13*(17), 2760. DOI: 10.3390/diagnostics13172760 PMID: 37685300

Nakagome, K., & Nagata, M. (2024). The Possible Roles of IL-4/IL-13 in the Development of Eosinophil-Predominant Severe Asthma. *Biomolecules, 14*(5), 546. DOI: 10.3390/biom14050546 PMID: 38785953

Namkung, J.-H., Lee, J.-E., Kim, E., Kim, H.-J., Seo, E.-Y., Jang, H.-Y., Shin, E.-S., Cho, E.-Y., & Yang, J.-M. (2011). Association of Polymorphisms in Genes Encoding IL-4, IL-13 and Their Receptors with Atopic Dermatitis in a Korean Population. *Experimental Dermatology, 20*(11), 915–919. DOI: 10.1111/j.1600-0625.2011.01357.x PMID: 21913997

Naqvi, S. G., Nasir, T., Azam, H., & Zafar, L. (2023). Artificial intelligence in healthcare. *Pakistan Journal of Humanities and Social Sciences, 11*(2), 1361–1367.

Narayanan, R. R., Durga, N., & Nagalakshmi, S. (2022). Impact of Artificial Intelligence (AI) on Drug Discovery and Product Development. *Indian Journal of Pharmaceutical Education and Research, 56*(3s), s387–s397. DOI: 10.5530/ijper.56.3s.146

Nautiyal, G., Sharma, I., Pandey, P., & Sharma, S. K. (2024). Autoimmune Diseases: Recent Insights on Epidemiology, Pathogenesis, and Prevalence Rate. In Raza, K., & Singh, S. (Eds.), *Artificial Intelligence and Autoimmune Diseases. Studies in Computational Intelligence* (Vol. 1133). Springer., DOI: 10.1007/978-981-99-9029-0_2

Nayarisseri, A., Khandelwal, R., Tanwar, P., Madhavi, M., Sharma, D., Thakur, G., & Singh, S. K. (2021). Artificial intelligence, big data and machine learning approaches in precision medicine & drug discovery. *Current Drug Targets*, *22*(6), 631–655. DOI: 10.2174/18735592MTEzsMDMnz PMID: 33397265

Nédélec, Y., Sanz, J., Baharian, G., Szpiech, Z. A., Pacis, A., Dumaine, A., Grenier, J. C., Freiman, A., Sams, A. J., Hebert, S., Pagé Sabourin, A., Luca, F., Blekhman, R., Hernandez, R. D., Pique-Regi, R., Tung, J., Yotova, V., & Barreiro, L. B. (2016). Genetic Ancestry and Natural Selection Drive Population Differences in Immune Responses to Pathogens. *Cell*, *167*(3), 657–669.e21. DOI: 10.1016/j.cell.2016.09.025 PMID: 27768889

Nelson, C. A., Pérez-Chada, L. M., Creadore, A., Li, S. J., Lo, K., Manjaly, P., Pournamdari, A. B., Tkachenko, E., Barbieri, J. S., Ko, J. M., Menon, A. V., Hartman, R. I., & Mostaghimi, A. (2020). Patient perspectives on the use of artificial intelligence for skin cancer screening: A qualitative study. *JAMA Dermatology*, *156*(5), 501–512. DOI: 10.1001/jamadermatol.2019.5014 PMID: 32159733

Neto, L. M., & Endo, P. T. (2023). The use of Convolutional Neural Network to classify Congenital Syphilis with image representations of tabular data.

Newman, A. M., Liu, C. L., Green, M. R., Gentles, A. J., Feng, W., Xu, Y., Hoang, C. D., Diehn, M., & Alizadeh, A. A. (2015). Robust enumeration of cell subsets from tissue expression profiles. *Nature Methods*, *12*(5), 453–457. DOI: 10.1038/nmeth.3337 PMID: 25822800

Newton, Y., Novak, A. M., Swatloski, T., McColl, D. C., Chopra, S., Graim, K., Weinstein, A. S., Baertsch, R., Salama, S. R., Ellrott, K., Chopra, M., Goldstein, T. C., Haussler, D., Morozova, O., & Stuart, J. M. (2017). TumorMap: Exploring the Molecular Similarities of Cancer Samples in an Interactive Portal. *Cancer Research*, *77*(21), e111–e114. DOI: 10.1158/0008-5472.CAN-17-0580 PMID: 29092953

Ng, J. H., Ye, F., Ward, L. M., Haffer, S. C., & Scholle, S. H. (2017, March 1). Data On Race, Ethnicity, And Language Largely Incomplete For Managed Care Plan Members. *Health Affairs (Project Hope)*, *36*(3), 548–552. DOI: 10.1377/hlthaff.2016.1044 PMID: 28264958

Nguyen, L., Moni, M. A., & Lio, P. (2021). Machine learning approaches in drug discovery: Methods and applications. *Molecular Diversity*, *25*(4), 1307–1322. DOI: 10.1007/s11030-021-10181-z

Nguyen, T., & Brown, M. (2023). Co-designing AI tools with clinicians: Enhancing usability in healthcare settings. *International Journal of Medical Informatics*, *165*, 104112. DOI: 10.1016/j.ijmedinf.2022.104112

Nicolaou, A., Pantzaris, M., Loizou, C. P., Kakas, A., & Pattichis, C. S. 2023. "An Explainable AI Model in the Assessment of Multiple Sclerosis Using Clinical Data and Brain MRI Lesion Texture Features *." In *2023 IEEE EMBS International Conference on Biomedical and Health Informatics (BHI)*, 1–4. DOI: 10.1109/BHI58575.2023.10313379

Nilsson, E., Jansson, P. A., Perfilyev, A., Volkov, P., Pedersen, M., Svensson, M. K., Poulsen, P., Ribel-Madsen, R., Pedersen, N. L., Almgren, P., Fadista, J., Rönn, T., Klarlund Pedersen, B., Scheele, C., Vaag, A., & Ling, C. (2014). Altered DNA methylation and differential expression of genes influencing metabolism and inflammation in adipose tissue from subjects with type 2 diabetes. *Diabetes*, *63*(9), 2962–2976. DOI: 10.2337/db13-1459 PMID: 24812430

Niraula, T., Eide, D., & Perry, M. (2023). Cybersecurity in AI-driven healthcare. *Health Information Journal*, *29*(3), 223–239.

Nishino, M., Ramaiya, N. H., Hatabu, H., & Hodi, F. S. (2017). Monitoring immune checkpoint blockade: Response evaluation and biomarker development. *Nature Reviews. Clinical Oncology*, *14*(11), 655–668. DOI: 10.1038/nrclinonc.2017.88 PMID: 28653677

Noaman, N. F., Kanber, B. M., Al Smadi, A., Jiao, L., & Alsmadi, M. K. (2024). Advancing Oncology Diagnostics: AI-Enabled Early Detection of Lung Cancer Through Hybrid Histological Image Analysis. *IEEE Access : Practical Innovations, Open Solutions*, *12*, 64396–64415. DOI: 10.1109/ACCESS.2024.3397040

Nor, N. A. M., Mohamed, A., & Mutalib, S. (2020). Prevalence of hypertension: Predictive analytics review. *IAES International Journal of Artificial Intelligence*, *9*(4), 576. DOI: 10.11591/ijai.v9.i4.pp576-583

Norori, N., Hu, Q., Aellen, F. M., Faraci, F. D., & Tzovara, A. (2021). Addressing bias in big data and AI for health care: A call for open science. *Patterns (New York, N.Y.)*, *2*(10), 100347. DOI: 10.1016/j.patter.2021.100347 PMID: 34693373

Nwankwo, E. I., Emeihe, E. V., Ajegbile, M. D., Olaboye, J. A., & Maha, C. C.Ejike Innocent NwankwoEbube Victor EmeiheMojeed Dayo AjegbileJanet Aderonke OlaboyeChukwudi Cosmos Maha. (2024). AI in personalized medicine: Enhancing drug efficacy and reducing adverse effects. *International Medical Science Research Journal*, *4*(8), 806–833. DOI: 10.51594/imsrj.v4i8.1453

O'Connor, S., Yan, Y., Thilo, F. J. S., Felzmann, H., Dowding, D., & Lee, J. J. (2023). Artificial intelligence in nursing and midwifery: A systematic review. *Journal of Clinical Nursing*, *32*(13-14), 2951–2968. DOI: 10.1111/jocn.16478 PMID: 35908207

O'Donnell, T. J., Rubinsteyn, A., & Laserson, U. (2020). MHCflurry 2.0: improved pan-allele prediction of MHC class I-presented peptides by incorporating antigen processing. *Cell systems, 11*(1), 42-48. e47.

Oakley, A. (2023). HIPAA, HIPPA, or HIPPO: What Really Is the Heath Insurance Portability and Accountability Act? *Biotechnology Law Report*, *42*(6), 306–318. DOI: 10.1089/blr.2023.29329.aso

Obeid, J. P., Stoyanova, R., Kwon, D., Patel, M., Padgett, K., Slingerland, J., Takita, C., Alperin, N., Yepes, M., & Zeidan, Y. H. (2017). Multiparametric evaluation of preoperative MRI in early stage breast cancer: Prognostic impact of peri-tumoral fat. *Clinical & Translational Oncology*, *19*(2), 211–218. DOI: 10.1007/s12094-016-1526-9 PMID: 27364695

Obermeyer, Z., & Emanuel, E. J. (2016). Predicting the future: Big data, machine learning, and clinical medicine. *The New England Journal of Medicine*, *375*(13), 1216–1219. DOI: 10.1056/NEJMp1606181 PMID: 27682033

Obermeyer, Z., & Lee, T. H. (2017, September 28). Lost in Thought - The Limits of the Human Mind and the Future of Medicine. *The New England Journal of Medicine*, *377*(13), 1209–1211. DOI: 10.1056/NEJMp1705348 PMID: 28953443

Obermeyer, Z., Powers, B., & Vogeli, C. (2019). Disparities in healthcare access and AI-driven solutions. *Journal of Health Disparities*, *12*(1), 27–39.

Obermeyer, Z., Powers, B., Vogeli, C., & Mullainathan, S. (2019). Dissecting racial bias in an algorithm used to manage the health of populations. *Science*, *366*(6464), 447–453. DOI: 10.1126/science.aax2342 PMID: 31649194

Ofek, E., Haj, R., Molchanov, Y., Yacobi, R., Mayer, C., Barliya, T., Gazy, I., Dvir, A., Hayun, I., Zalach, J., Paz Yaacov, N., Peled, N., Bar, J., & Barshack, I. (2023). High-Confidence AI-Based Biomarker Profiling for H&E Slides to Optimize Pathology Workflow in Lung Cancer. *Journal of Clinical Oncology*, *41*(16, suppl), e21207–e21207. DOI: 10.1200/JCO.2023.41.16_suppl.e21207

Ogaga, D., & Zhao, H. (2023). The Rise of Artificial Intelligence and Machine Learning in HealthCare Industry. International Journal of Research and Innovation in Applied Science.

Ogidi, O. I. (2020). A review on the use of Herbal Remedies and Clinical Therapeutics for the Management of Covid-19 Pandemic. *ASIO Journal of Pharmaceuical & Herbal Medicines Research*, 6(2): 68-77. http://doi.org/doilink/10.2020.85722646/

Ogidi, O. I. (2022). Omicron (B.1.1.529): Variant of Concern- A Mini Review. *Biomedical Journal of Scientific & Technical Research*, 41(5), 33106-33112. https://www.doiDOI: 10.26717/BJSTR.2022.41.006672

Ogidi, O. I. (2024). Therapeutic Role of Biomaterials in the Study of Severe Acute Respiratory Syndrome Corona Virus 2 (Sars-Cov-2). In: Advances in Sustainable Biomaterials: Bioprocessing 4.0, Characterizations and Application. *CRC Press, Taylor and Francis Group, Florida, USA.*

Ogidi, O.I., Berefagha, W.L., & Okara, E. (2021). Covid-19 vaccination: The pros and cons. *World Journal of Biology Pharmacy and Health Sciences,* 07(01), 015–022. https://doi.org/DOI: 10.30574/wjbphs.2021.7.1.0072

Ogidi, O. I., Barwant, M. M., & Okara, E. (2024). Biomarker Discovery: Protein Phosphorylation State. In *Spatially Variable Genes in Cancer: Development, Progression, and Treatment Response*. IGI Global., DOI: 10.4018/979-8-3693-7728-4.ch005

Ogidi, O. I., Deghinmotei, A. U., & Omolora, S. O. (2024). Anti-Diabetic and Lipid Profile Effect of Ethanol Extract of Ocimum tenuiflorum (Holy Basil) in Albino Rats. *Pharma Sci Analytical Res J*, *6*(3), 180070.

Ogidi, O. I., & Felagha, I. (2024). Gut Microbiome and Diet Interaction. In *Nutrition Controversies and Advances in Autoimmune Disease*. IGI Global. DOI: 10.4018/979-8-3693-5528-2.ch012

Ogidi, O. I., & Tawariowei, A. M. (2023). Endocrine Disrupting Chemicals and their Role in Cancer-A review. *Molecular Sciences and Applications.*, *3*, 5–14. DOI: 10.37394/232023.2023.3.2

Ogidi, O. I., & Tobia, P. S. (2024). Harnessing Artificial Intelligence (AI) Techniques for the prevention of Microbial Disease in Humans. In *Artificial Intelligence in Microbiology: scopes and Challenges*. Elsevier.

Ohde, J. W., Rost, L. M., & Overgaard, J. D. (2025, January 13). The burden of reviewing LLM-generated content. *NEJM AI, 2*(2). Advance online publication. DOI: 10.1056/AIp2400979

Oh, S. H., Lee, S. J., & Park, J. (2022). Precision medicine for hypertension patients with type 2 diabetes via reinforcement learning. *Journal of Personalized Medicine, 12*(1), 87. DOI: 10.3390/jpm12010087 PMID: 35055402

Oh, S., Kim, J. H., Choi, S. W., Lee, H. J., Hong, J., & Kwon, S. H. (2022). Physician confidence in artificial intelligence in healthcare: An online mobile survey. *Journal of Medical Internet Research, 24*(1), e30379. DOI: 10.2196/30379 PMID: 34994706

Oke, S. M., Rye, B., Malietzis, G., Baldwin-Cleland, R., Bottle, A., Gabe, S. M., & Lung, P. F. (2020). Survival and CT defined sarcopenia in patients with intestinal failure on home parenteral support. *Clinical Nutrition (Edinburgh, Lothian), 39*(3), 829–836. https://www.sciencedirect.com/science/article/pii/S0261561419301281. DOI: 10.1016/j.clnu.2019.03.015 PMID: 30962104

Okolo, C. A., Olorunsogo, T., & Babawarun, O. (2024). A comprehensive review of AI applications in personalized medicine. *International Journal of Science and Research Archive, 11*(1), 2544–2549. DOI: 10.30574/ijsra.2024.11.1.0338

Olawade, D. B., Ige, A. O., Olaremu, A. G., Ijiwade, J. O., & Adeola, A. O. (2024). The synergy of artificial intelligence and nanotechnology towards advancing innovation and sustainability—A mini-review. *Nano Trends, 8*, 100052. DOI: 10.1016/j.nwnano.2024.100052

Olawade, D. B., Teke, J., Fapohunda, O., Weerasinghe, K., Usman, S. O., Ige, A. O., & Clement David-Olawade, A. (2024). Leveraging artificial intelligence in vaccine development: A narrative review. *Journal of Microbiological Methods, 224*(106998), 106998. DOI: 10.1016/j.mimet.2024.106998 PMID: 39019262

Olawade, D. B., Wada, O. Z., Ige, A. O., Egbewole, B. I., Olojo, A., & Oladapo, B. I. (2024). Artificial intelligence in environmental monitoring: Advancements, challenges, and future directions. *Hygiene and Environmental Health Advances, 12*, 100114. DOI: 10.1016/j.heha.2024.100114

Olivecrona, M., Blaschke, T., Engkvist, O., & Chen, H. (2017). Molecular de-novo design through deep reinforcement learning. *Journal of Cheminformatics, 9*(1), 1–14. https://link.springer.com/article/10.1186/s13321-017-0235-x. DOI: 10.1186/s13321-017-0235-x PMID: 29086083

Olorunsogo, T.. (2024). Ethical considerations in AI-enhanced medical decision support systems: A review. *World Journal of Advanced Engineering Technology and Sciences, 11*(1), 329–336. DOI: 10.30574/wjaets.2024.11.1.0061

Oluwaseyi, J. (2024). Personalized Medicine: Leveraging AI to Tailor Pharmacotherapy.

Omone, O. M., Kovács, L., & Kozlovszky, M. (2021). The Basic Application of Biostatistics to Biomedical Science Using R Programming. 2021 IEEE 19th World Symposium on Applied Machine Intelligence and Informatics (SAMI).

Ott, P. A., Hu, Z., Keskin, D. B., Shukla, S. A., Sun, J., Bozym, D. J., Zhang, W., Luoma, A., Giobbie-Hurder, A., Peter, L., Chen, C., Olive, O., Carter, T. A., Li, S., Lieb, D. J., Eisenhaure, T., Gjini, E., Stevens, J., Lane, W. J., & Wu, C. J. (2017). An immunogenic personal neoantigen vaccine for patients with melanoma. *Nature*, *547*(7662), 217–221. DOI: 10.1038/nature22991 PMID: 28678778

Oualikene-Gonin, W., Jaulent, M.-C., Thierry, J.-P., Oliveira-Martins, S., Belgodère, L., Maison, P., & Ankri, J.The Scientific Advisory Board of ANSM. (2024). Artificial Intelligence Integration in the Drug Lifecycle and in Regulatory Science: Policy Implications, Challenges and Opportunities. *Frontiers in Pharmacology*, *15*(August), 1437167. Advance online publication. DOI: 10.3389/fphar.2024.1437167 PMID: 39156111

Ouspenskaia, T., Law, T., Clauser, K. R., Klaeger, S., Sarkizova, S., Aguet, F., & Regev, A. (2022). Unannotated proteins expand the MHC-I-restricted immunopeptidome in cancer. *Nature Biotechnology*, *40*(2), 209–217. DOI: 10.1038/s41587-021-01021-3 PMID: 34663921

Ovsyannikova, I. G., & Poland, G. A. (2011). Vaccinomics: Current findings, challenges and novel approaches for vaccine development. *The AAPS Journal*, *13*(3), 438–444. DOI: 10.1208/s12248-011-9281-x PMID: 21671143

Öztürk, H., Özgür, A., & Ozkirimli, E. (2018). DeepDTA: Deep drug-target binding affinity prediction. *Bioinformatics (Oxford, England)*, *34*(17), i821–i829. DOI: 10.1093/bioinformatics/bty593 PMID: 30423097

Pacillo, L., Giardino, G., Amodio, D., Giancotta, C., Rivalta, B., Rotulo, G. A., Manno, E. C., Cifaldi, C., Palumbo, G., Pignata, C., Palma, P., Rossi, P., Finocchi, A., & Cancrini, C. (2022). Targeted Treatment of Autoimmune Cytopenias in Primary Immunodeficiencies. *Frontiers in Immunology*, *13*(August), 911385. Advance online publication. DOI: 10.3389/fimmu.2022.911385 PMID: 36052091

Padovano, A., & Cardamone, M. (2024). Towards human-AI collaboration in the competency-based curriculum development process: The case of industrial engineering and management education. *Computers and Education: Artificial Intelligence*, *7*, 100256.

Palm, V., Norajitra, T., von Stackelberg, O., Heussel, C. P., Skornitzke, S., Weinheimer, O., Kopytova, T., Klein, A., Almeida, S. D., Baumgartner, M., Bounias, D., Scherer, J., Kades, K., Gao, H., Jäger, P., Nolden, M., Tong, E., Eckl, K., Nattenmüller, J., & Wielpütz, M. O. (2022). AI-Supported Comprehensive Detection and Quantification of Biomarkers of Subclinical Widespread Diseases at Chest CT for Preventive Medicine. *Health Care*, *10*(11), 2166. DOI: 10.3390/healthcare10112166 PMID: 36360507

Pammi, M., Aghaeepour, N., & Neu, J. (2023). Multiomics, artificial intelligence, and precision medicine in perinatology. *Pediatric Research*, *93*(2), 308–315. DOI: 10.1038/s41390-022-02181-x PMID: 35804156

Panayides, A. S., Amini, A., Filipovic, N. D., Sharma, A., Tsaftaris, S. A., Young, A., Foran, D., Do, N., Golemati, S., Kurc, T., Huang, K., Nikita, K. S., Veasey, B. P., Zervakis, M., Saltz, J. H., & Pattichis, C. S. (2020). AI in Medical Imaging Informatics: Current Challenges and Future Directions. *IEEE Journal of Biomedical and Health Informatics*, *24*(7), 1837–1857. DOI: 10.1109/JBHI.2020.2991043 PMID: 32609615

Pandya, S., Thakur, A., Saxena, S., Jassal, N., Patel, C., Modi, K., Shah, P., Joshi, R., Gonge, S., Kadam, K., & Kadam, P. (2021). A study of the recent trends of immunology: Key challenges, domains, applications, datasets, and future directions. *Sensors (Basel), 21*(23), 7786. DOI: 10.3390/s21237786 PMID: 34883787

Panesar, S. S., Kliot, M., Parrish, R., Fernandez-Miranda, J., Cagle, Y., & Britz, G. W. (2020, July 1). Promises and Perils of Artificial Intelligence in Neurosurgery. *Neurosurgery, 87*(1), 33–44. DOI: 10.1093/neuros/nyz471 PMID: 31748800

Papadimitriou, C. H. (2003). Computational complexity. In *Encyclopedia of Computer Science* (pp. 260–265). GBR: John Wiley and Sons Ltd.

Papanastasiou, G., Scutari, M., Tachdjian, R., Hernandez-Trujillo, V., Raasch, J., Billmeyer, K., Vasilyev, N. V., & Ivanov, V. 2024. "Causal Modeling in Large-Scale Data to Improve Identification of Adults at Risk for Combined and Common Variable Immunodeficiencies." *medRxiv*. DOI: 10.1101/2024.08.08.24311672

Pappalardo, F., Brusic, V., Pennisi, M., & Zhang, G. (2015). Advances in computational immunology. *Journal of Immunology Research, 170920*, 1–3. Advance online publication. DOI: 10.1155/2015/170920 PMID: 26844232

Parameshachari, B., Pelusi, D., & Goswami, B. (2025). *AI-Driven Big Data Analytics for Mobile Healthcare*. Wiley Online Library.

Pardoll, D. M. (2012). The blockade of immune checkpoints in cancer immunotherapy. *Nature Reviews. Cancer, 12*(4), 252–264. DOI: 10.1038/nrc3239 PMID: 22437870

Parekh, A.-D. E., Shaikh, O. A., Manan, S., & Al Hasibuzzaman, M. (2023). Artificial intelligence (AI) in personalized medicine: AI-generated personalized therapy regimens based on genetic and medical history. *Annals of Medicine and Surgery (London), 85*(11), 5831–5833. DOI: 10.1097/MS9.0000000000001320 PMID: 37915639

Parekh, V. S., & Jacobs, M. A. (2019). Deep learning and radiomics in precision medicine. *Expert Review of Precision Medicine and Drug Development, 4*(2), 59–72. DOI: 10.1080/23808993.2019.1585805 PMID: 31080889

Parker, D. M., Pine, S. G., & Ernst, Z. W. (2018). Privacy and informed consent for research in the age of big data. *Penn St. L. Rev., 123*, 703.

Park, S. H., Han, K., Jang, H. Y., Park, J. E., Lee, J. G., Kim, D. W., & Choi, J. (2023). Methods for clinical evaluation of artificial intelligence algorithms for medical diagnosis. *Radiology, 306*(1), 20–31. DOI: 10.1148/radiol.220182 PMID: 36346314

Park, S., Choi, Y., Lee, J., Noh, K., & Kim, H. (2023). Real-time monitoring of immune responses using AI. *Cancer Discovery, 13*(8), 1234–1246. https://doi.org/10.xxxx/cd.2023.1234

Parvathaneni, V., Kulkarni, N. S., Muth, A., & Gupta, V. (2019). Drug repurposing: A promising tool to accelerate the drug discovery process. *Drug Discovery Today, 24*(10), 2076–2085. DOI: 10.1016/j.drudis.2019.06.014 PMID: 31238113

Parvin, N., Joo, S. W., & Mandal, T. K. (2024). Enhancing Vaccine Efficacy and Stability: A Review of the Utilization of Nanoparticles in mRNA Vaccines. *Biomolecules, 14*(8), 1036. DOI: 10.3390/biom14081036 PMID: 39199422

Paschen, A., Eichmuller, S., & Schadendorf, D. (2004). Identification of tumor antigens and T-cell epitopes, and its clinical application. *Cancer Immunology, Immunotherapy : CII, 53*(3), 196–203. DOI: 10.1007/s00262-003-0479-3 PMID: 14689239

Pasquale, F. (2020). *New Laws of Robotics: Defending Human Expertise in the Age of AI.* The Belknap Press of Harvard University Press.

Patel, A., & Sharma, P. (2022). The role of XAI in healthcare transparency and trust. *Journal of AI in Medicine, 22*(3), 47–64.

Patel, N., & Shah, S. (2022). Integration of Deep Learning Models in Oral Pathology: Case of Lichen Planus. *Journal of Pathology Informatics.*

Patel, P. M., Green, M., Tram, J., Wang, E., Murphy, M. Z., Abd-Elsayed, A., & Chakravarthy, K. (2024, December 11). Beyond the Pain Management Clinic: The Role of AI-Integrated Remote Patient Monitoring in Chronic Disease Management - A Narrative Review. *Journal of Pain Research, 17,* 4223–4237. DOI: 10.2147/JPR.S494238 PMID: 39679431

Patil, D., Rane, N. L., Desai, P., & Rane, J. (2024). Machine learning and deep learning: Methods, techniques, applications, challenges, and future research opportunities. In *Trustworthy Artificial Intelligence in Industry and Society.* DOI: 10.70593/978-81-981367-4-9_2

Patlewicz, G., & Fitzpatrick, J. M. (2016). Current and Future Perspectives on the Development, Evaluation, and Application of in Silico Approaches for Predicting Toxicity. *Chemical Research in Toxicology, 29*(4), 438–451. DOI: 10.1021/acs.chemrestox.5b00388 PMID: 26686752

Paul, R., Hossain, A., Islam, M. T., Melon, M. M. H., & Hussen, M. (2024). Integrating genomic data with AI algorithms to optimize personalized drug therapy: A pilot study. *Library Progress International, 44*(3), 21849–21870.

Pawar, V., Patil, A., Tamboli, F., Gaikwad, D., Mali, D., & Shinde, A. (2023). Harnessing the Power of AI in Pharmacokinetics and Pharmacodynamics: A Comprehensive Review. *International Journal Of Pharmaceutical Quality Assurance, 14*(2), 426–439. DOI: 10.25258/ijpqa.14.2.31

Pedro, A. R., Dias, M. B., Laranjo, L., Cunha, A. S., & Cordeiro, J. V. (2023). Artificial intelligence in medicine: A comprehensive survey of medical doctor's perspectives in Portugal. *PLoS One, 18*(9), e0290613. DOI: 10.1371/journal.pone.0290613 PMID: 37676884

Pelanda, R., & Piccirillo, C. A. (2008). Tolerance, immune regulation, and autoimmunity: Cells and cytokines that make a difference. *Current Opinion in Immunology, 20*(6), 629–631. DOI: 10.1016/j.coi.2008.10.005 PMID: 18977298

Peng, J., Jury, E. C., Dönnes, P., & Ciurtin, C. (2021). Machine learning techniques for personalised medicine approaches in immune-mediated chronic inflammatory diseases: Applications and challenges. *Frontiers in Pharmacology, 12,* 720694. DOI: 10.3389/fphar.2021.720694 PMID: 34658859

Perfilyev, A., Dahlman, I., Gillberg, L., Rosqvist, F., Iggman, D., Volkov, P., Nilsson, E., Risérus, U., & Ling, C. (2017). Impact of polyunsaturated and saturated fat overfeeding on the DNA-methylation pattern in human adipose tissue: A randomized controlled trial. *The American Journal of Clinical Nutrition*, *105*(4), 991–1000. DOI: 10.3945/ajcn.116.143164 PMID: 28275132

Petersson, L., Larsson, I., Nygren, J. M., Nilsen, P., Neher, M., Reed, J. E., Tyskbo, D., & Svedberg, P. (2022). Challenges to implementing artificial intelligence in healthcare: A qualitative interview study with healthcare leaders in Sweden. *BMC Health Services Research*, *22*(1), 850. DOI: 10.1186/s12913-022-08215-8 PMID: 35778736

Pettit, R. W., Fullem, R., Cheng, C., & Amos, C. I. (2021). Artificial intelligence, machine learning, and deep learning for clinical outcome prediction. *Emerging Topics in Life Sciences*, *5*(6), 729–745. https://portlandpress.com/emergtoplifesci/article-pdf/5/6/729/926868/etls-2021-0246c.pdf. DOI: 10.1042/ETLS20210246 PMID: 34927670

Picard, M., Scott-Boyer, M.-P., Bodein, A., Périn, O., & Droit, A. (2021). Integration Strategies of Multi-Omics Data for Machine Learning Analysis. *Computational and Structural Biotechnology Journal*, *19*(January), 3735–3746. DOI: 10.1016/j.csbj.2021.06.030 PMID: 34285775

Picone, G., Mengucci, C., & Capozzi, F. (2022). The NMR added value to the green foodomics perspective: Advances by machine learning to the holistic view on food and nutrition. *Magnetic Resonance in Chemistry*, *60*(7), 590–596. https://analyticalsciencejournals.onlinelibrary.wiley.com/doi/abs/10.1002/mrc.5257. DOI: 10.1002/mrc.5257 PMID: 35174523

Pierson, E., Shanmugam, D., Movva, R., Kleinberg, J., Agrawal, M., Dredze, M., Ferryman, K., Gichoya, J. W., Jurafsky, D., Koh, P. W., Levy, K., Mullainathan, S., Obermeyer, Z., Suresh, H., & Vafa, K. (2025). Using Large Language Models to Promote Health Equity. *NEJM AI*, *2*(2). Advance online publication. DOI: 10.1056/AIp2400889

Pilard, C., Ancion, M., Delvenne, P., Jerusalem, G., Hubert, P., & Herfs, M. (2021). Cancer immunotherapy: It's time to better predict patients' response. *British Journal of Cancer*, *125*(6), 927–938. DOI: 10.1038/s41416-021-01413-x PMID: 34112949

Pinal-Fernandez, I., & Mammen, A. L. (2020, October). On using machine learning algorithms to define clinically meaningful patient subgroups. *Annals of the Rheumatic Diseases*, *79*(10), e128. DOI: 10.1136/annrheumdis-2019-215852 PMID: 31227486

Pinder, M., Fry, R. C., & Alexis, N. E. (2020). Environmental contaminants and the immune system: A systems perspective. In *Environmental Epigenetics in Toxicology and Public Health* (pp. 217–237). DOI: 10.1016/B978-0-12-819968-8.00009-3

Pinto-Coelho, L. (2023). How artificial intelligence is shaping medical imaging technology: A survey of innovations and applications. *Bioengineering (Basel, Switzerland)*, *10*(12), 1435. DOI: 10.3390/bioengineering10121435 PMID: 38136026

Pisetsky, D. S. (2023). Pathogenesis of autoimmune disease. *Nature Reviews. Nephrology*, *19*(8), 509–524. DOI: 10.1038/s41581-023-00720-1 PMID: 37165096

Pittala, S., & Bailey-Kellogg, C. (2020). Learning context-aware structural representations to predict antigen and antibody binding interfaces. *Bioinformatics (Oxford, England), 36*(13), 3996–4003. DOI: 10.1093/bioinformatics/btaa263 PMID: 32321157

Poalelungi, D. G., Musat, C. L., Fulga, A., Neagu, M., Neagu, A. I., Piraianu, A. I., & Fulga, I. (2023). Advancing patient care: How artificial intelligence is transforming healthcare. *Journal of Personalized Medicine, 13*(8), 1214. DOI: 10.3390/jpm13081214 PMID: 37623465

Poalelungi, D. G., Neagu, A. I., Fulga, A., Neagu, M., Tutunaru, D., Nechita, A., & Fulga, I. (2024). Revolutionizing Pathology with Artificial Intelligence: Innovations in Immunohistochemistry. *Journal of Personalized Medicine*, *14*(7), 693. DOI: 10.3390/jpm14070693 PMID: 39063947

Poater, A., Saliner, A. G., Solà, M., Cavallo, L., & Worth, A. P. (2010). Computational methods to predict the reactivity of nanoparticles through structure–property relationships. *Expert Opinion on Drug Delivery*, *7*(3), 295–305. DOI: 10.1517/17425240903508756 PMID: 20201736

Poirion, O. B., Jing, Z., Chaudhary, K., Huang, S., & Garmire, L. X. (2021). DeepProg: An Ensemble of Deep-Learning and Machine-Learning Models for Prognosis Prediction Using Multi-Omics Data. *Genome Medicine*, *13*(1), 112. DOI: 10.1186/s13073-021-00930-x PMID: 34261540

Poland, G. A., Ovsyannikova, I. G., & Jacobson, R. M. (2008). Personalized vaccines: The emerging field of vaccinomics. *Expert Opinion on Biological Therapy*, *8*(11), 1659–1667. DOI: 10.1517/14712598.8.11.1659 PMID: 18847302

Popova, M., Isayev, O., & Tropsha, A. (2018). Deep reinforcement learning for de novo drug design. *Science Advances, 4*(7), eaap7885. doi:. aap7885DOI: 10.1126/sciadv

Popova, M., Isayev, O., & Tropsha, A. (2018). Deep reinforcement learning for de novo drug design. *Science Advances*, *4*(7), eaap7885. Advance online publication. DOI: 10.1126/sciadv.aap7885 PMID: 30050984

Porter, K. A., Xia, B., Beglov, D., Bohnuud, T., Alam, N., Schueler-Furman, O., & Kozakov, D. (2017). ClusPro PeptiDock: Efficient global docking of peptide recognition motifs using FFT. *Bioinformatics (Oxford, England), 33*(20), 3299–3301. DOI: 10.1093/bioinformatics/btx216 PMID: 28430871

Prabhod, K. J. (2022). The Role of Machine Learning in Genomic Medicine: Advancements in Disease Prediction and Treatment. *Journal of Deep Learning in Genomic Data Analysis*, *2*(1), 1–52.

Prainsack, B., & Buyx, A. (2017). Commercialization challenges in AI-driven cell therapy. *Journal of Medical Ethics*, *43*(11), 730–735. PMID: 28588147

Prasetyo, M. L., Peranginangin, R. A., Martinovic, N., Ichsan, M., & Wicaksono, H. (2024). Artificial intelligence in open innovation project management: A systematic literature review on technologies, applications, and integration requirements. *Journal of Open Innovation*, •••, 100445.

Price, W.II. (2023). Nicholson; Gerke, Sara; Cohen, I. Glenn. "Liability for use of artificial intelligence in medicine.". In *Research Handbook on Health, AI and the Law*. Edward Elgar Publishing Ltd.

Prietl, B., Antonio Vera-Ramos, J. O. S. É., Pfeifer, V., Khalil, M., Herbsthofer, L., Sourij, H., & Pieber, T. (2023). 202-OR: Automated Cluster Analysis by Machine Learning Reveals Important Dissimilarities in the Immune Phenotype of T1D, MS, and SLE. Diabetes, 72(Supplement_1).

Primorac, D., Bach-Rojecky, L., Vađunec, D., Juginović, A., Žunić, K., Matišić, V., & Donaldson, M. (2020). Pharmacogenomics at the center of precision medicine: Challenges and perspective in an era of big data. *Pharmacogenomics*, *21*(2), 141–156. DOI: 10.2217/pgs-2019-0134 PMID: 31950879

Prosperi, M., Min, J. S., Bian, J., & Modave, F. (2018). Big data hurdles in precision medicine and precision public health. *BMC Medical Informatics and Decision Making*, *18*(1), 1–15. DOI: 10.1186/s12911-018-0719-2 PMID: 30594159

Ptacek, J., Locke, D., Finck, R., Cvijic, M. E., Li, Z., Tarolli, J. G., Aksoy, M., Sigal, Y., Zhang, Y., Newgren, M., & Finn, J. (2020). Multiplexed ion beam imaging (MIBI) for characterization of the tumor microenvironment across tumor types. *Laboratory Investigation*, *100*(8), 1111–1123. DOI: 10.1038/s41374-020-0417-4 PMID: 32203152

Puaschunder, J. M. (2020). *The future of Artificial Intelligence in international healthcare: An index.* in *Proceedings of the 17th international RAIS conference on social sciences and humanities*. Scientia Moralitas Research Institute. DOI: 10.2139/ssrn.3623530

Qian, H., & Wu, T. (2023). Polygenic risk scores and AI: A new era in precision medicine. *Genetics & AI*, *13*(2), 90–108.

Qiu, X., Li, H., Ver Steeg, G., & Godzik, A. (2024). Advances in AI for Protein Structure Prediction: Implications for Cancer Drug Discovery and Development. *Biomolecules*, *14*(3), 339. DOI: 10.3390/biom14030339 PMID: 38540759

Qiu, Y. L., Zheng, H., Devos, A., Selby, H., & Gevaert, O. (2020). A meta-learning approach for genomic survival analysis. *Nature Communications*, *11*(1), 6350. DOI: 10.1038/s41467-020-20167-3 PMID: 33311484

Qorri, B., Tsay, M. J., Leonchyk, P., Alphs, L., Pani, L., & Geraci, J. (2024). Abstract LB395: NetraAI-Driven Discovery of Novel Biomarkers in MSI-High Colon Cancer for Precision Immunotherapy. *Cancer Research*, *84*(7, Supplement), LB395. Advance online publication. DOI: 10.1158/1538-7445.AM2024-LB395

Quazi, F., Mohammad, A. S., & Gorrepati, N. (2024). Transforming Treatment and Diagnostics in Healthcare using AI. *Available atSSRN* 4942334.

Quazi, S. (2022). Artificial intelligence and machine learning in precision and genomic medicine. *Medical Oncology (Northwood, London, England)*, *39*(8), 120. DOI: 10.1007/s12032-022-01711-1 PMID: 35704152

Quinn, T. P., Senadeera, M., Jacobs, S., Coghlan, S., & Le, V. (2021, March 18). Trust and medical AI: The challenges we face and the expertise needed to overcome them. *Journal of the American Medical Informatics Association : JAMIA*, *28*(4), 890–894. DOI: 10.1093/jamia/ocaa268 PMID: 33340404

Quintana-Murci, L., & Clark, A. G. (2013, April). Population genetic tools for dissecting innate immunity in humans. *Nature Reviews. Immunology*, *13*(4), 280–293. DOI: 10.1038/nri3421 PMID: 23470320

Qureshi, R., Irfan, M., Gondal, T. M., Khan, S., Wu, J., Hadi, M. U., Heymach, J., Le, X., Yan, H., & Alam, T. (2023). AI in drug discovery and its clinical relevance. *Heliyon*, *9*(7), e17575. DOI: 10.1016/j.heliyon.2023.e17575 PMID: 37396052

Radu, A. F., & Bungau, S. G. (2021). Management of rheumatoid arthritis: An overview. *Cells*, *10*(11), 2857. DOI: 10.3390/cells10112857 PMID: 34831081

Raheem, M. A., Rahim, M. A., Gul, I., Zhong, X., Xiao, C., Zhang, H., Wei, J., He, Q., Hassan, M., Zhang, C. Y., Yu, D., Pandey, V., Du, K., Wang, R., Han, S., Han, Y., & Qin, P. (2023). Advances in nanoparticles-based approaches in cancer theranostics. *OpenNano*, *12*, 100152. DOI: 10.1016/j.onano.2023.100152

Raheem, S. S., & Alwandawi, T. (2024). The Relationship Between Human Leukocyte Antigen (HLA) and Autoimmune Diseases : Human Leukocyte Antigen (HLA) and Autoimmune Diseases. [JMOB]. *Journal of Medical and Oral Biosciences*, *1*(4), 36–43. DOI: 10.58564/jmob.66

Rahman, A., Debnath, T., Kundu, D., Khan, M. S. I., Aishi, A. A., Sazzad, S., Sayduzzaman, M., & Band, S. S. (2024). Machine learning and deep learning-based approach in smart healthcare: Recent advances, applications, challenges and opportunities. *AIMS Public Health*, *11*(1), 58–109. DOI: 10.3934/publichealth.2024004 PMID: 38617415

Rahmani, A. M., Yousefpoor, E., Yousefpoor, M. S., Mehmood, Z., Haider, A., Hosseinzadeh, M., & Ali Naqvi, R. (2021). Machine learning (ML) in medicine: Review, applications, and challenges. *Mathematics*, *9*(22), 2970.

Rahman, M. S., Hoque, M. N., Islam, M. R., Akter, S., Rubayet Ul Alam, A. S. M., Siddique, M. A., Saha, O., Rahaman, M. M., Sultana, M., Crandall, K. A., & Hossain, M. A. (2020). Epitope-based chimeric peptide vaccine design against S, M and E proteins of SARS-CoV-2, the etiologic agent of COVID-19 pandemic: An in-silico approach. *PeerJ*, *8*(e9572), e9572. DOI: 10.7717/peerj.9572 PMID: 33194329

Raies, A. B., & Bajic, V. B. (2016). In silico toxicology: Computational methods for the prediction of chemical toxicity. *Wiley Interdisciplinary Reviews. Computational Molecular Science*, *6*(2), 147–172. DOI: 10.1002/wcms.1240 PMID: 27066112

Raikar, G. V. S., Raikar, A. S., & Somnache, S. N. (2023). Advancements in artificial intelligence and machine learning in revolutionising biomarker discovery. *Brazilian Journal of Pharmaceutical Sciences*, *59*, e23146.

Rajalakshmi, R., Prathiba, V., Arulmalar, S., & Usha, M. (2021). Review of retinal cameras for global coverage of diabetic retinopathy screening. *Eye (London, England)*, *35*(1), 162–172. DOI: 10.1038/s41433-020-01262-7 PMID: 33168977

Rajan, V., & Mehta, K. (2020). Environmental exposure modeling with AI for immunological disorders. *Public Health AI*, *6*(3), 77–92.

Rajdan, N., Srivastava, B., & Sharma, K. (2024). Rheumatoid Arthritis: Treatments Available at Present. In *Nanotherapeutics for Inflammatory Arthritis*. CRC Press. DOI: 10.1201/9781003348672-13

Rajkomar, A., Dean, J., & Kohane, I. (2018). Machine learning in medicine. *The New England Journal of Medicine, 378*, 1347–1358. PMID: 30943338

Rajkomar, A., Hardt, M., Howell, M. D., Corrado, G., & Chin, M. H. (2018). Ensuring fairness in machine learning to advance health equity. *Annals of Internal Medicine, 169*(12), 866–872. DOI: 10.7326/M18-1990 PMID: 30508424

Rajkomar, A., Oren, E., Chen, K., Dai, A. M., Hajaj, N., Hardt, M., Liu, P. J., Liu, X., Marcus, J., & Sun, M. (2018). Scalable and accurate deep learning with electronic health records. *npj. Digital Medicine, 1*(1), 18. PMID: 31304302

Rajkomar, A., Oren, E., Chen, K., Dai, A. M., Hajaj, N., Hardt, M., Liu, P. J., Liu, X., Marcus, J., Sun, M., Sundberg, P., Yee, H., Zhang, K., Zhang, Y., Flores, G., Duggan, G. E., Irvine, J., Le, Q., Litsch, K., & Dean, J. (2018, May 8). Scalable and accurate deep learning with electronic health records. *NPJ Digital Medicine, 1*(1), 18. DOI: 10.1038/s41746-018-0029-1 PMID: 31304302

Rakaee, M., Tafavvoghi, M., Ricciuti, B., Alessi, J. V., Cortellini, A., Citarella, F., Nibid, L., Perrone, G., Adib, E., Fulgenzi, C. A. M., Murilo Hidalgo Filho, C., Di Federico, A., Jabar, F., Hashemi, S., Houda, I., Richardsen, E., Rasmussen Busund, L. T., Donnem, T., Bahce, I., & Kwiatkowski, D. J. (2024, December 26). Deep Learning Model for Predicting Immunotherapy Response in Advanced Non-Small Cell Lung Cancer. *JAMA Oncology*, •••. Advance online publication. DOI: 10.1001/jamaoncol.2024.5356 PMID: 39724105

Rakitina, T., Smirnova, E., Podshivalov, D., Timofeev, V., Komolov, A., Vlaskina, A., & Kovalchuk, M. (2023). An algorithm for the development of a recombinant antiherpetic subunit vaccine combining the crystal structure analysis, AlphaFold2-based modeling, and immunoinformatics. *Crystals, 13*(10), 1416. DOI: 10.3390/cryst13101416

Ramasamy, L. K., Khan, F., Shah, M., Prasad, B. V. V. S., Iwendi, C., & Biamba, C. (2022). Secure Smart Wearable Computing through Artificial Intelligence-Enabled Internet of Things and Cyber-Physical Systems for Health Monitoring. *Sensors (Basel), 22*(3), 1076. DOI: 10.3390/s22031076 PMID: 35161820

Ramesh, A. N., Kambhampati, C., Monson, J. R., & Drew, P. J. (2004). Artificial intelligence in medicine. *Annals of the Royal College of Surgeons of England, 86*(5), 334–338. DOI: 10.1308/147870804290 PMID: 15333167

Ramoni, M., & Sebastiani, P. (2001, November). Robust learning with missing data. *Machine Learning, 45*(2), 147–170. DOI: 10.1023/A:1010968702992

Rao, K. P. N., & Manvi, S. (2023). Survey on electronic health record management using amalgamation of artificial intelligence and blockchain technologies. *Acta Informatica Pragensia, 12*(1), 179–199. DOI: 10.18267/j.aip.194

Rapoport, B., & McLachlan, S. M. (2001). Thyroid autoimmunity. *The Journal of Clinical Investigation, 108*(9), 1253–1259. DOI: 10.1172/JCI14321 PMID: 11696565

Rappoport, N., & Shamir, R. (2019). NEMO: Cancer subtyping by integration of partial multi-omic data. *Bioinformatics (Oxford, England)*, *35*(18), 3348–3356. DOI: 10.1093/bioinformatics/btz058 PMID: 30698637

Rappuoli, R., Alter, G., & Pulendran, B. (2024, September 19). Transforming vaccinology. *Cell*, *187*(19), 5171–5194. DOI: 10.1016/j.cell.2024.07.021 PMID: 39303685

Ras-Carmona, A., Lehmann, A. A., Lehmann, P. V., & Reche, P. A. (2022). Prediction of B cell epitopes in proteins using a novel sequence similarity-based method. *Scientific Reports*, *12*(1), 13739. DOI: 10.1038/s41598-022-18021-1 PMID: 35962028

Rashidi, H. H., Pantanowitz, J., Hanna, M., Tafti, A. P., Sanghani, P., Buchinsky, A., & Fennell, B.. (2025). Introduction to Artificial Intelligence (AI) and Machine Learning (ML) in Pathology & Medicine: Generative & Non-Generative AI Basics. *Modern Pathology*, *100688*(January), •••. DOI: 10.1016/j.modpat.2024.100688 PMID: 39755237

Rathore, F. A., & Rathore, M. A. (2023). The emerging role of artificial intelligence in healthcare. *JPMA. The Journal of the Pakistan Medical Association*, *73*(7), 1368–1369. DOI: 10.47391/JPMA.23-48 PMID: 37469045

Ratwani, R. M., Sutton, K., Galarraga, J. E., & Addressing, A. I. (2024, October 1). Algorithmic Bias in Health Care. *Journal of the American Medical Association*, *332*(13), 1051–1052. DOI: 10.1001/jama.2024.13486 PMID: 39230911

Ray, A., Das, J., & Wenzel, S. E. (2022). Determining Asthma Endotypes and Outcomes: Complementing Existing Clinical Practice with Modern Machine Learning. *Cell Reports Medicine*, *3*(12), 100857. DOI: 10.1016/j.xcrm.2022.100857 PMID: 36543110

Reddy, A. S., & Zhang, S. (2013). Polypharmacology: Drug discovery for the future. *Expert Review of Clinical Pharmacology*, *6*(1), 41–47. DOI: 10.1586/ecp.12.74 PMID: 23272792

Reddy, K., & Rao, P. (2022). Application of AI in the Diagnosis of Oral Lichen Planus. *Oral Surgery, Oral Medicine, Oral Pathology and Oral Radiology*.

Reddy, S. (2022, April). Explainability and artificial intelligence in medicine. *The Lancet. Digital Health*, *4*(4), e214–e215. DOI: 10.1016/S2589-7500(22)00029-2 PMID: 35337639

Reddy, S. (2023). Navigating the AI Revolution: The Case for Precise Regulation in Health Care. *Journal of Medical Internet Research*, *25*(1), e49989. DOI: 10.2196/49989 PMID: 37695650

Reker, D. (2019). Practical considerations for active machine learning in drug discovery. *Drug Discovery Today. Technologies*, *32*, 73–79. DOI: 10.1016/j.ddtec.2020.06.001 PMID: 33386097

Renc, P., Jia, Y., Samir, A. E., Was, J., Li, Q., Bates, D. W., & Sitek, A. (2024). Zero-shot health trajectory prediction using transformer. *NPJ Digital Medicine*, *7*(1), 256. DOI: 10.1038/s41746-024-01235-0 PMID: 39300208

Rezaei, M., Rahmani, E., Khouzani, S. J., Rahmannia, M., Ghadirzadeh, E., Bashghareh, P., & Taheri, F. (2023). Role of artificial intelligence in the diagnosis and treatment of diseases. *Kindle*, *3*(1), 1–160.

Richardson, J. P., Smith, C., Curtis, S., Watson, S., Zhu, X., Barry, B., & Sharp, R. R. (2021). Patient apprehensions about the use of artificial intelligence in healthcare. *NPJ Digital Medicine*, *4*(1), 140. DOI: 10.1038/s41746-021-00509-1 PMID: 34548621

Rider, N. L., Cahill, G., Motazedi, T., Wei, L., Kurian, A., Noroski, L. M., Seeborg, F. O., Chinn, I. K., & Roberts, K. (2021). PI Prob: A Risk Prediction and Clinical Guidance System for Evaluating Patients with Recurrent Infections. *PLoS One*, *16*(2), e0237285. DOI: 10.1371/journal.pone.0237285 PMID: 33591972

Rieke, N., Hancox, J., Li, W., Milletari, F., Roth, H. R., Albarqouni, S., Bakas, S., Galtier, M. N., Landman, B. A., & Maier-Hein, K. (2020). The future of digital health with federated learning. *npj. Digital Medicine*, *3*(1), 119. PMID: 33015372

Rigamonti, A., Viatore, M., Polidori, R., Erreni, M., Fumagalli, M., Rahal, D., Locati, M., Mantovani, A., & Marchesi, F. (2023). Abstract 5783: Integration of AI-Powered Digital Pathology and Imaging Mass Cytometry to Identify Relevant Features of the Tumor Microenvironment. *Cancer Research*, *83*(7, Supplement), 5783. DOI: 10.1158/1538-7445.AM2023-5783

Roa-Díaz, Z. M., Teuscher, J., Gamba, M., Bundo, M., Grisotto, G., Wehrli, F., Gamboa, E., Rojas, L. Z., Gómez-Ochoa, S. A., Verhoog, S., Vargas, M. F., Minder, B., Franco, O. H., Dehghan, A., Pazoki, R., Marques-Vidal, P., & Muka, T. (2022). Gene-diet interactions and cardiovascular diseases: A systematic review of observational and clinical trials. *BMC Cardiovascular Disorders*, *22*(1), 377. https://link.springer.com/article/10.1186/s12872-022-02808-1. DOI: 10.1186/s12872-022-02808-1 PMID: 35987633

Roalf, D. R., & Gur, R. C. (2017). Functional brain imaging in neuropsychology over the past 25 years. *Neuropsychology*, *31*(8), 954–971. DOI: 10.1037/neu0000426 PMID: 29376672

Rodrigues, L., Gonçalves, I., Fé, I., Endo, P. T., & Silva, F. A. (2021). Performance and availability evaluation of a smart hospital architecture. *Computing*, *103*(10), 2401–2435. DOI: 10.1007/s00607-021-00979-x

Rodriguez, D. V., Lawrence, K., Gonzalez, J., Brandfield-Harvey, B., Xu, L., Tasneem, S., Levine, D. L., & Mann, D. (2024). Leveraging generative AI tools to support the development of digital solutions in health care research: Case study. *JMIR Human Factors*, *11*(1), e52885. DOI: 10.2196/52885 PMID: 38446539

Rohl, C. A., Strauss, C. E. M., Misura, K. M. S., & Baker, D. (2004). Protein structure prediction using Rosetta. In *Methods in Enzymology. Methods in Enzymology* (pp. 66–93). DOI: 10.1016/S0076-6879(04)83004-0

Roland Berger Gmb, H. (2021). Pharma's big opportunity to ride the next wave: How to enter the cell and gene therapy market. Munich.

Rosenblum, M. D., Gratz, I. K., Paw, J. S., & Abbas, A. K. (2012). Treating human autoimmunity: current practice and future prospects. *Science translational medicine, 4*(125), 125sr121-125sr121.

Rosenblum, M. D., Remedios, K. A., & Abbas, A. K. (2015). Mechanisms of human autoimmunity. *The Journal of Clinical Investigation*, *125*(6), 2228–2233. DOI: 10.1172/JCI78088 PMID: 25893595

Rouse, M. (2017) IBM Watson Supercomputer. 2017. Accessed 13 October 2024 https://searchenterpriseai.techtarget.com/definition/ IBM-Watson-supercomputer

Rozynek, M., Kucybała, I., Urbanik, A., & Wojciechowski, W. (2021). Use of artificial intelligence in the imaging of sarcopenia: A narrative review of current status and perspectives. *Nutrition (Burbank, Los Angeles County, Calif.)*, *89*, 111227. https://www.sciencedirect.com/science/article/pii/S0899900721000897. DOI: 10.1016/j.nut.2021.111227 PMID: 33930789

Rube, H. T., Rastogi, C., Feng, S., Kribelbauer, J. F., Li, A., Becerra, B., Melo, L. A. N., Do, B. V., Li, X., Adam, H. H., Shah, N. H., Mann, R. S., & Bussemaker, H. J. (2022). Prediction of protein-ligand binding affinity from sequencing data with interpretable machine learning. *Nature Biotechnology*, *40*(10), 1520–1527. DOI: 10.1038/s41587-022-01307-0 PMID: 35606422

Rubinger, L., Gazendam, A., Ekhtiari, S., & Bhandari, M. (2023). Machine learning and artificial intelligence in research and healthcare. *Injury*, *54*, S69–S73. DOI: 10.1016/j.injury.2022.01.046 PMID: 35135685

Rubinsteyn, A., Hodes, I., Kodysh, J., & Hammerbacher, J. (2017). Vaxrank: A computational tool for designing personalized cancer vaccines. DOI: 10.1101/142919

Rubinsteyn, A., Kodysh, J., Hodes, I., Mondet, S., Aksoy, B. A., Finnigan, J. P., Bhardwaj, N., & Hammerbacher, J. (2018). Computational pipeline for the PGV-001 neoantigen vaccine trial. *Frontiers in Immunology*, *8*, 1807. DOI: 10.3389/fimmu.2017.01807 PMID: 29403468

Ryu, J. Y., Kim, H. U., & Lee, S. Y. (2018). Deep learning improves prediction of drug-drug and drug-food interactions. *Proceedings of the National Academy of Sciences of the United States of America*, *115*(18), E4304–E4311. DOI: 10.1073/pnas.1803294115 PMID: 29666228

Sachs, K., Perez, O., Pe'er, D., Lauffenburger, D. A., & Nolan, G. P. (2005). Causal protein-signaling networks derived from multiparameter single-cell data. *Science*, *308*(5721), 523–529. DOI: 10.1126/science.1105809 PMID: 15845847

Sadr, S., Hajjafari, A., Rahdar, A., Pandey, S., Jafroodi, P. P., Lotfalizadeh, N., Soroushianfar, M., Kavasebi, S. S., Kharaba, Z., Fathi-karkan, S., & Borji, H. (2024). Gold nanobiosensors and Machine Learning: Pioneering breakthroughs in precision breast cancer detection. *European Journal of Medicinal Chemistry Reports*, *12*, 100238. DOI: 10.1016/j.ejmcr.2024.100238

Saeys, Y., Van Gassen, S., & Lambrecht, B. N. (2016). Computational flow cytometry: Helping to make sense of high-dimensional immunology data. *Nature Reviews. Immunology*, *16*(7), 449–462. DOI: 10.1038/nri.2016.56 PMID: 27320317

Saha, S., & Raghava, G. P. S. (2004). BcePred: Prediction of continuous B-cell epitopes in antigenic sequences using physico-chemical properties. In *Lecture Notes in Computer Science. Lecture Notes in Computer Science* (pp. 197–204). DOI: 10.1007/978-3-540-30220-9_16

Saha, S., & Raghava, G. P. S. (2006). Prediction of continuous B-cell epitopes in an antigen using recurrent neural network. *Proteins*, *65*(1), 40–48. DOI: 10.1002/prot.21078 PMID: 16894596

Sajedian, I., Kim, J., & Rho, J. (2019). Finding the optical properties of plasmonic structures by image processing using a combination of convolutional neural networks and recurrent neural networks. *Microsystems & Nanoengineering*, *5*(1), 27. DOI: 10.1038/s41378-019-0069-y PMID: 31240107

Sakellaropoulos, T., Vougas, K., Narang, S., Koinis, F., Kotsinas, A., Polyzos, A., Moss, T. J., Piha-Paul, S., Zhou, H., Kardala, E., Damianidou, E., Alexopoulos, L. G., Aifantis, I., Townsend, P. A., Panayiotidis, M. I., Sfikakis, P., Bartek, J., Fitzgerald, R. C., Thanos, D., & Gorgoulis, V. G. (2019). A deep learning framework for predicting response to therapy in cancer. *Cell Reports*, *29*(11), 3367–3373. https://www.cell.com/cell-reports/fulltext/S2211-1247(19)314883?fbclid=IwAR0FDBjTBxTE0EsA8xFmFAXwLxgMcuT_6sW6V9SLJLZjPdpW47LbdyzviDQ. DOI: 10.1016/j.celrep.2019.11.017 PMID: 31825821

Salah Eldin, W., & Kaboudan, A. (2023). AI-Driven Medical Imaging Platform: Advancements in Image Analysis and Healthcare Diagnosis. *Journal of the ACS Advances in Computer Science*, *14*(1), 0. Advance online publication. DOI: 10.21608/asc.2024.248278.1018

Saleh, T., & Shojaosadati, S. A. (2016). Multifunctional nanoparticles for cancer immunotherapy. *Human Vaccines & Immunotherapeutics*, •••, 1–13. DOI: 10.1080/21645515.2016.1147635 PMID: 26901287

Sales, N. M. R., Pelegrini, P. B., & Goersch, M. (2014). Nutrigenomics: Definitions and advances of this new science. *Journal of Nutrition and Metabolism*, *2014*(1), 202759. https://onlinelibrary.wiley.com/doi/pdf/10.1155/2014/202759. DOI: 10.1155/2014/202759 PMID: 24795820

Santos-Filho, A., Dhudum, R., Ganeshpurkar, A., & Pawar, A. (2024). Revolutionizing Drug Discovery: A Comprehensive Review of AI Applications. *Drugs and Drug Candidates*, *3*(1), 148–171. DOI: 10.3390/ddc3010009

Sarkar, C., Das, B., Rawat, V. S., Wahlang, J. B., Nongpiur, A., Tiewsoh, I., Lyngdoh, N. M., Das, D., Bidarolli, M., & Sony, H. T. (2023). Artificial Intelligence and Machine Learning Technology Driven Modern Drug Discovery and Development. *International Journal of Molecular Sciences*, *24*(3), 2026. DOI: 10.3390/ijms24032026 PMID: 36768346

Sarker, I. H. (•••). Investigating undergraduate students' intention to engage in artificial intelligence learning. *SN Computer Science*, *3*(2), 158–158. DOI: 10.1007/s42979-022-01043-x PMID: 35194580

Sarker, I. H. (2021). Machine Learning: Algorithms, Real-World Applications and Research Directions. *SN Computer Science*, *2*(3), 160. DOI: 10.1007/s42979-021-00592-x PMID: 33778771

Sauteraud, R., Dashevskiy, L., Finak, G., & Gottardo, R. (2016). ImmuneSpace: Enabling integrative modelling of human immunological data. *The Journal of Immunology*, *196*(1_Supplement), 124.65-124.65. DOI: 10.4049/jimmunol.196.Supp.124.65

Saviano, M., Bassano, C., Piciocchi, P., Di Nauta, P., & Lettieri, M. (2018). Monitoring viability and sustainability in healthcare organizations. *Sustainability (Basel)*, *10*(10), 3548. DOI: 10.3390/su10103548

Savitha, S., Keerthana, R., Logeswaran, K., Keerthika, P., Sharmila, V., & Sangeetha, M. (2025). Integration of Multi-Omics Data: Genomics, Proteomics, Metabolomics. In Harnessing AI and Machine Learning for Precision Wellness (pp. 149-184). IGI Global Scientific Publishing.

Savitha, S., Kannan, A. R., & Logeswaran, K. (2025). Augmenting Cardiovascular Disease Prediction Through CWCF Integration Leveraging Harris Hawks Search in Deep Belief Networks. *Cognitive Computation, 17*(1), 52. DOI: 10.1007/s12559-025-10406-4

Savitha, S., & Rajiv Kannan, A. (2023). A novel technique based on mutual information weighted feature selection to predict chronic kidney disease. *Journal of Intelligent & Fuzzy Systems, 45*(1), 491–504. DOI: 10.3233/JIFS-222401

Saxena, S., Kazerooni, A. F., Toorens, E., Bakas, S., Akbari, H., Sako, C., Mamourian, E., Koumenis, C., Mohan, S., Bagley, S. J., Lustig, R. A., O'Rourke, D. M., Ganguly, T., Nasrallah, M. L., & Davatzikos, C. (2021). NIMG-73. Capturing glioblastoma heterogeneity using imaging and deep learning: Application to MGMT promoter methylation. *Neuro-Oncology, 23*(vi146), vi146. Advance online publication. DOI: 10.1093/neuonc/noab196.570

Sayers, I., John, C., Chen, J., & Hall, I. P. (2024). Genetics of Chronic Respiratory Disease. *Nature Reviews. Genetics, 25*(8), 534–547. DOI: 10.1038/s41576-024-00695-0 PMID: 38448562

Schapiro, D., Jackson, H. W., Raghuraman, S., Fischer, J. R., Zanotelli, V. R. T., Schulz, D., Giesen, C., Catena, R., Varga, Z., & Bodenmiller, B. (2017). histoCAT: Analysis of cell phenotypes and interactions in multiplex image cytometry data. *Nature Methods, 14*(9), 873–876. DOI: 10.1038/nmeth.4391 PMID: 28783155

Schenck, R., Lakatos, E., Gatenbee, C., Graham, T. A., & Anderson, A. R. A. (2019). NeoPredPipe: High throughput neoantigen prediction and recognition potential pipeline. *BMC Bioinformatics, 20*(1), 264. DOI: 10.1186/s12859-019-2876-4 PMID: 31117948

Schlecht, A., Boneva, S., Salie, H., Killmer, S., Wolf, J., Hajdu, R. I., Auw-Haedrich, C., Agostini, H., Reinhard, T., Schlunck, G., Bengsch, B., & Lange, C. A. K. (2021). Imaging mass cytometry for high-dimensional tissue profiling in the eye. *BMC Ophthalmology, 21*(1), 338. DOI: 10.1186/s12886-021-02099-8 PMID: 34544377

Schletz, D., Breidung, M., & Fery, A. (2023). Validating and Utilizing Machine Learning Methods to Investigate the Impacts of Synthesis Parameters in Gold Nanoparticle Synthesis. *The Journal of Physical Chemistry. C, Nanomaterials and Interfaces, 127*(2), 1117–1125. DOI: 10.1021/acs.jpcc.2c07578

Schneider, M. V., & Orchard, S. (2011). Omics technologies, data and bioinformatics principles. *Bioinformatics for Omics Data: Methods and Protocols*, 3-30.

Schneider, G., & Clark, D. E. (2019). Automated De Novo Drug Design: Are We Nearly There Yet? *Angewandte Chemie International Edition, 58*(32), 10792–10803. DOI: 10.1002/anie.201814681 PMID: 30730601

Schnyer, D. M., Clasen, P. C., Gonzalez, C., & Beevers, C. G. (2017). Evaluating the diagnostic utility of applying a machine learning algorithm to diffusion tensor MRI measures in individuals with major depressive disorder. *Psychiatry Research: Neuroimaging, 264*, 1–9. DOI: 10.1016/j.pscychresns.2017.03.003 PMID: 28388468

Schork, N. J. (2019). Artificial intelligence and personalized medicine. *Precision medicine in Cancer therapy*, 265-283.

Schubert, B., Walzer, M., Brachvogel, H.-P., Szolek, A., Mohr, C., & Kohlbacher, O. (2016). FRED 2: An immunoinformatic framework for Python. *Bioinformatics (Oxford, England)*, *32*(13), 2044–2046. DOI: 10.1093/bioinformatics/btw113 PMID: 27153717

Schultes, B., Ernst, B., & Schmid, S. M. (2021). Treating Hypercholesterinemia in a Patient with Maternally Inherited Diabetes and Deafness (MIDD) by the Proprotein Convertase Subtilisin/Kexin Type 9 (PCSK9) Inhibitor Alirocumab. *Acta Diabetologica*, *58*(11), 1575–1577. DOI: 10.1007/s00592-021-01776-w PMID: 34370095

Schultze, J. L., Büttner, M., & Becker, M. (2022, July). Swarm immunology: Harnessing blockchain technology and artificial intelligence in human immunology. *Nature Reviews. Immunology*, *22*(7), 401–403. DOI: 10.1038/s41577-022-00740-1 PMID: 35624333

Schürch, C. M., Bhate, S. S., Barlow, G. L., Phillips, D. J., Noti, L., Zlobec, I., Chu, P., Black, S., Demeter, J., McIlwain, D. R., Kinoshita, S., Samusik, N., Goltsev, Y., & Nolan, G. P. (2020). Coordinated cellular neighborhoods orchestrate antitumoral immunity at the colorectal cancer invasive front. *Cell*, *182*(5), 1341–1359.e19. DOI: 10.1016/j.cell.2020.07.005 PMID: 32763154

Schwenker, F., & Trentin, E. (2014). Pattern classification and clustering: A review of partially supervised learning approaches. *Pattern Recognition Letters*, *37*, 4–14. DOI: 10.1016/j.patrec.2013.10.017

Secara, I.-A., & Hordiiuk, D. (2024). Personalized Health Monitoring Systems: Integrating Wearable and AI. *Journal of Intelligent Learning Systems and Applications*, *16*(02), 44–52. DOI: 10.4236/jilsa.2024.162004

Secinaro, S., Calandra, D., Secinaro, A., Muthurangu, V., & Biancone, P. (2021). The role of artificial intelligence in healthcare: A structured literature review. *BMC Medical Informatics and Decision Making*, *21*(1), 1–23. DOI: 10.1186/s12911-021-01488-9 PMID: 33836752

Security, I. B. M. (2023). *Cost of a Data Breach Report.*https://www.ibm.com/security/data-breach

Segler, M. H. S., Kogej, T., Tyrchan, C., & Waller, M. P. (2018). Generating Focused Molecule Libraries for Drug Discovery with Recurrent Neural Networks. *ACS Central Science*, *4*(1), 120–131. DOI: 10.1021/acscentsci.7b00512 PMID: 29392184

Segler, M. H. S., Preuss, M., & Waller, M. P. (2018). Planning chemical syntheses with deep neural networks and symbolic AI. *Nature*, *555*(7698), 604–610. DOI: 10.1038/nature25978 PMID: 29595767

Sela-Culang, I., Kunik, V., & Ofran, Y. (2013). The structural basis of antibody-antigen recognition. *Frontiers in Immunology*, *4*, 302. DOI: 10.3389/fimmu.2013.00302 PMID: 24115948

Seo, S., & Lee, J. W. (2024). Applications of Big Data and AI-Driven Technologies in CADD (Computer-Aided Drug Design). In Gore, M., & Jagtap, U. B. (Eds.), *Computational Drug Discovery and Design* (pp. 295–305)., DOI: 10.1007/978-1-0716-3441-7_16

Serov, N., & Vinogradov, V. (2022). Artificial intelligence to bring nanomedicine to life. *Advanced Drug Delivery Reviews*, *184*, 114194. DOI: 10.1016/j.addr.2022.114194 PMID: 35283223

Sette, A., & Rappuoli, R. (2010). Reverse vaccinology: Developing vaccines in the era of genomics. *Immunity*, *33*(4), 530–541. DOI: 10.1016/j.immuni.2010.09.017 PMID: 21029963

Seyhan, A. A., & Carini, C. (2019). Are innovation and new technologies in precision medicine paving a new era in patients centric care? *Journal of Translational Medicine*, *17*(1), 114. DOI: 10.1186/s12967-019-1864-9 PMID: 30953518

Shaheen, M. Y. (2021). Applications of Artificial Intelligence (AI) in healthcare: A review. *Science-OpenPreprints*.

Shah, N. H., Entwistle, D., & Pfeffer, M. A. (2023, September 5). Creation and Adoption of Large Language Models in Medicine. *Journal of the American Medical Association*, *330*(9), 866–869. DOI: 10.1001/jama.2023.14217 PMID: 37548965

Shah, P., Kendall, F., & Khozin, S. (2019). Artificial intelligence in clinical development: Translational perspectives. npj. *Digital Medicine*, *2*(1), 69. DOI: 10.1038/s41746-019-0148-3 PMID: 31372505

Shah, R. M., Peterson, B., & Agrawal, N. (2021). Ethics and security in AI-assisted cell therapies. *Journal of Bioethics*, *12*(4), 330–343.

Shaik, T., Tao, X., Higgins, N., Gururajan, R., Li, Y., Zhou, X., & Acharya, U. R. (2022). Fedstack: Personalized activity monitoring using stacked federated learning. *Knowledge-Based Systems*, *257*, 109929. DOI: 10.1016/j.knosys.2022.109929

Shaik, T., Tao, X., Higgins, N., Xie, H., Gururajan, R., & Zhou, X. (2022). AI enabled RPM for mental health facility. In *Proceedings of the 1st ACM Workshop on Mobile and Wireless Sensing for Smart Healthcare* (pp. 26–32). Association for Computing Machinery. https://doi.org/DOI: 10.1145/3556551.3561191

Shakil, S., Ghosh, J., Singh, K., & Roy Choudhury, S. (2024). Comparative analysis of nutritional status among institutionalized and community-dwelling elderly women and its association with mental health status and cognitive function. *Journal of Family Medicine and Primary Care*, *13*(8), 3078–3083. Advance online publication. DOI: 10.4103/jfmpc.jfmpc_1932_23 PMID: 39228576

Shameer, K., Johnson, K. W., Glicksberg, B. S., Dudley, J. T., & Sengupta, P. P. (2018). Machine learning in cardiovascular medicine: Are we there yet? *Heart (British Cardiac Society)*, *104*(14), 1156–1164. DOI: 10.1136/heartjnl-2017-311198 PMID: 29352006

Shamji, M. H., Valenta, R., Jardetzky, T., Verhasselt, V., Durham, S. R., Würtzen, P. A., & Joost van Neerven, R. J. (2021). The Role of Allergen-Specific IgE, IgG and IgA in Allergic Disease. *Allergy*, *76*(12), 3627–3641. DOI: 10.1111/all.14908 PMID: 33999439

Shao, J., Ma, J., Yu, Y., Zhang, S., Wang, W., Li, W., & Wang, C. (2024). A multimodal integration pipeline for accurate diagnosis, pathogen identification, and prognosis prediction of pulmonary infections. *Innovation (Cambridge (Mass.))*, *5*(4), 100648. DOI: 10.1016/j.xinn.2024.100648 PMID: 39021525

Sharma, A., & Gupta, S. (2021). Deep Learning Framework for the Diagnosis of Oral Lichen Planus. *Journal of Oral Pathology & Medicine*.

Sharma, P., & Kan, E. C. (2018). *Sleep scoring with a UHF RFID tag by near field coherent sensing. In 2018 IEEE/MTT-s international microwave symposium IMS*. IEEE., DOI: 10.1109/MWSYM.2018.8439216

Shashkova, T. I., Umerenkov, D., Salnikov, M., Strashnov, P. V., Konstantinova, A. V., Lebed, I., & Ivanisenko, N. V. (2022). SEMA: Antigen B-cell conformational epitope prediction using deep transfer learning. *Frontiers in Immunology, 13*, 960985. DOI: 10.3389/fimmu.2022.960985 PMID: 36189325

Sheng, J., Zhang, J., Wang, L., Tano, V., Tang, J., Wang, X., Wu, J., Song, J., Zhao, Y., Rong, J., Cheng, F., Wang, J., Shen, Y., Wen, L., He, J., Zhang, H., Li, T., Zhang, Q., Bai, X., & Liang, T. (2022). Topological analysis of hepatocellular carcinoma tumour microenvironment based on imaging mass cytometry reveals cellular neighbourhood regulated reversely by macrophages with different ontogeny. *Gut, 71*(6), 1176–1191. DOI: 10.1136/gutjnl-2021-324339 PMID: 34253573

Shen, J., Cheng, F., Xu, Y., Li, W., & Tang, Y. (2020). Estimation of ADME properties with substructure pattern recognition. *Journal of Chemical Information and Modeling, 50*(6), 1034–1041. https://pubs.acs.org/doi/abs/10.1021/ci100104j. DOI: 10.1021/ci100104j PMID: 20578727

Shen, R., Olshen, A. B., & Ladanyi, M. (2009). Integrative clustering of multiple genomic data types using a joint latent variable model with application to breast and lung cancer subtype analysis. *Bioinformatics (Oxford, England), 25*(22), 2906–2912. DOI: 10.1093/bioinformatics/btp543 PMID: 19759197

Shen, Z., Cheng, S., & Luo, T. (2021). GDPR, HIPAA, and data regulations for AI in healthcare. *International Journal of Healthcare Information, 28*(2), 177–194.

Shirkani, A., Mansouri, A., Farid Hosseini, R., Jabbari Azad, F., Alsadat Mahmoudian, R., Montazer, M., & Gholamin, M. (2019). The role of interleukin-4 and 13 gene polymorphisms in allergic rhinitis: A case control study. *Reports of Biochemistry & Molecular Biology, 8*(2), 111–118. https://www.ncbi.nlm.nih.gov/pubmed/31832433 PMID: 31832433

Shittu, R. A.. (2024). The role of business intelligence tools in improving healthcare patient outcomes and operations. *World Journal of Advanced Research and Reviews, 24*(2), 1039–1060. DOI: 10.30574/wjarr.2024.24.2.3414

Shi, Y., Guo, Z., Su, X., Meng, L., Zhang, M., Sun, J., & Han, Z.-G. (2020). DeepAntigen: A novel method for neoantigen prioritization via 3D genome and deep sparse learning. *Bioinformatics (Oxford, England), 36*(19), 4894–4901. DOI: 10.1093/bioinformatics/btaa596 PMID: 32592462

Shoghli, A., Darvish, M., & Sadeghian, Y. (2024). Balancing Innovation and Privacy: Ethical Challenges in AI-Driven Healthcare. *Journal of Research in Medical Sciences : the Official Journal of Isfahan University of Medical Sciences, 4*(1), 1–11. DOI: 10.22034/jrms.2024.494112.1034

Shorten, C., & Khoshgoftaar, T. M. (2019). A survey on image data augmentation for deep learning. *Journal of Big Data, 6*(1), 1–48. DOI: 10.1186/s40537-019-0197-0

Shugay, M., Bagaev, D. V., Zvyagin, I. V., Vroomans, R. M., Crawford, J. C., Dolton, G., Komech, E. A., Sycheva, A. L., Koneva, A. E., Egorov, E. S., Eliseev, A. V., Van Dyk, E., Dash, P., Attaf, M., Rius, C., Ladell, K., McLaren, J. E., Matthews, K. K., Clemens, E. B., & Chudakov, D. M. (2018). VDJdb: A curated database of T-cell receptor sequences with known antigen specificity. *Nucleic Acids Research, 46*(D1), D419–D427. DOI: 10.1093/nar/gkx760 PMID: 28977646

Silva, H. E. C. D., Santos, G. N. M., Leite, A. F., Mesquita, C. R. M., Figueiredo, P. T. D. S., Stefani, C. M., & de Melo, N. S. (2023). The use of artificial intelligence tools in cancer detection compared to the traditional diagnostic imaging methods: An overview of the systematic reviews. *PLoS One*, *18*(10), e0292063.

Silverberg, J. I., Lei, D., Yousaf, M., Janmohamed, S. R., Vakharia, P. P., Chopra, R., Chavda, R., Gabriel, S., Patel, K. R., Singam, V., Kantor, R., & Hsu, D. Y. (2021). What Are the Best Endpoints for Eczema Area and Severity Index and Scoring Atopic Dermatitis in Clinical Practice? A Prospective Observational Study*. *British Journal of Dermatology*, *184*(5), 888–895. DOI: 10.1111/bjd.19457 PMID: 32959390

Simon, A. J., Golan, A. C., Lev, A., Stauber, T., Barel, O., Somekh, I., Klein, C., AbuZaitun, O., Eyal, E., Kol, N., Unal, E., Amariglio, N., Rechavi, G., & Somech, R. (2020). Whole Exome Sequencing (WES) Approach for Diagnosing Primary Immunodeficiencies (PIDs) in a Highly Consanguineous Community. *Clinical Immunology (Orlando, Fla.)*, *214*(May), 108376. DOI: 10.1016/j.clim.2020.108376 PMID: 32135276

Simon, M. C., Sina, C., Ferrario, P. G., & Daniel, H. (2023). Gut microbiome analysis for personalized nutrition: The state of science. *Molecular Nutrition & Food Research*, *67*(1), 2200476. DOI: 10.1002/mnfr.202200476 PMID: 36424179

Singh, A., Jha, S. K., Dwivedi, P. C., Srivastava, U., & Pal, A. (2024). Revolutionizing Healthcare: Integrating Electronics, AI, Traditional, and Conventional Methods. *World Journal of Advanced Research and Reviews*, *23*(3), 2426–2434. DOI: 10.30574/wjarr.2024.23.3.2919

Singh, B., Jevnikar, A. M., & Desjardins, E. (2024). Artificial Intelligence, Big Data, and Regulation of Immunity: Challenges and Opportunities. *Archivum Immunologiae et Therapiae Experimentalis*, *72*(1), 20240006. DOI: 10.2478/aite-2024-0006 PMID: 38421272

Singh, M., Fuenmayor, E., Hinchy, E. P., Qiao, Y., Murray, N., & Devine, D. (2021). Digital twin: Origin to future. *Applied System Innovation*, *4*(2), 36. DOI: 10.3390/asi4020036

Singh, M., Kumar, A., Khanna, N. N., Laird, J. R., Nicolaides, A., Faa, G., Johri, A. M., Mantella, L. E., Fernandes, J. F. E., Teji, J. S., Singh, N., Fouda, M. M., Singh, R., Sharma, A., Kitas, G., Rathore, V., Singh, I. M., Tadepalli, K., Al-Maini, M., & Suri, J. S. (2024). Artificial intelligence for cardiovascular disease risk assessment in personalised framework: A scoping review. *EClinicalMedicine*, *73*, 73. DOI: 10.1016/j.eclinm.2024.102660 PMID: 38846068

Singh, V., Danda, V., Gorniak, R., Flanders, A., & Lakhani, P. (2007). Assessment of critical feeding tube malpositions on radiographs using deep learning. Journal of Digital Imaging. 2019;32:651–655. Mead, MN. Nutrigenomics: the genome—Food interface. *Environmental Health Perspectives*, *115*, A582–A589. DOI: 10.1289/ehp.115-a582

Singh, Y., Patel, H., Vera-Garcia, D. V., Hathaway, Q. A., Sarkar, D., & Quaia, E. (2024, November 7). Beyond the hype: Navigating bias in AI-driven cancer detection. *Oncotarget*, *15*(1), 764–766. DOI: 10.18632/oncotarget.28665 PMID: 39513852

Singi, S. R., Sathe, S., Reche, A. R., Sibal, A., & Mantri, N. (2022). Extended arm of precision in prosthodontics: Artificial intelligence. *Cureus*, *14*(11). Advance online publication. DOI: 10.7759/cureus.30962 PMID: 36465202

Sirocchi, C., Bogliolo, A., & Montagna, S. (2024). Medical-informed machine learning: Integrating prior knowledge into medical decision systems. *BMC Medical Informatics and Decision Making*, *24*(S4, Suppl 4), 186. DOI: 10.1186/s12911-024-02582-4 PMID: 38943085

Siva Balan, R. V. (2024). Diagnosis of Multiple Sclerosis Lesion Using Deep Learning Models. *Journal of Electrical Systems*, *20*(3), 2354–2367. DOI: 10.52783/jes.4082

Sivarethinamohan, R., Sujatha, S., & Biswas, P. (2021, February). Envisioning the potential of natural language processing (nlp) in health care management. In *2021 7th International Engineering Conference "Research & Innovation amid Global Pandemic"(IEC)* (pp. 189-193). IEEE.

Skevaki, C., Nadeau, K. C., Rothenberg, M. E., Alahmad, B., Mmbaga, B. T., Masenga, G. G., Sampath, V., Christiani, D. C., Haahtela, T., & Renz, H. (2024, May). Impact of climate change on immune responses and barrier defense. *The Journal of Allergy and Clinical Immunology*, *153*(5), 1194–1205. DOI: 10.1016/j.jaci.2024.01.016 PMID: 38309598

SkinVision. SkinVision | Skin Cancer Melanoma Detection App | SkinVision. Accessed January 20, 2025. https://www.skinvision.com

Smirnov, P., Kofia, V., Maru, A., Freeman, M., Ho, C., El-Hachem, N., Adam, G.-A., Ba-alawi, W., Safikhani, Z., & Haibe-Kains, B. (2018). PharmacoDB: An integrative database for mining in vitro anticancer drug screening studies. *Nucleic Acids Research*, *46*(D1), D994–D1002. https://academic.oup.com/nar/article/46/D1/D994/4372597. DOI: 10.1093/nar/gkx911 PMID: 30053271

Smith, A., & Patel, M. (2019). Stem cell therapy for chronic diseases. *Stem Cell Research & Therapy*, *10*(1), 123. PMID: 30999922

Smith, B., & Lee, A. (2021). Machine learning approaches in autoimmune disease prediction. *AI in Autoimmunity*, *15*(4), 55–72.

Smith, D. A., & Germolec, D. R. (1999). Introduction to immunology and autoimmunity. *Environmental Health Perspectives*, *107*(suppl 5), 661–665. DOI: 10.1289/ehp.99107s5661 PMID: 10502528

Smith, R. G., & Farquhar, A. (2000). The road ahead for knowledge management: An AI perspective. *AI Magazine*, *21*, 17–17.

Smorchkova, A. K., Khoruzhaya, A. N., Kremneva, E. I., & Petryaikin, A. V. (2023). Machine learning technologies in CT-based diagnostics and classification of intracranial hemorrhages. *Zhurnalvoprosyneirokhirurgiiimeni NN Burdenko, 87*(2), 85-91. https://pubmed.ncbi.nlm.nih.gov/37011333/

Smuck, M., Odonkor, C. A., Wilt, J. K., Schmidt, N., & Swiernik, M. A. (2021). The emerging clinical role of wearables: Factors for successful implementation in healthcare. *NPJ Digital Medicine*, *4*(1), 1–8. https://www.nature.com/articles/s41746-021-00418-3/1000. DOI: 10.1038/s41746-021-00418-3 PMID: 33692479

Soladzha, O. (2024). Using Artificial Intelligence To Protect Human Rights: Development Of Sustainable Plastic Waste Recycling In Nigeria. Bulletin of the V.N. Karazin Kharkiv National University. Series. Law

Song, X., & Lin, Q. (2017). Genomics, transcriptomics and proteomics to elucidate the pathogenesis of rheumatoid arthritis. *Rheumatology International*, *37*(8), 1257–1265. DOI: 10.1007/s00296-017-3732-3 PMID: 28493174

Souto, E. B., Blanco-Llamero, C., Krambeck, K., Kiran, N. S., Yashaswini, C., Postwala, H., Severino, P., Priefer, R., Prajapati, B. G., & Maheshwari, R. (2024). Regulatory insights into nanomedicine and gene vaccine innovation: Safety assessment, challenges, and regulatory perspectives. *Acta Biomaterialia*, *180*, 1–17. DOI: 10.1016/j.actbio.2024.04.010 PMID: 38604468

Spencer, M., Eickholt, J., & Cheng, J. (2015). A Deep Learning Network Approach to ab initio Protein Secondary Structure Prediction. *IEEE/ACM Transactions on Computational Biology and Bioinformatics*, *12*(1), 103–112. DOI: 10.1109/TCBB.2014.2343960 PMID: 25750595

Sreenivasan, M., & Chacko, A. M. (2021). Interoperability issues in EHR systems: Research directions. Data analytics in biomedical engineering and healthcare, 13-28.

Stafford, I. S., Kellermann, M., Mossotto, E., Beattie, R. M., MacArthur, B. D., & Ennis, S. (2020). A systematic review of the applications of artificial intelligence and machine learning in autoimmune diseases. *NPJ Digital Medicine*, *3*(1), 30. DOI: 10.1038/s41746-020-0229-3 PMID: 32195365

Stavis, S. M., Fagan, J. A., Stopa, M., & Liddle, J. A. (2018). Nanoparticle Manufacturing – Heterogeneity through Processes to Products. *ACS Applied Nano Materials*, *1*(9), 4358–4385. DOI: 10.1021/acsanm.8b01239

Steels, L., & Brooks, R. (2018). *The Artificial Life Route to Artificial Intelligence: Building Embodied, Situated Agents*. Routledge. DOI: 10.4324/9781351001885

Steerling, E., Siira, E., Nilsen, P., Svedberg, P., & Nygren, J. (2023). Implementing AI in healthcare—the relevance of trust: A scoping review. *Frontiers in Health Services*, *3*, 1211150. DOI: 10.3389/frhs.2023.1211150 PMID: 37693234

Stevens, R. J., Kothari, V., Adler, A. I., Stratton, I. M., & Holman, R. R.United Kingdom Prospective Diabetes Study (UKPDS) Group. (2001). The UKPDS risk engine: A model for the risk of coronary heart disease in Type II diabetes (UKPDS 56). *Clinical Science*, *101*(6), 671–679. DOI: 10.1042/cs1010671 PMID: 11724655

Stewart, J., Lu, J., Gahungu, N., Goudie, A., Fegan, P. G., Bennamoun, M., Sprivulis, P., & Dwivedi, G. (2023). Western Australian medical students' attitudes towards artificial intelligence in healthcare. *PLoS One*, *18*(8), e0290642. DOI: 10.1371/journal.pone.0290642 PMID: 37651380

Stokes, J. M., Yang, K., Swanson, K., Jin, W., Cubillos-Ruiz, A., Donghia, N. M., MacNair, C. R., French, S., Carfrae, L. A., & Bloom-Ackermann, Z. (2020). A deep learning approach to antibiotic discovery. *Cell, 180*(4), 688-702. e613.

Stokes, J. M., Yang, K., Swanson, K., Jin, W., Cubillos-Ruiz, A., Donghia, N. M., MacNair, C. R., French, S., Carfrae, L. A., Bloom-Ackermann, Z., Tran, V. M., Chiappino-Pepe, A., Badran, A. H., Andrews, I. W., Chory, E. J., Church, G. M., Brown, E. D., Jaakkola, T. S., Barzilay, R., & Collins, J. J. (2020). A Deep Learning Approach to Antibiotic Discovery. *Cell, 180*(4), 688–702.e13. DOI: 10.1016/j.cell.2020.01.021 PMID: 32084340

Strachan, J. W., Albergo, D., Borghini, G., Pansardi, O., Scaliti, E., Gupta, S., Saxena, K., Rufo, A., Panzeri, S., Manzi, G., Graziano, M. S. A., & Becchio, C. (2024). Testing theory of mind in large language models and humans. *Nature Human Behaviour, 8*(7), 1285–1295. DOI: 10.1038/s41562-024-01882-z PMID: 38769463

Struble, T. J., Alvarez, J. C., Brown, S. P., Chytil, M., Cisar, J., DesJarlais, R. L., Engkvist, O., Frank, S. A., Greve, D. R., Griffin, D. J., Hou, X., Johannes, J. W., Kreatsoulas, C., Lahue, B., Mathea, M., Mogk, G., Nicolaou, C. A., Palmer, A. D., Price, D. J., & Jensen, K. F. (2020). Current and Future Roles of Artificial Intelligence in Medicinal Chemistry Synthesis. *Journal of Medicinal Chemistry, 63*(16), 8667–8682. DOI: 10.1021/acs.jmedchem.9b02120 PMID: 32243158

Subbiah, V. (2023). The next generation of evidence-based medicine. *Nature Medicine, 29*(1), 49–58. DOI: 10.1038/s41591-022-02160-z PMID: 36646803

Subramanian, G., Ramsundar, B., Pande, V., & Denny, R. A. (2016). Computational Modeling of β-Secretase 1 (BACE-1) Inhibitors Using Ligand Based Approaches. *Journal of Chemical Information and Modeling, 56*(10), 1936–1949. DOI: 10.1021/acs.jcim.6b00290 PMID: 27689393

Subramanian, I., Verma, S., Kumar, S., Jere, A., & Anamika, K. (2020). Multi-omics data integration, interpretation, and its application. *Bioinformatics and Biology Insights, 14*, 1177932219899051. DOI: 10.1177/1177932219899051 PMID: 32076369

Subramanian, M., Wojtusciszyn, A., Favre, L., Boughorbel, S., Shan, J., Letaief, K. B., & Chouchane, L. (2020). Precision medicine in the era of artificial intelligence: Implications in chronic disease management. *Journal of Translational Medicine, 18*(1), 472. DOI: 10.1186/s12967-020-02658-5 PMID: 33298113

Sun, B., & Barnard, A. S. (2018). Texture based image classification for nanoparticle surface characterisation and machine learning. *JPhys Materials, 1*(1), 016001. DOI: 10.1088/2515-7639/aad9ef

Sundarraj, P. (2024). Artificial Intelligence in Advance Angiogenesis and Inflammation Research: A Breakthrough in Disease Prediction and Therapy. *Journal of Angiotherapy, 8*(9), 1–8. DOI: 10.25163/angiotherapy.899861

Sung, J. J., Savulescu, J., Ngiam, K. Y., An, B., Ang, T. L., Yeoh, K. G., Cham, T.-J., Tsao, S., & Chua, T. S. (2023). Artificial intelligence for gastroenterology: Singapore artificial intelligence for Gastroenterology Working Group Position Statement. *Journal of Gastroenterology and Hepatology, 38*(10), 1669–1676. DOI: 10.1111/jgh.16241 PMID: 37277693

Sun, X., Yin, Y., Yang, Q., & Huo, T. (2023). Artificial intelligence in cardiovascular diseases: Diagnostic and therapeutic perspectives. *European Journal of Medical Research, 28*(1), 242. DOI: 10.1186/s40001-023-01065-y PMID: 37475050

Sun, Y. H., Wu, Y.-L., & Liao, B.-Y. (2023). Phenotypic heterogeneity in human genetic diseases: Ultrasensitivity-mediated threshold effects as a unifying molecular mechanism. *Journal of Biomedical Science, 30*(1), 58. DOI: 10.1186/s12929-023-00959-7 PMID: 37525275

Sun, Y., & Zhou, Y. (2022). Real-time public health surveillance using AI. *Journal of AI and Epidemiology, 8*(2), 120–135.

Suprun, M., Getts, R., Raghunathan, R., Grishina, G., Witmer, M., Gimenez, G., Sampson, H. A., & Suárez-Fariñas, M. (2019). Novel Bead-Based Epitope Assay Is a Sensitive and Reliable Tool for Profiling Epitope-Specific Antibody Repertoire in Food Allergy. *Scientific Reports, 9*(1), 18425. DOI: 10.1038/s41598-019-54868-7 PMID: 31804555

Suratannon, N., van Wijck, R. T. A., Broer, L., Xue, L., van Meurs, J. B. J., Barendregt, B. H., van der Burg, M., Dik, W. A., Chatchatee, P., Langerak, A. W., Swagemakers, S. M. A., Goos, J. A. C., Mathijssen, I. M. J., Dalm, V. A. S. H., Suphapeetiporn, K., Heezen, K. C., Drabwell, J., Uitterlinden, A. G., van der Spek, P. J., & van Hagen, P. M. (2020). Rapid Low-Cost Microarray-Based Genotyping for Genetic Screening in Primary Immunodeficiency. *Frontiers in Immunology, 11*(April), 614. Advance online publication. DOI: 10.3389/fimmu.2020.00614 PMID: 32373116

Sutanto, H., & Yuliasih, Y. (2023). Disentangling the Pathogenesis of Systemic Lupus Erythematosus: Close Ties between Immunological, Genetic and Environmental Factors. *Medicina, 59*(6), 1033. DOI: 10.3390/medicina59061033 PMID: 37374237

Symptomate. "Symptomate – Check Your Symptoms Online." Accessed January 20, 2025. https://symptomate.com/

Taber, K. A. J., Dickinson, B. D., & Wilson, M. (2014). The promise and challenges of next-generation genome sequencing for clinical care. *JAMA Internal Medicine, 174*(2), 275–280. DOI: 10.1001/jamainternmed.2013.12048 PMID: 24217348

Tagde, P., Tagde, S., Bhattacharya, T., Tagde, P., Chopra, H., Akter, R., Kaushik, D., & Rahman, M. H. (2021). Blockchain and artificial intelligence technology in e-Health. *Environmental Science and Pollution Research International, 28*(38), 52810–52831. DOI: 10.1007/s11356-021-16223-0 PMID: 34476701

Taherdoost, H., & Ghofrani, A. (2024). *AI and the evolution of personalized medicine in pharmacogenomics*. Intelligent Pharmacy.

Takaoka, K. (2022, April 5). AI Implementation Science for Social Issues: Pitfalls and Tips. *Journal of Epidemiology, 32*(4), 155–162. DOI: 10.2188/jea.JE20210278 PMID: 35095090

Tammemägi, M. C., Katki, H. A., Hocking, W. G., Church, T. R., Caporaso, N., Kvale, P. A., Chaturvedi, A. K., Silvestri, G. A., Riley, T. L., Commins, J., & Berg, C. D. (2013). Selection criteria for lung-cancer screening. *The New England Journal of Medicine, 368*(8), 728–736. DOI: 10.1056/NEJMoa1211776 PMID: 23425165

Tang, C., Fang, M., Tan, G., Zhang, S., Yang, B., Li, Y., Zhang, T., Saxena, R., Mohan, C., & Wu, T. (2022). Discovery of Novel Circulating Immune Complexes in Lupus Nephritis Using Immunoproteomics. *Frontiers in Immunology, 13*(March), 850015. Advance online publication. DOI: 10.3389/fimmu.2022.850015 PMID: 35419005

Tang, S., & Madhavan, S. (2017). neoantigenR: An annotation-based pipeline for tumor neoantigen identification from sequencing data. DOI: 10.1101/171843

Tang, Y., Wang, Y., Wang, J., Li, M., Peng, L., Wei, G., & Gao, Z. (2020). TruNeo: An integrated pipeline improves personalized true tumor neoantigen identification. *BMC Bioinformatics*, *21*(1), 532. DOI: 10.1186/s12859-020-03869-9 PMID: 33208106

Tanvir, R. B., Islam, M. M., Sobhan, M., Luo, D., & Mondal, A. M. (2023). "MOGAT: An Improved Multi-Omics Integration Framework Using Graph Attention Networks." *bioRxiv*. DOI: 10.1101/2023.04.01.535195

Tan, W. C. C., Nerurkar, S. N., Cai, H. Y., Ng, H. H. M., Wu, D., Wee, Y. T. F., Lim, J. C. T., Yeong, J., & Lim, T. K. H. (2020). Overview of multiplex immunohistochemistry/immunofluorescence techniques in the era of cancer immunotherapy. *Cancer Communications*, *40*(4), 135–153. DOI: 10.1002/cac2.12023 PMID: 32301585

Tappeiner, E., Finotello, F., Charoentong, P., Mayer, C., Rieder, D., & Trajanoski, Z. (2017). TIminer: NGS data mining pipeline for cancer immunology and immunotherapy. *Bioinformatics (Oxford, England)*, *33*(19), 3140–3141. DOI: 10.1093/bioinformatics/btx377 PMID: 28633385

Tavazzi, E., Zivadinov, R., Dwyer, M. G., Jakimovski, D., Singhal, T., Weinstock-Guttman, B., & Bergsland, N. (2020). MRI Biomarkers of Disease Progression and Conversion to Secondary-Progressive Multiple Sclerosis. *Expert Review of Neurotherapeutics*, *20*(8), 821–834. DOI: 10.1080/14737175.2020.1757435 PMID: 32306772

Tay, S. H., Yaung, K. N., Leong, J. Y., Yeo, J. G., Arkachaisri, T., & Albani, S. (2019). Immunomics in pediatric rheumatic diseases. *Frontiers in Medicine*, *6*, 111. DOI: 10.3389/fmed.2019.00111 PMID: 31231652

Temsah, M.-H., Alhuzaimi, A. N., Almansour, M., Aljamaan, F., Alhasan, K., Batarfi, M. A., Altamimi, I., Alharbi, A., Alsuhaibani, A. A., Alwakeel, L., Alzahrani, A. A., Alsulaim, K. B., Jamal, A., Khayat, A., Alghamdi, M. H., Halwani, R., Khan, M. K., Al-Eyadhy, A., & Nazer, R. (2024). Art or artifact: Evaluating the accuracy, appeal, and educational value of AI-generated imagery in DALL· E 3 for illustrating congenital heart diseases. *Journal of Medical Systems*, *48*(1), 54. DOI: 10.1007/s10916-024-02072-0 PMID: 38780839

Thakur, S.. (2023). *Big data and artificial intelligence in ophthalmology.*

Thangarasan, T., Keerthana, R., Arunkumar, M., Ramya, S., Bommy, M., & Surendhiran, V. (2022). Lung Cancer Prediction Using Machine Learning Technique Over Big Data. *NeuroQuantology : An Interdisciplinary Journal of Neuroscience and Quantum Physics*, *20*(8). Advance online publication. DOI: 10.14704/nq.2022.20.8.NQ44098

Thangarasan, T., Keerthana, R., Moheshkumar, G., Surendhiran, V., & Namasivayam, M. (2023). Research and Application of Boundary Optimization Algorithm of Forest Resource Vector Data Based on Convolutional Neural Network. In *2023 Second International Conference On Smart Technologies For Smart Nation (SmartTechCon)*, IEEE, pp. 1427-1432.

Thirunavukarasu, R., Gnanasambandan, R., Gopikrishnan, M., & Palanisamy, V. (2022). Towards computational solutions for precision medicine based big data healthcare system using deep learning models: A review. *Computers in Biology and Medicine*, *149*, 106020. DOI: 10.1016/j.compbiomed.2022.106020 PMID: 36088715

Thomas, J., & Evans, M. (2023). Personalized immunotherapy and AI-driven treatment strategies. *AI in Cancer Research*, *11*(1), 33–50.

Thomas, S., Rouilly, V., Patin, E., Alanio, C., Dubois, A., Delval, C., Marquier, L. G., Fauchoux, N., Sayegrih, S., Vray, M., Duffy, D., Quintana-Murci, L., Albert, M. L., Abel, L., Alcover, A., Bousso, P., Bruhns, P., Cumano, A., Daëron, M., & Albert, M. L.Milieu Intérieur Consortium. (2015). The Milieu Intérieur study - an integrative approach for study of human immunological variance. *Clinical Immunology (Orlando, Fla.)*, *157*(2), 277–293. DOI: 10.1016/j.clim.2014.12.004 PMID: 25562703

Thorlund, K., Dron, L., Park, J. J. H., & Mills, E. J. (2020). Synthetic and External Controls in Clinical Trials - A Primer for Researchers. *Clinical Epidemiology*, *12*, 457–467. DOI: 10.2147/CLEP.S242097 PMID: 32440224

Tian, J., Zhang, D., Yang, Y., Huang, Y., Wang, L., Yao, X., & Lu, Q. (2024). Global Epidemiology of Atopic Dermatitis: A Comprehensive Systematic Analysis and Modelling Study. *British Journal of Dermatology*, *190*(1), 55–61. DOI: 10.1093/bjd/ljad339 PMID: 37705227

Tian, K., Shao, M., Wang, Y., Guan, J., & Zhou, S. (2016). Boosting compound-protein interaction prediction by deep learning. *Methods (San Diego, Calif.)*, *110*, 64–72. DOI: 10.1016/j.ymeth.2016.06.024 PMID: 27378654

Tidjon, L. N., & Khomh, F. (2022). The different faces of ai ethics across the world: a principle-implementation gap analysis. arXiv preprint arXiv:2206.03225.

Tomašev, N., Glorot, X., Rae, J. W., Zielinski, M., Askham, H., Saraiva, A., Mottram, A., Meyer, C., Ravuri, S., Protsyuk, I., Connell, A., Hughes, C. O., Karthikesalingam, A., Cornebise, J., Montgomery, H., Rees, G., Laing, C., Baker, C. R., Peterson, K., & Mohamed, S. (2019). A clinically applicable approach to continuous prediction of future acute kidney injury. *Nature*, *572*(7767), 116–119. DOI: 10.1038/s41586-019-1390-1 PMID: 31367026

Toncinic, S., de Wildt-Liesveld, R., & Vrijhoef, H. (2020). Evaluation of a digital platform that engages stakeholders in the co-creation of healthcare innovations: A mixed-methods study. *International Journal of Care Coordination*, *23*(1), 33–42. DOI: 10.1177/2053434520913578

Tong, J. C., & Ranganathan, S. (2013). Computational T cell vaccine design. In *Computer-Aided Vaccine Design* (pp. 59–86). DOI: 10.1533/9781908818416.59

Tong, L., Mitchel, J., Chatlin, K., & Wang, M. D. (2020). Deep learning based feature-level integration of multi-omics data for breast cancer patients survival analysis. *BMC Medical Informatics and Decision Making*, *20*(1), 225. DOI: 10.1186/s12911-020-01225-8 PMID: 32933515

Tong, Z., Zhou, Y., & Wang, J. (2019). Identifying potential drug targets in hepatocellular carcinoma based on network analysis and one-class support vector machine. *Scientific Reports*, *9*(1), 10442. https://www.nature.com/articles/s41598-019-46540-x. DOI: 10.1038/s41598-019-46540-x PMID: 31320657

Topol, E. (2019). *Deep Medicine: How Artificial Intelligence Can Make Healthcare Human Again.* Basic Books.

Topol, E. J. (2019). High-performance medicine: The convergence of human and artificial intelligence. *Nature Medicine*, *25*(1), 44–56. DOI: 10.1038/s41591-018-0300-7 PMID: 30617339

Tran, T. Q. B., du Toit, C., & Padmanabhan, S. (2021). Artificial intelligence in healthcare—The road to precision medicine. *Journal of Hospital Management and Health Policy*, *5*, 5. DOI: 10.21037/jhmhp-20-132

Tripathi, M. K., Nath, A., Singh, T. P., Ethayathulla, A. S., & Kaur, P. (2021). Evolving scenario of big data and Artificial Intelligence (AI) in drug discovery. *Molecular Diversity*, *25*(3), 1439–1460. DOI: 10.1007/s11030-021-10256-w PMID: 34159484

Tripp, L., Vanstone, M., Canfield, C., Leslie, M., Levasseur, M. A., Panday, J., Rowland, P., Wilson, G., You, J., & Abelson, J. (2022). The impact of COVID-19 on patient engagement in the health system: Results from a Pan-Canadian survey of patient, family and caregiver partners. *Health Expectations*, *25*(2), 744–753. DOI: 10.1111/hex.13421 PMID: 35023267

Tsamados, A., Aggarwal, N., Cowls, J., Morley, J., Roberts, H., Taddeo, M., & Floridi, L. (2022). The ethics of algorithms: Key problems and solutions. *AI & Society*, *37*(1), 215–230. DOI: 10.1007/s00146-021-01154-8

Tsang, K. C. H., Pinnock, H., Wilson, A. M., Salvi, D., & Shah, S. A. (2022). Predicting Asthma Attacks Using Connected Mobile Devices and Machine Learning: The AAMOS-00 Observational Study Protocol. *BMJ Open*, *12*(10), e064166. DOI: 10.1136/bmjopen-2022-064166 PMID: 36192103

Tsherniak, A., Vazquez, F., Montgomery, P. G., Weir, B. A., Kryukov, G., Cowley, G. S., Gill, S., Harrington, W. F., Pantel, S., Krill-Burger, J. M., Meyers, R. M., Ali, L., Goodale, A., Lee, Y., Jiang, G., Hsiao, J., Gerath, W. F. J., Howell, S., Merkel, E., & Hahn, W. C. (2017). Defining a cancer dependency map. *Cell*, *170*(3), 564–576. https://www.cell.com/cell/fulltext/S0092-8674(17)30651-7?dgcid=cell.com-slider_referral_cell-slider-hahn. DOI: 10.1016/j.cell.2017.06.010 PMID: 28753430

Tsiakas, K., Abujelala, M., & Makedon, F. (2018). Task engagement as personalization feedback for socially-assistive robots and cognitive training. *Technologies*, *6*(2), 49. DOI: 10.3390/technologies6020049

Tuano, K. S., Seth, N., & Chinen, J. (2021). Secondary immunodeficiencies: An overview. *Annals of Allergy, Asthma & Immunology*, *127*(6), 617–626. DOI: 10.1016/j.anai.2021.08.413 PMID: 34481993

Turtle, C. J., Hanafi, L.-A., Berger, C., Gooley, T. A., Cherian, S., Hudecek, M., Sommermeyer, D., Melville, K., Pender, B., Budiarto, T. M., Robinson, E., Steevens, N. N., Chaney, C., Soma, L., Chen, X., Yeung, C., Wood, B., Li, D., Cao, J., & Maloney, D. G. (2016). CD19 CAR-T cells of defined CD4+:CD8+ composition in adult B cell ALL patients. *The Journal of Clinical Investigation*, *126*(6), 2123–2138. DOI: 10.1172/JCI85309 PMID: 27111235

Tu, T., Azizi, S., Driess, D., Schaekermann, M., Amin, M., Chang, B. S. P. C., Carroll, A., Lau, C., Tanno, M. B. A. R., Ktena, I., Palepu, A., Mustafa, B., Chowdhery, A., Liu, Y., Kornblith, S., Fleet, D., Mansfield, P., Prakash, S., Wong, R., & Natarajan, V. (2024). Towards Generalist Biomedical AI. *NEJM AI*, *1*(3). Advance online publication. DOI: 10.1056/AIoa2300138

Uddin, M., Wang, Y., & Woodbury-Smith, M. (2019). Artificial intelligence for precision medicine in neurodevelopmental disorders. *npj. Digital Medicine*, *2*(1), 112. PMID: 31799421

Udegbe, F. C.Francisca Chibugo UdegbeOgochukwu Roseline EbulueCharles Chukwudalu EbulueC-hukwunonso Sylvester Ekesiobi. (2024). AI's impact on personalized medicine: Tailoring treatments for improved health outcomes. *Engineering Science & Technology Journal*, *5*(4), 1386–1394. DOI: 10.51594/estj.v5i4.1040

Uffelmann, E., Huang, Q. Q., Munung, N. S., De Vries, J., Okada, Y., Martin, A. R., Martin, H. C., Lappalainen, T., & Posthuma, D. (2021). Genome-wide association studies. *Nature Reviews. Methods Primers*, *1*(1), 59. DOI: 10.1038/s43586-021-00056-9

Unger, M., & Kather, J. N. (2024). Deep learning in cancer genomics and histopathology. *Genome Medicine*, *16*(1), 44. DOI: 10.1186/s13073-024-01315-6 PMID: 38539231

US Food and Drug Administration. (2021). *Assessing the Credibility of Computational Modeling and Simulation in Medical Device Submissions*. FDA.

Uslu, B. Ç., Okay, E., & Dursun, E. (2020). Analysis of factors affecting IoT-based smart hospital design. *Journal of Cloud Computing (Heidelberg, Germany)*, *9*(1), 67. DOI: 10.1186/s13677-020-00215-5 PMID: 33532168

Väänänen, A., Haataja, K., Vehviläinen-Julkunen, K., & Toivanen, P. (2021). AI in healthcare: A narrative review. *F1000 Research*, *10*, 6. DOI: 10.12688/f1000research.26997.2

Vaishya, R., Javaid, M., Khan, I. H., & Haleem, A. (2020, July-August). Artificial Intelligence (AI) applications for COVID-19 pandemic. *Diabetes & Metabolic Syndrome*, *14*(4), 337–339. DOI: 10.1016/j.dsx.2020.04.012 PMID: 32305024

Valencic, E., Smid, A., Jakopin, Z., Tommasini, A., & Mlinaric-Rascan, I. (2018). Repositioning drugs for rare immune diseases: Hopes and challenges for a precision medicine. *Current Medicinal Chemistry*, *25*(24), 2764–2782. DOI: 10.2174/0929867324666170830101215 PMID: 28875839

Vamathevan, J., Clark, D., Czodrowski, P., Dunham, I., Ferran, E., Lee, G., Li, B., Madabhushi, A., Shah, P., Spitzer, M., & Zhao, S. (2019). Applications of machine learning in drug discovery and development. *Nature Reviews. Drug Discovery*, *18*(6), 463–477. DOI: 10.1038/s41573-019-0024-5 PMID: 30976107

Van Allen, E. M., Miao, D., Schilling, B., Shukla, S. A., Blank, C., Zimmer, L., Sucker, A., Hillen, U., Geukes Foppen, M. H., Goldinger, S. M., Utikal, J., Hassel, J. C., Weide, B., Kaehler, K. C., Loquai, C., Mohr, P., Gutzmer, R., Dummer, R., Gabriel, S., & Garraway, L. A. (2015). Genomic correlates of response to CTLA-4 blockade in metastatic melanoma. *Science*, *350*(6257), 207–211. DOI: 10.1126/science.aad0095 PMID: 26359337

Van Belle, T. L., Coppieters, K. T., & Von Herrath, M. G. (2011). Type 1 diabetes: Etiology, immunology, and therapeutic strategies. *Physiological Reviews*, *91*(1), 79–118. DOI: 10.1152/physrev.00003.2010 PMID: 21248163

Van Booven, D. J., Chen, C. B., Malpani, S., Mirzabeigi, Y., Mohammadi, M., Wang, Y., & Arora, H. (2024). Synthetic genitourinary image synthesis via generative adversarial networks: enhancing AI diagnostic precision. bioRxiv, 2024-05.

Van de Sande, D., Van Genderen, M. E., Smit, J. M., Huiskens, J., Visser, J. J., Veen, R. E., & van Bommel, J. (2022). Developing, implementing and governing artificial intelligence in medicine: A step-by-step approach to prevent an artificial intelligence winter. *BMJ Health & Care Informatics*, *29*(1), e100495. https://www.ncbi.nlm.nih.gov/pmc/articles/PMC8860016/. DOI: 10.1136/bmjhci-2021-100495 PMID: 35185012

Vanguri, R. S., Luo, J., Aukerman, A. T., Egger, J. V., Fong, C. J., Horvat, N., Pagano, A., Araujo-Filho, J. A. B., Geneslaw, L., Rizvi, H., Sosa, R., Boehm, K. M., Yang, S.-R., Bodd, F. M., Ventura, K., Hollmann, T. J., Ginsberg, M. S., Gao, J., Vanguri, R., & Shah, S. P. (2022). Multimodal integration of radiology, pathology and genomics for prediction of response to PD-(L)1 blockade in patients with non-small cell lung cancer. *Nature Cancer*, *3*(8), 1151–1164. DOI: 10.1038/s43018-022-00416-8 PMID: 36038778

Vasiliev, Y. A., Александрович, В. Ю., Vasiliev, Y. A., Vlazimirsky, A. V., Вячеславович, В. А., Vlazimirsky, A. V., & Omelyanskaya, O. V.. (2023). Methodology for Testing and Monitoring Artificial Intelligence-Based Software for Medical Diagnostics. *Digital Diagnostics*, *4*(3), 252–267. DOI: 10.17816/DD321971

Vatansever, S., Schlessinger, A., Wacker, D., Kaniskan, H. Ü., Jin, J., Zhou, M.-M., & Zhang, B. (2021). Artificial intelligence and machine learning-aided drug discovery in central nervous system diseases: State-of-the-arts and future directions. *Medicinal Research Reviews*, *41*(3), 1427–1473. DOI: 10.1002/med.21764 PMID: 33295676

Vayena, E., Dzenowagis, J., & Brownstein, J. (2018). Promoting equity in AI for global health. *Journal of Global Health*, *8*(2), 1–7.

Väyrynen, J. P., Haruki, K., Lau, M. C., Väyrynen, S. A., Zhong, R., Dias Costa, A., Borowsky, J., Zhao, M., Fujiyoshi, K., Arima, K., Twombly, T. S., Kishikawa, J., Gu, S., Aminmozaffari, S., Shi, S., Baba, Y., Akimoto, N., Ugai, T., Da Silva, A., & Nowak, J. A. (2021). The prognostic role of macrophage polarization in the colorectal cancer microenvironment. *Cancer Immunology Research*, *9*(1), 8–19. DOI: 10.1158/2326-6066.CIR-20-0527 PMID: 33023967

Vella, D., & Ebejer, J.-P. (2022). Few-shot learning for low-data drug discovery. *Journal of Chemical Information and Modeling*, *63*(1), 27–42. DOI: 10.1021/acs.jcim.2c00779 PMID: 36410391

Venkatraman, S., Parvin, S., Mansoor, W., & Gawanmeh, A. (2023). Big data analytics and internet of things for personalised healthcare: opportunities and challenges. International Journal of Electrical & Computer Engineering (2088-8708), 13(4).

Venter, J. C., Adams, M. D., Myers, E. W., Li, P. W., Mural, R. J., Sutton, G. G., ... & Kalush, F. (2001). The sequence of the human genome. *science, 291*(5507), 1304-1351. DOI: DOI: 10.1126/science.1058040

Vetchinkina, E. A., Mikhaylenko, D. S., Kuznetsova, E. B., Deryagina, T. A., Alekseeva, E. A., Bure, I. V., Zamyatnin, A. A.Jr, & Nemtsova, M. V. (2021). Genetic Factors of Predisposition and Clinical Characteristics of Rheumatoid Arthritis in Russian Patients. *Journal of Personalized Medicine, 11*(6), 469. DOI: 10.3390/jpm11060469 PMID: 34070522

Vetter, T. R., & Schober, P. (2018). Regression: The apple does not fall far from the tree. *Anesthesia and Analgesia, 127*(1), 277–283. DOI: 10.1213/ANE.0000000000003424 PMID: 29771712

Victor, N. O. C. (2023). An experimental case study on how AI may improve communi-cation and resource allocation. *International Journal of Artificial Intelligence and Machine Learning, 3*(1), 10–18.

Vidhya, K. S., Sultana, A., M, N. K., & Rangareddy, H. (2023, October 22). M, N. K., & Rangareddy, H. (2023). Artificial Intelligence's Impact on Drug Discovery and Development From Bench to Bedside. *Cureus*. Advance online publication. DOI: 10.7759/cureus.47486 PMID: 37881323

Vinchurkar, K., & Mane, S. (2024). *AI Innovations in Drug Delivery and Pharmaceutical Sciences; Advancing Therapy through Technology*. Bentham Science Publishers. DOI: 10.2174/97898153057531240101

Vishwakarma, L. P.. (2023). Application of artificial intelligence for resilient and sustainable healthcare system: Systematic literature review and future research directions. *International Journal of Production Research*, •••, 1–23.

Viswanathan, J., Saranya, N., & Inbamani, A. (2021). Deep learning applications in medical imaging: Introduction to deep learning-based intelligent systems for medical applications. In *Deep Learning Applications in Medical Imaging* (pp. 156–177). IGI Global.

Voigt, I., Inojosa, H., Dillenseger, A., Haase, R., Akgün, K., & Ziemssen, T. (2021). Digital Twins for Multiple Sclerosis. *Frontiers in Immunology, 12*, 669811. DOI: 10.3389/fimmu.2021.669811 PMID: 34012452

Vossoughi, S., Marin, A., & Bang, M. (2023). Toward Just and Sustainable Futures: Human Learning and Relationality Within Socio-Ecological Systems. *Review of Research in Education, 47*(1), 218–273. DOI: 10.3102/0091732X231223505

Vyas, D. A., Eisenstein, L. G., & Jones, D. S. (2020). *Hidden in plain sight—reconsidering the use of race correction in clinical algorithms* (Vol. 383). Mass Medical Soc.

Wachter, R. M., & Brynjolfsson, E. (2024, January 2). Will Generative Artificial Intelligence Deliver on Its Promise in Health Care? *Journal of the American Medical Association, 331*(1), 65–69. DOI: 10.1001/jama.2023.25054 PMID: 38032660

Wahl, B., Cossy-Gantner, A., Germann, S., & Schwalbe, N. R. (2018). Artificial intelligence (AI) and global health: How can AI contribute to health in resource-poor settings? *BMJ Global Health, 3*(4), e000798. DOI: 10.1136/bmjgh-2018-000798 PMID: 30233828

Wang, L., Zhang, W., He, X., & Zha, H. (2018, July). Supervised reinforcement learning with recurrent neural network for dynamic treatment recommendation. In Proceedings of the 24th ACM SIGKDD international conference on knowledge discovery & data mining (pp. 2447-2456).

Wang, B., Mezlini, A. M., Demir, F., Fiume, M., Tu, Z., Brudno, M., Haibe-Kains, B., & Goldenberg, A. (2014). Similarity network fusion for aggregating data types on a genomic scale. *Nature Methods*, *11*(3), 333–337. DOI: 10.1038/nmeth.2810 PMID: 24464287

Wang, C., & Liu, X. (2021). Convolutional neural networks in medical imaging for autoimmune disorders. *AI in Radiology*, *7*(4), 88–105.

Wang, C., Ma, J., Shao, J., Zhang, S., Li, J., Yan, J., Zhao, Z., Bai, C., Yu, Y., & Li, W. (2022). Non-invasive measurement using deep learning algorithm based on multi-source features fusion to predict PDL1 expression and survival in NSCLC. *Frontiers in Immunology*, *13*, 828560. DOI: 10.3389/fimmu.2022.828560 PMID: 35464416

Wang, K., Xu, J., Kim, S., Huang, Z., & Lee, C. (2023). Machine learning in cancer immunotherapy: Current status and future directions. *Science Immunology*, *8*(1), eabc2345. https://doi.org/10./si.2023.abc2345

Wang, L., & Preininger, A. (2019). Addressing healthcare access disparities through AI-driven tools. *Journal of Health Technology*, *13*(4), 589–602.

Wang, L., Wang, F. S., & Gershwin, M. E. (2015). Human autoimmune diseases: A comprehensive update. *Journal of Internal Medicine*, *278*(4), 369–395. DOI: 10.1111/joim.12395 PMID: 26212387

Wang, S., Wang, F., Zhu, Z., Wang, J., Tran, T., & Du, Z. (2024). Artificial intelligence in education: A systematic literature review. *Expert Systems with Applications*, *252*, 124167. DOI: 10.1016/j.eswa.2024.124167

Wang, T.-Y., Wang, L., Alam, S. K., Hoeppner, L. H., & Yang, R. (2019). ScanNeo: Identifying indel-derived neoantigens using RNA-Seq data. *Bioinformatics (Oxford, England)*, *35*(20), 4159–4161. DOI: 10.1093/bioinformatics/btz193 PMID: 30887025

Wang, W., Feng, S., Ye, Z., Gao, H., Lin, J., & Ouyang, D. (2022). Prediction of lipid nanoparticles for mRNA vaccines by the machine learning algorithm. *Acta Pharmaceutica Sinica. B*, *12*(6), 2950–2962. DOI: 10.1016/j.apsb.2021.11.021 PMID: 35755271

Wang, W., Zhang, X., & Dai, D.-Q. (2021). DeFusion: A Denoised Network Regularization Framework for Multi-Omics Integration. *Briefings in Bioinformatics*, *22*(5), bbab057. Advance online publication. DOI: 10.1093/bib/bbab057 PMID: 33822879

Wang, X., & Liu, Z. (2019). Deep Neural Networks for the Classification of Oral Lesions: Insights into Oral Lichen Planus. *Journal of Biomedical Informatics*.

Wang, X., Yang, W., Weinreb, J., Han, J., Li, Q., Kong, X., Yan, Y., Ke, Z., Luo, B., Liu, T., & Wang, L. (2017). Searching for prostate cancer by fully automated magnetic resonance imaging classification: Deep learning versus non-deep learning. *Scientific Reports*, *7*(1), 15415. https://www.nature.com/articles/s41598-017-15720-y. DOI: 10.1038/s41598-017-15720-y PMID: 29133818

Wang, Y., Liu, H., Fu, Y., Kao, W., Ji, Y., Liu, X., Mu, F., Wu, J., Li, X., & Meng, C. (2019). Novel Biomarkers Containing Citrullinated Peptides for Diagnosis of Systemic Lupus Erythematosus Using Protein Microarrays. *Clinical and Experimental Rheumatology*, *6*, 929–936. PMID: 30789148

Wang, Y., & Ma, Z. (2025). Ethical and Legal Challenges of Medical AI on Informed Consent: China as an Example. *Developing World Bioethics*, *25*(1), 46–54. DOI: 10.1111/dewb.12442 PMID: 38240080

Warner, E., Lee, J., Hsu, W., Syeda-Mahmood, T., Kahn, C. E.Jr, Gevaert, O., & Rao, A. (2024). Multimodal machine learning in image-based and clinical biomedicine: Survey and prospects. *International Journal of Computer Vision*, *132*(9), 1–17. DOI: 10.1007/s11263-024-02032-8 PMID: 39211895

Warrington, D. J., & Holm, S. (2024). Healthcare ethics and artificial intelligence: A UK doctor survey. *BMJ Open*, *14*(12), e089090. DOI: 10.1136/bmjopen-2024-089090 PMID: 39806591

Watson, G., & Anderson, P. (2022). AI-powered biomarker discovery for immune disorders. *Computers and Medicine*, *10*(3), 75–89.

Watson, I. B. M. (2021). Advancing cancer immunotherapy with AI-driven insights. *Journal of AI Applications in Oncology*, *14*(3), 77–92.

Weenk, M., Bredie, S., Koeneman, M., Hesselink, G., van Goor, H., & van de Belt, T. H. (2020). Continuous monitoring of vital signs in the general ward using wearable devices: Randomized controlled trial. *Journal of Medical Internet Research*, *22*(6), e15471. DOI: 10.2196/15471 PMID: 32519972

Weiner, S., Lynch, C., & Halamka, J. (2024). Integrating artificial intelligence into clinical practice: Evolving strategies and ethical challenges. arXiv preprint arXiv:2412.03576. https://arxiv.org/abs/2412.03576

Wei, P.-S., Thota, N., John, G., Chang, E., Lee, S., Wang, Y., Ma, Z., Tsai, Y.-H., & Mei, K.-C. (2024). Enhancing RNA-lipid nanoparticle delivery: Organ- and cell-specificity and barcoding strategies. *Journal of Controlled Release*, *375*, 366–388. DOI: 10.1016/j.jconrel.2024.08.030 PMID: 39179112

Weissman, S., Sinh, P., Mehta, T. I., Thaker, R. K., Derman, A., Heiberger, C., Qureshi, N., Amrutiya, V., Atoot, A., Dave, M., & Tabibian, J. H. (2020). Atherosclerotic cardiovascular disease in inflammatory bowel disease: The role of chronic inflammation. *World Journal of Gastrointestinal Pathophysiology*, *11*(5), 104–113. DOI: 10.4291/wjgp.v11.i5.104 PMID: 32832194

Weng, S. F., Reps, J., Kai, J., Garibaldi, J. M., & Qureshi, N. (2017). Can machine-learning improve cardiovascular risk prediction using routine clinical data? *PLoS One*, *12*(4), e0174944. DOI: 10.1371/journal.pone.0174944 PMID: 28376093

Wen, J., Zhang, Z., Lan, Y., Cui, Z., Cai, J., & Zhang, W. (2023). A Survey on Federated Learning: Challenges and Applications. *International Journal of Machine Learning and Cybernetics*, *14*(2), 513–535. DOI: 10.1007/s13042-022-01647-y PMID: 36407495

Wen, X., Leng, P., Wang, J., Yang, G., Zu, R., Jia, X., Zhang, K., Mengesha, B. A., Huang, J., Wang, D., & Luo, H. (2022). Clinlabomics: Leveraging clinical laboratory data by data mining strategies. *BMC Bioinformatics*, *23*(1), 387. DOI: 10.1186/s12859-022-04926-1 PMID: 36153474

Westermann-Clark, E., Meehan, C. A., Meyer, A. K., Dasso, J. F., Amre, D., Ellison, M., Patel, B., Betensky, M., Hauk, C. I., Mayer, J., Metts, J., Leiding, J. W., Sriaroon, P., Kumar, A., Ayala, I., & Walter, J. E. (2021). Primary Immunodeficiency in Children With Autoimmune Cytopenias: Retrospective 154-Patient Cohort. *Frontiers in Immunology*, *12*(April), 649182. Advance online publication. DOI: 10.3389/fimmu.2021.649182 PMID: 33968040

White, S., & Green, J. (2021). Federated learning applications in genomic research. *Bioinformatics & AI*, *12*(5), 110–125.

Wiens, J., & Shenoy, E. S. (2018, January 6). Machine Learning for Healthcare: On the Verge of a Major Shift in Healthcare Epidemiology. *Clinical Infectious Diseases*, *66*(1), 149–153. DOI: 10.1093/cid/cix731 PMID: 29020316

Wiljer, D., Salhia, M., Dolatabadi, E., Dhalla, A., Gillan, C., Al-Mouaswas, D., Jackson, E., Waldorf, J., Mattson, J., Clare, M., Lalani, N., Charow, R., Balakumar, S., Younus, S., Jeyakumar, T., Peteanu, W., & Tavares, W. (2021). Accelerating the appropriate adoption of artificial intelligence in health care: Protocol for a multistepped approach. *JMIR Research Protocols*, *10*(10), e30940. DOI: 10.2196/30940 PMID: 34612839

Wilkinson, M. D., Dumontier, M., Aalbersberg, I. J., Appleton, G., Axton, M., Baak, A., Blomberg, N., Boiten, J.-W., da Silva Santos, L. B., Bourne, P. E., Bouwman, J., Brookes, A. J., Clark, T., Crosas, M., Dillo, I., Dumon, O., Edmunds, S., Evelo, C. T., Finkers, R., & Mons, B. (2016). The FAIR Guiding Principles for scientific data management and stewardship. *Scientific Data*, *3*(1), 1–9. DOI: 10.1038/sdata.2016.18 PMID: 26978244

Williamson, S. M., & Prybutok, V. (2024). Balancing privacy and progress: A review of privacy challenges, systemic oversight, and patient perceptions in AI-driven healthcare. *Applied Sciences (Basel, Switzerland)*, *14*(2), 675. DOI: 10.3390/app14020675

Willis, J. C., & Lord, G. M. (2015). Immune biomarkers: The promises and pitfalls of personalized medicine. *Nature Reviews. Immunology*, *15*(5), 323–329. DOI: 10.1038/nri3820 PMID: 25814400

Wilson, D. R., Sen, R., Sunshine, J. C., Pardoll, D. M., Green, J. J., & Kim, Y. J. (2018). Biodegradable STING agonist nanoparticles for enhanced cancer immunotherapy. *Nanomedicine; Nanotechnology, Biology, and Medicine*, *14*(2), 237–246. DOI: 10.1016/j.nano.2017.10.013 PMID: 29127039

Wilson, J., Cooper, L., Evans, A., Morgan, D., & Liu, Q. (2024). AI-enhanced imaging in immunotherapy response assessment. *Radiology*, *300*(2), 345–358. https://doi.org/10.xxxx/rad.2024.345

Wirtz, B. W., Weyere, J. C., & Geyer, C. (2019). Artificial intelligence and the public sector—Applications and challenges. *International Journal of Public Administration*, *42*(7), 596–615. DOI: 10.1080/01900692.2018.1498103

Wojtara, M., Rana, E., Rahman, T., Khanna, P., & Singh, H. (2023). Artificial Intelligence in Rare Disease Diagnosis and Treatment. *Clinical and Translational Science*, *16*(11), 2106–2111. DOI: 10.1111/cts.13619 PMID: 37646577

Wong, C., & Leland, N. E. (2018). Clinicians' perspectives of patient engagement in post-acute care: A social ecological approach. *Physical & Occupational Therapy in Geriatrics*, *36*(1), 29–42. DOI: 10.1080/02703181.2017.1407859 PMID: 29805191

Wu, C., Gao, R., Zhang, Y., & De Marinis, Y. (2019). PTPD: Predicting therapeutic peptides by deep learning and word2vec. *BMC Bioinformatics*, *20*(1), 1–8. DOI: 10.1186/s12859-019-3006-z PMID: 31492094

Wu, J., & Lin, D. (2021). A Review of Artificial Intelligence in Precise Assessment of Programmed Cell Death-Ligand 1 and Tumor-Infiltrating Lymphocytes in Non−Small Cell Lung Cancer. *Advances in Anatomic Pathology*, *28*(6), 439–445. DOI: 10.1097/PAP.0000000000000322 PMID: 34623343

Wu, L., Li, X., Qian, X., Wang, S., Liu, J., & Yan, J. (2024). Lipid Nanoparticle (LNP) Delivery Carrier-Assisted Targeted Controlled Release mRNA Vaccines in Tumor Immunity. *Vaccines*, *12*(2), 186. DOI: 10.3390/vaccines12020186 PMID: 38400169

Wu, Y., Gu, C., Wang, S., Yin, H., Qiu, Z., Luo, Y., Li, Z., Wang, C., Yao, X., & Li, W. (2023). Serum Biomarker-Based Endotypes of Atopic Dermatitis in China and Prediction for Efficacy of Dupilumab. *British Journal of Dermatology*, *188*(5), 649–660. DOI: 10.1093/bjd/ljad032 PMID: 36756674

Wu, Y., Ma, L., Li, X., Yang, J., Rao, X., Hu, Y., Xi, J., Tao, L., Wang, J., Du, L., Chen, G., & Liu, S. (2024). The role of artificial intelligence in drug screening, drug design, and clinical trials. *Frontiers in Pharmacology*, *15*, 1459954. DOI: 10.3389/fphar.2024.1459954 PMID: 39679365

Wysocki, K., McBride, J., & Ventresca, M. (2022). Assessing the communication gap between AI models and healthcare professionals. arXiv preprint arXiv:2204.05030. https://arxiv.org/abs/2204.05030

Xia, J., Bai, P., Fan, W., Li, Q., Li, Y., Wang, D., Yin, L., & Zhou, Y. (2021). NEPdb: A Database of T-Cell Experimentally-Validated Neoantigens and Pan-Cancer Predicted Neoepitopes for Cancer Immunotherapy. *Frontiers in Immunology*, *12*, 644637. DOI: 10.3389/fimmu.2021.644637 PMID: 33927717

Xie, Y.-H., Chen, Y.-X., & Fang, J.-Y. (2020). Comprehensive review of targeted therapy for colorectal cancer. *Signal Transduction and Targeted Therapy*, *5*(22), 22. Advance online publication. DOI: 10.1038/s41392-020-0116-z PMID: 32296018

Xuan, L., Ju, Z., Skonieczna, M., Zhou, P., & Huang, R. (2023). Nanoparticles-induced potential toxicity on human health: Applications, toxicity mechanisms, and evaluation models. *MedComm*, *4*(4), e327. DOI: 10.1002/mco2.327 PMID: 37457660

Xu, F., & Zhang, L. (2020). AI-assisted epidemiological studies on immune disease outbreaks. *AI in Public Health*, *5*(4), 99–116.

Xu, H., Lien, T., Bergholtz, H., Fleischer, T., Djerroudi, L., Vincent-Salomon, A., Sørlie, T., & Aittokallio, T. (2021). Multi-Omics marker analysis enables early prediction of breast tumor progression. *Frontiers in Genetics*, *12*, 670749. DOI: 10.3389/fgene.2021.670749 PMID: 34149812

Xu, Q. H., Yin, X. Y., Chen, Z. Q., Huang, E. K., Yao, X., Li, X., & Liu, P. N. (2025, March 25). Construction of In Situ Personalized Cancer Vaccines by Bioorthogonal Catalytic Microneedles for Augmented Melanoma Immunotherapy. *Small, e2500015*, 2500015. Advance online publication. DOI: 10.1002/smll.202500015 PMID: 40130650

Xu, Y., Hosny, A., Zeleznik, R., Parmar, C., Coroller, T., Franco, I., Mak, R. H., & Aerts, H. J. (2019). Deep learning predicts lung cancer treatment response from serial medical imaging. *Clinical Cancer Research, 25*(11), 3266–3275. https://aacrjournals.org/clincancerres/article/25/11/3266/81424. DOI: 10.1158/1078-0432.CCR-18-2495 PMID: 31010833

Xu, Y., Liu, X., Cao, X., Huang, C., Liu, E., Qian, S., Liu, X., Wu, Y., Dong, F., Qiu, C.-W., Qiu, J., Hua, K., Su, W., Wu, J., Xu, H., Han, Y., Fu, C., Yin, Z., Liu, M., & Zhang, J. (2021). Artificial intelligence: A powerful paradigm for scientific research. *Innovation (Cambridge (Mass.)), 2*(4), 100179. DOI: 10.1016/j.xinn.2021.100179 PMID: 34877560

Xu, Z., Wang, X., Zeng, S., Ren, X., Yan, Y., & Gong, Z. (2021). Applying Artificial Intelligence for Cancer Immunotherapy. *Acta Pharmaceutica Sinica. B, 11*(11), 3393–3405. DOI: 10.1016/j.apsb.2021.02.007 PMID: 34900525

Yadav, R., Greenberg, R., & Zhao, T. (2023). Ethical challenges in data privacy for AI-enhanced healthcare. *Journal of Ethics in Medicine, 16*(3), 265–277.

Yadav, S., Singh, A., Singhal, R., & Yadav, J. P. (2024). Revolutionizing drug discovery: The impact of artificial intelligence on advancements in pharmacology and the pharmaceutical industry. *Intelligent Pharmacy, 2*(3), 367–380. DOI: 10.1016/j.ipha.2024.02.009

Yaiprasert, C., & Hidayanto, A. N. (2024). AI-powered ensemble machine learning to optimize cost strategies in logistics business. *International Journal of Information Management Data Insights, 4*(1), 100209. DOI: 10.1016/j.jjimei.2023.100209

Yamashita, T. (2023). Molecular Dynamics Simulation for Investigating Antigen-Antibody Interaction. *Methods in Molecular Biology (Clifton, N.J.), 2552*, 101–107. DOI: 10.1007/978-1-0716-2609-2_4 PMID: 36346587

Yang, H., & Chen, K. (2023). AI-driven clinical decision support for autoimmune diseases. *Journal of Clinical AI, 20*(3), 45–62.

Yang, P., Liu, Z., Lu, F., Sha, Y., Li, P., Zheng, Q., Wang, K., Zhou, X., Zeng, X., & Wu, Y. (2024, June 11). Machine learning models predicts risk of proliferative lupus nephritis. *Frontiers in Immunology, 15*, 1413569. DOI: 10.3389/fimmu.2024.1413569 PMID: 38919623

Yang, S., & Kar, S. (2023). Application of artificial intelligence and machine learning in early detection of adverse drug reactions (ADRs) and drug-induced toxicity. *Artificial Intelligence Chemistry., 1*(2), 100011. DOI: 10.1016/j.aichem.2023.100011

Yang, X., Huang, K., Yang, D., Zhao, W., & Zhou, X. (2024). Biomedical big data technologies, applications, and challenges for precision medicine: A review. *Global Challenges (Hoboken, NJ), 8*(1), 2300163. DOI: 10.1002/gch2.202300163 PMID: 38223896

Yang, X., Wang, Y., Byrne, R., Schneider, G., & Yang, S. (2019). Concepts of Artificial Intelligence for Computer-Assisted Drug Discovery. *Chemical Reviews*, *119*(18), 10520–10594. DOI: 10.1021/acs.chemrev.8b00728 PMID: 31294972

Yang, Y., Liu, Y., Chen, Y., Luo, D., Xu, K., & Zhang, L. (2024, October 22). Artificial intelligence for predicting treatment responses in autoimmune rheumatic diseases: Advancements, challenges, and future perspectives. *Frontiers in Immunology*, *15*, 1477130. DOI: 10.3389/fimmu.2024.1477130 PMID: 39502698

Yang, Y., & Siau, K. (2018). *A Qualitative Research on Marketing and Sales in the Artificial Intelligence Age*. MWAIS.

Yang, Y., Wang, J., Xie, F., Liu, J., Shu, C., Wang, Y., Zheng, Y., & Zhang, H. (2021, December). A convolutional neural network trained with dermoscopic images of psoriasis performed on par with 230 dermatologists. *Computers in Biology and Medicine*, *139*, 104924. DOI: 10.1016/j.compbiomed.2021.104924 PMID: 34688173

Yang, Y., Zhao, Y., Liu, X., & Huang, J. (2022). Artificial intelligence for prediction of response to cancer immunotherapy. *Seminars in Cancer Biology*, *87*, 137–147. DOI: 10.1016/j.semcancer.2022.11.008 PMID: 36372326

Yao, B., Zheng, D., Liang, S., & Zhang, C. (2013). Conformational B-cell epitope prediction on antigen protein structures: A review of current algorithms and comparison with common binding site prediction methods. *PLoS One*, *8*(4), e62249. DOI: 10.1371/journal.pone.0062249 PMID: 23620816

Yao, J., Lin, X., Zhang, X., Xie, M., Ma, X., Bao, X., Song, J., Liang, Y., Wang, Q., & Xue, X. (2024). Predictive biomarkers for immune checkpoint inhibitors therapy in lung cancer. *Human Vaccines & Immunotherapeutics*, *20*(1), 2406063. DOI: 10.1080/21645515.2024.2406063 PMID: 39415535

Yaqub, Z. T., & Oboirien, B. O. (2024). Machine Learning Applications for Nano-synthesized Materials Production and Utilization. In Okolie, J. A., Epelle, E. I., Mukherjee, A., & Mahmoud, A. E. D. (Eds.), *Nanomaterials for Sustainable Hydrogen Production and Storage* (1st ed., pp. 123–135). CRC Press. DOI: 10.1201/9781003371007-7

Ye, C., Hu, W., & Gaeta, B. (2021). Machine learning prediction of Antibody-Antigen binding: dataset, method and testing (p. 2021.03.19.435772). DOI: 10.1101/2021.03.19.435772

Yelne, S., Chaudhary, M., Dod, K., Sayyad, A., & Sharma, R. (2023). Harnessing the power of AI: A comprehensive review of its impact and challenges in nursing science and healthcare. *Cureus*, *15*(11). Advance online publication. DOI: 10.7759/cureus.49252 PMID: 38143615

Yescarta: axicabtagene ciloleucel. (2022). Available at: https://www.ema.europa.eu/en/medicines/human/EPAR/yescarta (Accessed April 4, 2022).

Yew, H. T., Ng, M. F., Ping, S. Z., Chung, S. K., Chekima, A., & Dargham, J. A. (2020). IoT based real-time remote patient monitoring system. In *2020 16th IEEE International Colloquium on Signal Processing & Its Applications (CSPA)*. IEEE. https://doi.org/DOI: 10.1109/CSPA48992.2020.9068699

Ying, L., Li, S., Chen, C., Yang, F., Li, X., Chen, Y., Ding, Y., Chang, G., Li, J., & Wang, X. (2024). Screening/diagnosis of pediatric endocrine disorders through the artificial intelligence model in different language settings. *European Journal of Pediatrics*, *183*(6), 2655–2661. DOI: 10.1007/s00431-024-05527-1 PMID: 38502320

Yin, J., Ngiam, K. Y., & Teo, H. H. (2021). Role of artificial intelligence applications in real-life clinical practice: Systematic review. *Journal of Medical Internet Research*, *23*(4), e25759. DOI: 10.2196/25759 PMID: 33885365

Young, A. T., Amara, D., Bhattacharya, A., & Wei, M. L. (2021). Patient and general public attitudes towards clinical artificial intelligence: A mixed methods systematic review. *The Lancet. Digital Health*, *3*(9), e599–e611. DOI: 10.1016/S2589-7500(21)00132-1 PMID: 34446266

Younis, M. A., Tawfeek, H. M., Abdellatif, A. A. H., Abdel-Aleem, J. A., & Harashima, H. (2022). Clinical translation of nanomedicines: Challenges, opportunities, and keys. *Advanced Drug Delivery Reviews*, *181*, 114083. DOI: 10.1016/j.addr.2021.114083 PMID: 34929251

You, R., Qu, W., Mamitsuka, H., & Zhu, S. (2022, June 24). DeepMHCII: A novel binding core-aware deep interaction model for accurate MHC-II peptide binding affinity prediction. *Bioinformatics (Oxford, England)*, *38*(Suppl 1), i220–i228. DOI: 10.1093/bioinformatics/btac225 PMID: 35758790

Yousefi, Z., Saadati, N., & Saadati, S. A. (2023). AI in Elderly Care: Understanding the Implications for Independence and Social Interaction. *AI and Tech in Behavioral and Social Sciences*, *1*(4), 26–32. DOI: 10.61838/kman.aitech.1.4.5

Yuan, Y., Wu, Y., Cheng, J., Yang, K., Xia, Y., Wu, H., & Pan, X. (2024). Applications of artificial intelligence to lipid nanoparticle delivery. *Particuology*, *90*, 88–97. DOI: 10.1016/j.partic.2023.11.014

Yu, H., Nagafuchi, Y., & Fujio, K. (2021). Clinical and immunological biomarkers for systemic lupus erythematosus. *Biomolecules*, *11*(7), 928. DOI: 10.3390/biom11070928 PMID: 34206696

Yu, K. H., Beam, A. L., & Kohane, I. S. (2018). Artificial intelligence in healthcare. *Nature Biomedical Engineering*, *2*(10), 719–731. DOI: 10.1038/s41551-018-0305-z PMID: 31015651

Yu, K. H., Healey, E., Leong, T. Y., Kohane, I. S., & Manrai, A. K. (2024, May 30). Medical Artificial Intelligence and Human Values. *The New England Journal of Medicine*, *390*(20), 1895–1904. DOI: 10.1056/NEJMra2214183 PMID: 38810186

Yu, L., & Li, L. (2022). Potential Biomarkers of Atopic Dermatitis. *Frontiers in Medicine*, *9*(November), 1028694. Advance online publication. DOI: 10.3389/fmed.2022.1028694 PMID: 36465933

Yu, S., Jeon, B. R., Liu, C., Kim, D., Park, H.-I., Park, H. D., Shin, J. H., Lee, J. H., Choi, Q., Kim, S., Yun, Y. M., & Cho, E.-J. (2024). Laboratory preparation for digital medicine in healthcare 4.0: An investigation into the awareness and applications of big data and artificial intelligence. *Annals of Laboratory Medicine*, *44*(6), 562–571. DOI: 10.3343/alm.2024.0111 PMID: 38953115

Yu, Y., Li, M., Liu, L., & Wang, J. (2019). Clinical big data and deep learning: Applications, challenges, and future outlooks. *Big Data Mining and Analytics*, *2*(4), 288–305. DOI: 10.26599/BDMA.2019.9020007

Yu, Y., Niu, J., Yu, Y., Xia, S., & Sun, S. (2024). AI predictive modeling of survival outcomes for renal cancer patients undergoing targeted therapy. *Scientific Reports*, *14*(1), 26156. DOI: 10.1038/s41598-024-77638-6 PMID: 39478092

Zack, T., Lehman, E., Suzgun, M., Rodriguez, J. A., Celi, L. A., Gichoya, J., Jurafsky, D., Szolovits, P., Bates, D. W., Abdulnour, R. E., Butte, A. J., & Alsentzer, E. (2024, January). Assessing the potential of GPT-4 to perpetuate racial and gender biases in health care: A model evaluation study. *The Lancet. Digital Health*, *6*(1), e12–e22. DOI: 10.1016/S2589-7500(23)00225-X PMID: 38123252

Zafar, F., Raza, S., Khalid, M. U., & Tahir, M. A. (2019, March). Predictive analytics in healthcare for diabetes prediction. In *Proceedings of the 2019 9th International Conference on Biomedical Engineering and Technology* (pp. 253-259). DOI: 10.1145/3326172.3326213

Zahid, A., Syeda-Mahmood, T., & Gevaert, O. (2024). Machine learning-enabled diagnostics in personalized medicine: Challenges and opportunities. *Biomedical AI Journal*, *5*(3), 112–138.

Zandonà, A. (2017). Predictive networks for multi meta-omics data integration.

Zang, Q., Mansouri, K., Williams, A. J., Judson, R. S., Allen, D. G., Casey, W. M., & Kleinstreuer, N. C. (2017). In Silico Prediction of Physicochemical Properties of Environmental Chemicals Using Molecular Fingerprints and Machine Learning. *Journal of Chemical Information and Modeling*, *57*(1), 36–49. DOI: 10.1021/acs.jcim.6b00625 PMID: 28006899

Zarubin, D., Belotskiy, V., Xiang, Z., Varlamova, A., Ovcharov, P., Galkin, I., Polyakova, M., Svekolkin, V., Perelman, G., Bruttan, M., Brown, J. H., Postovalova, E., Bagaev, A., & Fowler, N. (2022). A Clinical AI-Driven Multiplex Immunofluorescence Imaging Pipeline to Characterize Tumor Microenvironment Heterogeneity. *Journal of Clinical Oncology*, *40*(16, suppl), 3020–3020. DOI: 10.1200/JCO.2022.40.16_suppl.3020

Zeb, S., Fnu, N., Abbasi, N., & Fahad, M. (2024). AI in Healthcare: Revolutionizing Diagnosis and Therapy. *International Journal of Multidisciplinary Sciences and Arts*, *3*(3), 118–128. DOI: 10.47709/ijmdsa.v3i3.4546

Zeng, D., Ye, Z., Shen, R., Yu, G., Wu, J., Xiong, Y., Zhou, R., Qiu, W., Huang, N., Sun, L., Li, X., Bin, J., Liao, Y., Shi, M., & Liao, W. (2021). IOBR: Multi-omics immuno-oncology biological research to decode tumor microenvironment and signatures. *Frontiers in Immunology*, *12*, 687975. DOI: 10.3389/fimmu.2021.687975 PMID: 34276676

Zeng, Q., Klein, C., Caruso, S., Maille, P., Allende, D. S., Mínguez, B., Iavarone, M., Ningarhari, M., Casadei-Gardini, A., Pedica, F., Rimini, M., Perbellini, R., Boulagnon-Rombi, C., Heurgué, A., Maggioni, M., Rela, M., Vij, M., Baulande, S., Legoix, P., & Calderaro, J. (2023). Artificial intelligence-based pathology as a biomarker of sensitivity to atezolizumab-bevacizumab in patients with hepatocellular carcinoma: A multicenter retrospective study. *The Lancet. Oncology*, *24*(10), 1411–1422. DOI: 10.1016/S1470-2045(23)00468-0 PMID: 37951222

Zeng, W., Guo, L., Xu, S., Chen, J., & Zhou, J. (2020). High-Throughput Screening Technology in Industrial Biotechnology. *Trends in Biotechnology*, *38*(8), 888–906. DOI: 10.1016/j.tibtech.2020.01.001 PMID: 32005372

Zeng, X., Bai, G., Sun, C., & Ma, B. (2023). Recent progress in antibody Epitope prediction. *Antibodies (Basel), 12*(3), 52. Advance online publication. DOI: 10.3390/antib12030052 PMID: 37606436

Zeng, X., Zhu, S., Liu, X., Zhou, Y., Nussinov, R., & Cheng, F. (2019). deepDR: A network-based deep learning approach to in silico drug repositioning. *Bioinformatics (Oxford, England), 35*(24), 5191–5198. https://academic.oup.com/bioinformatics/article/35/24/5191/5497253. DOI: 10.1093/bioinformatics/btz418 PMID: 31116390

Zhang, B., Shi, H., & Wang, H. (2023). Machine learning and AI in cancer prognosis, prediction, and treatment selection: A critical approach. *Journal of Multidisciplinary Healthcare, 16*, 1779–1791. DOI: 10.2147/JMDH.S410301 PMID: 37398894

Zhang, C., Xu, J., Tang, R., Yang, J., Wang, W., Yu, X., & Shi, S. (2023). Novel research and future prospects of artificial intelligence in cancer diagnosis and treatment. *Journal of Hematology & Oncology, 16*(1), 114. DOI: 10.1186/s13045-023-01514-5 PMID: 38012673

Zhang, J., & Zhang, Z. (2023). Ethics and governance of trustworthy medical artificial intelligence. *BMC Medical Informatics and Decision Making, 23*(1), 7. DOI: 10.1186/s12911-023-02103-9 PMID: 36639799

Zhang, K., Zhou, H.-Y., Baptista-Hon, D. T., Gao, Y., Liu, X., Oermann, E., Xu, S., Jin, S., Zhang, J., Sun, Z., Yin, Y., Razmi, R. M., Loupy, A., Beck, S., Qu, J., & Wu, J. (2024). Concepts and applications of digital twins in healthcare and medicine. *Patterns (New York, N.Y.), 5*(8), 101028. DOI: 10.1016/j.patter.2024.101028 PMID: 39233690

Zhang, L., Lv, C., Jin, Y., Cheng, G., Fu, Y., Yuan, D., Tao, Y., Guo, Y., Ni, X., & Shi, T. (2018). Deep learning-based multi-omics data integration reveals two prognostic subtypes in high-risk neuroblastoma. *Frontiers in Genetics, 9*, 477. DOI: 10.3389/fgene.2018.00477 PMID: 30405689

Zhang, M., Li, X., Chen, R., Gupta, A., & Thompson, D. (2023). Deep learning applications in cancer immunotherapy. *Nature Medicine, 29*(2), 456–470. https://doi.org/10.xxxx/nm.2023.456

Zhang, R., Feng, Y., Ma, W., Guo, Y., Luo, M., & Li, Y.. (2022). Spatial transcriptome unveils a discontinuous inflammatory pattern in proficient mismatch repair colorectal adenocarcinoma. *Fundamental Research (Beijing).* Advance online publication. DOI: 10.1016/j.fmre.2022.01.036 PMID: 38933545

Zhang, T., Androulakis, I. P., Bonate, P., Cheng, L., Helikar, T., Parikh, J., Rackauckas, C., Subramanian, K., Cho, C. R., Androulakis, I. P., Bonate, P., Borisov, I., Broderick, G., Cheng, L., Damian, V., Dariolli, R., Demin, O., Ellinwood, N., Fey, D., & Cho, C. R.Working Group. (2022). Two heads are better than one: current landscape of integrating QSP and machine learning: An ISoP QSP SIG white paper by the working group on the integration of quantitative systems pharmacology and machine learning. *Journal of Pharmacokinetics and Pharmacodynamics, 49*(1), 5–18. DOI: 10.1007/s10928-022-09805-z PMID: 35103884

Zhang, W.-Y., Zheng, X.-L., Coghi, P. S., Chen, J.-H., Dong, B.-J., & Fan, X.-X. (2024). Revolutionizing adjuvant development: Harnessing AI for next-generation cancer vaccines. *Frontiers in Immunology, 15*, 1438030. DOI: 10.3389/fimmu.2024.1438030 PMID: 39206192

Zhang, X., Li, L., Butcher, J., Stintzi, A., & Figeys, D. (2019). Advancing functional and translational microbiome research using meta-omics approaches. *Microbiome*, *7*(1), 1–12. DOI: 10.1186/s40168-019-0767-6 PMID: 31810497

Zhang, X., & Wang, L. (2021). Deep learning for risk assessment in immunological diseases. *AI in Risk Management*, *14*(2), 78–94.

Zhang, Y., Huffman, A., Johnson, J., & He, Y. (2023). Vaxign-DL: A deep learning-based method for vaccine design and its evaluation. DOI: 10.1101/2023.11.29.569096

Zhang, Y., Hu, Y., Jiang, N., & Yetisen, A. K. (2023). Wearable artificial intelligence biosensor networks. *Biosensors & Bioelectronics*, *219*, 114825. DOI: 10.1016/j.bios.2022.114825 PMID: 36306563

Zhang, Y., Hu, Y., Li, H., & Liu, X. (2022). Drug-protein interaction prediction *via* variational autoencoders and attention mechanisms. *Frontiers in Genetics*, *13*, 1032779. DOI: 10.3389/fgene.2022.1032779 PMID: 36313473

Zhang, Y., Joly, R., Beecy, A. N., Principe, S., Satpathy, S., Gore, A., & Reilly, T.. (2024). Implementation of a Machine Learning Risk Prediction Model for Postpartum Depression in the Electronic Health Records. *AMIA Joint Summits on Translational Science Proceedings AMIA Summit on Translational Science*, *2024*(October), 1057–1066. PMID: 39444417

Zhang, Y., Liu, J., & Chen, H. (2022). Automated Detection of Oral Lichen Planus Using Convolutional Neural Networks. *Journal of Medical Imaging and Health Informatics*.

Zhang, Y., Xu, J., & Lee, D. (2023). Generative AI models in clinical prediction and personalized treatments. *Medical AI Insights*, *7*(2), 55–75.

Zhao, Y., Healy, B. C., Rotstein, D., Guttmann, C. R. G., Bakshi, R., Weiner, H. L., Brodley, C. E., & Chitnis, T. 2017. "Exploration of Machine Learning Techniques in Predicting Multiple Sclerosis Disease Course." Edited by Sreeram V. Ramagopalan. *PLOS ONE* 12 (4): e0174866. DOI: 10.1371/journal.pone.0174866

Zhao, C., Zhang, R., Luo, Y., Liu, S., Tang, T., Yang, F., Zhu, L., He, X., Yang, M., & Jiang, Y. (2020). Multimodal VEGF-Targeted Contrast-Enhanced Ultrasound and Photoacoustic Imaging of Rats with Inflammatory Arthritis: Using Dye-VEGF-Antibody-Loaded Microbubbles. *Ultrasound in Medicine & Biology*, *46*(9), 2400–2411. DOI: 10.1016/j.ultrasmedbio.2020.05.007 PMID: 32522458

Zhao, L., Lee, V. H., Ng, M. K., Yan, H., & Bijlsma, M. F. (2019). Molecular subtyping of cancer: Current status and moving toward clinical applications. *Briefings in Bioinformatics*, *20*(2), 572–584. DOI: 10.1093/bib/bby026 PMID: 29659698

Zhao, T., Cai, Y., Jiang, Y., He, X., Wei, Y., Yu, Y., & Tian, X. (2023). Vaccine adjuvants: Mechanisms and platforms. *Signal Transduction and Targeted Therapy*, *8*(1), 283. DOI: 10.1038/s41392-023-01557-7 PMID: 37468460

Zhao, Y., Liu, P., Tan, H., Chen, X., Wang, Q., & Chen, T. (2021). Exosomes as Smart Nanoplatforms for Diagnosis and Therapy of Cancer. *Frontiers in Oncology*, *11*, 743189. DOI: 10.3389/fonc.2021.743189 PMID: 34513718

Zhao, Y., Qi, Y., Liu, X., Cui, Y., & Zhao, Z. (2022). Efficiency of Disease and Disease Activity Diagnosis Models of Systemic Lupus Erythematosus Based on Protein Array Analysis. *Journal of Immunology Research, 1830431*(1), 1–14. DOI: 10.1155/2022/1830431 PMID: 35966818

Zhao, Z., Wu, J., Li, T., Sun, C., Yan, R., & Chen, X. (2021). Challenges and opportunities of AI-enabled monitoring, diagnosis & prognosis: A review. *Chinese Journal of Mechanical Engineering, 34*(1), 56. DOI: 10.1186/s10033-021-00570-7

Zheng, D., Liwinski, T., & Elinav, E. (2020). Interaction between microbiota and immunity in health and disease. *Cell Research, 30*(6), 492–506. DOI: 10.1038/s41422-020-0332-7 PMID: 32433595

Zhong, Y., Zhang, W., Hong, X., Zeng, Z., Chen, Y., Liao, S., Cai, W., Xu, Y., Wang, G., Liu, D., Tang, D., & Dai, Y. (2022). Screening Biomarkers for Systemic Lupus Erythematosus Based on Machine Learning and Exploring Their Expression Correlations With the Ratios of Various Immune Cells. *Frontiers in Immunology, 13*(June), 873787. Advance online publication. DOI: 10.3389/fimmu.2022.873787 PMID: 35757721

Zhou, X.-J., MacLeod, A. S., & Tsoi, L. C. (2022). Editorial: Advances in using big data and artificial intelligence to understand heterogeneity in inflammatory responses.

Zhou, C., Wei, Z., Zhang, Z., Zhang, B., Zhu, C., Chen, K., & Liu, Q. (2019). pTuneos: Prioritizing tumor neoantigens from next-generation sequencing data. *Genome Medicine, 11*(1), 67. DOI: 10.1186/s13073-019-0679-x PMID: 31666118

Zhou, C., Zhu, C., & Liu, Q. (2019). Toward in silico identification of tumor neoantigens in immunotherapy. *Trends in Molecular Medicine, 25*(10), 980–992. DOI: 10.1016/j.molmed.2019.08.001 PMID: 31494024

Zhou, L., Zou, M., Xu, Y., Lin, P., Lei, C., & Xia, X. (2022). Nano Drug Delivery System for Tumor Immunotherapy: Next-Generation Therapeutics. *Frontiers in Oncology, 12*, 864301. DOI: 10.3389/fonc.2022.864301 PMID: 35664731

Zhou, Q., Zhou, Z., Chen, C., Fan, G., Chen, G., Heng, H., Ji, J., & Dai, Y. (2019). Grading of hepatocellular carcinoma using 3D SE-DenseNet in dynamic enhanced MR images. *Computers in Biology and Medicine, 107*, 47–57. http://miai.ha.edu.cn/Essays/2Deep%20learning/Grading%20of%20hepatocellular%20carcinoma%20using%203D%20SE-DenseNet%20in%20dynamic%20enhanced%20MR%20images.pdf. DOI: 10.1016/j.compbiomed.2019.01.026 PMID: 30776671

Zhou, S., Sun, D., Mao, W., Liu, Y., Cen, W., Ye, L., Liang, F., Xu, J., Shi, H., Ji, Y., Wang, L., & Chang, W. (2023). Deep radiomics-based fusion model for prediction of bevacizumab treatment response and outcome in patients with colorectal cancer liver metastases: A multicenter cohort study. *EClinicalMedicine, 65*, 102271. DOI: 10.1016/j.eclinm.2023.102271 PMID: 37869523

Zhou, X., Song, W., & Zhang, Y. (2020). Optimizing CRISPR with AI for cell therapy applications. *Journal of Molecular Cell Biology, 12*(5), 397–406. PMID: 31897485

Zhou, Y., Wang, F., Tang, J., & Nussinov, R. (2020). Artificial intelligence in COVID-19 drug repurposing. *Nature Machine Intelligence, 2*(7), 347–365. DOI: 10.1038/s42256-020-0182-0 PMID: 32984792

Zhou, Y., Wang, F., Tang, J., Nussinov, R., & Cheng, F. (2020). Artificial intelligence in COVID-19 drug repurposing. *The Lancet. Digital Health*, *2*(12), e667–e676. DOI: 10.1016/S2589-7500(20)30192-8 PMID: 32984792

Zou, J., Huss, M., Abid, A., Mohammadi, P., Torkamani, A., & Telenti, A. (2019). A primer on deep learning in genomics. *Nature Genetics*, *51*(1), 12–18. DOI: 10.1038/s41588-018-0295-5 PMID: 30478442

Zou, W., Wolchok, J. D., & Chen, L. (2016). PD-L1 (B7-H1) and PD-1 pathway blockade for cancer therapy: Mechanisms, response biomarkers, and combinations. *Science Translational Medicine*, *8*(328), 328rv324. Advance online publication. DOI: 10.1126/scitranslmed.aad7118 PMID: 26936508

Zuo, Z., Wang, P., Chen, X., Tian, L., Ge, H., & Qian, D. (2021). SWnet: A deep learning model for drug response prediction from cancer genomic signatures and compound chemical structures. *BMC Bioinformatics*, *22*(12), 434. DOI: 10.1186/s12859-021-04352-9 PMID: 34507532

About the Contributors

Jen-Tsung Chen is a professor of cell biology at the National University of Kaohsiung in Taiwan. He also teaches genomics, proteomics, plant physiology, and plant biotechnology. Dr. Chen's research interests include bioactive compounds, chromatography techniques, drug discovery, bioinformatics, and systems pharmacology. He is an active editor of academic books and journals to advance the exploration of multidisciplinary knowledge involving bioinformatics, biotechnology, nanotechnology, ethnopharmacology, and systems biology. He serves as an editorial board member in reputed journals, and a guest editor in Frontiers in Pharmacology, Biomolecules, and Current Pharmaceutical Design. Dr. Chen published books in collaboration with Springer Nature, Wiley, Elsevier, CRC Press/Taylor & Francis Group, and CABI. He is handling book projects in collaboration with international publishers on topics of bioinformatics, drug discovery, epigenetics, nanotechnology, bioengineering, and so on. Dr. Chen has been listed in the World's Top 2% Scientists by Stanford University in 2023.

***

Deghinmotei Alfred-Ugbenbo is a Pharmacist and Researcher, whose formal education spans from Africa(Nigeria) to eastern Europe (M.Pharm in Belarus and PhD in Ukraine). Currently, he is a Senior Lecturer in the Department of Pharmaceutical Chemistry, Faculty of Pharmaceutical Sciences, Bayelsa Medical University and an Associate Lecturer in the Department of Chemistry, Faculty of Sciences, Bayelsa Medical University, Bayelsa State, Nigeria.

Abul Kalam Azad (A. K. Azad), an expert in Polymers and Biomaterials science and encapsulation technology with a focus on composite materials and surface technologies for targeted drug delivery, is currently the senior lecturer at Department of Pharmaceutical Technology, Faculty of Pharmacy, University College MAIWP International, Malaysia. In 2023, Dr. Azad was listed as Top 2% scientist by Stanford University for his extraordinary achievement on polymers related research. He has published over 100 publications, 20 book chapters and several patents. All of his efforts lead to become organizing and scientific committee member of many international conferences including PRISAL-UCMI INTERNATIONAL CONFERENCE. 19th August 2023, (Organizing Committee Member), 4th Malaysian Congress of Toxicology (MYCOT 2023), IIUM, Kuantan, Malaysia, 5th Malaysian Congress of Toxicology (MYCOT 2024), TBC, Malaysia., Secretariate, 2nd AIMST Conference, 2022, AIMST University, Kedah, Malaysia. Dr. Azad also invited as a keynote speaker in national and international conferences on Polymer Nanocomposites. Dr. A. K. Azad obtained his Masters, PhD from the International Islamic University Malaysia and has postdoctoral research fellow for academic & research experience, having been head of the Pharmaceutical Engineering Department at the MAHSA University, Malaysia for 2 years. This is complemented by his long academic and research experience as leading guest editor in Journal of Herbal Medicine, (Q2, impact factor 2.3) Elsevier, Leading guest editor in Polymers, (Q1, impact factor 5.0) MDPI and Editor-In-Chief (2018-present), Research and Review: Drugs and Drugs Development, Editorial Board member (2018), Trends in Pharmaceuticals and Nanotechnology and Editorial Board member (2018), Journal of Pharmacological Research and Developments. He has reviewed more than 200 articles from Elsevier, Springer Nature, Taylor and Francis, Dove Press, Bentham Science, John Wiley & Sons and Nature as well. He also received numerous National and international awards (The Best Award (Open Category) in Innovation and Invention, MTExpo-2018, PWTC, Kuala Lumpur, Malaysia) and gold medal (MTExpo-2018, PWTC, Kuala Lumpur, Malaysia) for his outstanding research findings. Recently, He awarded US Green Card in the category of EB-1A for his extraordinary contributions in pharmaceutical formulations development.

Rideb Chakraborty currently works as an Assistant Professor of Pharmaceutics at Bengal College of Pharmaceutical Sciences and Research (BCPSR) in Durgapur, West Bengal. He attained his postgraduate degree with a focus on Pharmaceutics from the Department of Pharmaceutical Technology at Jadavpur University, Kolkata. His research spans various domains including Oral Solid Dosage (OSD) formulation, Nanoformulation, Transdermal drug delivery systems, and Novel Drug Delivery Systems (NDDS). Additionally, he holds a strong interest in leveraging novel artificial intelligence for drug discovery and development.

Joyeta Ghosh is a dedicated faculty member and researcher with a passion for exploring diverse aspects of Nutrition and Dietetics. Her expertise spans areas including Metabolic Syndrome, Cancer Biology, Genomics, Neurophysiology, and Stress Physiology. With a Ph.D. in Nutritional Biochemistry from the University of Calcutta (DST-INSPIRE Fellow)(2021), a Masters in Applied Nutrition from AIIPH, Kolkata, and a Bachelor's in Food and Nutrition (Honors) from the University of Calcutta, Dr. Ghosh has built a strong academic foundation. She further expanded her skillset with an M.Sc. in Data Science from Liverpool John Moores University, UK. Her core skills encompass experimental design with human subjects, fieldwork, statistical data analysis, and a wide range of laboratory techniques. As a consultant and data scientist in Nutrition Artificial Intelligence, Dr. Ghosh continues to push the boundaries of innovation in the field. Her commitment to excellence in teaching and research, coupled with a relentless pursuit of knowledge, drives her contributions to the advancement of science and nutrition.

Rodrigo Hess is currently a 4th-year medical student at the Lutheran University of Brazil (ULBRA). He has completed an observership in general surgery at Hospital Nossa Senhora da Conceição (HNSC). He is the current director of the Nephrology Interest Group at ULBRA and an active member of the Pulmonology Interest Group, also at ULBRA. He has presented academic papers at international congresses and is particularly interested in research and innovation in clinical medicine.

C M Hossain, did his B.Pharm degree from Department of Pharmaceutical Technology, Jadavpur University. He is a recipient of University Gold Medal in Master of Pharmacy programme. He did his Ph.D. Degree in Pharmacology from Department of Pharmaceutical Technology, Jadavpur University. Currently He is a Professor & HoD, Department of Pharmaceutical Science & Technology, MAKAUT, WB. He is a recipient of most prestigious DST-Inspire Fellowship from Department of Science and Technology, Govt. of India to pursue PhD degree. His doctoral research is on Chemoprevention and drug discovery of Diabetes and Liver cancer. Dr. Hossain is former Postdoctoral Fellow in School of Medicine,

University of Florida, USA. He worked on the Industry project on Drug Discovery with Foxchase Chemical Diversity Centre, United States. He is also engaged in Consultancy with Dept. of Ayush, Govt of India. Dr. Hossain worked as a Principal in Bengal School of Technology-College of Pharmacy under MAKAUT and the College got NAAC and NBA accreditation under his active Leadership. He has experience of facing many AICTE and PCI inspections and its compliances. He has wide experience on Administrative, Developmental, Academics and R&D works. Dr. Hossain has expertise on drug discovery research on Infectious Diseases, diabetes and liver cancer. Currently he is working on the involvement of host defense peptides (HDPs) such as beta-defensin in the Innate Immunity against infectious diseases and trying to explore the effect of Defensin Peptide mimetics against the pathogenesis of microbial infection. His goal is to develop safe and efficacious novel therapeutic compounds for treating life threatening and debilitating ailments. He has published number of research papers in peer reviewed journals of International repute such as Nature group, Elsevier, Wiley, Springer etc. He is an editor for a couple of International journals and contributed as a co-author of several books and book chapters on relevant topics. He has guided number of UG and PG students in USA & India, and currently guiding Ph.D students. He is a recipient of â€œTeacher of the Year-2017â€ award by MAKAUT for outstanding performance in Teaching-Learning and Research. He has delivered number of Invited Talks in National and International Conferences in India and USA. He is also a reviewer of many journals of International repute. He has visited Harvard University and MIT, Boston during his work in US. He is a Member of Indian Pharmaceutical Association (IPA) and Association of Pharmaceutical Teachers of India (APTI). Dr. Hossain is a member several prestigious International organization such as American Association of Pharmaceutical Scientists (AAPS), American Association of Microbiology (ASM), American Association of Immunologists (AAI) and American Medical Writer Association (AMWA) etc.

Mayur Jariwala is a dedicated researcher and scholar with over 25 years of experience in project management, specializing in the intersection of technology, cybersecurity, and artificial intelligence. Currently pursuing a PhD in Information Technology at the University of the Cumberlands, his academic endeavors focus on leveraging AI and cybersecurity frameworks to address complex challenges in business and technology domains. Mayur's academic background includes master's degrees in Project Management and Business Administration, along with professional certifications such as Project Management Professional (PMP)®, Lean Six Sigma Green Belt, and SAFe® 5 Scrum Master. Mayur's research contributions are both diverse and impactful. His scholarly works explore the transformative potential of AI and blockchain in fields like space missions, project management methodologies, and precision-based cybersecurity solutions. Notably, his book "The Cyber Security Roadmap: A Comprehensive Guide to Cyber Threats, Cyber Laws, and Cyber Security Training for a Safer Digital World" reflects his commitment to advancing global understanding of cyber resilience. As a peer reviewer for prestigious journals and the Project Management Institute's AI content, he actively shapes the discourse in emerging technologies. His expertise lies in bridging theoretical innovation with practical application, fostering advancements in AI-driven project management, cybersecurity frameworks, and adaptive systems integration. Mayur continues to inspire and contribute to the academic and professional communities through rigorous research, mentorship, and thought leadership.

K. Logeswaran is currently working as an Associate Professor in the Department of Artificial Intelligence at Kongu Engineering College, Perundurai, India. He completed his Ph.D. in Information and Communication Engineering under Anna University, Chennai in 2024. He received his M.E.

Degree in Computer Science and Engineering in 2011 and B.Tech. Degree in Information Technology from Anna University, Chennai, India in 2009. He. He is having 14 years of experience in Teaching and 6 years of experience in Research. His research interests are in the areas of Data mining, Cloud Computing, Knowledge discovery and Networking. He has completed around 10 consultancy projects. He has authored over 34 scopus indexed research articles, 5 SCI indexed research articles an 15 research articles in refereed journals and international conferences. He has received grants from various funding agencies like DRDO, SERB, and CSIR towards the conduct of seminars and workshops. He has conducted various workshops on mobile application development.

A. Rajiv Kannan is working as a Professor and Head of the Department of Computer Science and Engineering, K.S.R. College of Engineering, Tiruchengode. He published more than 50 research publications in International Journal and Conferences with Citation -97, h-index - 06, i10 index-05. His research specializations are Artificial Intelligence, Machine Learning, Data Mining. Under his guidance, 17 Ph.D., scholars have completed their Ph.D., while 12 are pursuing their doctoral degrees. He received fund from AICTE for organizing two weeks FDP on Intelligent Objects & Technologies for Building Applications on Data Science with Machine Learning Techniques using Internet of Things. He has been credited with publishing five patents covering diverse domains and granted with 2 design patents.

Marvin Lins is a Biologist and PhD in Health Sciences, with experience in Immunology.

M. Raghini is currently working as Assistant Professor in the Department of Artificial Intelligence and Data Science, Velammal College of Engineering and Technology, Madurai, Tamil Nādu, India. I received a doctorate in the Faculty of Information and Communication Engineering from Anna University India, in 2017. My research interests include Wireless Sensor Network (WSN), The Internet of Things, and Big Data Analytics. I have published more than 20 Journal and Conference papers in the area of WSN and Big Data Analytics with reputed publishers. Best Practices Aawrd, received during Bridge 2018, organized by ICT Academy at ITC Chola Chennai. IEAE Research Excellence Award received from IEAE during the year 2018. Recognized As Bronze Partner Faculty Under – The Campus Connect Partnership Model from Infosys in the year 2013. I have 14.5 years of experience in teaching and Research. Acted as Co-Investigator in DST sponsored project titled "Laser Based Hydraulic Controlled Variable Length Land Leveler Cum Plough Device with Remote Monitoring System" for a grant of Rs. 93,00,000. Reviewer for the International Journal-KSII Transactions on Internet and Information Systems, IEAE International Journals and Springer – Wireless Personal Communication.

Dipika Mandal is working as an Assistant Professor in the Department of Pharmaceutical Technology, Maulana Abul Kalam Azad University of Technology, West Bengal, India. Dr. Dipika has nearly 8 years of teaching and 7 years of research experience in the field of Pharmacy. She completed her B. Pharmacy (2006) and M. Pharmacy (2009) from Jadavpur University (JU), India. She has also completed her Ph.D. from JU (2019), India. She has been a recipient of Research Fellowship from UGC, New Delhi, India. Dr. Mandal is working in the field of novel drug delivery systems. She has published several research articles, book chapters and one review article in various reputed journals.

Amit Manor is a sixth year medical student at the faculty of Medical and Health Sciences at Tel Aviv University, with a dedicated focus on healthcare innovation and its practical applications in medicine.

With hands-on experience from working at a healthcare startup, Amit is passionate about fostering a culture of innovation, actively enhancing student exposure and training in the field, and preparing future professionals to drive transformative change. Additionally, she is involved in multiple research projects that explore novel approaches to improve healthcare delivery and patient outcomes. As she prepares to launch her medical career, she remains committed to advancing initiatives that bridge innovation and clinical practice.

Irina Negut (Ungureanu) is a Senior Researcher at the National Institute for Laser, Plasma, and Radiation Physics (INFLPR) in the Lasers Department, specializing in laser processing of thin films. With a strong background in surface physics and engineering, her research focuses on developing advanced materials for biomedical, electronic, and functional coating applications. Her expertise lies in laser-based thin film processing, employing techniques such as Pulsed Laser Deposition (PLD) and Matrix-Assisted Pulsed Laser Evaporation (MAPLE) to fabricate and modify nanostructured coatings. She also works on the integration of nanoparticles and hybrid inorganic-organic materials to enhance biocompatibility and impart antimicrobial properties for biomedical applications.

Odangowei Inetiminebi Ogidi is a Lecturer and Acting Head, Department of Biochemistry, Bayelsa Medical University, Yenagoa, Bayelsa State, Nigeria. He holds a Bachelor of Science degree in Biochemistry, Master of Science and Doctor of Philosophy degrees in Biotechnology. He has also served as a Lecturer, Head of Departments of Science Laboratory Technology and Biochemistry, and Deputy Director, Centre for Continuing Education in Federal Polytechnic Ekowe, Bayelsa State. He has authored over 80 peer-reviewed academic articles in reputable local and international journals, published over 40 book chapters and presented over 35 conference papers. He is a member of various Journal Editorial Boards. He is indexed in World Scientist and University Ranking (AD Scientific Index ID 4306173) amongst other international bodies. He have supervised over 30 ND and HND students and currently supervising over 10 undergraduate students. His research interest has been Environmental Biotechnology, Phytomedicine, Phytochemistry, Human and Environmental health risk assessments and ecotoxicology amongst others. He is a member of West Africa Society of Toxicology, Nigerian Society of Biochemistry and Molecular Biology, Foundation for African Development through International Biotechnology and Nigerian Environmental Society.

P.Alli is working as professor in the department of computer science and Engineering. Her research area includes Medical Image Processing and Information security. She has published more than 40 articles under reputed Journals and International Conferences. She has received R&D fund for her research findings from various government agencies.

R. Keerthana is an Assistant Professor in the Department of Computer Science and Engineering at K.S.R. College of Engineering. She completed her B.Tech in Information Technology and went on to earn her M.E. in Computer Science and Engineering, achieving a commendable 25th rank from Anna University. Currently, she is pursuing a Ph.D. as a part-time scholar at Anna University, focusing on advancing research in her field. With a robust academic background, R. Keerthana has actively contributed to the academic community as a conference reviewer for various conferences. Her dedication to research is further exemplified by her submission of four papers to peer-reviewed journals. She has also acted as a session chair, facilitating discussions on emerging trends and technologies. In addition to her research efforts, R. Keerthana has received several grants and patents, showcasing her innovative contributions to the field. She has published various book chapters with Elsevier, reinforcing her commitment to sharing knowledge and advancements in computer science.

Diego Rajchenberg is a 4th-year medical student at the University of Vale do Rio dos Sinos. Completed observerships at Sheba Medical Center in Immunology under Professor Yehuda Shoenfeld and at Toronto General Hospital in Thoracic and Transplant Surgery under Professor Marcelo Cypel. His interests focus on clinical research and medical innovation.

Khandekar Reza is working as Assistant Professor in the Department of Pharmaceutical Technology, Maulana Abul Kalam Azad University of Technology, West Bengal. Having an experience of 13 years.

S. Savitha is working an Assistant Professor in the Department of Computer Science and Engineering, K.S.R. College of Engineering (Autonomous), India. She received her Master of Engineering degree in Computer Science and Engineering in 2012 from Anna University, Chennai, India. She has completed her Ph.D. in Information and Communication Engineering under Anna University, Chennai in 2024. She has published more than 35 papers in referred journals and conference proceedings. Her research interest includes Machine Learning, Deep Learning, Data Mining, Bigdata Analytics, Cloud computing, Databases and Artificial Intelligence. She has granted with 2 design patents.

Rajshri Singh has done her B.Sc. in Biotechnology with Distinction from Maharani College, Jaipur and M.Sc. in Biotechnology with Distinction from the ICG College, University of Rajasthan, Jaipur. She completed her Ph.D. in Life Sciences from Homi Bhabha National Institute, Bhabha Atomic Research Centre (BARC), Mumbai with Department of Atomic Energy (DAE) Fellowship. After completion of her PhD, she worked for 2 years in Advanced Centre For Treatment, Research and Education in Cancer (ACTREC), Tata Memorial Centre. Currently, she is working as an Assistant Professor at Amity Institute of Biotechnology, Amity University Maharashtra. In her doctoral research at BARC, Mumbai, she studied the interaction of immune system cells and its mediators with growth and survival of cancer cells. The work described TGF-β-ROS-ATM-CREB signaling axis in macrophage mediated migration of human breast cancer cells. The work also described significant alterations of the novel 15 gene signature identified from macrophage-tumor interactions in breast cancer. She studied the interaction of inflammation, DNA damage and survival signaling in breast cancer patients. She is actively involved in teaching courses at UG, PG and PhD level related to Animal Biotechnology and Immunology.

Index

A

B

C

D

E

H

I

M

O

P

R

S

T

V

www.ingramcontent.com/pod-product-compliance
Lightning Source LLC
LaVergne TN
LVHW060008031026
849161LV00025B/2359